General microbiolo_

General microbiology

Hans G. Schlegel

assisted by C. Zaborosch

translated by M. Kogut

Seventh Edition

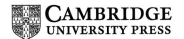

CAMBRIDGE
UNIVERSITY PRESS

Published by the Press Syndicate of the University of Cambridge
The Pitt Building, Trumpington Street, Cambridge CB2 1RP
40 West 20th Street, New York, NY 10011–4211, USA
10 Stamford Road, Oakleigh, Melbourne 3166, Australia

Originally published in German as *Allgemeine Mikrobiologie*
by Georg Thieme Verlag, Stuttgart 1969, seventh edition 1992 and
© Georg Thieme Verlag, Stuttgart 1969, 1972, 1974, 1976, 1981, 1985, 1992

First published in English by Cambridge University Press 1986
as *General microbiology*

Reprinted 1987, 1988 (twice), 1990
Second edition 1993
English translation © Cambridge University Press 1986, 1993

Printed in Great Britain at the University Press, Cambridge

A catologue record of this book is available from the British Library

Library of Congress cataloguing in publication data

Schlegel, Hans Günter, 1924–
    [Allgemeine Mikrobiologie.   English]
    General microbiology   Hans G. Schlegel; translated by M. Kogut.
    – 7th ed.
        p.   cm.
    Translation of: Allgemeine Mikrobiologie.
    Includes bibliographical references and index.
    ISBN 0 521 43372 X. – ISBN 0 521 43980 9 (pbk.)
    1. Microbiology.   I. Title.
  QR41.2.S3413   1992
  576–dc20   92-39911   CIP

ISBN 0 521 43372 X hardback
ISBN 0 521 43980 9 paperback

K S

Contents

Preface to the seventh edition

For the last 25 years this book has addressed two tasks: namely, to survey the field of microbiology and demarcate it from other biological areas; and to confront the question of the depth to which a first presentation should encompass the abundance of material and its detailed contents. I am convinced that the main task of a textbook such as this must be the presentation of essentials, leaving out excess information as ballast which cannot advance basic understanding. I have also tried not to give too much weight to the currently fashionable, since 'fruitful branches may arise from inconspicuous buds'. It has thus been possible to keep the volume of this new edition within reasonable limits. The increased number of pages is largely due to improved instructional content; the advances made in all fields of microbiology have necessitated a large number of additions as well as some alterations and condensations of the text and rearrangements of some chapters, with the inclusion of new illustrations and alterations to some well-established diagrams.

Two lines of thought which could affect motivation for studying microbiology have also been extended and explored. These concern on the one hand, the evolution of prokaryotes and on the other, the ecology of microorganisms. Comparisons of the nucleotide sequences in ribosomal RNA have undoubtedly produced impressive insight into evolution, and allowed the recognition, even among prokaryotes, of a phylogenetic tree which is in agreement with a considerable amount of biochemical data. The discovery of new bacterial species as well as of novel metabolic pathways and their regulation has furthered the study of microbial ecology, whilst the now recognised necessity to reach a better understanding of relations in the biosphere – not least as a precondition for conservation – has underlined its increasing importance.

Again I have to thank colleagues and students for stimulating and critical comments. Especially helpful – apart from those already mentioned in the preface to the first edition – have been the contributions by Barbel Friedrich and Margot Kogut, and from Jan R. Andreesen and Botho Bowien. Mrs B. Friedrich is largely responsible for the extensive revision of Chapter 15, 'Constancy, change, recombination and transfer of genetic characters', which contains much new information. I am grateful to Mrs Christiane Zaborosch for valuable support with editorial work.

The book has also benefited from new diagrams, illustrations and tables, and for these, and the agreeable and understanding collaboration, I thank Mr Gunther Bosch. My appreciation expressed already in 1968 to the publisher, G. Thieme, can be repeated in full and without reservations.

Finally, my family, my wife and children, have learned to live with *Microbiology*, and have always shown full understanding for the priorities. For this I acknowledge my heartfelt thanks.

Hans Gunter Schlegel
Göttingen, July 1991

Preface to the first edition

Microbiology deals mostly with the large groups of fungi, bacteria and viruses which equal in diversity and physiological phenomena the more traditional group of organisms within the disciplines of botany and zoology. During recent years the study of microorganisms has contributed important insights into the basic problems of biology. Because of their ease of manipulation, rapid growth, highly developed capacity for adaptation, and other properties, microorganisms have become one of the preferred objects of research in biochemistry and genetics.

Students of microbiology have many excellent textbooks at their disposal (many mentioned in the bibiliography) such as *General Microbiology* by Stanier *et al.*, *Microbiology* by Davis *et al.*, *Biology of Microorganisms* by Brock, as well as many others, including reference works (both in English and in German). There is a lack, however, of a concise presentation that gives an overview of the field to students of microbiology and also presents the required basic knowledge of general microbiology to students of botany, zoology, pharmacy, medicine, agriculture, nutrition, chemistry, etc. This book is designed to appeal to such a wide spectrum of readers. Its aim is to convey a general view as well as specific knowledge and to stimulate.

The book does presuppose a certain knowledge of biology, such as is contained in basic texts of botany and zoology. It should also stimulate further study in adjoining disciplines, especially in general biochemistry. Apart from an outline of the basic biochemistry of metabolism, only those metabolic reactions and pathway that are specific to microorganisms are dealt with in any detail.

Because our present knowledge of molecular details and interactions has made biological phenomena more easily understood, this book concentrates on the physiological aspects of microorganisms and the presentation of basic relationships at the expense of a more descriptive approach. The diversity of living beings and processes, as well as of metabolism, can be derived from common origins and a limited number of elementary structures and processes, i.e. architectural and metabolic plans. Their knowledge in turn also yields valuable heuristic principles for the descriptive domain. Thus penetration into depths is also fruitful for an understanding of breadth.

Acknowledgments

I would like to thank especially my colleagues, D. Claus, U. Eberhardt, G. Gottschalk, and N. Pfennig for their extensive support, advice, and criticism. A considerable part of the work on the book was shared with Dr Karin Schmidt. Without her collaboration in the design of illustrations, drafting of the manuscript, and many editorial tasks, the manuscript could not have been made ready for publication. My thanks are also due to Mr L. Schnellbächer for the careful and faithful execution of the drawings, and to Mrs M. Welskop for the typing of the manuscript and producing the index.

My thanks are also due to all my colleagues who supplied unpublished photographs or high quality reproductions from published work. The generous consent for the reproduction of such pictures by the respective publishers is also gratefully acknowledged.

The G. Thieme publishing house which undertook to publish a series of very reasonably priced, well-endowed, introductory texts for the benefit of biological sciences merits special acknowledgement.

H. G. Schlegel
Göttingen, November, 1968

Translator's preface

My wish to translate Professor Schlegel's book arose from the realisation that some of the aims he states in the preface to the first edition are not adequately served by any of the existing textbooks in English.

These aims were to provide a comprehensive, yet concise, general textbook that would 'transmit the required basic knowledge of microbiology' not only to students who take Microbiology as their major subject, but also to those studying medicine, agriculture, nutrition, biochemistry, pharmacy, food technology, etc. On reading this German textbook on General Microbiology, I found that it largely fulfils these aims by the breadth and depth of coverage, as well as by the way the contents are organised. This allows assembly of the required information without too much overlap, whilst avoiding topics also dealt with in other courses, such as basic metabolic pathways (Chapter 7) for those who have already studied biochemistry, or photosynthesis and nitrogen fixation (Chapters 12 and 13) for medical students. The handy format and reasonable price should also prove a great attraction for this body of readers.

I would like here to express my appreciation to Cambridge University Press and their Biological Sciences editor, Dr F. Bendall, and later, Mr P. Silver, for agreeing to take up my suggestion of an English edition, and for the support and help they gave me in accomplishing this task. Next, I gratefully acknowledge the agreement and cooperation of Professor Schlegel and the George Thieme Verlag. To Professor Schlegel especially I would like to express my thanks for his freely given support, advice and extensive cooperation. He has read the whole of my drafts for the sixth and the seventh editions, and supplied many technical terms and felicitous renderings, as well as his own revisions. In addition, I am also greatly indebted to my colleague, Dr N. J. Russel of University College, Cardiff, who read the whole of my draft for the sixth edition and made many valuable suggestions.

Finally, all the above named have contributed to make the translation a pleasant and often stimulating task. I hope that similar pleasure and stimulation will also be experienced by the readers.

Margot Kogut

Use of technical terms, conventions and nomenclature

The author of the German text states that it is customary to leave the use of conventions and spellings of technical terms to the decisions of author and publisher. He therefore stated the following guidelines for the original text.

In the designation of microorganisms abbreviations of generic names should be rarely used, and then only where misinterpretations are excluded by the context. Similarly, abbreviations for chemical compounds should also be avoided. However, certain abbreviations have been used in this book, especially in the many diagrammatic schemes for metabolic routes.

To make the reading of the text simple for microbiologists without a biochemistry background, it was decided to continue with certain now-incorrect conventions in the use of some terms. In particular, the indication of charge on the nicotinamide adenine nucleotides has been omitted (i.e. NAD(P) is used throughout instead of NAD(P)$^+$). Similarly, the formulae of organic acids and phosphate esters are given for the undissociated form, whereas they are referred to in the text as salts, i.e. lactate, pyruvate, succinate, etc.

as undissociated acid	as present under physiological conditions
COOH | C=O | CH$_3$	COO$^-$ C$\diagup^O_{O^-}$ | or | C=O C=O | | CH$_3$ CH$_3$

Pyruvate

Commonly used abbreviations

1. Amino acids

Ala	alanine	Ile	isoleucine
Arg	arginine	Leu	leucine
Asn	asparagine	Lys	lysine
Asp	aspartic acid	Met	methionine
Cys	cysteine	Phe	phenylalanine
Dab	diaminobutyric acid	Pro	proline
Dpm	diaminopimelic acid	Ser	serine
Gln	glutamine	Thr	threonine
Glu	glutamic acid	Trp	tryptophan
Gly	glycine	Tyr	tyrosine
His	histidine	Val	valine

2. Nucleoside phosphates

AMP, ADP, ATP	adenosine mono-, di- and triphosphates
CMP, CDP, CTP	cytidine mono-, di- and triphosphates
GMP, GDP, GTP	guanosine mono-, di- and triphosphates
IMP, IDP, ITP	inosine mono-, di- and triphosphates
TMP, TDP, TTP	thymidine mono-, di- and triphosphates
UMP, UDP, UTP	uridine mono-, di- and triphosphates
NuMP, NuDP, NuTP	nucleoside mono-, di- and triphosphates

3. Other abbreviations in alphabetical order

CoA	coenzyme A	Glc	glucose
Cyt	cytochrome	GlcN	glucosamine
DH	dehydrogenase	GlcNAc	*N*-acetylglucosamine
DNA	deoxyribonucleic acid	GSH	glutathione, reduced form
EDTA	ethylenediamino-tetraacetate		
FAD	flavine adenine dinucleotide	KDPG	2-keto-3-deoxy-6-phosphogluconic acid
FBP	fructose-1,6-bisphosphate		
FMN	flavine mononucleotide	M	molar (concentration)
F-6-P	fructose-6-phosphate	mol	mole (amount)
G-6-P	glucose-6-phosphate	MurNAc	*N*-acetyl muramic acid
GAP	glyceraldehyde-3-phosphate	NAD(P)	nicotinamide adenine dinucleotide (phosphate)
Gal-6-P	galactose-6-phosphate		

NAD(P)H$_2$	reduced nicotinamide adenine dinucleotide (phosphate)	RuBP	ribulose-1,5-bisphosphate
		RNA	ribonucleic acid
		Shu-7-P	sedoheptulose-7-phosphate
PEP	phospheoenol-pyruvate		
3-PG	3-phosphoglyceric acid	ShuBP	sedoheptulose-1,7-bisphosphate
6-PG	6-phosphogluconic acid		
PHB	polyhydroxy-butyric acid	TA	transaldolase
P$_i$	orthophosphate	TCA	tricarboxylic acid cycle
Ⓟ	PO$_3$H$_2$	TK	transketolase
PK	phosphoketolase	TPP	thiamine diphosphate
PP$_i$	pyrophosphate	UQ	ubiquinone
R-5-P	ribose-5-phosphate	Xu-5-P	xylulose-5-phosphate
Ru-5-P	ribulose-5-phosphate		

1   The place of microorganisms in nature

1.1   The three kingdoms: animals, plants and protista

Until the last century, living organisms were classified as animals or plants by their obvious differences in form and constitution. These differences can be explained by the basic differences in their modes of nutrition. Animals (carbon-heterotrophs) feed on complex organic substances which are hydrolysed, digested and absorbed from the intestinal tract inside the body. During embryonic development these body cavities arise from invagination of the blastula. Indeed, the development of animals seem to aim at the creation of large, absorbing, internal surfaces. This principle of construction appears to apply to a large range of animals, from the Hydrozoa (freshwater polyps) to the highest vertebrates.

In accord with their entirely different nutritional mode, plants (carbon-autotrophs) are constructed on a completely different plan. They synthesise the substances needed for growth and maintenance from inorganic materials and utilise sunlight as a source of energy. The photosynthetically active cells and tissues, which contain the light-absorbing pigments (Chlorophylls and carotenoids), and orientated towards the environment and form large external surfaces. Other general differences between plants and animals concern the presence of cell walls, the capacity for active movement and change of position within the environment, and abilities to synthesise various substances.

Thus, it was easy to make sharp distinctions between plant and animal kingdoms as long as little was known about microorganisms. Even fungi had so many properties in common with higher plants that they could be included in the plant kingdom despite their generally heterotrophic nutrition. Much more difficult decisions arose in assigning bacteria, slime moulds, and other unicellular organisms to one of the two kingdoms. Hence, a third division of living organisms with the collective name of **Protista** was established by Haeckel (1866). Based on the selection and evolutionary theory of Charles Darwin (1859), Haeckel unified the then known genera and species of plants and animals from the viewpoint of their possible evolutionary development. In a **'phylogenetic tree'** he tried to show how the contemporary organisms could have evolved from a common 'root', the 'Radix Communis Organisatorum'. However, Haeckel does not seem to have had a very clear idea about the division of the Protista.

The kingdom Protista contains those organisms that are differentiated from plants and animals by their lack of morphological specialisation, most of them being unicellular. The protists can then be further subdivided into two clearly differentiated groups on the basis of their cellular structure. The higher protists resemble plants and animals in their cell composition: they are eukaryotes. This group includes algae, fungi and protozoa. The lower protists include the bacteria and cyanobacteria (blue-green algae): they are prokaryotes and their cellular structure is very different from that of all other organisms. The term microorganisms is derived from the minute size of the various organisms mentioned above and corresponds in its meaning and application to that of Protista. Viruses are non-cellular particles, different from all other organisms in that they are not capable of self-replication and can proliferate only in living cells.

1.2   Prokaryotes and eukaryotes

The basic physical unit of living organisms is the cell, the smallest unit capable of life. Its material composition is the same in all organisms; DNA, RNA, proteins, lipids, and phospholipids are the fundamental components of all cells. However, investigations of the details of composition and the fine structure of different cell types have revealed significant differences between bacteria and cyanobacteria, on the one hand, and animals and plants, including their microscopically small representatives, on the other. These differences are so fundamental that the two groups are sharply differentiated as prokaryotes and eukaryotes. The **prokaryotes** are regarded as relics from the earliest time of biological evolution, and the development of eukaryotes represents the greatest discontinuity in the evolution of living organisms. The division of living organisms into the above three main groups, and the distinctions between the two great divisions of **prokaryotes** and **eukaryotes** are shown schematically in Fig. 1.1.

The **eukaryotes** possess a true nucleus (karyon) which contains the major part of the genome distributed on a set of chromosomes. These chromosomes are replicated by a process known as mitosis. In the chromosomes, DNA is associated with histones (basic proteins). The eukaryotic cell also contains organelles such as mitochondria and (in plants) chloroplasts that contain a small portion of the genome in the

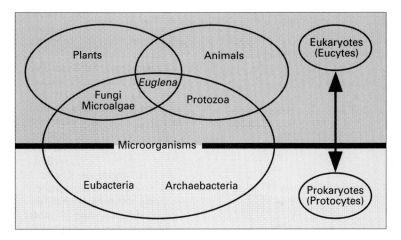

Fig. 1.1. *The three kingdoms: plants, animals and microorganisms, and the differences between eukaryotes and prokaryotes.*

form of closed circular DNA molecules. The ribosomes of eukaryotes are relatively large (80S).

The prokaryotes lack a true, membrane-bounded nucleus. DNA exists as a closed circular molecule in the cytoplasm. This single 'bacterial chromosome' contains all the information necessary for reproduction of the cell. In addition to this, there may be one or more small, circular DNA molecules, called plasmids; these are, however, dispensable. The prokaryotic cell does not contain distinct membrane-bounded organelles. Any subdivision of the cell interior into compartments is less definite than in eukaryotes. Prokaryotic ribosomes are relatively small (70S). The properties of prokaryotic ribosomes and enzymes involved in protein synthesis, as well as the structure of prokaryotic cell walls, are the bases for the selective effects of several antibiotics. Further differences will be discussed later (Chapter 2).

There is relatively little morphological differentiation among prokaryotes. Only a few basic shapes can be distinguished, derived from spheres and straight or curved cylinders. Such 'uniformity' in shape, however, is accompanied by a remarkable diversity and flexibility in metabolic properties. Whilst plants and animals all need oxygen, there are several groups of prokaryotes that can live anaerobically (in the absence of O_2) and can obtain the energy necessary for growth by means of fermentation reactions or by anaerobic respiration. Other groups are able to utilise light energy and can synthesise their cell materials either from organic compounds or from carbon dioxide. Yet other groups of bacteria are able to obtain their energy from oxidation of inorganic compounds or elements, whilst the ability to fix atmospheric nitrogen is also widely distributed.

This physiological versatility and flexibility, high rates of growth and synthesis, as well as the simple architecture of the cell and uncomplicated structure of its genetic material, have made the prokaryotes the preferred experimental objects of general biology over the last three decades or more. Because of these considerations and also the limitations of space this introductory text on microbiology deals mainly with the biology of bacteria.

1.3   Evolution of organisms

As long as little was known about the diversity of bacteria, and practically nothing about the molecular structure of their components, it seemed pointless to think along the lines that Haeckel had proposed. Indeed, the evolution of microorganisms was for a long time the subject of speculation and controversy. A phylogenetic tree could be constructed only after C. Woese had isolated and sequenced the ribosomal RNA of a large number of bacteria. The degree of relatedness of the base sequences from different bacteria then led to the conclusion that all prokaryotes could have arisen from a common precursor (sometimes designated the 'progenote'), and that the prokaryotes split very early into two large groups: the **Archaebacteria** and the **Eubacteria** (Chapters 3 and 17.4).

Some facts can now be established about the very early period of biological evolution, during which individual groups of bacteria developed from the progenote. Thus, the development of basic metabolic routes in bacteria must have occurred at a very early time. This can be concluded from the $^{13}C/^{12}C$ ratios in organic carbon compounds (C_{org}) which were deposited in sediments more than 3000 million years ago. The isotopic composition of these organic compounds (also known as 'kerogen') is the same as that of the recent autotrophic bacteria and plants. It can therefore be concluded that the C_{org} deposited in the early archaic period must stem from autotrophic bacteria. Whether these early producers of biomass were phototrophic bacteria, or anaerobically respiring methane bacteria (Ch. 9.4) cannot be determined from the isotope data.

Stromatolites.   Biogenic sedimentary rocks contain the oldest clues for the dating of biological activities in the earth's history. Their origins

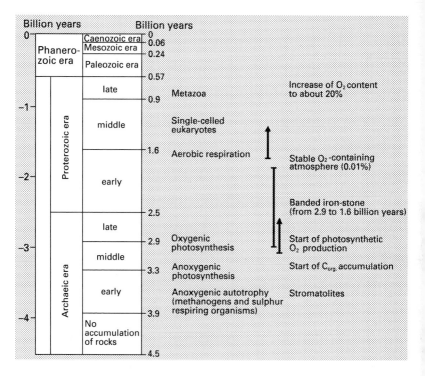

Fig. 1.2. *Chronological history of the earth.*
Time scale in billion years.

must also have involved participation of autotrophic organisms. Photosynthetic cyanobacteria apparently existed some 2.8 thousand million (10^9) years ago. Their activities gave rise to the evolution of oxygen. However, this early oxygen was captured by reduced iron compounds, which were thereby oxidised to insoluble iron oxides which, in turn, were deposited around the edges of the earth's oceans as 'banded iron formations' (BIFs) (Fig. 1.2). These discoveries have led to the hypothesis that the then living prokaryotes were the offspring of the oldest organisms, and that general cellular metabolism developed at the prokaryotes level. Evolution of the eukaryotes could occur only after the cyanobacteria provided a stable oxygen-containing atmosphere.

1.4   Participation in the elementary cycles of nature

Living organisms can be divided into three groups according to their role and function in the economy of nature. Green plants utilise the energy of sunlight to produce organic matter from carbon dioxide and are called primary producers. Animals are the consumers; they utilise the major part of the primary biomass for synthesis of their specific body substances. Eventually, both plants and animals are subject to degradative processes that convert organic material back to inorganic and mineral compounds. In this process, called mineralisation, bacteria and fungi are the main participants; they function as the degradative agents in the economy of nature. The bioelements are thus subject to cyclical processes. Here we will briefly elucidate the main features of the carbon, nitrogen, phosphate and sulphur cycles.

The carbon cycle. In this cycle, microorganisms carry out their most important function in the maintenance of life on earth. They effect the mineralisation of the organic carbon compounds produced by photosynthesis and thereby maintain a delicate equilibrium (Fig. 1.3). Atmospheric air contains hardly more than 0.03% carbon dioxide ($12\ \mu mol/l$). The photosynthetic activity of green plants is of such magnitude that the whole CO_2 content of the atmosphere would be exhausted in about 20 years. This is a relatively short period in our time span; it is estimated that the energy and carbon sources of the earth should suffice for another 1000–3000 years. Even with the oceans included, the carbon dioxide sources would last for only 2000 years. The green plants would soon have to relinquish their CO_2 fixation if lower animals and microorganisms did not constantly replenish the CO_2 reserves by mineralisation of organic compounds. Thus, the bacteria and fungi in soil are no less important than the photosynthetic green plants in the economy of matter. Indeed, the mutual dependence of all life forms on this earth is most clearly demonstrated in the carbon cycle.

> A special aspect of the mineralisation process of carbon is that a small part (1–1.5%) of mineralised carbon reaches the atmosphere not in the form of carbon dioxide, but as methane. This gas is produced from organic matter in situations where atmospheric oxygen is excluded (tundra, rice fields, rumen of ruminants) and is then oxidised by OH radicals in the atmosphere, via CO, to CO_2. The formation of methane, as well as other trace gases (H_2, CO, N_2O, NO_2) is mainly due to bacteria.
>
> The oceans would at first glance seem to constitute an enormous reservoir of carbon dioxide. However, one has to consider that the exchange rate between atmospheric carbon dioxide and the carbon dioxide of the sea – over 90% of which exists as HCO_3^- – is very low. Only one tenth of

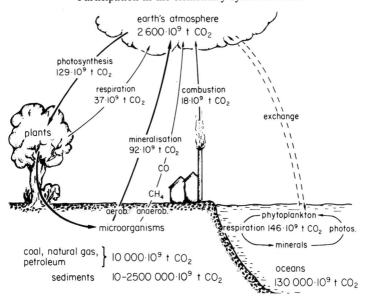

Fig. 1.3. *The carbon cycle in the biosphere.*

The quantities given in the arrowed lines refer to the conversion of carbon dioxide (fixation, production and exchange) per annum. The photosynthetic fixation of carbon dioxide by green plants would exhaust atmospheric carbon dioxide in a short time if organic material were not degraded and oxidised to CO_2 by microorganisms so that the atmospheric level of CO_2 is maintained. The burning of fossil carbon (petroleum, coal, natural gas) leads to a gradual increase in the CO_2 content of the atmosphere.

the CO_2 in the air is exchanged with that in the sea per annum. In addition, only a very shallow surface layer participates in such gaseous exchange. The large quantities of CO_2 present in seawater below this layer get to the surface in only a few areas of upwelling currents (West Africa, Chile) where they do enrich the CO_2 content of the atmosphere (to 0.05%). In recent years, however, it has been found that the CO_2 content of the atmosphere is steadily increasing. This increase is due, on the one hand, to the burning of oil, petroleum, and coal; during 1976 the whole earth's consumption of crude oil amounted to 3.2×10^9 tonnes, the major part of which was burned. On the other hand, the increase in atmospheric CO_2 is probably also due to decline in photosynthetic CO_2 fixation and soil erosion. However, it should be mentioned in this connection that the oceans do constitute a powerful CO_2 buffering system and help to maintain the CO_2 content of the atmosphere.

The biochemical pathways of photosynthetic CO_2 fixation by green plants are concerned primarily with sugars and related compounds. Thus most of the fixed carbon dioxide is deposited as polymeric sugars in the form of wood and grasses; almost 60% of the terrestrially fixed CO_2 consists of wood. Wood consists of about 75% polysaccharides (cellulose, hemicellulose, starch, pectins and arabinoglycans) and only a little more than 20% lignin and lignans, whilst the protein content is very low (1%). In grasses and shrubby plants the polysaccharide content is even higher. This predominance of polysaccharides in the assimilation products of green plants determines the overwhelming importance of sugars for all living organisms that depend on organic nutrients. Glucose and other sugars in the form of polymers are, therefore, not only the major substrates for the mineralisation processes of nature, but they are also, as monomers, the preferred nutrients for most heterotrophic microorganisms.

The nitrogen cycle.   Central to the nitrogen cycle is ammonia. This is the end-product of the degradation of proteins and amino acids that reach the soil in the form of dead animal and vegetable matter. In well-aerated soils ammonia undergoes 'nitrification'. The bacterial genera *Nitrosomonas* and *Nitrobacter* can oxidise ammonium to nitrite and nitrate. Ammonium, as well as nitrate, can be utilised and assimilated as a nitrogen source by green plants. When nitrate is present (in soil) under anaerobic conditions, 'denitrification' takes place. Certain bacteria can use nitrate as a hydrogen acceptor, that is, they respire with NO_3^- instead of O_2, and thus this process is also referred to as 'nitrate respiration'. Such denitrification causes loss of nitrogen from the soil. Other bacteria are able to carry out nitrogen fixation. Some nitrogen-fixing bacteria are free-living in the soil (non-symbiotic) whereas others exist only symbiotically with higher plants (symbiotic nitrogen fixers). Thus animals, plants and bacteria participate in the nitrogen cycle (Fig. 1.4).

The phosphate cycle.   Phosphorus is present in the biosphere almost exclusively in the form of phosphates. In living organisms phosphoric acid is bound as phosphate esters. These esters are easily hydrolysed after death, and phosphate ions are liberated. Plants assimilate phosphorus in the soil as phosphoric acid ions (H_3PO_4). The concentration of these ions is often very low and growth limitation is mostly due to accumulation of insoluble phosphate compounds such as apatite or heavy metal complexes and not to lack of total phosphorus in the soil. The reserves of phosphates are large and are unlikely to limit agricultural production in the foreseeable future; however, the phosphates must be converted to their soluble forms. Phosphates from fertilisers often get

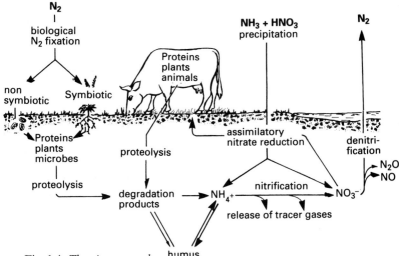

Fig. 1.4. *The nitrogen cycle.*

into streams and lakes. Since concentrations of iron, calcium, and aluminium in such waters are usually rather low, the phosphates remain soluble and lead to eutrophication of such waters, which is advantageous for the nitrogen-fixing cyanobacteria. In soils, on the other hand, phosphates are often rapidly deposited as insoluble salts.

The sulphur cycle. Sulphur is present in living cells mainly as the mercapto group in sulphur-containing amino acids (methionine, cysteine, homocysteine). It constitutes about 1% of the dry matter. The mercapto groups are cleaved by sulphurases during anaerobic degradation of organic matter; the formation of hydrogen sulphide during anaerobic mineralisation is also referred to as 'desulphuration'. The major part of the hydrogen sulphide that occurs in nature, however, is produced in the course of dissimilatory sulphate reduction by sulphate-reducing bacteria (Fig. 9.4). Anaerobic phototrophic bacteria (Chromatiaceae: Chapter 12) can oxidise the hydrogen sulphide produced in anoxic sediments to elementary sulphur and sulphates. If the hydrogen sulphide reaches aerobic situations, it is oxidised either abiotically or by aerobic sulphur bacteria to sulphates (Ch. 12.1, 12.1.2). The sulphur necessary for synthesis of sulphur-containing amino acids is obtained by plants and microorganisms via assimilatory sulphate reduction. Animals, on the other hand, depend on the uptake of compounds containing reduced sulphur in their diet (Fig. 1.5).

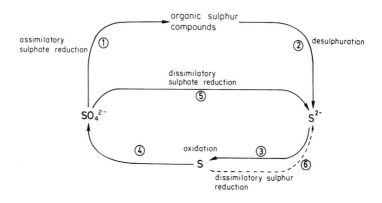

Fig. 1.5. *The sulphur cycle.*

(1) Assimilatory sulphate reduction converts sulphate to the reduction level of sulphide and fixes it in organic form in the proteins of living organisms. (2) Sulphur is liberated from amino acids by degradation of proteins and release of S^{2-}, (3, 4) Under aerobic conditions sulphide can be oxidised to sulphur and sulphate, either abiotically or by bacteria (*Beggiatoa, Thiothrix*). Free sulphur is oxidised aerobically to sulphate by *Thiobacilli*. (4) Under anaerobic conditions sulphide can be oxidised by phototrophic bacteria to sulphur (*Chlorobium*) or sulphate (*Chromatium*). (5) Under anaerobic conditions sulphate can be reduced to sulphide by dissilatory reduction (*Desulfovibrio, Desulfotomaculum*) and sulphur can be reduced by dissimilatory reduction (6) to sulphide by *Desulfuromonas*.

Limitations of biomass production by supplies of phosphorus and nitrogen.   The elements that limit the growth of plants, and hence production of biomass, are phosphorus and nitrogen. They are the growth-limiting factors on land and in the sea. Accurate figures are available for seawater. Table 1.1 shows how much biomass (in terms of gram dry weight) can be obtained from the elements present in 1 m^3 of seawater: 28 g of carbon can yield 60–100 g of biomass; 0.3 g of nitrogen can give 6 g, and 0.03 g of phosphorus can give only 5 g of biomass. These calculations show that the production of biomass is finally limited by phosphates. In seawater, therefore, even the nitrogen-fixing organisms like cyanobacteria have no selective advantage.

Table 1.1. *Distribution of bioelements in seawater*

Element	g/100 g dry organisms (N)	g/m³ seawater (A)	Ratio A/N
Potassium	1	390	390
Carbon	30	28	~ 1
Silicon	0.5	0.5	1
Nitrogen	5.0	0.3	0.06
Phosphorus	0.6	0.03	0.05
Sulphur	1	900	900
Iron	1	0.05	0.05
Vanadium	0.003	0.0003	0.1

1.5   Useful microorganisms

The naïve observer first realises the practical importance of microorganisms by the damage they cause to man, animals, and plants. These disease-producing or pathogenic microorganisms are the subjects of human and veterinary medicine, as well as phytopathology. However, whilst there are even more processes in nature and industry where microorganisms can cause damage, their useful roles overshadow all of these. They have long played useful parts in domestic and industrial processes, where they have become indispensible. Their application ranges from processing of primary agricultural products to the catalysis of complicated chemical reactions.

Classical microbial processes.   Beer and wine production by yeasts, bread making, the processing of milk to dairy products by lactic acid bacteria, and the formation of vinegar by acetic acid bacteria show that microbes are among the oldest domesticated organisms. In Japan and Indonesia, soybeans are treated by a process involving moulds, yeast and lactic acid bacteria. On the other hand, with the exception of alcohol production, microorganisms have been applied to industrial processes for only the last six decades or so. During the First World War, controlled fermentation by yeast was used to obtain glycerol. Cheap carbohydrate-containing wastes can be converted to acetone, butanol, 2-propanol, butanediol and other basic chemicals via fermentations carried out by clostridia and bacilli, whilst in the food industry large amounts of lactic and citric acids are obtained by the use of lactic acid bacteria and the fungus *Aspergillus*, respectively.

Antibiotic production.   A new era in medical therapy and the pharmaceutical industry was opened by the discovery of antibiotics. Penicillin and other secondary products of fungi, actinomycetes and some bacteria have provided the most powerful tools in the fight against bacterial infections. The search for new antibiotics continues successfully. Even the fight against viral infections and diseases due to tumour viruses can be conceived (at present theoretically) by the use of antibiotics.

New microbiological processes.   The classic fermentations mentioned above are now complemented by newer microbial reactions and processes. Carotenoids and steroids can be obtained from fungi. Following the discovery that *Corynebacterium glutamicum* can produce large yields of glutamic acid from sugar and ammonium salts, the development of microbial mutants and processes has led to the possibility of large-scale production of various amino acids, nucleotides, and other biochemical products. Microorganisms can also be used for catalysis of certain steps in extensive synthetic chains; microbial reactions often exceed chemical ones in specificity and yield. Amylases for the hydrolysis of starch, proteinases for curing leathers, pectinases for producing fruit juices, and many other industrially used enzymes are obtained from microbial cultures.

The monopoly position of microorganisms.   It should be emphasised that a number of major primary raw materials, such as crude oil, gases, or cellulose, can be utilised only by microorganisms, which convert these to either biomass or intermediary products that are secreted by the cells. Because of this, microorganisms can be regarded as occupying a 'monopoly position' in the processing of these raw materials, though the application of microbiological methods to such processes is just beginning.

Gene technology.   Elucidation of the mechanisms of gene transmission in bacteria, and the participation of extrachromosomal elements in this, have opened the possibility of transferring foreign DNA into bacteria. This, 'gene technology', means that small pieces of a carrier of genetic information, for example from man, could be inserted into bacteria, which could then synthesise the corresponding proteins. Thus, hormones, antigens, antibodies and other proteins can be produced with the help of bacteria. Further, various properties conferring resistance, such as against insects (potato beetle), or fungal infection, can be induced in economic crops by gene technology. There are also attempts to transfer the capacity for molecular nitrogen fixation to higher plants. Finally, gene technology allows the production of 'DNA probes' which can be used to recognise defective or altered sections of DNA and RNA. Gene technology, with bacteria as tools, thus opens a new era of biological evolution.

Immediate applicability of basic scientific knowledge.   It would be inappropriate here even to attempt to list all the processes and products of industrial microbiology and to speculate on the possibilities of further applications. The relationship between basic scientific research and the applicability of its results in practical processes is close, in microbiology as in other sciences: 'Il n'y a pas des sciences appliqués … mais il y a des applications de la science' (Pasteur).

1.6   General properties of microorganisms

The defining property of microorganisms, incorporated in the very name of the group, is the microscopic size of the individual. These small dimensions are not only the original motive for placing them in a special group, separate from plant and animal kingdoms, but they also have important consequences for their morphology, activity, diversity and flexibility of metabolism, ecological distribution, and manipulation in the laboratory.

> *Units of measurement and surface–volume relationships.*   The diameter of most bacteria is not much greater than one thousandth of a millimetre; the yardstick for microbiologists is therefore the unit 1 micrometre (micron) or $1 \mu m = 10^{-3}$ mm; observations regarding fine structure are reported in nanometres: $1 \text{ nm} = 10^{-3} \mu m = 10^{-6}$ mm. Dimensions of the smaller corynebacteria, yeasts and protozoa are usually less than $10 \mu m$. In all these tiny organisms the ratio of surface area to volume is very large (division of a 1 cm³ cube into cubes of $1 \mu m^3$ produces 10^{12} cubes of this size, and their combined surfaces are 10000 times that of the original 1 cm³ cube). The volume of a medium-sized bacterium is $1 \mu m^3$.

The high surface-to-volume ratio leads to extensive interactions with the environment and is the reason for the high metabolic rates of many microorganisms. The 'surface rule' of Rubner (1893) established that energy consumption of animals at rest is not proportional to their mass, but their surface area. Extrapolation of this rule to the dimensions of tissues and small cells would yield metabolic rates ranging over several orders of magnitude. Table 1.2 shows the expected correlation between metabolic rates, measured as oxygen consumption, and the dimensions of tissues and cells. Similar relationships can be found for the growth rates of microorganisms. The reader who is interested in the problems of feeding the growing world population could reflect that a cow weighing

Table 1.2. *Specific respiratory rates of microorganisms and tissues* (Q_{O_2} *in* μl O_2/mg *dry weight per hour) and generation times (doubling times) of bacteria at their optimal growth rates*

Biological material	Temp. (°C)	$- Q_{O_2}$	Organism	Temp. (°C)	Generation time (min)
Azotobacter	28	2000	*Bacillus megaterium*	40	22
Acetobacter	30	1800	*B. subtilis*	40	26
Pseudomonas	30	1200	*Escherichia coli*	40	21
Baker's yeast	28	100	*B. stearothermophilus*	60	11
Kidney, liver	37	10–20	*B. megaterium*	70	13
Roots, leaves	20	0.5–4	*B. coagulans*	70	14
			B. circulans	70	14

500 kg will produce 0.5 kg protein in 24 hours, whilst 500 kg of yeast would be making 50 000 kg of protein.

Metabolic flexibility.   Higher plants and animals are rather inflexible in their enzymatic equipment; their enzyme complement may change somewhat during individual development but cannot respond much to changes in the environment. Metabolic flexibility in microorganisms is far greater. In bacteria, extensive adaptability is a necessity determined by their small size: a micrococcal cell has space for only some 100 000 molecules of protein. Enzymes that are not currently being used cannot be held in reserve, and therefore certain catabolic enzymes are produced only if the appropriate substrate is present. Such inducible enzymes can constitute up to 10% of the cellular protein under some conditions. Therefore regulatory mechanisms play a far greater part in microbial cells and are more easily recognisable than in other organisms.

Distribution of microorganisms.   The small dimensions of microorganisms are also of ecological significance. Before humans helped to distribute them, many species of animals and plants were limited in distribution to one of the continents. Bacteria and cyanobacteria, however, are ubiquitous. They are found in arctic conditions, in all waters, and in the upper strata of the atmosphere. Species distribution in these places is generally similar to that in soils. Because of their low mass, microorganisms can be transported by air currents. Under natural conditions, therefore, no substrate or location needs to be inoculated. This situation can be exploited for the isolation of specific microorganisms by enrichment culture. Usually only 1 g of garden soil is needed to find any bacterium that utilises a given natural substrate. Microorganisms are virtually omnipresent; only the environment determines which species can reproduce. By application of selective conditions in a test tube or flask, one can cultivate most common microorganisms from a bit of soil or mud or some other natural sample, via enrichment culture techniques, to eventual isolation in pure culture.

Quantitative investigations and the progress of genetic research. The methodology for cultivation of microorganisms in the laboratory was developed in the 19th century by O. Brefeld and R. Koch, and their schools. The introduction of clear solid media, using gelatin and agar, enabled them to isolate single cells, follow their growth into colonies, and obtain pure cultures. Standardisation of sterile techniques, cultivation media, and conditions resulted in the rapid development of medical and diagnostic microbiology. Although Koch had already described some quantitative methods, the real advantages of quantitative techniques in microbiology became established only during the last 50 years. The small dimensions of microorganisms allow populations of 10^8 or 10^9 cells to be worked with in a single test tube or petri dish, so that such rare events as mutations or transfer of genetic characters can be studied with simple apparatus and limited space. The enormous progress of biochemical and genetic research is thus due, at least in part, to the easy manipulation of bacteria.

2 The cell and its structure

Until recently, our knowledge of detailed cell structure depended entirely on direct visual observation and light microscopy and was limited by the availability of optical instruments and the development of preparative methods. Gradually, improvements in microscopical techniques and instruments have resulted in increasingly detailed information about micromorphology and the fine structure of cells. More recently, extension of light microscopy has brought about dramatic reductions in the limits of resolution. However, most methods of microscopy, especially electron microscopy, involve the preparation of biological materials by complicated procedures which are still indispensible; dark-field and phase-contrast microscopy, on the other hand, allow observations of living cells. Less direct physical and chemical methods can also be used to complement optical investigations and allow isolation and characterisation of cell components at the molecular level. Differential centrifugation of homogenates, for example, has led to isolation and biochemical investigations of cell fractions and organelles, whilst the combination of optical and biochemical methods has facilitated rapid and increasingly detailed elucidation of function and structure in cells, their organelles, and components. These investigations have shown that eukaryotes and prokaryotes differ in a large number of properties.

All cells consist of cytoplasmic and nuclear material and are surrounded and separated from the environment by the cytoplasmic membrane. In some cases such protoplasts are further enveloped by a cell wall, which has mainly mechanical functions. This is the case in most plant cells and bacteria.

A brief description of the fundamental properties of eukaryotic cells (eucytes) and prokaryotic cells (protocytes) follows. The embryonic plant cell (Fig. 2.1) is taken as a representative example of the eucyte.

2.1 The eukaryotic cell (eucyte)

The nucleus. The structure of the nucleus and the type of nuclear division are the most striking and fundamental differences between eukaryotic and prokaryotic cells (Fig. 2.2).

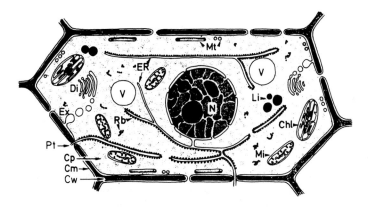

Fig. 2.1. *Longitudinal section of a eukaryotic (plant) cell.*

Chl; chloroplasts:
Cm; cytoplasmic membrane;
Cp; cytoplasm; Di; dictyosomes;
ER; endoplasmic reticulum;
Ex; secretory vesicles (exocytosis);

Li; lipid droplet; Mi; mitochondria;
Mt; microtubules; N; nucleus;
Pt; pit with plasmodesma;
Rb; ribosomes; V; vacuoles; Cw; cell
wall.

  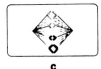 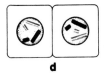

Fig. 2.2. *Mitosis in a dipoid cell.*

The nucleus contains two chromosomes from each of the two parents. Mitosis results in the equal distribution of the chromosomes to the two daughter cells. (a) During prophase the chromosomes, already longitudinally split, become visible and the nuclear membrane dissolves; (b) during metaphase the chromosomes become arranged in the equatorial plane; (c) during anaphase the separate halves of the chromosomes are drawn apart by the spindle threads, towards the poles of the cell; (d) during telophase the choromosomes, again longitudinally divided, are surrounded by the nuclear membrane and the nucleus assumes the functional form.

The interphase nucleus is surrounded by the nuclear envelope, a membrane composed of two lipid bilayers, perforated by nuclear pores. Nuclear DNA, which constitutes the genome, is distributed among a number of structures called chromosomes, which become visible only during nuclear division. Nuclear division occurs by mitosis (Fig. 2.2), which serves two functions; (1) the accurate replication of the genetic material, which eventually becomes visible in the lengthwise separation of the duplicated chromosomes, and (2) the equal distribution of the two complete sets of chromosomes to each of the two daughter nuclei. How the duplication of chromosomes is accomplished is not yet fully understood, though much of the process of DNA replications has been elucidated in prokaryotes. The separation and distribution of the chromosomes can be observed with the light microscope and has been known for a long time. Although in the light microscope the interphase nucleus appears to be an undifferentiated mass, the chromosomes shorten and become visible with the onset of the division phase. They arrange themselves in an equatorial plane with the pairs of duplicated chromosomes in parallel. The two paired sets of chromosomes are then pulled apart by means of a contractile spindle. Following this, the spindle disappears, the chromosomes lose their visibility, and the two daughter nuclei are again bounded by a nuclear membrane.

All higher plants and animals undergo a nuclear rearrangement as part of sexual reproduction. At fertilisation the gametes (germ cells) and their nuclei fuse to give rise to the zygote. The male and female nucleus contribute equal numbers (n) of chromosomes during fertilisation. The zygote nucleus therefore has two sets of chromosomes (and genomes) ($2n$). Thus, whilst the gametes are haploid, with one set of chromosomes each, all somatic cells are diploid, with two sets of chromosomes. For the next sexual generation, therefore, the normal diploid ($2n$) chromosome complement has to be reduced to the haploid number (n). The process leading to the halving of the chromosome number is called meiosis or reduction division (Fig. 2.3). Meiosis is a fundamental process in all sexually reproducing organisms. It fulfils two functions: (1) the recombination of paternal and maternal genetic material, and (2) the reduction in the chromosome number. Meiosis starts with the pairing of chromosomes. Each chromosome aligns itself with the homologous chromosome derived from the other parent. At this stage, breaks can occur in the chromosomes, and the joining of the broken strands may involve crossing over between two chromosomes. In this way exchange of segments between the homologous chromosomes may be achieved. The pairing of the chromosomes is followed by two sequential separations (spindle formation) of the paired and divided chromosomes. As a result, cells with haploid nuclei are produced. Thus, in the course of meiosis, there is not only a reassortment of the chromosome sets derived from the paternal and maternal gametes, but also the possibility of exchange of segments between homologous chromosomes. Both these processes lead to a recombination of genetic material. In many of the lower plants (including algae) and in protozoa, meiosis occurs immediately after the

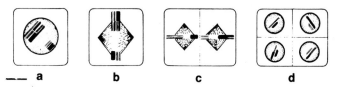

Fig. 2.3. *Meiosis.*

Meiosis leads to recombination of paternal and maternal genes, and to the reduction in chromosome number. (a) At first the homologous chromosomes pair; crossing over has produced an exchange of segments between the homologous chromosomes; (b, c) a double spindle formation draws the chromosomes apart, separating the homologous chromosomes; (d) four cells with haploid nuclei result.

formation of the zygote, so that the organism is actually haploid. In plants with heterophasic generation changes, such as mosses and ferns, haploid and diploid generations alternate.

Eukaryotic chromosomes consist of DNA strands associated with numerous proteins; some of these are basic proteins known as histones. Histones and DNA are apparently associated in a highly ordered manner, forming nucleosomes, which are regarded as the subunits of chromosomes.

During interphase a nucleolus is visible inside the nucleus. This contains the information for ribosomal RNA (rRNA) and probably also for transfer RNA (tRNA). Messenger RNA (mRNA) is made on the chromosomal DNA in the nucleus and then transported through the pores of the nuclear membrane into the cytoplasms, whereas ribosomal and tRNA are apparently synthesised in the nucleolus and then transported into the cytoplasm. Embryonic cells and ova may contain numerous nucleoli. The eukaryotic nucleus, although the most important carrier of genetic information for the cell, is not the only one. Some of the information is contained in the DNA of mitochondria and chloroplasts.

The cytoplasm.   The protoplast is surrounded by the cytoplasmic membrane. The eucyte is characterised by extensive subdivision of the cytoplasm into a large number of compartments. This compartmentation is achieved to some extent by invaginations of the cytoplasmic membrane, which forms vesicles and cisternae. In addition the eukaryotic cytoplasm contains mitochondria and (in photosynthetic organisms) chloroplasts which are themselves surrounded by complete membranes. The cytoplasmic membrane is contiguous in the interior of the cytoplasm with the endoplasmic reticulum (ER). This endoplasmic reticulum also forms the nuclear membrane, which surrounds the nucleus and contains numerous pores to allow easy transfer of nucleic acids, proteins, and metabolites between the nucleus and cytoplasm. Part of the endoplasmic reticulum has many ribosomes attached to it, and this is known as the rough or granular ER. Ribosomes are the sites of protein synthesis. The ribosomes attached to the endoplasmic reticulum and those that are free in the cytoplasm of the eucyte both belong to the 80S type.

A special membraneous organelle of the animal cells is the Golgi apparatus. Similar organelles found in plant cells are called dictyosomes. They consist of bundles of flattened membrane vesicles, so-called cisternae. Both the Golgi apparatus and dictyosomes have important functions in secretion of, mainly, enzymes that are synthesised on the cisternae and collected inside them. Eventually one of the vesicles detaches itself, moves to and fuses with the cytoplasmic membrane whilst emptying its content to the cell exterior. This process is called exocytosis.

Mitochondria and chloroplasts.   The eucyte contains two further membrane-bounded organelles, the mitochondria and (in photosynthetic organisms) chloroplasts. The mitochondria function in respiration. They are pleiomorphic, lipid-rich structures which consist of two membranes, an external one and a much-folded inner one that constitutes what are known as cristae. The infoldings contain the components of the electron-transport chain and ATP synthase. The cells of algae and green plants contain chloroplasts in addition to mitochondria. The inner membrane of chloroplasts (thylakoids) are the sites of photosynthetic pigments and components of photosynthetic electron transport.

Endocytosis.   Another characteristic property of eucytes is the ability to take up solid as well as liquid nutrients from the environment. The uptake of solid particles is known as phagocytosis, for example by leucocytes in the blood, or by amoebae. Fluid uptake is called pinocytosis. Both kinds of uptake of extracellular material are known collectively as endocytosis. The capacity of eukaryotes to take up solid matter, including living cells, is of fundamental biological importance. Such endocytosis can be regarded as a precursor and mechanism for the origin of endosymbiosis. In the normal course of events, a solid particle taken up by an amoeba via phagocytosis would be completely digested and assimilated. However, in some cases such endocytosis results in intracellular symbiosis. The best-known example of this is leguminous root nodules with rhizobia (Chapter 13). Such endosymbioses are fairly widespread among eukaryotes (Ch. 17.2.1). The capacity of eukaryotic cells for endocytosis supports the hypothesis for the endosymbiotic origins of mitochondria and chloroplasts.

The endosymbiotic hypothesis.   The subcellular organelles of eukaryotes show many important features of prokaryotic cells. They contain a circular closed DNA molecule, ribosomes of the 70S type, and a membrane containing the components of the electron-transport chain (flavoproteins, quinones, iron-sulphur proteins and cytochromes) which function in respiratory or photosynthetic energy conversion. The endosymbiotic hypothesis proposes that mitochondria are derived from a colourless, aerobic prokaryote and chloroplasts are derived from cyanobacteria that established endosymbiotic relationships with a primitive eukaryotic cells. Subsequently a pronounced specialisation must have occurred in which ATP generation became delegated to the intracellular organelle; the membrane surrounding the eukaryotic protoplast does not contain components of the electron transport chain. On the other hand, the intracellular organelles are not independent either: although they have their own molecule of DNA, a considerable amount of the information necessary for the synthesis of their proteins is located in the eukaryotic cell nucleus. An example is the enzyme ribulose-bisphosphate carboxylase, a key element in autotrophic CO_2 fixation by green plants. It consists of eight major and eight minor subunits. The information for the major subunits is located on the chloroplast DNA, but that for the minor subunits is part of the nuclear DNA. These organelles, therefore, are not able to multiply outside the eucyte and the endosymbiotic hypothesis is not susceptible to conclusive proof or disproof.

Organelles of locomotion.   The known flagella or cilia of eukaryotes, i.e. in algae, protozoa, spermatozoa or epithelia, are of uniform structure. Transverse sections show nine peripheral double filaments with two central single filaments (the 9 + 2 pattern). They are surrounded by the cytoplasmic membrane. The flagella are inserted in the outer layer of the cytoplasm via a basal plate or 'blepharoplast', which itself arises from a self-duplicating organelle, the centriole.

2.2   The prokaryotic cell (protocyte)

The structure and functions of prokaryotic cells will be described in detail. Before embarking on this, however, it is desirable first to outline the most important characteristics by which prokaryotic cells differ from eucytes.

As already mentioned, prokaryotic cells are rather small. Most bacterial species are rod-shaped, usually not more than 1 μm wide and 5 μm long. Many pseudomonads have a diameter of 0.4–0.7 μm and a length of 2–3 μm. The diameter of micrococci is only 0.5 μm. There are only a

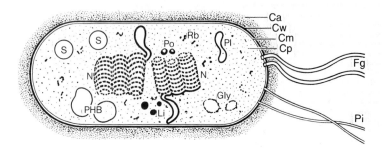

Fig. 2.4. *Longitudinal section of a prokaryotic (bacterial) cell.*

Cm; Cytoplasmic membrane;	Pi; pili; Pl; plasmid;
Cp; cytoplasm; Fg; flagella;	Po; polyphosphate granules;
Gly; glycogen granules; Ca; capsule;	Rb; ribosomes (and polysomes);
Li; lipid droplets; N; nucleoid;	S; sulphur inclusions; Cw; cell wall.
PHB; poly-β-hydroxybutyrate;	

few large forms among bacterial species (*Chromatium okenii, Thiospirillum jenense, Achromatium,* etc). These giant bacteria generally grow relatively slowly. Compartmentation in prokaryotic cells is far less pronounced than in the eucyte (Fig. 2.4). There are no organelles of the kind exemplified by mitochondria and chloroplasts, nor is the DNA surrounded by a nuclear membrane. A nuclear region, visible in electron micrographs of ultrathin sections of bacteria as a network of very fine threads, borders directly on the cytoplasm, which contains large quantities of ribosomes (Fig. 2.5). These ribosomes are smaller than the ribosomes of eukaryotes. They belong to the 70S type. The cytoplasmic membranes of many bacteria extend into the interior of the cytoplasm (intracytoplasmic membrane). In prokaryotes the cytoplasmic membrane is the site of respiratory and photosynthetic energy generation. Analogous functions in eukaryotes are localised in the membranes of mitochondria and chloroplasts.

The entire genetic information of the protocyte is contained in a single thread of DNA, the bacterial chromosome. This DNA molecule exists as a circular strand (0.25–3 mm long) in all bacteria so far examined. No histones are present. However, in many bacteria, extrachromosomal DNA has been identified; it is found as small DNA molecules which are also circular and are called plasmids. Some linear plasmids have also been found. The information localised in the plasmids is apparently not essential for the organism.

Bacteria generally multiply by binary fission. After the appropriate

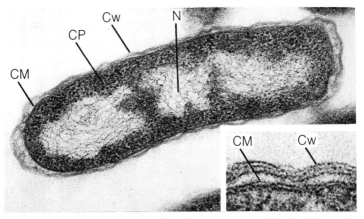

Fig. 2.5. *Electron micrograph of an ultrathin section of* Escherichia coli.

Due to slight plasmolysis, the protoplast has drawn away from the cell wall, and the cell wall (Cw) and the cytoplasmic membrane (CM) can be easily recognised. CP, cytoplasm with ribosomes; N, nuclear region. Magnification of whole cell, × 56 200; of the inset, × 216 000. (Photograph: H. Frank, Max-Planck Institute for Virus Research, Tübingen.)

increases in cell dimensions, septa appear, starting at the circumference and proceeding inwards, until eventually the two daughter cells separate. In many types of bacteria, however, and under appropriate conditions the daughter cells remain attached in characteristic patterns. According to the number of cell divisions and the division plane, pairs of bacteria (diplococci), chains (streptococci), packets or plates (sarcina) and grape-like bunches (staphylococci) can be distinguished among the spherical bacteria. Rod-shaped bacteria also occur as pairs or chains. Multiplication by budding or sprouting is rare in prokaryotes. Cell division is preceded by the doubling and replicating of the bacterial chromosome. A diploid phase is therefore limited to a very short stage of the cell division cycle. Prokaryotes are haploid.

The cells of prokaryotes (with very few exceptions, such as *Mycoplasma*) are surrounded by a cell wall. This contains a skeleton of peptidoglycan (also called murein), which is a heteropolymer characteristic of prokaryotes and not found in eukaryotic cells.

Many prokaryotes are motile, moving by either swimming or gliding. The organs of locomotion in swimming bacteria are the bacterial flagella. These are much simpler in structure than eukaryotic flagella and contain a single kind of fibril.

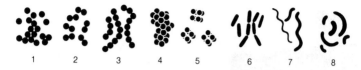

Fig. 2.6. *Shapes of unicellular bacteria*

The shape of nearly all bacteria, with very few exceptions, can be derived from spheres, cylinders and curved cylinders. The basic forms therefore are cocci, straight rods and curved rods (Fig. 2.6). Among the straight rods, one can identify members of the genera *Pseudomonas* and *Bacillus*. Spirilla have the form of a corkscrew. Curved rods are called vibrios. Deviations from these basic forms are characteristic of some bacteria. A club-shaped form and a tendency to vary in shape characterise the genus *Corynebacterium* and coryneform bacteria. Many species of the genus *Mycobacterium* show tendencies for cell branching. In streptomycetes there is formation of mycelia, similar to those in fungi, but distinguishable by their much smaller diameter (less than 1 μm. compared with 5 μm in fungi).

Material composition of the cell.   The wet or fresh weight (mass) of unicellular organisms can be determined after centrifugation from the nutrient medium and washing. The sedimented cell mass has a water content of 70–86%. The dry weight, therefore, constitutes 15–30% of the wet weight. Bacteria containing a large amount of reserve material (lipids, polysaccharides, polyphosphates or sulphur) have higher percentage dry weights. The solid substance of bacteria, as a percentage of the dry mass, consists of: proteins, 50; cell wall, 10–20; RNA, 10–20; DNA, 3–4; lipids, about 10. The ten bioelements are represented in the composition of bacteria in the following approximate percentages: carbon, 50; oxygen, 20; nitrogen, 14; hydrogen, 8; phosphorus, 3; sulphur, 1; potassium, 1; calcium, 0.5; magnesium, 0.4; iron, 0.2.

2.2.1   The bacterial 'nucleus'

The small size of bacteria and the presence of two types of nucleic acid has made the cytochemical study of bacterial nuclear material very difficult. However, classical cytological methods and the development of ultrathin section techniques, allied to electron microscopy, eventually established that bacteria contain DNA that is not diffusely distributed within the cytoplasm, but occupies discrete regions and divides before each cell division.

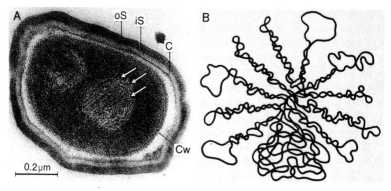

Fig. 2.7. *The bacterial chromosome.*

(A) As can be seen here in a germinating spore of *Bacillus megaterium*, the chromosome exists in a highly ordered condensed state. (oS, outer spore coat; iS, inner spore coat; C, cortex; Cw, cell wall. Photograph by Giesbrecht, Berlin). (B) Schematic representation of a chromosome isolated from a lysed cell and spread out. Most of the loops are highly ordered (supercoiled). In the lower domain, the double helix is in a relaxed state as the result of a single-strand break that allows free rotation.

The problem of the bacterial nuclear structure was further clarified by electron microscopy of ultrathin sections of bacterial cells. For optimal reproduction of what can be regarded as the natural fine structure of the nuclear region, a suitable fixation (with osmium tetroxide, uranyl acetate or phosphotungstate) is essential. This shows that the nuclear region of bacteria is filled with very fine strands. In electron micrographs, this nuclear region or nucleoplasm appears less dense than the ribosome-containing cytoplasm. No membrane structure dividing these two regions has ever been demonstrated (Fig. 2.7).

Autoradiography.   Cairns first demonstrated that the nuclear material in bacteria consists of DNA and, in the case of *Escherichia coli*, is in the form of a single closed, circular strand, approximately 1 mm long. He grew bacteria in the presence of tritiated thymidine, DNA being the only thymidine-containing substance in the cell. After such tritium-labelled cells have been lysed with lysozyme or lauryl sulphate on a membrane filter, the chromosomal material spreads out and can then be visualised by autoradiography. Such autoradiographs (Fig. 2.8) are impressive evidence for the existence of bacterial DNA as a closed, circular strand. This strand corresponds to a 'coupling group' in the genetic sense and is

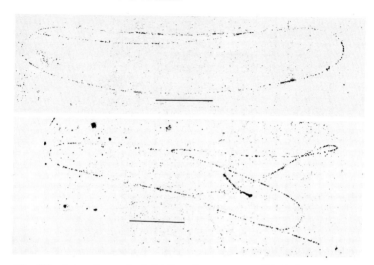

Fig. 2.8. *Autoradiograph of dividing chromosomes of* E. Coli.

The cells were grown for two generations in the presence of tritiated thymidine and were lysed with lysozyme (see text for details of procedure). (From Bleecken, S., Strohbach, E. & Sarfert, E. (1966). *Z. allg. Mikrobiol.* **6**, 121.)

called the bacterial chromosome. These autoradiographs also indicate how the process of chromosome division can be envisaged. The DNA of a bacteriophage, prepared by a different method, is shown in Fig. 2.9.

Structure of DNA.   Deoxyribonucleic acid (DNA) is a macromolecule, which upon acid hydrolysis yields equimolar amounts of its three components: deoxyribose, phosphoric acid and nitrogenous base. The DNA molecule contains four different bases: two purines (adenine and guanine) and two pyrimidines (cytosine and thymine). When DNA is digested by nucleases (pancreatic DNAase I or snake venom diesterase), the 3' and 5' nucleotides are liberated. Nucleic acids consist of long chains of such nucleotides with alternating pentose and phosphate groups with a base (one of the four) attached to each sugar molecule. Such a nucleotide chain has an orientation, i.e. a polarity, with a phosphate group in the 5' position at one end, and a free hydroxyl group in the 3' position at the other end.

By 1950 Chargaff had already derived some general laws about nucleic acid composition. Adenine and thymine, on the one hand, and guanine and cytosine, on the other, always occur in equal amounts (A = T; G = C).

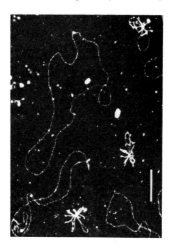

Fig. 2.9. *DNA molecules of bacteriophage PM2.*

DNA molecules are shown in two different states. The globular forms consist of covalently closed, circular (CCC) DNA. UV irradiation has caused breaks in one strand of some of the DNA molecules. This has resulted in the formation of open circular (OC) DNA which are seen as large rings with contour lengths of 3.02 μm. The DNA was covered with a quaternary ammonium compound and (positively) contrasted with uranyl acetate. Dark-field electron micrograph. (U. Hahn, Göttingen.)

The sum of the purines equals the sum of the pyrimidines. The base pair ratio $G + C/A + T$ varies from species to species over a wide range, but it is constant for a given species.

> The actual sequence of the building blocks in the large macromolecules and the secondary structure of DNA have been elucidated by **X-ray crystallography.** An X-ray diffraction diagram of DNA can be obtained by pulling it out to a thread, which is rotated in a beam of monochromatic X-rays, and imaging the refracted rays on film. Such diagrams obtained from different sources (sperm, thymus, bacteria, phage) are practically identical. The interpretation of these X-ray diffraction diagrams by Wilkins showed that the purine and pyrimidine rings are arranged at right angles to the longitudinal axis of the polynucleotide chain. The chain must have a helical conformation around a central axis with a turn of about 3.4 nm. On the basis of mass density it was assumed that there must be more than one strand.

All these data were combined by Watson and Crick in 1953 into a brilliant theory of DNA structure. According to the Watson and Crick model, the

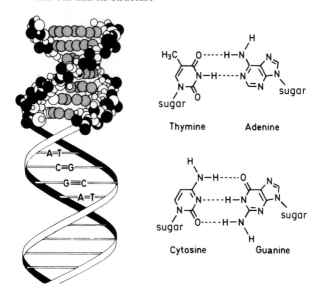

Thymine   Adenine

Cytosine   Guanine

Fig. 2.10. *Structure of DNA.*

The two strands of DNA are connected by hydrogen bridges. (*Left*) The double helix shown as a scale model (*top*) and as an arrangement of bases in a spiral staircase form (*bottom*). (*Right*) The pairing of adenine with thymine, and guanine with cytosine; the broken lines represent hydrogen bridges.

polynucleotide strands are wound like a double helix around an imaginary axis, the two strands being held together by hydrogen bridges between the internally located bases (Fig. 2.10). To account for the distances and relationships between the bases, each adenine must be paired with a thymine and each guanine with a cytosine. Each turn of the helix contains about ten base pairs (bp). The sequence of the bases in the two strands is therefore complementary, whilst the polarity of the strands is in opposite directions, i.e. $5' \rightarrow 3'$ and $3' \rightarrow 5'$. The contour length of *E. coli* DNA is about 1.4 mm. The relative mass of 1 μm of double-stranded DNA is approximately 2×10^6 or 3000 bp (3 kilobases (kb)). The chromosome of *E. coli*, therefore, has a relative mass of 2.9×10^9.

> The **hydrogen bridges** that connect adenine with thymine and guanine with cytosine are of unequal strengths. The H-bonds are largely electrostatic in nature; they are formed by OH and NH_2 groups. Oxygen and nitrogen are strongly electronegative elements; they thus exert an electron repulsion and confer a positive charge on the attached H-atoms. The protonated H-

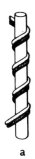 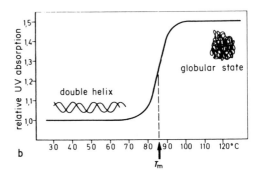

Fig. 2.11.

(a) *Model of a plectonemical double helix*. This can be made by winding two parallel strands of wire around a rod, and then pulling out the rod. The two single strands remain attached and can only be separated by twisting. (b) Melting curve of bacterial DNA. T_m is the temperature at which half the maximal increase in extinction occurs.

atoms can then be attracted by other electronegative groups that have a lone electron pair and, thus, form a hydrogen bridge. The strength of the H-bridge can be characterised by the acidity of the H-atoms and the basicity of the acceptor atom. Hydrogen bridges are stronger than van der Waals' forces; their bond energies may amount to 38 kJ (9 kcal)/mol. On average, they are not much greater than the energies of temperature variations around 37 °C. As shown in Fig. 2.10, there are two such bonds between thymine and adenine and three between guanine and cytosine. Because of these low bond energies, profound alterations or even severing of the bonds can be produced by elevated temperatures, small changes in magnesium concentrations, or addition of urea. Increases in temperature lead to destruction of these H-bonds and unwinding of the polynucleotide strands. This destruction of the secondary structure of DNA is accompanied by increased light absorption at 259 nm (hyperchromicity). The temperature at which the half-maximal increase in extinction occurs is called the T_m value. The temperature at which this destruction occurs increases with increased content of guanine and cytosine. It is therefore possible to determine the relative GC content of a given DNA sample, after suitable purification, by measuring the T_m value (Fig. 2.11). The **GC content** gives the number of moles of guanine and cytosine as a percentage of the total number of moles of the four bases in a given sample of DNA.

Bacterial species vary widely in their GC content, ranging from 30% in some staphylococci and the *Cytophaga* group to above 70% in certain representatives of the genus *Micrococcus* and some myxobacteria. The GC content is species-specific and is regarded as a taxonomic character.

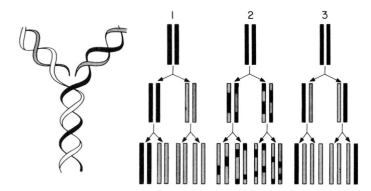

Fig. 2.12. *Model of DNA replication according to the semi-conservative mechanism and the three possible mechanisms of DNA replication.*
(1) Conservative method;   (3) semi-conservative. See text for
(2) dispersive method;   details.

Replication of DNA.   Because DNA contains the genetic information of the cell, its replication and division, which always precede cell division, must lead to the formation of two completely identical DNA chromosomes. Superficially, the increase in DNA, i.e. its identical reduplication or replication, is very simple. The two strands have merely to separate so that nucleotide building blocks can line up with the complementary bases of each polynucleotide strand, and then these can be joined. However, one of the main difficulties is already encountered in the conception of how the two strands of the double helix separate. According to the X-ray structure diagrams, DNA is a plectonemical and not a parenemical helix (Fig. 2.11a). To determine whether unwinding of the helix is a necessary assumption, three possible mechanisms of DNA replication were considered as heuristic hypotheses by Delbruck and Stent (1957) (Fig. 2.12).

> (1) Conservative mechanism. This does not involve unwinding of the helix. The parental helix serves as template for the synthesis of two daughter helices, so that the daughter double helix consists entirely of new material, and the parental helix continues to exist.
>
> (2) Dispersive mechanism. The parental helix is broken down during replication of each half turn by multiple fragmentation. The new synthesis then takes place on the parental fragments with crosswise annealing. Each polynucleotide strand then contains alternating segments of old and newly synthesised material.
>
> (3) Semi-conservative mechanism. The parental double helix is unwound, and each polynucleotide strand serves as the template for the synthesis of

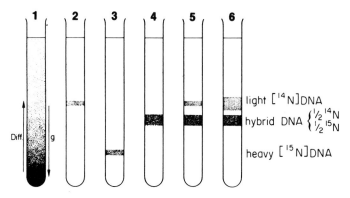

Fig. 2.13. *Semi-conservative replication of DNA: results of the Meselsohn–Stahl experiment.*

[^{15}N]- and [^{14}N]DNA were separated by equilibrium density gradient centrifugation in a 6 M CsCl solution. (1) The density gradient is the result of equilibrium between diffusion and sedimentation (g). (2) DNA from 'normal' ^{14}N-labelled cells (3) DNA from cells that were grown for several generations with ^{15}NH$_4$Cl. (4) DNA from ^{15}N-labelled cells that were grown for one generation in the presence of ^{14}NH$_4$Cl. (5) DNA from ^{15}N-labelled cells that were grown for two generations with ^{14}NH$_4$Cl. (6) DNA from ^{15}N-labelled cells that were grown for three generations with ^{14}NH4Cl.

a new complementary strand. The new helix is therefore a hybrid, consisting of one pre-existing and one newly synthesised strand.

To distinguish between these possibilities, Meselson and Stahl carried out experiments in which DNA was labelled with heavy isotope markers and subsequently separated in density gradients (Fig. 2.13).

A density gradient of CsCl can be produced by centrifugation of a 6 M CsCl solution for many hours at $100\,000$ g (due to equilibrium between diffusion and gravity). When such a solution contains DNA, the DNA collects at a certain position in the gradient. This position depends on the specific density of the DNA. If the DNA is obtained from bacteria grown with ^{15}NH$_4$Cl, it is 0.8% heavier than corresponding DNA from bacteria grown in the normal ^{14}NH$_4$Cl. The heavy DNA forms a separate band in the CsCl gradient. A culture of *E. coli* was grown for several generations with ^{15}NH$_4$Cl as the nitrogen source, so that its DNA contained only ^{15}N. The growth medium was then enriched with ^{14}NH$_4$Cl. Before and after this addition, samples of DNA were prepared from parts of the culture and analysed in CsCl gradients. After one generation of growth with the ^{14}NH$_4$Cl, all the extracted DNA was intermediate between the heavy DNA

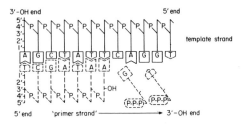

Fig. 2.14. *Biochemical basis for the function of DNA polymerases.*

The DNA double helix consists of two antiparallel polynucleotide strands. When a free (i.e. not connected with a neighbouring nucleotide) 3'-OH group is at the left-hand end of one of the strands, the same group is at the right-hand end of the other strand. The replication of DNA is catalysed by DNA polymerase. This enzyme needs a template in the form of a single-stranded piece of DNA, a primer, and a mixture of deoxy-nucleotide-5'-triphosphates. The DNA polymerases can attach the free nucleotide only to the free 3'-OH end of the nucleotide strand. Therefore the synthesis can only proceed in the direction 5' $\rightarrow$ 3' and not in the reverse direction.

containing ^{15}N and the light DNA containing only ^{14}N. The content of the intermediate DNA was maintained over several generations after addition of the $^{14}NH_4Cl$, whilst the proportion of the light DNA increased. To determine whether the intermediate DNA really consisted of a strand of [^{14}N]DNA and a strand of [^{15}N]DNA, a sample of the intermediate DNA was heated to 100 °C and cooled quickly to prevent re-formation of the double-stranded form by base pair hydrogen bonding. On subsequent centrifugation in a CsCl gradient, two bands appeared, corresponding to [^{14}N] and [^{15}N] single-stranded DNA.

The results of these experiments clearly contradict both the conservative and the dispersive mechanisms. They are entirely consistent with the hypothesis of a **semi-conservative mechanism of DNA replication.** During replication the two strands of the double helix unwind and separate. Each single strand then serves as a template for the synthesis of a new complementary strand. **DNA polymerases are involved** in this synthesis. They join the correct sequence of new nucleotides to the pre-existing template strand of DNA by base-pairing, thus producing a new polynucleotide strand. The biochemical aspects of DNA polymerase function are shown in Fig. 2.14. The synthesis of one new polynucleotide strand is therefore readily explained: DNA polymerase can join the nucleotides in the direction 5' $\rightarrow$ 3' in a continuous chain. However, since the double helix is antiparallel, the synthesis of the opposite strand would have to proceed in the opposite direction, i.e. 3' $\rightarrow$ 5'. The mech-

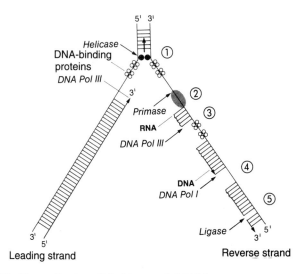

Fig. 2.15. *The replication of double-stranded DNA.*

Double-stranded DNA is first unwound by helicase so as to produce the replication fork. (1) The single strands of the DNA are stabilised by DNA-binding (SSB = single-strand binding) proteins. The leading strand is replicated by Polymerase III (DNA Pol III) in the direction 5' to 3' (**continuous replication**). (2) The synthesis of the other strand has to proceed in the reverse direction and hence must be **discontinuous**. It starts with the synthesis of a short piece of RNA which serves as a starter molecule (RNA primer) by a primase. (3) DNA Pol III synthesises an attaching piece of DNA. (4) The RNA primer is removed by an endonuclease and the gap is filled by DNA polymerase I, and closed by DNA ligase. (From Wehner, R. & Gehring, W. (1990). *Zoologie*, 22nd edn. Stuttgart: Thieme).

anism of discontinuous synthesis of the second strand, based on the above considerations and on experimental results is shown in Fig. 2.15. At first only short sequences (perhaps 1000 nucleotides long), the so-called Okazaki fragments, are formed. Their synthesis starts with the formation of a short strand of RNA which serves as a primer. A DNA polymerase III then proceeds to join a DNA chain of 100-2000 bases onto the RNA primer. Subsequently, the RNA primer is removed and the gap is filled by DNA polymerase I, and the product is joined to the rest of the newly synthesised segment by a ligase. This discontinuous method of polynucleotide synthesis can explain the replication of the second strand in the 5' → 3' direction. Figure 2.16 shows how the repli-

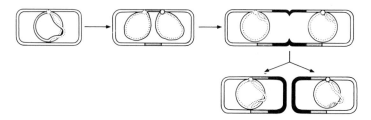

Fig. 2.16. *Replication of the circular bacterial chromosome and division of the bacterial cell.*

This presentation is based on the unidirectional mechanism of DNA replication, i.e. with the presence of only one replication centre.

cation of the bacterial chromosome and the division of the cell can be visualised, assuming that the replication mechanism is unidirectional. It has been found, however, that this is not necessarily the case. Synthesis of the two new strands does not only take place unidirectionally, but it can also proceed from an initiation point in both directions on either or both of the two strands. Such a bidirectional mechanism implies the existence of two replication centres on each molecule of DNA. The synthesis of the two new single strands thus takes place at each of the two branches of the replication fork formed by the unwinding of the double helix. Duplication of the *E. coli* chromosome takes about 40 minutes, but under favourable conditions *E. coli* cells have a doubling time of about 20 minutes. These facts can be reconciled by observations that indicate that the two daughter chromosomes can start a new replication cycle before the first cycle has been completed.

Considerably more details about the replication mechanism of bacterial DNA are available than can be discussed in this context. There are, for example, considerable differences between the replication of chromosomal, plasmid and phage DNA.

Genome size and number. The size of the bacterial genome differs in different species within a range of approximately 0.6×10^6–13×10^6 base pairs (bp). Most bacterial genomes have a size similar to that of *E. coli*, i.e. about 4×10^6 bp. The number of genomes per cell also differs in different species, but this number also depends on cultural conditions. *E. coli*, growing in batch culture, show 2–4 genomes/cell; *Azotobacter chroococcum* show 20–40 genomes/cell; *Desulfovibrio gigas* show 10–15 genomes/cell. (Genome sizes in eukaryotic organisms are: *Neurospora crassa*, 19×10^6 *Aspergillus niger*, 40×10^6 bp; *Zea mays*, 7×10^9 bp; *Homo sapiens*, 2.9×10^9 bp.)

DNA–DNA hybridisation: sequence homologies among DNAs of different species.   As described earlier, the heating of isolated DNA results in separation of the two polynucleotide strands, due to destruction of the hydrogen bridges. This denaturation of DNA by strand separation is reversible by slow cooling, which allows pairing and reassociation of complementary segments. Such reassociation can also take place when short pieces of denatured DNA derived from different, though related, bacteria are mixed above their melting temperature and allowed to cool slowly. DNA doublets formed from single strands derived from different organisms are called heteroduplex molecules. To follow the formation of heteroduplex molecules, the DNA from one of the bacterial species must be labelled with either heavy or radioactive isotope.

> If a bacterial culture is grown, for instance, in heavy water (D_2O), it will produce heavy DNA, and the formation of a heteroduplex can be shown by centrifugation in a CsCl density gradient in the same way that Meselson and Stahl demonstrated hybrid [^{14}N] and [^{15}N]DNA. It is also possible to culture one of the partners in medium containing ^{14}C or ^{32}P to label its DNA. Long pieces of denatured DNA from the unlabelled culture are then combined with short pieces of denatured DNA from the labelled cultured. This mixture is allowed to cool slowly (a process known as annealing) and it is then filtered through a membrane that retains only the long strands; thus heteroduplex molecules are fixed to the filter. The radioactivity retained by the filter is determined by the number of short labelled pieces annealed to the long unlabelled DNA strands and is therefore proportional to the base sequence homology between the two DNAs. Such DNA–DNA reassociation methods allow determination of the degree of sequence homology between DNAs of different origins. A control experiment with DNA samples from the same bacterial strain, one of which is labelled and one unlabelled, allows this degree of association to be designated 100. The degree of reassociation of DNA molecules of this strain with those of different strains can then be expressed as a percentage of complete homology. Various methods for the determination of DNA homology have been developed and used; they are all based on the same principle of heteroduplex formation between two samples of DNA, one of which is suitably labelled.

DNA sequence homology, i.e. similarities in the base sequence of DNA molecules from different bacteria, is greatest in the most closely related strains. These homology comparisons have been useful for comparison and study of related genera and species. There is rarely enough homology between unrelated species to show any heteroduplex formation. Single-stranded DNA can also associate with complementary RNA, and the above methods can therefore also be used to measure base homologies between DNA and RNA.

Plasmids.   In addition to chromosomal DNA, many bacteria contain extrachromosomal DNA in closed, circular, double-stranded form. These autonomously replicating DNA elements are called plasmids. Linear plasmids have been found in some bacteria.

2.2.2   Cytoplasm, proteins and ribosomes

The cytoplasm is separated from the cell wall by the cytoplasmic membrane and contains various inclusions (vesicle, grana) as well as the nuclear material. With the advent of the electron microscope and the development of biochemical techniques it has become clear that the cytoplasm is not a homogenous protein solution, but is traversed by various membraneous bodies and invaginations; apart from these, the cytoplasm consists largely of plasma ground substance and ribosomes. An aqueous dilution of bacterial cytoplasm can be separated by centrifugation at $100\,000\ g$ into a 'soluble' fraction, which mainly contains soluble enzymes and RNA, and a particulate fraction, which consists mostly of ribosomes and membraneous material. The soluble enzymes catalyse a variety of catabolic and synthetic reactions, whereas the soluble RNAs (messenger RNA and transfer RNAs), as well as the ribosomes, take part in protein synthesis.

Proteins.   Proteins consist of amino acids that are joined by peptide bonds in a specific sequence to form a polypeptide chain. Such polypeptide chains have specific conformations which are stabilised by additional bonds, both covalent and non-covalent (Fig. 2.17). Several levels of structure in proteins are associated with the different varieties of bonds. The **primary structure** of a protein is defined by the number and sequences of the covalently linked amino acids. Parts of the polypeptide chain may then assume a **secondary structure**, either an a-helix or a 'pleated sheet', by virtue of hydrogen bonds between carbonyl oxygen and amide nitrogen atoms of constituent amino acids. Further interactions between various side chains and groups of the polypeptide chain result in a characteristic overall conformational form, the **tertiary structure**. The bonds involved in this include hydrogen bonds, ionic bonds, and hydrophobic interactions. In addition, there may be covalent cross-linking between different parts of the chain, such as the disulphide bonds produced by oxidation of sulphydryl groups. Finally, intermolecular interactions between different polypeptide chains may occur to form characteristic aggregate structures. This assembly of a protein from a definite number of polypeptide chains is called its **quarternary structure**. Under physiological conditions, soluble proteins exist in an aqueous phase. As a conse-

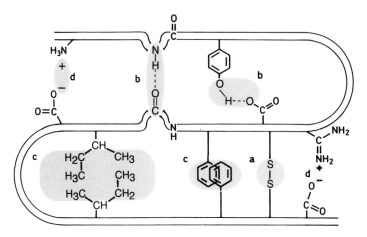

Fig. 2.17. *Possible intramolecular bonds between different sections of polypeptide chains.*

(a) Covalent disulphide bonds; (b) hydrogen bonds; (c) hydrophobic bonds; (d) ionic bonds.

(After Lynen, F. (1970). *Naturw. Rdsch.* **23**, 266.)

quence, there are also interactions between proteins and water dipoles. Polar groups are hydrated, and factors which influence the charge of a protein also determine its degree of hydration, and hence its conformation and colloidal form.

Ribosomes.   The ribosomes are the sites of protein synthesis. They are seen in electron micrographs as particles in the cytoplasm. Bacterial ribosomes are about 16×18 nm in size and contain about 80–85% of the bacterial RNA. Since intact bacterial ribosomes sediment in the ultracentrifuge with a sedimentation velocity of about 70 svedberg units, they are referred to as 70S ribosomes. The cytoplasmic ribosomes of eukaryotes are (with a few exceptions) somewhat larger and are called 80S ribosomes. Ribosomes consist of two subunits. In bacteria, these are 30S and 50S particles, which combine to give the 70S ribosome (Fig. 2.18). Bacterial ribosomes resemble those of mitochondria and chloroplasts in size and many other properties.

Bacterial cells contain about 5000–50 000 ribosomes. The number varies with the growth rate and is highest in the fastest growing cells. Regular chains of ribosomes can be seen on electron micrographs of thin sections from cells engaged in active protein synthesis. These chains

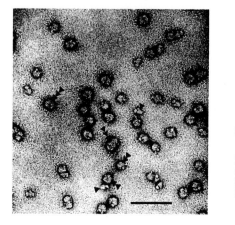

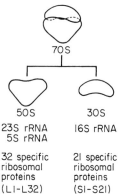

70S

50S
23S rRNA
5S rRNA

32 specific
ribosomal
proteins
(LI-L32)

30S
I6S rRNA

2I specific
ribosomal
proteins
(SI-S2I)

Fig. 2.18. *Bacterial ribosomes.*

(*Left*) The electron micrograph shows ribosomes of *E. coli.* The intact 70S ribosomes are indicated with three arrows, the 50S particles with two arrows, and the 30S appear threaded on strands of mRNA, like pearls in a necklace, and are referred to as polyribosomes or polysomes. particles with single arrows. Scale bar, 100 nm. (Picture: E. Spiess.) (*Right*) Composition of the ribosomes.

appear threaded on strands of mRNA, like pearls in a necklace, and are referred to as polyribosomes or polysomes.

The differences between bacterial ribosomes (70S) and eukaryotic ribosomes (80S) are of great importance in the effective treatment of infection. Several antibiotics inhibit protein synthesis carried out by 70S ribosomes, without affecting the function of 80S ribosomes.

Composition of RNA.   RNA differs from DNA with regard to its building blocks as well as its secondary structure. The backbone of the polynucleotide strand consists of ribose and phosphate (analogous to the deoxyribose and phosphate backbone of DNA) and three of the bases are the same as in DNA: adenine, guanine and cytosine. However, RNA contains uracil instead of thymine. In addition, RNA molecules may contain rare bases, such as pseudouracil. Cellular RNA is usually single stranded; base-pairing generally occurs only in segments.

The genetic code.   Each gene is represented by a specific sequence of DNA. The specific information of the gene resides in the base sequence of this DNA. The script in which this genetic information is encoded has four characters: the bases adenine (A), guanine (G), thymine (T) and

Table 2.1. *The genetic code. The triplets or codons UAA (ochre), UAG (amber), and UGA are the 'stop' signals for termination of synthesis and release of the growing polypeptide chain from the ribosome. The symbols for amino acids are detailed in the list of abbreviations at the beginning of the book*

Triplet	Amino acid	Triplet	Amino acid	Triplet	Amino acid	Triplet	Amino acid
UUU	Phe	UCU	Ser	UAU	Tyr	UGU	Cys
UUC	Phe	UCC	Ser	UAC	Tyr	UGC	Cys
UUA	Leu	UCA	Ser	UAA	Stop	UGA	Stop
UUG	Leu	UCG	Ser	UAG	Stop	UGG	Trp
CUU	Leu	CCU	Pro	CAU	His	CGU	Arg
CUC	Leu	CCC	Pro	CAC	His	CGC	Arg
CUA	Leu	CCA	Pro	CAA	Gln	CGA	Arg
CUG	Leu	CCG	Pro	CAG	Gln	CGG	Arg
AUU	Ileu	ACU	Thr	AAU	Asn	AGU	Ser
AUC	Ileu	ACC	Thr	AAC	Asn	AGC	Ser
AUA	Ileu	ACA	Thr	AAA	Lys	AGA	Arg
AUG	Met	ACG	Thr	AAG	Lys	AGG	Arg
GUU	Val	GCU	Ala	GAU	Asp	GGU	Gly
GUC	Val	GCC	Ala	GAC	Asp	GGC	Gly
GUA	Val	GCA	Ala	GAA	Glu	GGA	Gly
GUG	Cal	GCG	Ala	GAG	Glu	GGG	Gly

cytosine (C). In the script of RNA, uracil (U) replaces thymine. The specificity of the enzyme proteins, whose synthesis is scripted by the genes, is based on the amino acid sequence in the polypeptide chains. The amino acid sequence also determines the spatial organisation, that is the conformation of the protein (its secondary, tertiary and quarternary structure).

The information transfer from the nucleotide script to the amino acid script is mediated by a code. A sequence of three nucleotides, a triplet or codon, determines an amino acid, so that the sequence of triplets in the nucleic acid determines the sequence of amino acids in a polypeptide chain. This also means that the polypeptide chain is a co-linear reflection of the nucleic acid. The arrangement of the nucleic acid bases in triplets permits 64 combinations (Table 2.1). If only one triplet were to code for each of the 20 amino acids, 44 possible combinations would remain unused (redundant). It has been found that many amino acids are coded by two or more triplets. The triplets are read in the order 1,2,3, starting from the initiation codon of mRNA. Some triplets have special meanings. UAG codes for the amino acid methionine and functions as the start codon. The triplets UAA, UAG and UGA are 'nonsense' or 'stop' codons. They do not code for an amino acids, but signal the end of the mRNA segment being translated.

The triplets are 'read' by a complex procedure that involves a 'decoding' step and results in the translation of the nucleotide script of the mRNA into the amino acid script of the protein.

Transcripton of DNA.   The information contained in the sequence of DNA is not transferred directly during the synthesis of proteins that occurs on ribosomes which are not localised in the immediate vicinity of DNA. Rather, the transfer of information to the site of protein synthesis is mediated by an 'RNA messenger'. The resulting molecule of RNA is called '**messenger RNA**' or **mRNA**, and the process is called **transcription**. The mRNA is single-stranded and its synthesis occurs on only one strand of DNA, the **codogenic** or transcription strand, starting from the 3' end. The base sequence of mRNA is therefore directly complementary to the (codogenic) transcription strand of DNA. The enzyme carrying out the synthesis of RNA is a relatively large protein, consisting of a number of subunits. In *E. coli* it is composed of 2 α subunits, a β and a β' subunit. In addition, this RNA polymerase needs a further subunit, the sigma factor (σ factor) for the initiation of RNA synthesis. The σ factor is involved in the recognition of the promoter, that is the start sequence, of the DNA being transcribed. Following the initiation, the σ factor becomes superfluous. During transcription the DNA double helix has to unwind. Figure 2.19a illustrates the process of transcription. The synthesis of RNA is terminated when a certain base sequence of DNA the terminator codon   is reached.

Transcription is contrasted with the true '**translation**' of the nucleic acid base sequence into the amino acid sequence of a protein.

The translation of mRNA: protein synthesis.   The amino acids are joined into a polypeptide chain in the sequence determined by the triplet sequence of mRNA in a process that involves participation of transfer RNA (tRNA), the ribosomes, various enzymes, ATP, and several 'factors'.

As a first step, amino acids are activated by reaction with ATP to aminoacyl-AMP.

$$\text{amino acid} + \text{ATP} \rightarrow \text{aminoacyl-AMP} + \text{PP}_i$$

The aminoacyl residue is then transferred from the AMP to the terminal nucleotide of tRNA. The activation and coupling of an amino acid to its appropriate tRNA is carried out by a specific enzyme, the appro-

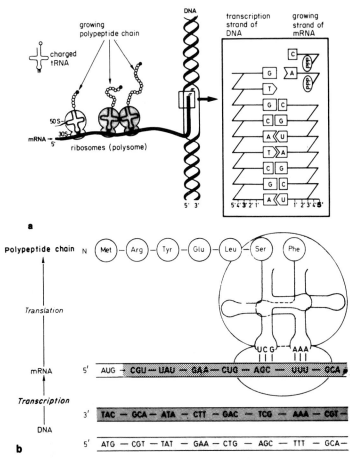

Fig. 2.19. *Protein biosynthesis.*

The transfer of genetic information (from the genome to proteins) occurs in two stages. In the first stage, mRNA is synthesised according to the codon sequence on the transcription strand of DNA. In the second stage, translation, amino acids are brought by their tRNA to the ribosomes, which move (from left to right) along the mRNA. The amino acids are brought in the sequence dictated by the triplet sequence of the mRNA and are joined by peptide bonds. (a) General view; (b) detailed presentation.

priate aminoacyl-tRNA synthetase. This recognises both the amino acid and its cognate tRNA. There are 20 different aminoacyl-tRNA synthetases, one for each amino acid. It follows that the different individual tRNAs must also have appropriate recognition sites for each of the aminoacyl-tRNA synthetases.

There are several codons for some of the amino acids (this is called degeneracy of the genetic code), and for these amino acids there are also several tRNAs. The different tRNAs that can accept the same amino acid are called iso-accepting tRNAs. In these cases the specific aminoacyl-tRNA synthetase can charge the several iso-accepting tRNAs (i.e. iso-accepting tRNAs recognise different codons, but the same aminoacyl-tRNA synthetase). Each tRNA contains a region, the anticodon, which is complementary to the appropriate triplet (codon) of the mRNA. The tRNA molecule is thus central to the translation process. It selects the specific amino acid by its recognition site for the appropriate aminoacyl-tRNA synthetase and recognises the appropriate codon by its anticodon triplet.

The joining of the amino acids (by peptide bonds) takes place on the ribosomes (Fig. 2.19a,b), the ribosomes moving along relative to the mRNA, starting at the 5'-OH end. This process of peptide chain synthesis has been divided into three stages: initiation, elongation and termination. The initiation process involves the dissociated ribosomal subunits (30S and 50S), a molecule of mRNA that has a special 'initiating sequence' with the codon for formyl-methionine as the initiating amino acid at its 5'-OH end, and the formyl-methionyl-tRNA, as well as several initiation factors.

There are two specific sites on the ribosomes for tRNAs, called the A-site (for aminoacyl-tRNA) and the P-site (for peptidyl-tRNA). The initiating, formyl-methionyl-tRNA moves into the P-site. The next aminoacyl-tRNA moves into the A-site for the process of elongation. The amino group of the amino acid attached to the tRNA in the A-site makes a peptide bond with the carboxyl group of the preceding amino acid in the growing peptide chain in the P-site. This is, of course, an enzyme-catalysed reaction and involves GTP and various factors, and it also liberates the tRNA from the P-site. The growing peptide chain is now attached to the last incoming tRNA in the A-site, which then moves to the P-site, in a step called translocation, at the same time as the ribosome moves relative to the mRNA (or the mRNA travels along the ribosome). This elongation process continues until the 'stop' codon is reached on the mRNA, when the peptide chain is released and the ribosome dissociates into its 30S and 50S subunits.

As already mentioned, the actual structure of the polypeptide chain, determined by the sequence of amino acids and the nature of various side chains (hydrophobic and hydrophilic groups), leads to the folding and coiling which determine its specific properties and function.

Several ribosomes can attach to a given mRNA strand so that this can bear several ribosomes simultaneously and function as the template for a number of polypeptide chains. The complex of mRNA with several ribosomes is called a polysome.

Thus, the nucleotide sequence of DNA constitutes the code that determines the structures of proteins via the mediation of mRNA. The transfer of information from DNA via mRNA to protein has been called the 'central dogma' of molecular biology. This kind of information transfer, as shown below, applies to all organisms that contain DNA as the genetic material.

This universal process of information transfer in DNA replication, transcription and translation is shown in the diagram. This applies to eukaryotes, prokaryotes and DNA-viruses.

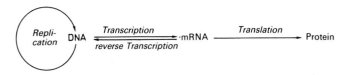

In some RNA viruses RNA can be replicated directly. However, in some oncogenic (tumour-producing) virus systems this is preceded by RNA-directed DNA synthesis, in which RNA acts as the template. The information contained in the RNA is thus transferred to DNA in a process preceeding in the opposite direction to transcription, by reverse transcriptase. This enzyme has been isolated from RNA-tumour cells and has found application in gene technology (see molecular cloning techniques: Chapter 15). Thus, when mRNA is isolated as the information carrier, rather than DNA, it must be transcribed into DNA for the information to be incorporated into a plasmid. By using reverse transcriptase, the desired DNA can be synthesised *in vitro*

Transcription and translation are targets for a number of antibiotics (see Ch. 6.6). The interesting property of antibiotics is their highly specific and selective action. Thus nalidixic acid and novobiocin inhibit the unwinding of DNA for replication and transcription. Rifamicin inhibits RNA polymerase in prokaryotes. Protein synthesis, especially the translation step in prokaryotes, is inhibited by streptomycin, neomycin, erythromycin, tetracyclines and chloramphenicol. In eukaryotes, inhibitors are cycloheximide and diptheria toxin. The extensive elucidation of the molecular processes in protein synthesis is due, to a large extent, to research on the mode of action of antibiotics.

2.2.3   Membranes

Cytoplasmic membranes.   In electron micrographs of ultrathin sections from osmium tetroxide-treated cells, the bacterial cytoplasmic membrane appears to consist of several layers. Two osmophilic (and hence dark) layers, each about 2–3 nm thick, surround a lighter layer that is 4–5 nm thick. The membranes of bacteria, plants and animals show considerable resemblance in their general structure; therefore it seems justified to refer to an 'elementary membrane' or 'unit membrane'.

The bacterial cytoplasmic membrane can be isolated from lysozyme protoplasts by osmotic shock. The membrane is rich in lipids, especially phospholipids (Table 2.2). Membrane lipids constitute about 70–90% of the cellular lipids, whereas the membrane constitutes only 8–15% of the cellular dry weight. The cytoplasmic membrane consists of a lipid bilayer, with the hydrophobic ends of the phospholipids in the interior and the hydrophilic head groups exposed on the exterior surfaces. The membrane is stabilised by hydrophobic forces between the fatty acid residues of the lipids and by electrostatic forces between the hydrophilic head groups. The bilayer has proteins incorporated into it; these are the integral membrane proteins, which can be considered as floating in the membrane matrix, some completely traversing it, whilst others are partially immersed. Other proteins are attached to the membrane and are described as peripheral membrane proteins (Fig. 2.20). Some membranes are apparently covered on one or both surfaces by a network of elongated proteins.

The membrane should be considered as a very soft, deformable, almost fluid structure. Isolated membranes have a tendency to round up into vesicles with fragments apparently fusing along their edges.

The cytoplasmic membrane has important metabolic functions. It con-

Table 2.2. *Membrane composition of* Micrococcus *luteus (lysodeikticus) and of phototrophic bacteria*

	Percentage of membrane dry weight	
Components	*M. luteus*	Purple bacteria
Lipids	28–37	40–50
neutral	9	10–20
phospholipids	28	30
Proteins	50	50
Hexose	15–20	5–30

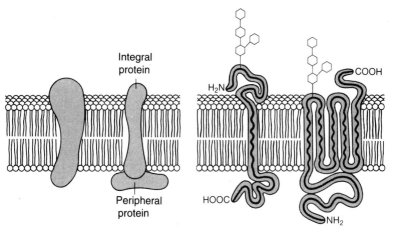

Fig. 2.20. *Model of the cytoplasmic membrane.*

Integral proteins are shown embedded in the lipid bilayer. Peripheral proteins are situated on the membrane surface. The poly- or oligosaccharide chains which are attached to the outer surface of some membranes are indicated at the top.

stitutes the osmotic barrier of the cell and exerts control over the influx and efflux of materials. It is the site of active transport mechanisms and of substrate-specific permease systems.

The continuous phospholipid bilayer of the cytoplasmic membrane shows different degrees of resistance to permeation of different substances. The diffusion rates shown in Fig. 2.21 demonstrate that the hydrophobic substances diffuse easily whilst ions practically not at all. The transport of substances into the cell (influx) and out of the cell (efflux) are mediated by integral membrane proteins, which are specific for one or a group of closely related substrates.

The enzymes of electron transport and oxidative phosphorylation, which in eukaryotes are localised in the mitochondrial membrane, are part of, or attached to, the bacterial cytoplasmic membrane. Thus cytochromes, iron–sulphur proteins, and other components of the electron transport chain are found solely in the cytoplasmic membrane,. Detailed investigations on the localisation of individual components have shown that the membrane has an asymmetric structure. Cytochrome c, for example, is arrange on the outer surface, and ATP synthase is on the inner surface. The membrane is characterised by a vectorial metabolism (Ch. 7.4). Various other biosynthetic processes, including the synthesis

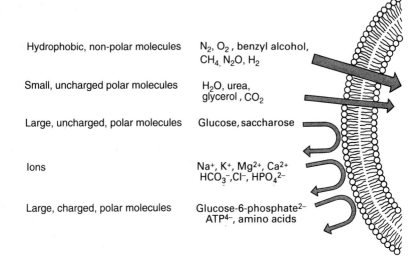

Hydrophobic, non-polar molecules N_2, O_2, benzyl alcohol, CH_4, N_2O, H_2

Small, uncharged polar molecules H_2O, urea, glycerol, CO_2

Large, uncharged, polar molecules   Glucose, saccharose

Ions Na^+, K^+, Mg^{2+}, Ca^{2+} HCO_3^-, Cl^-, HPO_4^{2-}

Large, charged, polar molecules   Glucose-6-phosphate^{2-} ATP^{4-}, amino acids

Fig. 2.21. *Permeabilities of an artificial lipid double-membrane for different molecules*

of cell wall and capsule components, and the secretion of exoenzymes, are most probably membrane functions. The replication centre of DNA is thought to be localised on the membrane. The membrane also provides the anchorage site for flagella.

Intracytoplasmic membranes and lamellae. In some bacteria, the membrane surrounds the cytoplasm without invaginations or folds. In others, the membrane is invaginated and may traverse the cytoplasm or form membraneous bodies. In some bacteria, bodies called mesosomes have been described. However, they are most probably artefacts of preparation. Other bacteria (e.g. *Nitrobacter, Nitrosomonas, Nitrosococcus*) have packets of lamellae that are formed by flat vesicles arranged in parallel, some of which are connected to the plasma membrane (Fig. 2.22).

Phototrophic purple bacteria are especially rich in intracytoplasmic membrane systems. In ultrathin sections these can be seen as tubules, vesicles, and plates. In *Rhodospirillum rubrum* and *Chromatium* species the cell lumen appears almost completely filled with closely packed spherical vesicles (Fig. 2.23). These vesicles seem to be formed by invagination and tubular accretion of the cytoplasmic membrane. Constrictions of the tubules at equal intervals interrupt the vesicular structure, without

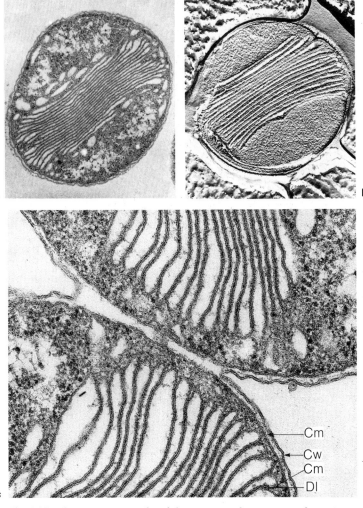

Fig. 2.22. *Electron micrographs of the nitrite-producing marine bacterium* Nitrosococcus oceanus.

(a,c) Ultrathin section after fixation with OsO₄; (b) preparation by freeze-etching technique. (a,b) × 22 000; (c) × 81 000. (From Remsen, C. C., Valois, F. W. & Watson, S. W. (1967). *J. Bacteriol.* **94**, 422.) Cm, cytoplasmic membrane; Dl, double lamella; Cw, cell wall.

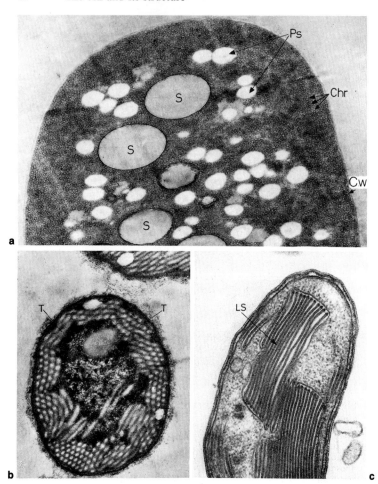

Fig. 2.23. *The photosynthetic pigments of phototrophic purple bacteria are bound to intracytoplasmic membranes.*

Enlargement of the membrane surface is achieved by different bacteria in different ways. In *Chromatium okenii*, the structures are vesicular and are known as vesicles or chromatophores (a).

Thiocapsa pfennigii contains tubular photosynthetic membranes (b). In *Ectothiorhodospira mobilis*, the membranes are multiply folded and present as lamellar stacks (c). Chr, chromatophores; LS, lamellar

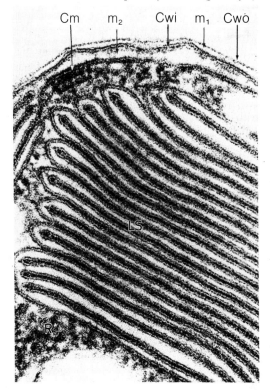

Fig. 2.24. Ectothiorhodspira mobilis *with stacks of photosynthetic lamellae.*

Electron micrograph of an ultrathin section ($\times$ 150 000). Cm, cytoplasmic membrane; LS, lamellar stacks; R, ribosomes; Cwo, cell wall, outer membrane; Cwi, cell wall, inner layer; m_1 and m_2, outer and inner electron-transparent layers. (From Remsen, C. C., Watson, S. W., Waterbury, J. B. & Trüper, H. G. (1968). *J. Bacteriol.* **95**, 2374.)

Fig. 2.23 (*cont.*)
stacks; Ps, polysaccharide granules; S, sulphur droplets; T, tubular photosynthetic membranes; Cw, cell wall; (Pictures: (a) G. Kran; (b) K. Eimhjellen; (c) from Remsen, C. C., Watson, S. W., Waterbury, J. B. & Trüper, H. G. (1968). *J. Bacteriol.* **95**, 2374.)

separating it completely. Upon cell breakage and as a result of homogenising procedures, these structures are liberated as isolated vesicles and have been called chromatophores. In other purple bacteria, the vesicular bodies are very flattened and stacked into regular plates (Figs 2.23, 2.24). They are often called thylakoid plates, in analogy to the structure of chloroplasts in green plants.

Photosynthetic membranes are similar in structure to the cytoplasmic membranes of non-photosynthetic organisms (Table 2.2). They carry the light-absorbing pigments (bacteriochlorophylls and carotenoids) as well as the components of the photosynthetic electron transport system (cytochromes, ubiquinone, etc.) and the phosphorylating systems.

2.2.4   The cell wall

The cell wall of bacteria is not like a rigid steel sphere, but rather elastic, like the leather cover of a football. The analogy is apt, in that the tautly stretched protoplast confers a certain rigidity on the cell, as does the well-filled inner balloon of the football. The interior pressure, or turgor, is osmotically determined. The cytoplasmic membrane is the osmotically active barrier; it is semi-permeable and controls the uptake and extrusion of dissolved materials. In contrast, the cell wall is freely permeable to salts and a number of other low molecular weight substances.

Plasmolysis.   Normally, the concentrations of osmotically active sugars and salts inside the cell are higher than those in the external medium. The osmotic pressure of the cell interior is equivalent to a 10–20% sucrose solution, and water is taken up by the cell, producing swelling to the extent permitted by the cell wall. If the osmotic value of the external medium is raised above that prevailing inside the cell, e.g. by addition of sugars or urea, water moves out of the cell so that the protoplast shrinks and the cytoplasmic membrane pulls away from the cell wall. This process, taking place in a hypertonic medium, is called plasmolysis. It is this shrinking of the protoplast which allowed the demonstration, in the larger bacteria, that the cytoplasmic membrane is separate from, and surrounded by, a cell wall. The cytoplasmic membrane and the cell wall can also be stained with the water-soluble dye Victoria blue.

The Gram stain.   The cell wall is responsible for the gram staining reaction. The property of being coloured dark violet, or not, by the staining procedure developed by Gram in 1884 is an important taxonomic feature which correlates with many other properties of bacteria. The Gram staining procedure begins with the addition of the basic dye crystal violet to the fixed bacteria. This is followed by treatment with an iodine solution. Iodine and crystal violet form a complex which is insoluble in water and only moderately soluble in ethanol or acetone. The cells are then treated with alcohol (differentiated): the gram-positive bacteria retain the dye-iodine complex and hence remain deep blue-purple, whereas the gram-negative cells are destained by the alcohol. A counterstain such as fuchsin then allows the latter to be visualised. If gram-positive cells are treated with lysozyme after being subjected to the Gram stain, the protoplasts appear blue but can be decolorised by alcohol. On the other hand, germinating spores of the gram-positive *Bacillus subtilis*, and the first cell generation after germination, appear gram-negative. The gram-positive character is acquired later on. These observations suggest that the colour complex is localised in or on the protoplast, but that it is the cell wall of gram-positive bacteria that exerts the strong resistance to extraction of the dye complex.

The basic skeleton of the bacterial cell wall.   To understand the structure of the bacterial cell wall it may be useful to consider its similarities with the skeletal structures formed by polymers of β-D-glucose, cellulose and chitin.

Cellulose is the basic constituent of cell walls in higher and lower plants, algae, and oomycetes. It is not usually found in bacterial cell walls, but it is the substance which keeps the cells of *Sarcina ventriculi* together in large packets or bunches. Also, *Acetobacter aceti* var. *xylinum* excretes cellulose into the medium in the form of fine threads and fimbriae which confer a leathery consistency on the 'mycoderma aceti', a structure that surrounds the cells.

Cellulose

Chitin is the supporting skeleton of arthropods and other animal groups. It is also a significant component in the cell walls of large groups of fungi (basidiomycetes, ascomycetes and zygomycetes). Chitin is made up of molecules of *N*-acetylglucosamine. These building blocks are linked together by 1,4-β-glycosidic bonds, as are the glucose molecules in cellulose.

Chitin

The supporting skeleton of the bacterial cell wall also consists of a regular polymer, the peptidoglycan **murein**. This macromolecule is a heteropolymer made up of chains of alternating molecules of N-acetyl-glucosamine (GlcNAc) and its lactic acid ether, N-acetyl muramic acid (MurNAc) linked by 1,4-β-glycosidic bonds. These heteropolymers are straight chains without branching and form the backbone of murein. The muramic acid units in the chain have short peptides attached to their lactyl residues by peptide bonds. The typical amino acids of these peptides are L-alanine, D-glutamic acid, m-diaminopimelic acid or L-lysine and D-alanine. The diamino acids m- (or LL-) diaminopimelic acid and L-lysine play an important role in the formation of an intramolecular network because both of their amino groups can take part in peptide bond formation. Thus, they can connect two of the straight hetero-polymer chains (Fig. 2.25). Diaminopimelic acid or lysine may be re-placed in some cases by ornithine or diaminobutyric acid. The heteropolymer chains, thus connected via their peptide side chains, form a sac-like molecule, the '**murein sacculus**'. The classic model that views the heteropolymer chains as circular closed strands enclosing the rod shaped bacteria like the hoops of a barrel is probably not correct. Ap-parently, the heteropolymer chains are only about one tenth the length of the bacterial circumference. It must be assumed, therefore, that chains of 50–500 disaccharides (GlcNAc and MurNAc) are connected by peptides to form a less regular network than was originally proposed. The space immediately contiguous to the cell wall, called the **periplasmic space**, is apparently of a gel-type consistency.

It should be emphasised that the bacterial cell wall contains unique structures and components that are not found in plants and animals. These include the alternating sequence of N-acetylglucosamine and N-acetyl muramic acid, and several amino acids not found in proteins, namely diaminopimelic acid and the D-isomers of alanine and glutamic acid. These unique components and structures of bacteria, along with the reactions of cell wall synthesis, offer an 'Achilles' heel' to medical therapy. Since bacteria differ fundamentally in these respects from plants and animals, therapeutic agents directed specifically at the bacterial cell

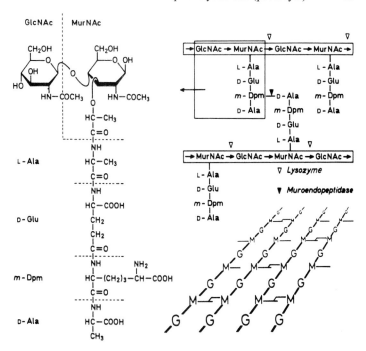

Fig. 2.25. *Structure of the murein in* E. coli.

Heteropolymer chains of alternating *N*-acetyl glucosamine (GlcNAc) and *N*-acetyl muramic acid (MurNAc) are connected by peptide bonds. Arrowheads show the bonds that can be split by lysozyme (muramidase) and by a specific muroendo-peptidase. (*Left*) the single muropeptide (framed in the upper right diagram) in detail. (*Lower right*) a perspective of the cross-linked GlcNAc (G) and Mur NAc (M) network.

wall and its synthesis should be non-toxic to the host. The presence of a peptidoglycan layer in the cell wall is a distinguishing feature of almost all eubacteria. The only exceptions to this are the archaebacteria and a few other groups and species.

The murein sacculus functions as the **supporting skeleton** of the cell wall and is penetrated and surrounded by a number of other substances. Both the detailed structure of the supporting skeleton and the participation of accessory substances differ between gram-positive and gram-negative bacteria.

The cell wall of gram-positive bacteria.   In gram-positive bacteria the murein network represents 30–70% of the dry weight of the cell wall and consists of about 40 layers. In many cases LL-diaminopimelic acid or L-lysine takes the place of *m*-diaminopimelic acid. In *Staphylococcus aureus*, the tetrapeptide side chains of the muramic acid are connected by interpeptide chains (such as pentaglycine) but the amino acids contained in these vary in different species. Indeed, the species-specific structural features of the supporting skeleton are of taxonomic importance. Polysaccharides, if present in the cell wall of gram-positive organisms, are covalently bound, whilst any protein content is very minor. The presence of teichoic acids is characteristic. These are chains of 8–50 glycerol or ribitol molecules connected by phosphate ester bridges. Some contain erythritol or mannitol. Teichoic acids may be bound to the murein via the phosphates in an amide-like fashion.

The cell wall of gram-negative bacteria.   In gram-negative bacteria the murein network is present as a single layer and represents less than 10% of the cell wall dry weight (in *E. coli*). The murein contains no lysine, only *m*-diaminopimelic acid, and has no interpeptide bridges. The structure of the sacculus appears similar in all gram-negative bacteria that have been examined. Apart from the supporting skeleton, there are large quantities of lipoproteins, lipopolysaccharides and other lipids, which appear attached to the outer surface of the murein skeleton. They are covalently bound and constitute up to 80% of the cell wall dry weight. The lipopolysaccharide layer appears to require calcium ions to maintain its stability. If calcium ions are removed by treatment with EDTA, a chelating agent, lipopolysaccharides are liberated, thus making the murein layer accessible to degradation by the enzyme lysozyme. So far, no teichoic acids have been found in any gram-negative organisms.

The action of lysozyme and penicillin.   Elucidation of the cell wall structure and murein composition of bacteria is based largely on studies of the action of lysozyme and penicillin. Lysozyme, discovered by A. Fleming in 1922, is an antibacterial enzyme found in egg white, tear secretions and nasal mucus. It has also been isolated from bacteria (*E. coli*, *Streptomyces*) and from bacteriophages. Treatment of gram-positive bacteria with lysozyme results in rapid clearing of the suspension, i.e. lysis of the organisms, although there are quantitative differences in the susceptibilities of different species. Equivalent suspensions of *Micrococcus luteus* (*lysiodeikticus*) can be lysed with 1 μg of lysozyme whereas *Bacillus megaterium* requires 50 μg of the enzyme per ml cell suspension. Many gram-negative bacteria are affected only in the presence of chelating agents such as EDTA. Lysozyme attacks the glycosidic bonds between

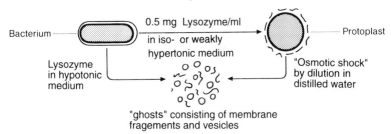

Fig. 2.26. *Production of protoplasts and membrane vesicles by treatment with lysozyme.*

the C-1 atom of *N*-acetylmuramate and the C-4 atom of *N*-acetyl-glucosamine in the murein, and thus degrades it to GlcNAc-MurNAc (Fig. 2.25). Lysozyme is therefore an acetyl muramidase. Lysis of the bacteria in the presence of lysozyme can be prevented by carrying out the treatment in an isotonic or weakly hypertonic (0.1–0.2 M) sucrose solution. Under these conditions the action of lysozyme produces osmotically fragile, spherical **protoplasts** (Fig. 2.26). These are stable in isotonic or hypertonic media, but burst in hypotonic media, leaving only 'ghosts', i.e. remains of the cytoplasmic membrane. The term **protoplasts** should be confined to those spherical bodies that are demonstrably free of cell wall components, i.e. do not contain any murein or diaminopimelic acid (which is absent from proteins). The dissolution of the cell wall does not affect metabolism; protoplasts respire in the same way as intact cells and can form spores (in the case of sporogenous bacteria) if sporulation has been initiated prior to destruction of the cell wall. However, they are unable to adsorb bacteriophages.

Apart from lysozyme there are a number of other enzymes that attack the murein skeleton. The mucoendopeptidases, found mainly in bacteria, are specific for hydrolysing peptide bonds involved in the cross-linking of the murein network. One of the endopeptidases isolated from *E. coli* splits the D-alanyl-*m*-diaminopimelic acid bond (indicated in Fig. 2.25). Other enzymes act at different places.

The antibiotic penicillin acts mainly on gram-positive bacteria (such as staphylococci, streptococci, pneumococci), but some penicillins can also act in a bactericidal manner on a number of gram-negative organisms (gonococci, meningococci, enterobacteria). The bactericidal effect is exerted only on growing bacteria; non-growing, resting cells are protected. The most obvious change observable during penicillin treatment of susceptible organisms is the production of so-called L-forms. This results from irregular growth in length and diameter of the treated cells, producing a manifold increase in volume compared with the original

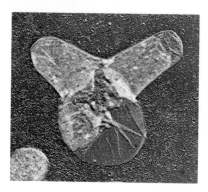

Fig. 2.27. E. coli *after treatment for 90 minutes with 100 units/ml of penicillin.*

Magnification, × 9000. (Picture: H. Frank.)

rods (Ch. 3.19). These giant cells remain viable for a time on solid media. If the penicillin treatment of growing cells is carried out in an isotonic or hypertonic medium, the rods change into spherical forms, which are called L-forms or spheroplasts (Fig. 2.27). The latter differ from the true protoplasts in their possession of cell wall fragments; the presence of murein and diaminopimelic acid can be demonstrated. Thus, penicillin interferes with cell wall synthesis.

Cell wall biosynthesis.   The biosynthesis and assembly of the building blocks into the peptidoglycan skeleton can be divided into three phases (Fig. 2.28). The first steps in the biosynthesis take place in the cytoplasm. This is where the muramic acid-pentapeptide is formed. The synthesis starts with N-acetylglucosamine-1-phosphate. In sequential enzymatic steps this is converted to the uridine diphosphate (UDP) derivative and then to the lactyl ether to which the five amino acids are attached. During this process the growing molecule of muramic acid remains attached to the UDP carrier. The second phase comprises the combination of the muramic acid-pentapeptide with N-acetylglucosamine and (in the case of *Staphylococcus aureus*) the attachment of the five glycyl residues. This takes place at the cytoplasmic membrane and is initiated by converting the hydrophilic molecule into a lipophilic entity by exchanging the UDP carrier for a C_{55}-polyisoprenoid, the undecaprenyl phosphate known as bactoprenol. Eventually, this combination also mediates the transport of the finished unit through the cytoplasmic membrane for the last (third) phase. This consists of the insertion of the nascent murein subunit into the pre-existing peptidoglycan skeleton and

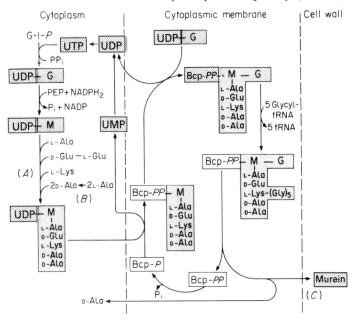

Fig. 2.28. *Biosynthesis of murein by* Staphylococcus aureus.

The three stages of synthesis (separated by dotted lines) occur in the cytoplasm, at the cytoplasmic membrane, and at the cell wall. G, GlcNAc (*N*-acetyl glucosamine); M, MurNAc (*N*-acetyl muramic acid); Bcp, bactoprenol. No synthesis of cell wall takes place under the following conditions: (A) when no diaminoacid (lysine) is available; (B) when the racemisation of L-alanine to D-alanine and its peptide bond formation are inhibited by *C*-cycloserine (oxamycin); (C) when the cross-linking of the peptide chains is inhibited by penicillin.

the cross-linking by peptide bonds. The cross-linking is carried out by a transpeptidation reaction; the bond between the two D-alanyl groups in the pentapeptide of the incoming unit is split and the liberated carboxyl group of the penultimate D-alanine is joined to the amino group of the lysing in the neighbouring oligopeptide. One D-alanyl residue is thereby liberated. During this assembly, one molecule of bactoprenol (undecaprenyl) diphosphate is also liberated, and it is then dephosphorylated to bactoprenol (undecaprenyl) monophosphate, which is available for another unit of murein being synthesised. The lipid bactoprenol also functions as a carrier in the synthesis of other extracytoplasmic membrane polymers, such as polysaccharides, lipopolysaccharides and cellulose.

Penicillin does not affect the synthesis of the murein building blocks or the transglycolysation that results in the elongation of the heteropolymer strands, but it inhibits their cross-linking by transpeptidation. Therefore, various bacterial strains excrete not only the precursor UDP-muramic acid-pentapeptide, but also non-cross-linked peptidoglycan strands during penicillin treatment. Penicillin derivatives, as well as cephalosporins, ristocetins, vancomycin, bacitracin, and D-cycloserine also interfere with cell wall synthesis. In addition **spheroplasts** can be formed under the influence of glycine and D-amino acids and by 'anaerobic lysis'.

The outer layers of gram-negative cell walls.   In gram-negative bacteria the monolayer or, at most, bilayer of the murein sacculus is surrounded by an outer cell wall layer, or envelope. In thin section this appears similar to the cytoplasmic membrane and is therefore often called the **outer membrane**. This outer layer has a complex composition of proteins, phospholipids and lipopolysaccharides (Fig. 2.29). The murein layer has lipoproteins attached to its diaminopimelic acids by covalent bonds. These lipoproteins have their lipophilic ends orientated away from the murein and embedded in a lipophilic double layer by hydrophobic interactions. This double layer contains the phospholipids and the hydrophobic ends of the lipopolysaccharides; the hydrophilic ends of the latter are orientated toward the outside of the cell.

The functions of the outer membrane.   The outer membrane of gram-negative bacteria has important physiological as well as mechanical functions. The lipid bilayer composed of lipid A (of the lipopolysaccharides) and phospholipids has proteins incorporated into it, which penetrate the whole of its thickness. These transmembrane proteins are thought to constitute water-filled channels or hydrophilic pores in the lipophilic membrane and are called porins. There are several different kinds of porins. They allow low molecular weight substances (up to a relative particle mass of about 600) to enter the cell.

The outer membrane is firmly attached to the murein layer and is connected to it by lipoproteins (see above). The murein layer apparently does not limit uptake of metabolites.

The periplasmic space.   In many bacteria the space between the outer membrane and the peptidoglycan layer, which is called the **periplasmic space**, contains a considerable number of enzymes. These include, for example, enzymes which break down substrates like ethanol and glucose, or those which initiate the actions of inorganic groups like SO_4^{2-} and NO_3^-, etc. Some of these enzymes are anchored in the cytoplasmic membrane, whilst others exist freely in solution. In addition, depolymerases for proteins, polysaccharides, nucleic acids and other biopolymers, as

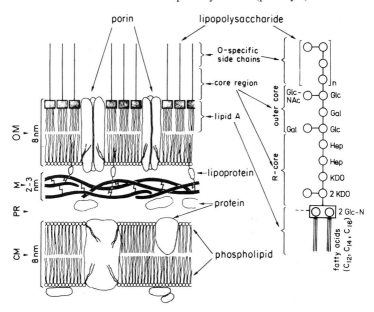

Fig. 2.29. *Model of the gram-negative cell envelope or outer membrane (OM).*

The murein layer (M) surrounds the cytoplasmic membrane (CM) and periplasmic space (PR) and has the hydrophilic ends of lipoproteins covalently bound to it. The lipophilic ends of the lipoproteins are embedded in a lipid bilayer which contains phospholipids and the lipid A zone of lipopolysaccharides. The hydrophilic,

O-specific, heteropolysaccharide side chains of the lipopolysaccharides point outwards (*top*).
(*Right*) detailed structure of a lipololysaccharide.
Glc, glucose; Glc-N, glucosamine; Glc-NAc, *N*-acetyl glucosamine; Gal, galactose; Hep, heptose; KDO, 2-keto-3-deoxyoctanoic acid.

well as binding proteins, which may act as receptors for chemotactic stimuli or function in the transport of various substrates, are found there. It is quite probable that the periplasm contains as high a concentration of proteins as does the cytoplasm.

Lipopolysaccharides   (LPS) are the endotoxins of gram-negative bacteria. They have achieved great importance in diagnostic bacteriology. Different strains of *Salmonella typhimurium*, *Shigella dysenteriae* and other causative organisms of intestinal infections are differentiated by

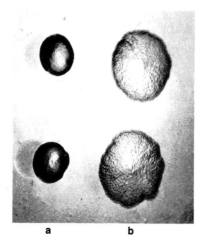

a   b

Fig. 2.30. *Colonial forms of* Salmonella paratyphi *B.*
(a) S-form; (b) R-form. (Picture: E. Kröger.)

their 'O-specific' side chains of lipopolysaccharides which constitute the outermost layer of the cell. Very slight differences in the composition of this layer can be recognised by immunological methods; more than 1000 species and strains of the genus *Salmonella* have been identified by such serological reactions and the differences have been confirmed by chemical analysis (Westphal). Because even local strain variations among *Salmonella* can be recognised by their immunochemical properties, the place of infection of a patient or the origin of an epidemic can be localised. It can be determined, for example, whether a patient contracted his diarrhoea in a given town during a South American journey, or in a Far Eastern city.

Many bacterial strains, freshly isolated from nature or from a patient, grow on agar medium as smooth, shiny colonies (S-forms). Their O-specific polysaccharides in the cell surface apparently retain water. These S-forms may mutate spontaneously to R-forms which show flat, rough colonies (Fig. 2.30). In the animal host these bacteria are very resistant to phagocytosis, and hence virulent. Only the formation of antibodies by the host and the combination of these antibodies with the polysaccharide chains render the bacteria susceptible to attack. The great diversity of O-specific polysaccharides in pathogenic bacteria could be the result of continuous selection of new O-antigenic types (mutants); these would have a selective advantage because the host can hardly be equipped with antibodies against hundreds of different antigens at the same time. The lipopolysaccharides also belong to the most effective endotoxins of bacteria, causing fever and diarrhoea.

> The lipopolysaccharides of *Salmonella typhimurium* and other enterobacteria have been examined in great detail. There are three main constituents: lipid A, a core, and the O-specific polysaccharides (Fig. 2.29). Lipid A consists of a glucosamine disaccharide whose hydroxyl groups are esterified with C_{12}, C_{14} and C_{16} fatty acids. This consists of a 2-keto-3-deoxyoctanoic acid (KDO) trisaccharide combined with phosphoethanolamine, two heptose molecules, and the outer core layer. The latter consists of a branched chain of glucose, galactose and *N*-acetylglucosamine. This basic structure is found in all *Salmonella* species and is apparently uniform. The O-specific side chains (polysaccharides) are attached to the core. They consist of long chains of repeating oligosaccharides, their sequence and composition being strain-specific. They may contain galactose, mannose, rhamnose, abequose, fucose, colitose and other sugars. The C-1, reducing ends of the sugars point inwards. These outer heteropolysaccharide chains, which are strain-specific, represent the somatic O-antigens and allow identification of a strain by immunological methods. In rough mutants, the KDO-trisaccharide constitutes the outer boundary of the cell.

2.2.5   Capsules and slimes

Many bacteria accumulate layers of water-rich materials on their outer surface. These are known as capsules and slimy envelopes. These envelopes are usually not essential for life, but the possession of capsules makes some pathogenic bacteria resistant to phagocytosis and enhances their virulence.

Capsules.   After addition of dyes that do not penetrate the capsular material, such as Chinese ink, nigrosin, or Congo red, it is easy to demonstrate the presence of the capsules with the light microscope. In this technique, called negative staining, the capsules appear light against a dark background (Figs 2.31, 2.32). The less dense capsules of pneumococci can be visualised after addition of homologous antiserum, which leads to accumulation of antibody protein. This procedure causes the cells to look swollen (Neufeld's swelling reaction).

Most capsules consist of polysaccharides (*Streptococcus mutans*, *S. salivarious*, *Xanthomonas*, corynebacteria) that contain, apart from glucose, aminosugars, rhamnose, 2-keto-3-deoxygalactonic acid, uronic acids of various sugars, and organic acids like pyruvate and acetate. However, the capsules of some bacilli (*Bacillus anthracis*, *B. subtilis*) consist of polypeptides, mainly polyglutamic acid.

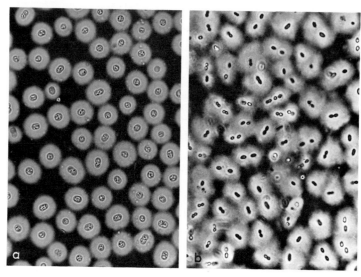

Fig. 2.31. *Bacterial capsules.*

(a) Of the purple sulphur bacterium *Amoebobacter roseus*, × 1200; (b) of the nitrogen-fixing bacterium *Azotobacter chroococcum*, × 500.

Negatively stained preparations. (Pictures: (a) N. Pfennig; (b) D. Claus.)

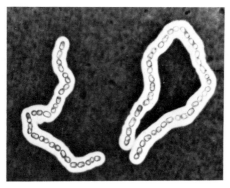

Fig. 2.32. *Bacterial capsules of cell chains of* Bacillus megaterium *suspended in Indian ink.*

The capsular material is contrasted as the light zone from the background of Indian ink. Phase contrast, × 1000. (Picture: Bohiken, G. (1965). Diss., Göttingen.)

Slimes. Much of the capsular material may be excreted into the medium as slime. In some cases the entire capsular material can be removed from the cell surface by shaking or homogenising the bacterial suspension, and it can then be recovered from the medium as slime. A more extensive slime formation occurs with many microorganisms when the medium contains saccharose. A well-known example of this is *Leuconostoc mesenteriodes*, a heterofermentative lactic acid bacterium known in sugar-refining plants as 'frogspawn bacterium', which rapidly converts a solution containing cane sugar to a stiff jelly consisting of dextran. This conversion takes place outside the cell and is catalysed by an extracellular hexosyl transferase called dextran saccharase:

$$n \text{ saccharose} + (1,6\text{-}\alpha\text{-glucosyl})_m \rightarrow n \text{ fructose} + (1,6\text{-}\alpha\text{-glucosyl})_{m+n}$$

Dextran is a polysaccharide consisting of $1,6$-α-D-glucose residues ($1,6$-α-glucan); parallel chains are joined to give a network. Dextran is used as a plasma substitute, as an agent to increase the viscosity of aqueous solutions, and as the basis of Sephadex. The streptococci that produce dental caries, among them *Streptococcus salivarious* and *S. mutans*, excrete another hexosyl transferase that converts saccharose to polyfructose (laevan). The polysaccharides attach to the dental surface and are the matrix in which the acidic products of streptococcal fermentation, mainly lactic acid, are accumulated.

Sheaths. Some filamentous bacteria form tubular envelopes, described as sheaths (*Sphaerotilus natans*, *Leptothrix ochracea*). These sheaths consist of a heteropolysaccharide containing glucose, glucuronic acid, galactose, and fucose. In a few bacteria, excretion of slime with a polar orientation, in the form of a pseudostem, facilitates a moderate change of position (*Gallionella ferruginea*). In others, slime may enable individual cells to stay associated in cell colonies (*Zoogloea ramigera*: Fig. 2.33) or invests them with a skin (*Bacteriogloea*). *Acetobacter aceti* var. *xylinum* secretes cellulose which forms the 'mycoderma aceti', a leather-like skin that surrounds the cells. The cells of *Sarcina ventriculi* and of *Lampropedia hyalina* are bound by the excreted cellulose in regular associations (aggregates). The cellulose in these cases serves as a kind of mortar and is quite different from capsules, both structurally and functionally. Loss of ability to form cellulose has no adverse effects on the growth of these bacteria (Fig. 2.34).

Biosynthesis. All of the polysaccharides that are localised outside the cell wall are known collectively as exopolysaccharides. Capsules and slimes are differentiated according to their physical properties. When the exopolysaccharides are bound relatively tightly to the cell surface, they

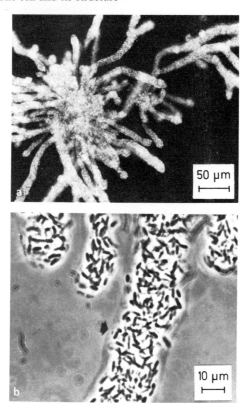

Fig. 2.33. *Colonial structure of* Zoogloea ramigera.

(a) Typical colony form; (b) single
cells suspended in the slimy matrix.

(From Unz, R. F. & Dondero. N. C.
(1967). *Can. J. Microbiol.* **13**, 1971.)

are called capsules; if they are loosely associated or free in the medium,
they are referred to as slimes.

Two mechanisms have been described for the biosynthesis of exopolysaccharides: (1) dextrans and laevans are formed from disaccharides by
extracellular enzymes; (2) the composition of most exopolysaccharides is
independent of the cell substrate. The pathways of their biosynthesis are
similar to that of murein and the lipopolysaccharides. In all these processes, uridine triphosphate (UTP) and the lipid bactoprenol (undecaprenyl)
diphosphate (C_{55}-polyisoprenoid) participate. After activation by UTP

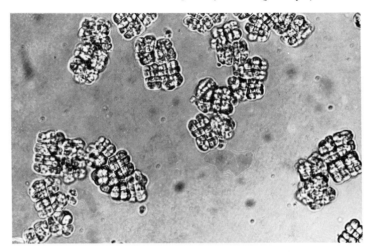

Fig. 2.34. Sarcina ventriculi *cell packets grown in nutrient solution.*
Bright-field illumination, × 750.   (Picture: D. Claus.)

(to UDP-sugars), the sugars are attached to the lipid carrier, combined to the homo- or heteropolymeric building blocks, and transported from the protoplast to the outer layers of the cell wall, where they are linked into the macromolecular exopolysaccharides.

2.2.6   Flagella and motility

Bacteria can achieve motility in a number of ways. In most of the actively motile, swimming bacteria, motility is brought about by the rotation of flagella. Motility without flagella is found in the gliding bacteria, a group which includes myxobacteria, cyanobacteria and a few other bacterial groups, as well as spirochaetes. The mechanisms of their motility will be described in the chapters discussing these organisms.

Arrangement of flagella.   The ways in which flagella are arranged on the bacterial cell are highly specific for different motile eubacteria and, hence, are of taxonomic value. In rod-shaped bacteria, insertion of flagella may be **polar** or **lateral** (Fig. 2.35).

Amongst the bacteria with monopolar flagellation, some have only a single but exceptionally thick flagellum (*Vibrio metchnikovii*, Fig. 2.36) and *Caulobacter* species. However, many of those that appear as and

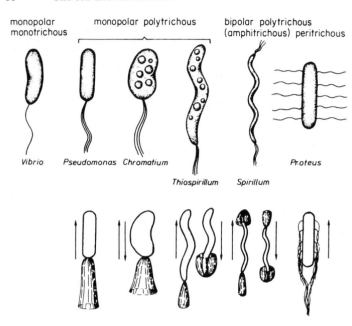

monopolar   monopolar polytrichous   bipolar polytrichous
monotrichous   (amphitrichous) peritrichous

Vibrio   Pseudomonas   Chromatium   Proteus

Thiospirillum   Spirillum

Fig. 2.35. *The most important types of flagellation and movement in bacteria.*

function as monopolar or bipolar flagella actually consist of bundles of from 2 to 50 single units (polytrichous). Monopolar polytrichous flagellation is also referred to as **lophotrichous** (*Pseudomonas*, *Chromatium*), and bipolar polytrichous flagellation is called **amphitrichous** (*Spirillum*). *Selenomonas* has a laterally inserted flagellar bundle (Fig. 2.37b). In peritrichously flagellated bacteria (Enterobacteriaceae, Bacillaceae and others) the flagella are inserted in the lateral walls or over the entire surface (Fig. 2.37a).

Recognition of flagella.   Flagella or flagellar bundles can be recognised in a few bacteria by ordinary bright-field or phase-contrast microscopy, e.g. in *Chromatium okenii*, *Bdellovibrio*, *Thiospirillum* (Fig. 2.38). In many other bacteria the flagella and their movements can only be demonstrated by dark-field illumination (*Pseudomonas*, *Spirillum*). In general, flagella can be visualised most easily by deposition of a specific dye or metal complex, or by electron microscopy (Fig. 2.39).

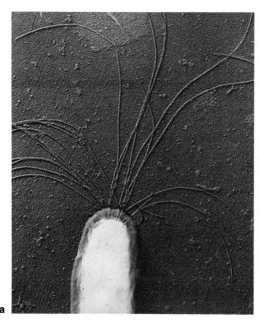
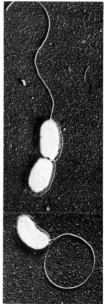

a   b

Fig. 2.36. *Types of flagellation.*

(a) *Spirillum serpens*, polar polytrichous flagellation, × 11 000.
(b) *Vibrio metchnikovii*, polar

monotrichous flagellation, × 7199.
(Electron micrographs: W. van
Iterson.)

Flagellar function.   In most cases of polar flagellation, the flagellum acts like a ship's screw and pushes the bacterial cell through the medium. The flagellum consists of helically wound threads which are driven by a 'rotation motor' localised at the site of flagellar insertion into the cytoplasmic membrane, so that they rotate around the fictitious axis of the screw. This movement can be carried out by a single flagellum or by flagellar bundles. Flagella rotate with relatively high frequencies, in the case of spirilla at about 3000 r.p.m., i.e. similar to the speed of a medium-sized electric motor. This flagellar rotation results in rotation of the bacterial body at about one third of this velocity in the opposite direction. Flagella can change the orientation of their rotation, either spontaneously or in response to external stimuli (Fig. 2.35). In some bacteria with polar flagellation, reversal of the orientation of rotation leads to reversal of direction of movement. In *Chromatium okenii*, for example, reversal of rotation in response to light stimuli induces the

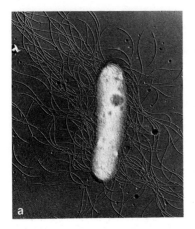

Fig. 2.37. *Types of flagellation.*

(a) *Proteus mirabilis*, peritrichous
flagellation; (b) *Selenomonas
ruminantium*, lateral flagellation.
Electron micrographs: (a) platinum–

palladium diagonal shadowing,
× 9500 (picture: H. Frank);
(b) negative-contrast preparation,
× 4080 (picture: V. Kingsley).

flagellar bundle to exert a pulling action. The velocity of this backward
motion is only about one quarter of that in the forward direction and
results in a tumbling movement. In *Thiospirillum jenense*, a phototrophic
giant spirillum with monopolar flagellation, the flagellar bundle does not
beat in a forward direction when the organism is moving backwards, but
appears inverted over the cell body, rather like an umbrella inverted by
a high wind. Spirilla which have amphitrichous flagellation generally
show such inversion of flagellar bundles over the bacterial body.

The peritrichously arranged flagella of *E. coli* function as a well-co-
ordinated helical bundle and push the cell through the medium. A
reversal of rotation by the flagella results in tumbling. Apparently,
peritrichously arranged flagella cannot pull the cell.

Flagellated bacteria can move with high velocities. *Bacillus megaterium*
can move 1.6 mm/min and *Vibrio cholerae* can move 12 mm/min, corresponding to 300–3000 times the cell length per minute.

Fine structure of flagella.   Flagella are helically wound protein threads.
Different bacteria have flagella that differ in diameter (12–18 nm), length
(up to 20 μm), and the length and amplitude of their helical axis. These
parameters are species-specific, although a few bacteria can have several
types of flagella. Flagellar filaments are made of subunits of a single

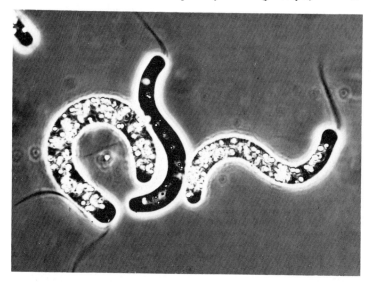

Fig. 2.38. Thiospirillum jenense.

Phase contrast, × 1200. (Picture: N. Pfennig.)

species of protein, flagellin, which has a relatively low molecular weight. These subunits are arranged in helical order around an axial cylinder (similar to the tobacco mosaic virus: Chapter 4.1). Therefore the structure of flagella is determined by the properties of the protein subunits. Flagella have three sections: the flagellar filament just described, a flagellar 'hook' near the cell surface, and a basal body which anchors the flagellum in the cytoplasmic membrane and cell wall. (Fig. 2.40). In gram-negative bacteria the basal body consists of a central core which carries two pairs of rings. The outer pair (L- and P-rings) are located at the levels of the outer and inner layers of the cell wall, whilst the inner pair (S- and M-rings) are situated at the level of the outer layer of the cytoplasmic membrane. Since gram-positive bacteria lack the outer pair of rings, it is assumed that only the inner pair is essential for flagellar motion. It is envisaged that the M-ring functions as a drive plate and the S-ring functions as a counterbalance on the inner surface of the peptidoglycan layer. The molecular mechanisms of the flagellar 'rotary' motor is not yet known.

O- and H-antigens. *Proteus vulgaris* often spreads over the whole of an agar surface as a thin film (in German, *Hauch*, hence H-form). This

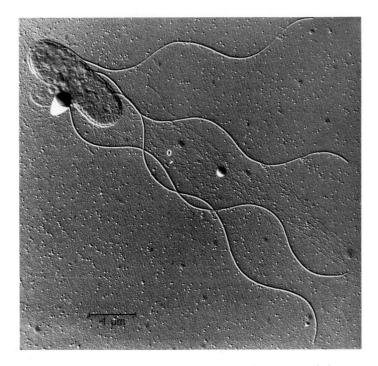

Fig. 2.39. Alcaligenes eutrophus, *a soil and water bacterium with degenerate peritrichous flagellation.*

(Electron micrograph after oblique shadowing with platinum/iridium: T. Hollemann.)

swarming behaviour reflects exceptional motility. Some strains do not spread like this (in German, 'ohne Hauch', hence O-form). These are non-motile strains lacking flagella. These observations led to some of the common nomenclature of bacterial serology: the antigens of the cell surface or body (somatic antigens) were referred to as O-antigens, whilst the flagellar antigens were called H-antigens.

Fimbriae and pili.   The surface of some bacteria is covered by a number (ten to several thousand) of long, thin, straight threads 3–25 nm in diameter and up to 12 μm in length. These are called fimbriae or pili, and they occur in flagellated and non-flagellated species and varieties. These type-1 pili differ from the sex pili (F-pili) that have been demonstrated in

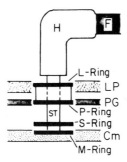

Fig. 2.40. *Anchoring of a bacterial flagellum in the cell wall and cytoplasmic membrane of a gram-negative bacterium.*

F, flagellum filament; H, hook;
Cm, cytoplasmic membrane;
LP, lipopolysaccharide layer;

PG, peptidoglycan layer; ST, basal
body (stem).

donor cells of *E. coli* K12, i.e. in strains that carry the mating factor F (F^+ and Hfr). Only two F-pili are found per cell; they resemble hollow protein tubes, 0.5–10 μm long.

Chemotaxis. Freely motile bacteria are able to move in definite directions: they exhibit taxis. According to which environmental factor governs such behaviour, it is referred to as chemotaxis, aerotaxis, phototaxis, or magnetotaxis.

When motile bacteria react to chemical stimuli, they accumulate in some areas or retreat from others. Such stimulus-response behaviour is called chemotaxis. The attraction of organisms by chemical stimuli is brought about in the following manner (Fig. 2.41). Peritrichously flagellated bacteria have two kinds of motile behaviour, straight-line swimming and tumbling, which interrupts the straight movement and causes reorientation. If the bacteria are placed in a concentration gradient of an attractant, the linear swimming movement will last many seconds if it is in the direction of the optimal concentration of the attractant, but in the opposite direction it is interrupted after only a few seconds. Whilst the tumbling movement leads to a completely random selection of the new swimming direction, the direction-dependent duration of the linear swimming motion results in accumulation of the organisms in the region of optimal substrate concentration. The sensing of, and response to, stimuli is due to specific chemoreceptors. In some cases these are independent of substrate assimilation. Thus, some mutants show unchanged chemotactic reactions to certain nutrients, though they have lost the capacity to utilise them.

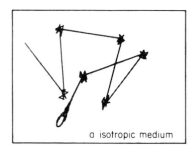
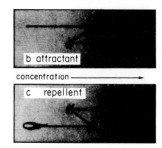
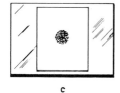

Fig. 2.41. *Chemotactic movement.*

(a) In a normal, isotropic medium, a bacterium swims linearly in a given direction for a certain time, before tumbling. (b) In a concentration gradient of an attractant, the frequency of tumbling decreases when the cell swims in the direction of the higher concentration. (c) In a concentration gradient of a repellent, the frequency of tumbling decreases when the cell swims away from the higher concentration.

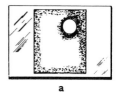
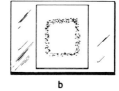

Fig. 2.42. *Aerotactic responses of motile bacteria.*

(a) Aerobic bacteria collect at the edges of a cover slip and around trapped air bubbles; (b) micro-aerophilic bacteria keep a certain distance from the edges of the cover slip; (c) strictly anaerobic bacteria collect in the centre. (After Beijerinck.)

Aerotaxis.   Some motile bacteria reveal their metabolic capacities relative to oxygen or air by their aerotactic movements and accumulation at certain distances from the edge of the coverslip. In bacterial suspensions placed between slide and coverslip, aerophilic organisms accumulate near the edge of the coverslip and in the vicinity of air bubbles, demonstrating their requirement for aerobic conditions and their dependence on aerobic respiration for energy (Fig. 2.42). Strictly anaerobic bacteria, on the other hand, tend to collect in the centre, whilst microaerophilic bacteria, such as some pseudomonads and spirilla, keep a certain distance from the air interface. Engelmann used positively aerotactic bacteria to demonstrate oxygen evolution by locally illuminated chloroplasts of the green alga *Spirogyra*.

Phototaxis.   The phototrophic purple bacteria depend on light for their energy supply. Therefore it is not surprising that they possess a phototactic mechanism and accumulate in illuminated areas. If one projects a small spot of light onto a thick suspension of *Chromatium* on a slide previously kept in the dark, the organisms can be seen to collect in the illuminated area. Moreover, it appears that the organisms cannot leave the illuminated area, once they have entered it, in the course of their random movements. On entering the dark zone, abrupt reversal of flagellar motion propels them back into the light zone. This reversal is so sudden that this response has been called 'phobotaxis' (shock reaction). Even slight differences in light intensity between areas of illumination can evoke this reaction. Some *Chromatium* species accumulate in areas that receive only 0.7% more light than the environment. This contrast sensitivity (with regard to illumination) is similar to that of the human eye (0.4%).

Magnetotaxis.   Recently a number of bacteria (rods, spirilla, cocci) isolated from the surface layers of sediments in freshwater ponds and the sea have been found to orientate themselves in a magnetic field and swim in the direction of the field lines. They contain unusual amounts of iron (0.4% of their dry weight) as ferromagnetic iron oxide (magnetite) in the form of grana (magnetosomes) which are localised close to the area of flagellar insertion. Bacteria isolated in the northern hemisphere seek the north; the field lines are directed downwards with a gradient of about 70°. Magnetotactic behaviour thus enables these bacteria to migrate downwards into the oxygen-poor or oxygen-free sediments. Since the magnetotactic bacteria are anaerobic or microaerophilic, this mechanism and behaviour finds a ready ecological explanation. When such organisms are transferred to the southern hemisphere, they cannot survive; a few 'wrongly polarised' cells, however, can grow and multiply. It seems that the polarity is not genetically fixed.

2.2.7   Reserve materials and other cellular inclusions

Under appropriate conditions many microorganisms contain intracellular inclusions that can be regarded as reserve or storage materials. Among these are polysaccharides, lipids, polyphosphates, and sulphur. These materials are accumulated when their precursors are present in the medium but microbial growth is inhibited or stopped by a growth-limiting factor or the presence of a growth-inhibitory agent. Such reserve materials are osmotically inert and insoluble in aqueous media. On restoration of favourable growth conditions, they can be mobilised for use in cell metabolism. Reserve polysaccharides, neutral lipids, and poly-β-hydroxybutyrate can serve as carbon and energy sources and, in the absence of external energy sources, they can thus extend the lifespan of the organism. In spore formers they can allow sporulation in the absence of extracellular substrates. Polyphosphates can be regarded as reserve phosphates, and elementary sulphur deposits can function as electron donors.

Polysaccharides. The chemical constitution of storage polysaccharides in microorganisms has been the subject of only a few investigations. In some microbes these polysaccharides have been characterised as **starch** or **glycogen** by their colour reaction with Lugol's iodine (blue and brown, respectively). Contrary to the cell wall polysaccharides, these storage polysaccharides are derived from α-D-glucose, the glucose molecules being linked via α-1,4-glycosidic bonds into chains which can form networks via multiple cross linkages (Fig. 14.3). Because of the α-glycosidic bonds, the chains are not straight but appear helically wound.

starch, glycogen

The starch granules of plants consist of amylose and amylopectin, amylose representing about 20–30% of the total and being responsible for the iodine-starch reaction (deep blue colour) caused by the entrapment of iodine in the helical turns. A substance resembling starch has been described in clostridia and referred to as 'granulose'. Cells of *Clostridium butyricum* are filled with small starch granules with only the spore-forming pole free of them. Starch is also found in *Acetobacter pasteurianus* and in many *Neisseria* species. Glycogen, also known as 'animal starch', is similar to amylopectin, although it is more extensively branched (in 1,6-linkage) and in bacteria it appears to be more common than starch. It is found in yeasts and other fungi as well as in bacilli (*Bacillus polymyxa*), in *Salmonella*, *E. coli* and other Enterobacteriaceae, in *Micrococcus luteus*, and in *Arthrobacter* (Fig. 2.43).

Lipid-like substances. Intracellular fat granules and droplets occur in many microorganisms. They can be stained with lipophilic dyes (Sudan

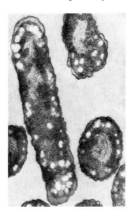

Fig. 2.43. *Glycogen inclusions in cells of* E. coli.

Accumulation of glycogen that occurred during a 15-hour aerobic incubation in a phosphate buffer containing glucose. Electron micrograph of ultrathin sections (osmium tetroxide-bichromate; uranyl acetate), × 8000. (Picture: F. Amelunxen.)

III or Sudan black B) and are also visible in unstained preparations under the light microscope by virtue of their high refractivity.

poly-β-hydroxybutyrate (n = 60)

Poly-β-hydroxybutyrate (PHB) is accumulated by aerobic and facultative bacteria when the cells are deprived of oxygen and must carry out fermentative metabolism; it can therefore also be regarded as a polymeric, intracellular fermentation product (Figs 2.44, 2.45). On return to aerobic conditions it can be used as an energy and carbon source and incorporated into the oxidative metabolism.

Some bacteria can also produce co-polymers together with PHB. Thus, for example, when propionic acid or β-hydroxyvaleric acid are provided as substrate, polymers can be formed which consist of β-hydroxybutyric acid and β-hydroxyvaleric acid. There may also be other γ-hydroxy fatty acids as well as long-chain hydroxyacids (C_8, C_{10}, C_{12}) so that these reserve materials are often referred to as poly (hydroxy) fatty acids, or poly-hydroxy-alkanoates (PHA). These PHAs can be thermoplastically moulded and can be used as new plastics which have the advantage over polypropylene or polyethylene of being biodegradable.

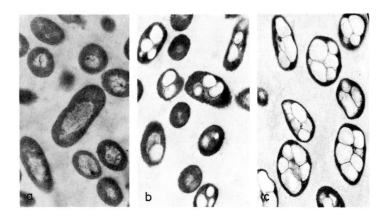

Fig. 2.44. *Accumulation of poly-β-hydroxybutyrate in cells of* Alcaligenes eutrophus.

(a) Cells during exponential growth; (b) cells after 1-hour assimilation of acetate in the absence of a nitrogen source; (c) cells after 24-hour assimilation of acetate in the absence of a nitrogen source, before fixation. Electron micrographs of ultrathin sections (osmium tetroxide–bichromate; uranyl acetate–lead citrate), × 6000. (Pictures: P. Hillmer and F. Amelunxen.)

Neutral lipids (triglycerides) that are frequently found in yeasts and other fungi, inside vacuoles, are of similar composition to the lipids of higher organisms. Up to 90% of the dry weight of yeasts such as *Candida* and *Rhodotorula* may be neutral lipids. Mycobacteria, Nocardiae and actinomycetes contain various other lipoid substances stored in vacuoles; these substances sometimes may be excreted into the medium. Up to 40% of the dry weight of mycobacteria may be wax, i.e. esters of long-chain fatty acids and alcohols. Whereas the cellular contents of storage lipids is dependent on nutritional factors (a high carbon:nitrogen ratio), the presence and amounts of other lipid fractions, though not their composition, are almost independent of environmental factors. These lipids are only liberated upon hydrolysis of proteins and polysaccharides and are components of lipoproteins (in the cytoplasmic and other membranes) and lipopolysaccharides.

Polyphosphates. Many bacteria and algae can accumulate phosphates in the form of polyphosphates. Because they were first described in *Spirillum volutans* and because they bring about characteristic changes in

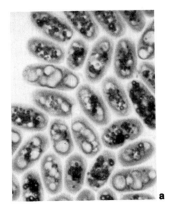
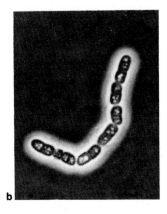

a   b

Fig. 2.45. *Cells with inclusions of poly-β-hydroxybutyrate.*
(a) *Chromatium okenii.* The dark inclusions are sulphur droplets. Bright-field illumination. × 1000; (b) *Bacillus megaterium.* Indian ink preparation. (From Schlegel, H. G. (1962). *Arch. Mikrobiol.* **42**, 110 and Bohlken, G. (1965). Diss., Göttingen.)

the pigmentation of certain dyes, they have been called 'volutin granules' and 'metachromatic granules'. Such granules consist predominantly of

polyphosphate

trimetaphosphate

long chains of polyphosphates of the 'Graham Salts' type. The metaphosphates that are often determined analytically are probably degradation artefacts.

These 'volutin granules' function as reserve phosphates and enable the cells to carry out some cell division even under conditions of relative phosphate starvation. The 'energy content' of the polyphosphates seems to be of minor importance.

Sulphur.   Many of the sulphide-oxidising bacteria show transient accumulations of elementary sulphur in the shape of highly refractive spheres. Such intracellularly stored, as well as excretory, sulphur is initially present in liquid form and is only slowly converted to the orthorhombic form.

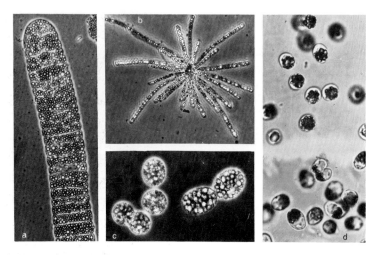

Fig. 2.46. *Colourless, hydrogen sulphide-oxidising bacteria.*

(a) *Beggiatoa gigantea* with sulphur inclusions. Bright-field illumination, × 300. (b) Rosette of *Thiothrix*. Phase contrast, × 300. (c) *Achromatium oxaliferum* with inclusions of calcium carbonate and sulphur, × 200. (d) *Thiovulum* with inclusions of sulphur, × 1000. (Pictures: (a, c) K. Schmidt; (b) D. Claus; (d) J. W. W. LaRiviere and H. Schuur.)

The extent of sulphur storage depends on the hydrogen sulphide content of the medium; in the absence of hydrogen sulphide, elementary sulphur is oxidised to sulphate. Sulphur can serve as an energy source for aerobic hydrogen sulphide-oxidising bacteria (*Beggiatoa*, *Thiothrix*, *Achromatium*, *Thiovulum*: Fig. 2.46), whilst it functions as an electron donor in anaerobic phototrophic purple sulphur bacteria (*Chromatium*). The sulphur inclusions occasionally found in cyanobacteria and *Sphaerotilus natans* can be regarded as detoxification products of the hydrogen sulphide often present in the habitats of these organisms.

Other cellular inclusions.   In *Bacillus thuringiensis* and related species (*B. laterosporus*, *B. medusa*), crystalline inclusion bodies have been observed next to spores (Fig. 3.9). These parasporal crystals consist of a protein toxin. The protein is dissolved by the intestinal juices of sensitive insects (the caterpillar stage of butterflies), and the liberated toxin destroys the intestinal epithelium and leads to the death of the caterpillar. The highly selective toxicity of bacillary preparations against a few groups of insects has led to their successful application as a biological pesticide.

Gas vacuoles.   Many aquatic bacteria, especially phototrophs but also non-pigmented species (*Pelonema, Peloploca*) and halobacteria (*Halobacterium halobium*) and a few clostridia contain gas vacuoles. These enable the cells to alter their specific mass and to float in water. The ability to float by virtue of intracellular gas vacuoles enables some bacteria to remain in a fixed stratum of water where growth conditions are optimal even though they lack the capacity for active movement by means of flagella. Anoxygenic phototrophs, including the red bacteria (*Lamprocystis, Amoebobacter, Thiodictyon*) and green bacteria (*Pelodictyon*) grow in the anaerobic zone (hypolimnion) just below the thermocline (Fig. 17.2). This buoyancy seems just adequate to keep the organisms in the cold (heavy) water layer of the hypolimnion but does not enable them to rise into the warmer lighter layer above. The oxygenic phototrophs, cyanobacteria (*Oscillatoria agardhi, Aphanizomenon flos-aquae, Microcystis aeruginosa*), flourish above the thermocline. The floating behaviour of these organisms seems to be regulated via photosynthesis, cellular turgor, and the number and size of gas vesicles.

Each gas vacuole consists of several or many vesicles which are spindle-shaped. Their walls do not have the usual membrane structure but consist of pure proteins in a leaflet arrangement. The walls are only 2 nm thick. In electron micrographs one can recognise an arrangement of ribs like the hoops around a barrel. The protein of the walls consists of subunits with a relative molecular mass of 14×10^3. Apparently, the proteins are arranged so that a hydrophobic surface is on the inside of the vesicle and a hydrophilic surface is on the outside. The intracellular gas vesicles are arranged in parallel, and in the light microscope the resulting vacuoles appear as highly refractive, optically empty spaces.

Carboxysomes.   Some autotrophic bacteria contain carboxysomes. These are polyhedrical bodies that are about the size of bacteriophages and contain, apart from a little DNA, the enzyme ribulose bisphosphate carboxylase. Carboxysomes have been found in *Nitrosomonas, Thiobacillus*, and in many cyanobacteria.

Cyanophycin granules.   Stores of bound nitrogen are found among the prokaryotes only in cyanobacteria. These contain cyanophycin granules which consist of a specific polypeptide (Ch. 3.2.1).

2.2.8   Endospores and other persistent (survival) forms

Only a small group of bacteria is capable of producing endospores. The importance of spores is largely due to their heat resistance. Whilst almost all other bacteria, as well as the vegetative cells of spore formers, are killed by heating to 80°C for 10 minutes (pasteurisation), the heat-resistance endospores can survive far greater thermal exposures; some spores are resistance to boiling water for several hours.

Expensive, labour-intensive, sterile techniques are aimed at the destruction of endospores. On the other hand, the thermal resistance of spores can also be used for isolation of spore formers by enrichment culture. Soil samples or other inocula from various habitats are heated for 10 minutes at 80 or 100°C to kill off all vegetative cells; only the heat resistant spores remain viable. These can then be induced to germinate by incubation on suitable media.

Classification of endospore-forming bacteria. With one exception, all spore formers are rod-shaped, gram-positive bacteria. Most are motile by virtue of peritrichous flagellation. The members of the genus *Bacillus* are all strict or facultative aerobes. The anaerobic spore formers are found in the genera *Clostridium* and *Desulfotomaculum*. Clostridia are dependent on fermentation for their energy requirements; *Desulfotomaculum* can derive its energy from anaerobic respiration, using sulphate as an electron acceptor. *Sporolactobacillus* belongs to the lactic acid bacteria. *Sporosarcina* has spherical cells, but its physiological characteristics would place it in the genus *Bacillus*. Spore formers have a remarkably low GC content; indeed, clostridia with a GC content of 20–27% have the lowest GC content of all prokaryotes.

Recognition of endospores. Spores are easily recognised by a microscopist because of their high refractivity, which corresponds to that of dehydrated proteins and indicates a high concentration of protein-rich material inside the spores. The spore contains almost the entire dry weight of the vegetative cell but occupies only about one tenth its volume. In doubtful cases, specific spore stains can be used to determine the presence of true endospores. When a heat-fixed bacterial smear is treated with boiling carbol fuchsin the spores absorb the stain and retain it after a washing with ethanol or 1 M acetic acid, which decolorises the rest of the cell.

Spore formation. Spores arise intracellularly, starting with the accumulation of protein-rich material, which increases the refractivity of the area. Numerous metabolic conversions occur at the expense of storage materials (poly-β-hydroxybutyrate in aerobes and polysaccharides in anaerobes). During the first 5 hours of sporulation much of the vegetative cell protein is degraded. A spore-specific substance not found in vegetative cells, dipicolinic acid (pyridine-2,6-dicarbonate), is formed. During the synthesis of dipicolinic acid, calcium ions are preferentially

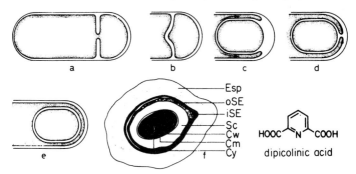

Fig. 2.47. *Spore formation and the structure of mature spores.*

(a,b) Septation of the spore protoplast; (c–e) formation of the forespore; (f) mature spore. Cy, cytoplasm with nuclear region; Cm, cytoplasmic membrane; Cw, cell wall of the vegetative cell; Sc, spore cortex; iSE, inner spore envelope; oSE, outer spore envelope; Esp, exosporium. (After W. G. Murrel.)

accumulated; in mature spores, dipicolinate apparently acts as a calcium chelate and can make up 10–15% of the spore dry weight. The dipicolinic acid is localised in the spore protoplast and is found only in endospores (Figs 2.47, 2.48).

Sporulation is one of the most complex processes of differentiation in bacteria. It starts with a **specific, unequal cell division** (Fig. 2.47). The cytoplasmic membrane divides off a portion of the cell protoplast. This (incipient) spore protoplast contains part of the nuclear material, namely, one genome. Contrary to normal cell division, the two protoplasts do not become separated by the cell wall; rather, the spore protoplast is gradually enveloped by the cytoplasmic membrane of the mother cell. As a result, the spore protoplast is eventually surrounded by two cytoplasmic membranes; both take part in the synthesis of the spore wall. The membrane of the spore protoplast forms the germination cell wall towards the outside; the membrane originating from the vegetative cytoplasmic membrane synthesises the spore cortex towards the inside. The cortex consists of a multilayered skeleton of peptidoglycan which differs from that of the vegetative cell in several respects, including the degree of cross-linking. The outer spore envelope is formed by the mother cell and consists mostly of polypeptides. In a few bacteria (e.g. *Bacillus cereus*), a further envelope, the exosporium, is formed by the mother cell. This remains as a loose, balloon-type envelope in the maturing spore. Because of these manifold layers, the envelope material can represent up to 50% of the volume or dry weight of the mature spore.

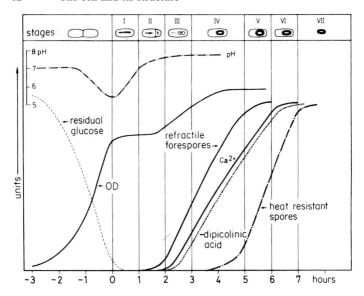

Fig. 2.48. *Microphological and physiological changes during spore forma-tion in aerobic spore-forming bacteria.*

The processes are initiated by the exhaustion of glucose (zero time). Spore formation can be followed by the increase in calcium and dipicolinic acid content, the increase in numbers of heat-resistant spores, and the increase in refractivity. Morphologi-cal changes can be aligned with the biochemical processes. Stages I–VII are shown at the top.

Initiation of sporulation.   Spores are not an obligate part of the 'life cycle' in bacteria; under favourable nutritional conditions even spore-forming bacilli can continue to grow indefinitely by division of vegeta-tive cells. Spore formation is initiated only when nutrients are exhausted or unfavourable metabolic products accumulate. Specific conditions fa-vourable to spore formation are required; drying or dehydration does not bring it about. However, transfer of vegetative cells into distilled water leads to an 'endotrophic' sporulation, i.e. spore formation at the expense of intracellular storage materials. Sporulation is apparently ini-tiated by lack of an external substrate. This induction of spore forma-tion is manifested over the course of several hours. If, for example, vegetative cells of *B. cereus* var. *mycoides* are suspended in water, and glucose is added at any time during the subsequent 5 hours, no spore formation takes place; apparently the added substrate can reverse the initiation of sporulation. Addition of glucose more than 6 hours after suspension in water is no longer (completely) effective in this repression; the induction (or derepression) of sporulation persists and between the tenth and thirteenth hour after transfer to water, about 90% of the cells have sporulated. It appears, therefore, that spore formation is regulated by environmental factors. The yield of sporulating cells can often be increased by the addition of manganese salts to the medium.

The capacity to form endospores can be lost gradually by repeated subculturing of vegetative cells (under non-sporulating conditions). Since suspensions of sporogenous organisms contain vegetative cells as well as spores (under appropriate conditions), they are usually briefly exposed to boiling water temperatures before subculturing. This treatment helps to maintain or even increases the capacity of the culture to form endospores.

Properties of mature spores.   Spores are liberated upon autolysis of the vegetative cell. The mature spores have no demonstrable metabolic activity and exhibit a high degree of resistance to heat, radiation, and chemicals. Their heat resistance is due to the low water content of spores. *Bacillus megaterium* spores, for example, have a water content of 15%, similar to that of wool or dry casein. Lyophilised vegetative bacteria are also very heat resistant. In addition, the heat resistance of spores appears to be proportional to their dipicolinic acid content. The radiation resistance of spores is also greater than that of vegetative cells, and it is approximately proportional to the number of disulphide bridges present in the outer protein layers. The spore envelope mainly contains a cysteine-rich protein which resembles keratin. The chemical resistance of spores is due to the impermeability of the spore envelope to many chemicals.

Spore germination.   In suitable nutrient media, most spores can be induced to germinate. However, certain pretreatments, such as storage and brief exposure to high temperature, can increase the percentage of germination of a spore population. For *Bacillus subtilis* spores, for instance, a 'rest period' of 7 days and heating for 5 minutes at 60 °C are regarded as optimal conditions for germination. Other spores can be 'activated' by exposing to boiling water temperature (100 °C) for 10 minutes. This heat-shock treatment must be carried out immediately before placing the spores on germination medium, since the activation process(es) appear to be reversible. Germination of spores is preceded by water uptake and swelling of the spores. In some cases it is dependent on the presence of glucose, amino acids, nucleosides, or other substances. During germination, fundamental physiological alterations take place: respiration and enzymatic activities increase rapidly; amino acids, dipicolinic acid, and peptides are excreted; and about 25–30% of the dry

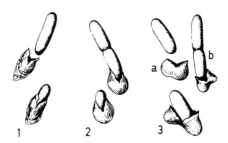

Fig. 2.49. *Germinating spores.*

(1) Polar germination of a *Clos-tridium* spore with its exosporium; (2) polar germination of a *Bacillus megaterium* spore, the spore coat remaining attached; (3) lateral germination of *Bacillus* spores; (a) *B. cereus*; (b) *B. subtilis*.

weight of the spore is lost. The heat resistance of the spores is also lost during germination.

A germination tube is extruded from the spore either polarly or later-ally and appears to be surrounded by a very thin and perhaps incom-plete cell wall, the cell envelope being torn or perforated by the extrusion of the tube (Fig. 2.49). During this stage, therefore, the uptake of DNA by the protoplast is facilitated (see Transformation, Ch. 15.2.2).

Survival of spores.   The formation of spores enables bacteria to survive in a latent state for a long time. A few viable spores of *Bacillus subtilis* and *B. licheniformis* were found in the soil attached to plants that had been stored under dry conditions at the Kew Gardens Herbarium for 200–300 years. Viable spores of *Bacillus coagulans* and *B. circulans* were also present in samples 50–100 years old. Extrapolation from these ob-servations suggests that during storage of a dry soil sample, about 90% of spores will lose viability within 50 years. This means, however, that in a tonne of dry soil some viable spores would be present after 1000 years!

> The viability of many, if not most, bacteria can be maintained for years in a dry state. **Maintenance of bacteria** in collections, for example, is achieved by drying vegetative cells from the frozen state (lyophilisation) and stor-ing them at room temperature, or at lower temperatures under vacuum. As Becquerel calculated, microorganisms could retain viability for mil-lions of years at temperatures of absolute zero. Extrapolation from short-term experiments using the temperature of liquid nitrogen seems to con-firm this prediction. Bacteria that are sensitive to lyophilisation can be stored for several years at the temperature of liquid nitrogen.

Other persistent forms: cysts, exospores, myxospores.   Of all the persistent forms produced by bacteria, endospores show the greatest resistance to heat, drying, radiation, and chemicals. A few bacteria, however, produce other kinds of persistent forms: cysts and exospores. The formation of exospores has only been observed in the methane-utilising bacterium *Methylosinus trichosporium.* These exospores are formed by the budding of the vegetative cell, and they have the same properties as *Bacillus* endospores. Some bacteria form spherical, thick-walled cells that are called cysts. This formation of cysts occurs when nutrients are exhausted. The whole rod-shaped vegetative cell is transformed into a cyst, rather than only a portion of the vegetative cell as in the formation of endospores. The cysts of *Azotobacter* and *Methylocystis* species are resistant to drying, mechanical stress, and radiation, but not to heat. A similar transformation occurs in the production of myxospores from the rod-shaped vegetative cells of the genera *Myxococcus* and *Sporocytophaga.*

The cells of the genus *Arthrobacter* (*A. globigormis*) are pleomorphic. When plenty of substrate is available, they grow as rods; when the substrate is exhausted, the cells become coccoid. *Arthrobacter* belongs to those bacteria that can survive dehydration for a time, in dried soil for instance. No structural differentiation is known, however.

2.2.9   Pigments of bacteria and fungi

Many bacterial and fungal colonies show distinct colorations because their cells are pigmented or because they secrete pigments into the medium. The ability to synthesis pigments is determined genetically and is thus a diagnostic character. Coloured organisms are easy to recognise and identify. Many of the pigments are derivatives of certain groups of chemicals such as carotenoids, phenazine or pyrollic dyes, azaquinones, and anthocyanates (Fig. 2.50).

Protection against light and UV irradiation.   When petri dishes containing complex nutrients are exposed to dusty air (so-called air plates) coloured colonies often arise. The colonies predominantly have yellow, orange, or reddish pigmentation based on **carotenoids.** In these colonies the bacteria are mostly members of the genera *Micrococcus*, *Corynebacterium*, *Myocobacterium* and *Nocardia*, and the yeast *Rhodotorula*. Pigmented forms are common among airborne inocula because the pigments protect against the rays of the visible and near-UV light ranges. Thus, on straw and dust and in other locations that are exposed to light, the ability to form such pigments confers a selective advantage over non-pigmented forms, which are more easily inactivated by light. This

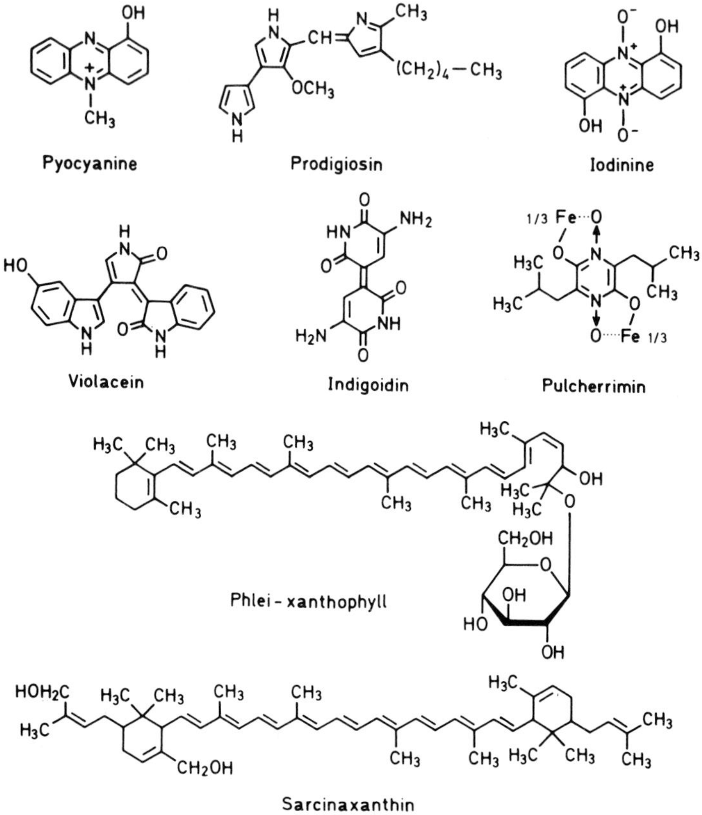

Pyocyanine   Prodigiosin   Iodinine

Violacein   Indigoidin   Pulcherrimin

Phlei - xanthophyll

Sarcinaxanthin

Fig. 2.50. *Some of the pigments produced by bacteria and yeasts.*

Pyocyanine is excreted by *Pseudomonas aeruginosa* and iodinine is excreted by *Chromobacterium iodinum.* Indigoidin is produced by several bacteria including *Pseudomonas indigofera*. Prodigiosin is the pigment of *Serratia marcescens* (formerly *Bacterium prodigiosum*). Violacein is formed by *Chromobacterium violaceum.* Pulcherrimin is the pigment of the yeast *Candida pulcherrima*. Phleixanthophyll is the main carotenoid of *Mycobacterium phlei* and is present as a glycoside. Sarcinaxanthin is the main carotenoid of yellow *Sarcina* species (including *Micrococcus luteus,* formerly called *Sarcina hitea*).

protection against photodynamic damage was demonstrated in a study of a normally orange-coloured, carotenoid-containing strain of a halophilic bacterium and its colourless mutant. Whilst both grew equally well under weak illumination, growth of the colourless mutant was greatly inhibited on exposure to bright sunlight, which did not affect the growth of the pigmented variant. The bactericidal effect of visible light occurred under aerobic conditions, i.e. in the presence of oxygen, and thus was apparently due to **photo-oxidation.** In photo-oxidation. several cellular pigments (flavins, cytochromes) apparently act as catalysts (photosensitisers); the carotenoids, localised in the cytoplasmic membrane, protect the sensitive regions of the cell from the effects of photo-oxidation.

> **Photosensitisation.**   The normal sensitivity to oxygen in visible light can be increased by treating bacteria with various vital stains, such as methylene blue, eosin, or acridine orange. The treated organisms are more rapidly inactivated by visible light than untreated controls. The dye molecules can absorb light and transfer its energy to an oxygen molecule, which is then converted from its normal ground state (triplet oxygen) to an excited state singlet oxygen. The singlet oxygen radical can cause oxidative reactions that do not occur in the case of the normal O_2 (namely cyclo-additions, en-reactions). Such photo-sensitisation is used to inactivate possibly pathogenic bacteria in zoological gardens, fur farms, etc. by adding methylene blue or other dyes to the drinking water. The photosensitised bacteria are then 'killed' by exposure to normal daylight.

Synthesis of carotenoids.   Red carotenoids (with 12 to 13 double bonds and methoxy and oxo groups) are responsible for the deep red coloration of the purple bacteria. In these bacteria, the carotenoids not only function as protective agents but they also absorb light for photosynthetic reactions and take part in the perception of light involved in phototaxis. Together with bacteriochlorophylls, the carotenoids are localised in the photosynthetically active membranes (thylakoids, chromatophores).

In many bacteria the synthesis of these pigments is light-dependent, as is the formation of photosynthetically active pigments in higher plants. Thus mycobacteria, including the pathogenic tubercle bacillus (*Mycobacterium tuberculosis*), produce carotenoids only when exposed to light. The same is true of many bacteria that commonly grow on bacon and cheese. In some cases, pigmentation can also depend on the composition of the medium and the temperature.

Pulcherrimin.   Whilst the coloration of many red yeasts (*Rhodotorula, Sporobolomyces salmonicolor*) is predominantly due to carotenoids, *Candida pulcherrima* produces the pigment pulcherrimin, which belongs to another class of compounds. *Candida pulcherrima* can be isolated, together with *Candida reukaufii*, from nectar-containing flowers, certain fruits, and the gut of bees. On iron-containing media, this species forms deep red colonies containing a red pyrazine pigment that is insoluble in water and organic solvents and contains complexed iron.

Prodigiosin.   *Serratia marcescens*, formerly known as *Bacterium prodigiosum*, is commonly encountered on carbohydrate-rich media. The deep red coloration of its colonies and suspensions is due to the presence of prodigiosin, a pigment whose basic skeleton contains three pyrrole rings. This pigment also occurs in actinomycetes.

Indigoidin.   This pigment belongs to the class of compounds called azaquinones (diazo-diphenoquinones). It is a blue, water-insoluble dye which is secreted into the medium by a number of bacteria (*Pseudomonas indigofera*, *Corrynebacterium indigiosum*, *Arthrobacter atrocyaneus*, *Arthrobacter polychromogenes*).

Violacein.   *Chromobacterium violaceum* can be isolated readily from soil by placing some grains of rice on wet soil. The colonies are easily recognised by their violet-blue coloration, which is caused by the water-insoluble purple pigment violacein. Violacein is an indole derivative produced via oxidation of tryptophan.

Phenazine dyes.   Many of the pigments excreted by aquatic bacteria are phenazines. The best known of these is pyocyanine, produced by *Pseudomonas aeruginosa* (formerly called *P. pyrocyanea*). Various pseudomonad strains also excrete, singly or together, phenazine-l-carbonic acid, oxychloraphin and iodinine.

Yellow-green fluorescing pigments.   The yellow-green pigments of fluorescent pseudomonads, which show marked fluorescence under UV light or neon tubes, functions as **siderophores.** They are formed and excreted into the medium when this is deficient in iron. They are used to bind and transport iron into the cell (Chapter 7). The yellow-green fluorescing siderophores of *Pseudomonas putida* and *P. aeruginosa* are characterised as pyoverdins (= pseudobactins). They are chromopeptides consisting of a peptide chain made of 6–10 amino acids and a chromophore which is a diamino-dihydroxyquinoline.

Secondary metabolites.   The microbial pigments are secondary metabolites (Ch. 10.4), that is, they are compounds not found in all organisms. It is clear from their structure that they are not derived from the normal building blocks and metabolites of cells. Some pigments are antibiotically active and many microorganisms that produce pigments also produce antibiotics or other active compounds.

3   The grouping of prokaryotes

3.1   Introduction

The groups of schizomycetes (bacteria in the wider sense, formerly called Schizophyta) and **Schizophycetes** (cyanobacteria) are classified together as the prokaryotes. As discussed in Chapter 2, **prokaryotes** all share important characteristics such as cell walls containing murein, nuclear regions without membrane and lack of cellular compartmentation. Their description and naming follows the **Bacteriologic Code**. This has been established by the International Committee of Systematic Bacteriology, which also supervised adherence to the code. The Bacteriologic Code is distinguished from the Botanical Code mainly by the rule that for each newly described strain a viable culture must be deposited with a recognised collection of type cultures to serve as a reference or type culture.

Description of bacteria.   Description of bacteria should contain their **morphological characters**, i.e. whether they are rod-shaped, coccoid or spirillar, whether capsules are present, whether they occur singly or in associations (chains, tetrads or packets), whether they are flagellated and the location of the flagella, whether they produce spores, and what their reaction is to the Gram stain. These descriptions are complemented by enumeration of physiological and biochemical characters: (1) whether the cells can grow under aerobic, anaerobic or both conditions; (2) whether energy is derived via respiration, fermentation or photosynthesis; (3) utilisable nutrients; (4) temperature and pH dependence of growth, with optima and tolerance limits; (5) habitat; (6) symbiotic or parasitic relationships with other organisms; (7) cell inclusions, pigmentation, and capsular materials; (8) composition of cell wall components (peptidoglycan skeleton, lipopolysaccharides, teichoic acids); (9) serological properties (surface antigens, homologous proteins); (10) base composition of DNA (GC content); (11) DNA–DNA hybridisation, transformability by interspecies transfer; (12) sequence of 16S or 5S rRNA; (13) antibiotic sensitivities.

Nomenclature.   The **binary system of nomenclature** used in the classification of plants and animals is also applied to prokaryotes; that is, they are identified by a generic and a specific name. The original custom of basing the generic name on morphological characteristics and the specific name on physiological characters has not been adhered to during periods of very rapid accumulation of newly discovered organisms. Beijerinck and Winogradsky, overwhelmed by the large number of metabolic types, used generic names based on ecological, physiological, and biochemical features. There are, therefore, genera that are named according to physiological properties (*Acetobacter, Nitrosomonas, Azotobacter*), pigmentation (*Chromobacterium, Rhodomicrobium*), pathogenic properties (*Pneumococcus, Phytomonas*), and specific nutrients (*Haemophilus, Amylobacter*). According to the rules of nomenclature, once names have been assigned to reliably identified new organisms, they are adhered to. The assignment and use of names is governed by definite rules.

Classification.   The classification of prokaryotic microorganisms is based mainly on practical considerations and is aimed at recognition and identification of the types that have been described. Classification means the ordering of groups into higher units. This is done in several stages. The basic unit, i.e. the pure culture of an isolated bacterium, is the strain. Strains are collected into species, and species are collected into genera (plural of genus). These are collected into families, which have names ending in -aceae. Such classification requires adequate description of strains and proceeds by comparing the properties of various groups. The creation of classification systems is the subject of **taxonomy**.

Two kinds of classification can be distinguished: **phylogenetic** (or natural) and artificial (or pragmatic). It is the overall aim of bacterial taxonomy to group related forms, i.e. those possessing common ancestors, together in a phylogenetic system. Eventually this goal will be reached on the basis of biochemical properties, such as amino acid sequences of functionally identical enzymes, or base sequences of nucleic acids in conserved cell components, such as ribosomal RNA.

Artificial classification.   A pragmatic, artificial classification of bacteria is less demanding than a phylogenetic system. It aims to group organisms according to their similarities so that they **can be recognised and identified**. Such a system is designed for use as a **determinative key**. The most complete work of descriptive bacteriology is *Bergey's Manual of Determinative Bacteriology* (1974), which contains names, descriptions of morphological and physiological properties with literature citations, and determinative keys for classification of new isolates. A new edition of *Bergey's Manual* is in preparation.

Numerical taxonomy. Numerical taxonomy aims at a more objective system of classification. This started originally with the adoption of the Adamson principle that all properties used for classification should be given equal weight. As many diagnostic characters as possible are used for numerical analysis, and these are formulated as yes or no alternatives (given + and – signs). Multiple correlations are worked out by computer; every diagnostic character of each strain is compared with every diagnostic character of all other strains. The degree of relatedness between strains is a function of the number of similar characters in proportion to the total number of characters examined. The similarities between pairs of strains is then expressed by a similarity **coefficient** (S value), which is defined as:

$$S = \frac{a+d}{a+b+c+d}$$

where a and d are the sums of the characters which are common to strains A and B (a, both positive, d, both negative), b is the sum of the characters in which A is positive and B is negative, and c is the sum of the characters in which A is negative and B is positive. The calculations yield values between 1 and 0; $S = 1$ means 100% similarity, i.e. identity, and $S < 0.02$ means complete unrelatedness. The values are entered on a similarity matrix, or they can be expressed as a dendogram (similar to a phylogenetic tree). Numerical taxonomy, however, is not related to phylogeny.

Bacterial phylogeny. The analysis and comparisons of highly conserved phylogenetic markers enabled C. Woese to develop a **phylogenetic tree of the prokaryotes**. The ribosomes, as the sites of protein synthesis, are present in all cells. Functionally they must be very conservative. This is also and especially true of ribosomal RNA (rRNA) because its base sequence is not affected by the degeneracy of the genetic code, nor by suppressor mutations. rRNA, therefore, provides the properties appropriate to a general phylogenetic marker.

The **16S rRNA** from the 30S ribosomes of all the organisms that are to be compared has now been isolated. For analysis the RNA is divided into large pieces (oligonucleotides) by use of specific restriction enzymes. The oligonucleotides are separated by electrophoresis and their base sequences determined. A catalogue of the characteristic base sequences for individual organisms can then be subjected to comparative analysis with the assistance of appropriate computer programmes. This yields, on the one hand, highly conserved sequences, which are largely the same in all bacteria, but differ significantly from those of the eukaryotes and those of other large groups of bacteria. On the other hand, differences

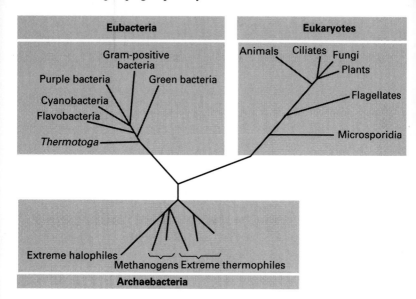

Fig. 3.1. *Phylogenetic tree without roots, derived from the base sequences of ribosomal RNA.*

for some oligonucleotide sequences are found even within genera and species. Certain 'signature' sequences have been identified which seem to be characteristic for groups of organisms.

These analyses have produced dendograms which can be considered as parts of a phylogenetic tree. They have revealed hitherto unrecognised relationships. One of the most exciting results from such 16S rRNA sequence analyses was the discovery that there was a much higher sequence homology between two such morphologically and physiologically distinct bacteria as *Escherichia coli* and a *Cyanobacterium*, than between *E. coli* and a morphologically very similar *Methanobacterium*. This led to the recognition of Methanobacteria as belonging to a large group of fundamentally very different prokaryotes. It has to be assumed that the prokaryotes split very early into two large groups, the so-called **Archaebacteria** (to which the Methanobacteria belong) and the other prokaryotes designated as **Eubacteria**. It is envisaged that the very early cells – the progenotes – gave rise to the Archaebacteria and Eubacteria. The third group that arose were the Eukaryotes. Their precursors must also have developed from the common root (Fig. 3.1).

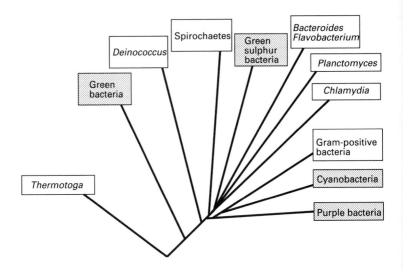

Fig. 3.2. *Phylogenetic tree of Eubacteria, derived from the base sequences of 16S RNA.*

Comparison of the representative Eubacteria leads to the recognition of 11 large groups (Fig. 3.2). One of these is the group of **anoxygenic phototrophic purple bacteria**. Further detailed comparisons of the members of this group of gram-negative bacteria with numerous **chemotrophic** gram-negative bacteria led to another surprising result: the purple bacteria can be divided into four groups which have been designated as **alpha, beta, gamma and delta purple bacteria**. Each of these groups – except the delta purple bacteria – contains a few well-known representatives of the purple bacteria as well as a large number of heterotrophic or **chemolithoautotrophic non-photosynthetic** bacteria (Fig. 3.3). Phylogenetically, this suggests that at least four groups of purple bacteria developed during the course of evolution. The heterotrophic respiratory or fermentative bacteria, as well as the chemolithoautotrophs and other bacteria with anaerobic respiratory systems, must then have developed from the representatives of these four branches by loss of the photosynthetic apparatus and metabolic specialisation. These non-photosynthetic bacteria, which are phylogenetically related to the purple bacteria, are collectively known as **Proteobacteria**. This leads to the general hypothesis that the majority of the soil and water bacteria, as well as many pathogenic organisms, are derived from the purple bacteria.

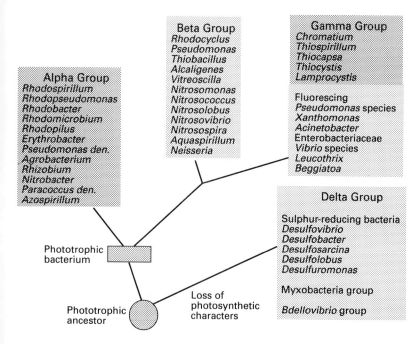

Fig. 3.3. *Phylogenetic tree of the purple bacteria and closely related gram-negative bacteria.*

Dark grey, phototrophic bacteria; light grey, non-phototrophic bacteria.

It can be readily appreciated that the taxonomic system, which is based mainly on phenotypic characters – shape, flagellation, gram-staining behaviour, etc., is very different from the phylogenetic system. Only a few groups which have been classified in families or higher units by classical taxonomic criteria appear to be phylogenetically related. This is the case, for example, in the sulphate-reducing bacteria of the delta group and in the case of the Enterobacteriaceae. In contrast, members of the pseudomonads are found in alpha, beta and gamma groups (of the phylogenetic branches) of the purple bacteria. It seems, therefore, that the cell type of *Pseudomonas* must be the result of convergent development.

A phylogenetically based classification system, however, does not replace the system based on the traditional taxonomy, or make it superfluous. The latter still has an important role in the **identification**, and in *de novo* **descriptions** of bacteria. The phylogenetic system, though, conveys a wealth of heuristic principles for evolutionary studies as well as for applied microbiology.

Survey of the diversity of prokaryotes.   The following aims to give an idea of the diversity of the prokaryotes. The treatment is similar to that in *Bergey's Manual of Determinative Bacteriology* (8th edition, 1974) and *Bergey's Manual of Systematic Bacteriology* (four volumes, 1954–89). Many recent discoveries make it highly probable that a number of modifications and additions will need to be introduced. The microscopic characters of the bacteria, however, remain unchanged, and the relationship of bacteria to oxygen and Gram staining properties are also relatively easy to determine. In the following list, the eubacteria are grouped according to their (1) shape, as cocci, rods, or curved rods (spirilla); (2) ability to grow aerobically or anaerobically; and (3) Gram staining reaction. Those bacteria that cannot be assigned easily to the three basic categories are listed here as 'Large Special Groups'.

Sections 3.3–3.21 of this chapter describe the groups of bacteria in the sequence in which they appear in the list. Some groups are mentioned only briefly in this chapter and the reader is referred to the chapters in which these bacteria are described with emphasis on their physiological and biochemical properties. The groups of bacteria described in detail in this chapter are not discussed in later chapters.

This overview of the prokaryotes does give some indications for the identification of bacteria. Every biologist has probably had the experience that a given determinative key allows him to identify only those organisms that are known to him. Identification of a bacterium presupposes some background knowledge; when the identification procedure yields *Methanobacterium* for a rod-shaped organism isolated from yoghurt, scepticism is justified.

3.2   Prokaryotic groups

The following survey of the prokaryotic system is arranged according to microscopic shape (cocci, rods, spirilla), Gram staining, and relationship to oxygen (aerobic or anaerobic).

1. Cocci (spherical bacteria)

A. Gram-positive cocci

AEROBES   *Micrococcus, Staphylococcus, Streptococcus, Leuconostoc, Pediococcus*

ANAEROBES *Peptococcus, Peptostreptococcus, Ruminococcus, Sarcina*

B. Gram-negative cocci

AEROBES   *Neisseria, Moraxella, Acinetobacter, Paracoccus, Lampropedia*

ANAEROBES *Veillonella, Acidaminococcus, Megasphaera*

2. Rods (straight, cylindrical bacteria)

A. Gram-positive bacteria

Gram-positive, non-spore-forming rods

AEROBES   *Lactobacillus, Listeria, Erysipelothrix, Caryophanon*

Coryneform bacteria and actinomycetes

AEROBES   *Corynebacterium, Arthrobacter, Brevibacterium, Cellulomonas, Propionibacterium, Eubacterium Bifidobacterium, Mycobacterium, Nocardia Actinomyces, Frankia, Actinoplanes, Dermatophilus, Micromonospora, Microbispora, Streptomyces, Streptosporangium*

Endospore-forming rods and cocci

AEROBES   *Bacillus, Sporolactobacillus, Sporosarcina, Thermoactinomyces*

ANAEROBES *Clostridium, Desulfotomaculum, Oscillospira*

B. Gram-negative bacteria

Gram-negative aerobic rods and cocci

AEROBES   *Pseudomonas, Xanthomonas, Zoogloea, Gluconobacter, Acetobacter Azotobacter, Azomonas, Beijerinckia, Derxia Rhizobium, Agrobacterium, Alcaligenes Brucella, Legionella, Thermus*

Gram-negative, aerobic, chemolithotrophic bacteria

AEROBES   *Nitrobacter, Nitrospina, Nitrococcus, Nitrosomonas, Nitrosospira, Nitrosococcus, Nitrosolobus Thiobacillus, Thiobacterium, Thiovulum*

Sheathed bacteria

AEROBES   *Sphaerotilus, Leptothrix, Streptothrix, Crenothrix*

Gram-negative, facultatively anaerobic rods

FACULTATIVE ANAEROBES   *Escherichia, Klebsiella, Enterobacter,*
Salmonella, Shigella, Proteus, Serratia, Erwinia
Yersinia
Vibrio, Aeromonas, Photobacterium

Gram-negative anaerobic bacteria

STRICT ANAEROBES   *Bacteroides, Fusobacterium, Leptotrichia,*
Fibrobacter

Archaebacteria

STRICT ANAEROBES   *Methanobacterium, Methanothermus,*
Methanosarcina, Methanothrix, Methanococcus
AEROBES   *Halobacterium, Haloferax, Halococcus*
Sulfolobus, Thermoplasma
ANAEROBES   *Thermoproteus, Pyrodictium, Desulfurococcus*
Pyrococcus, Thermococcus, Thermodiscus

3. Curved rods and flexible cells

Gram-negative spirillar and curved bacteria

AEROBES   *Spirillum, Aquaspirillum, Azospirillum, Oceanospirillum,*
Campylobacter, Helicobacter
Bdellovibrio, Microcyclus, Pelosigma

Gram-negative curved, anaerobic bacteria

ANAEROBES   *Desulfovibrio, Succinivibrio, Butyrivibrio, Selenomonas*

Spirochaetes

AEROBES AND ANAEROBES   *Spirochaeta, Cristispira, Treponema,*
Borrelia, Leptospira

4. Large special groups

Gliding bacteria (always gram-negative)

Myxococcus, Archangium, Cystobacter, Melittangium,
Stigmatella, Polyangium, Nannocystis, Chondromyces,
Cytophaga, Sporocytophaga, Flexibacter, Herpetosiphon,
Saprospira
Beggiatoa, Thiothrix, Thioploca, Achromatium, Leucothrix,
Vitreoscilla
Simonsiella, Alysiella

Bacteria with appendices, prosthecate bacteria, and budding bacteria

Hyphomicrobium, Hyphomonas
Caulobacter, Asticcacaulis, Planctomyces
Ancalomicrobium, Prosthecomicrobium, Blastobacter,
Seliberia, Gallionella, Nevskia

Obligate parasitic bacteria: rickettsiae and chlamydiae

Rickettisa, Coxiella, Chlamydia

Mycoplasma group (Mollicutes)

Mycoplasma, Acholeplasma, Spiroplasma, Metallogenium

Anaerobic, anoxygenic phototrophic bacteria

Rhodospirillum, Rhodopseudomonas, Rhodobacter,
Rhodomicrobium, Rhodocyclus, Rhodopilus
Chromatium, Thiocystis, Thiosarcina, Thiocapsa,
Thiospirillum, Thiopedia, Amoebobacter,
Ectothiorhodospira, Lamprocystis, Thiodictyon
Chlorobium, Prosthecochloris, Pelodictyon, Chloroherpeton,
Chloroflexus, Chloronema, Oscillochloris

Aerobic, oxygenic phototrophic bacteria: Cyanobacteria

Synechococcus, Gloeocapsa, Gloeothece, Gloeobacter
Pleurocapsa, Dermocarpa, Myxosarcina
Oscillatoria, Spirulina, Lyngbya, Phormidium, Plectonema
Anabaena, Nostoc, Calothrix, Fischerella

3.3   Gram-positive cocci

In the wider sense, gram-positive cocci include coccoid forms of lactic acid bacteria, such as *Streptococcus, Leuconostoc* and *Pediococcus* (see Table 8.2). These bacteria depend on fermentation reactions for their energy, are microaerotolerant, and most contain no haem pigments. Apart from these, there are the aerobic and facultatively anaerobic genera *Micrococcus* and *Staphylococcus*, and the obligately anaerobic genera *Sarcina, Peptococcus* and *Ruminococcus*. The genus *Micrococcus* contains those pigmented organisms whose yellow and orange colonies are often found on 'air plates' (Ch. 2.2). These were formerly assigned to the genus *Sarcina* because they form packets of cells or tetrads; the bacteria once known as *Sarcina lutea, S. flava, S. aurantiaca*, etc. are now classified together as *Micrococcus luteus*. This species also includes the organism that was named *Micrococcus lysodeikticus* by A. Fleming because of its high lysozyme sensitivity. *Micrococcus* species are obligately aerobic and characterised by a high GC content (66–72%).

The name of the genus *Staphylococcus* is based on the appearance of its cells under the microscope. The cells appear to be arranged in a grape-like cluster (Greek *staphyle*, grape), which results from an irregular pattern of cell division in different planes (Fig. 2.6). *Staphylococcus* is facultatively anaerobic, forms cytochromes only under aerobic conditions, and is relatively resistant to dehydration. *S. aureus* is pathogenic, producing toxins and exoenzymes, and is a pus former. Other strains cause food poisoning by excreting enterotoxins during their growth on non-refrigerated food.

Sarcina ventriculi (Ch. 2.2.5, Fig. 2.34) is a microaerotolerant, anaerobic organism which can be isolated easily from soil, but it is also found in the stomach contents of patients with gastric disease. It is unusual in its large size (diameter of 4 μm), in its formation of large cell clusters (more than 64 cells may be held together by cellulose), in its pH tolerance (it can grow in pH 0.9–9.8), and in its ability to produce endospores.

3.4   Gram-negative cocci

This group contains some cocci and very short rods that are gram-negative and non-motile. Included among these are aerobes and anaerobes, pathogens, soil bacteria, and some that inhabit the intestinal tract and mucous membranes of various mammals.

Aerobic cocci. The genus *Neisseria* is oxidase-positive and contains several animal and human pathogens. The species *N. gonorrhoeae* causes gonorrhoea, a venereal disease which had been almost eradicated in many countries because of the sensitivity of the organism to penicillin (even 1 μg penicillin is effective bacteriostatically). *N. gonorrhoeae* is difficult to cultivate in the laboratory; it needs aerobic conditions with 10% CO_2 and is extremely sensitive to light and dehydration, these being the reasons why infection is limited to direct intimate contact. *N. meningitidis* inhabits the nasopharyngeal tract but may penetrate into the vascular system and produce inflammation of the meninges. *Moraxella* is also oxidase-positive and very sensitive to penicillin. These are coccobacilli that are unable to utilise carbohydrates. *Acinetobacter* is an oxidase-negative soil and aquatic bacterium that is easily obtained and isolated by enrichment culture in a medium containing 0.2% acetate at pH 5.5–6.0. It does not normally utilise glucose, disaccharides, or polysaccharides, but it otherwise resembles the genus *Pseudomonas* with respect to its versatility in the utilisation of substrates. Within the species *A. calcoaceticus*, genetic markers can be exchanged by transformation. Since the bacterium is able to store a lot of polyphosphate it is hoped to use it for the removal of excess phosphates from effluents. The **oxidase reaction** that is used for differential diagnosis in this group is based on the formation of a coloured product from dimethyl-phenylene diamine (*N,N*-dimethyl-1,4-diaminobenzene) in the presence of cytochrome *c* (which is water-soluble); a few drops of the reagent are applied to agar colonies, and production of a red coloration is the diagnostic feature.

Anaerobic cocci. The best-known gram-negative anaerobic cocci are *Veillonella alcalescens* (formerly *Micrococcus lactilyticus*) and *Megasphaera* (formerly *Peptostreptococcus*) *elsdenii*. Both are unable to ferment carbohydrates. *V. alcalescens* is found in the saliva of humans and animals and in the rumen of ruminants. It ferments organic acids, especially lactate, to propionate, acetate, CO_2 and H_2 (Ch. 8.3). *M. elsdenii* ferments glutamic acid and other amino acids and is apparently a normal inhabitant of the intestinal tract of many animals.

3.5   Gram-positive, non-spore-forming rods

Gram-positive, non-sporing rods that can grow in the presence of oxygen and form mainly lactate by the fermentation of carbohydrates (glucose, lactose) are known collectively as 'lactic acid bacteria'. The genera *Lactobacillus, Lactococcus, Leuconostoc, Streptococcus, Pediococcus* and *Bifidobacterium* belong to these. The last is one of the few anaerobic lactic acid producers. The lactic acid bacteria are further discussed in Chapter 8.2. Here, we mention also a gram-positive aerobic rod, *Listeria monocytogenes*, which has recently been identified as a contaminant of soft cheeses that can cause listeriosis in consumers of such cheeses.

Gram-positive bacteria can be arranged in a sequence according to their cell shape and other morphological and physiological properties. The rod-shaped lactic acid bacteria are at the beginning of this sequence. Most of the lactic acid bacteria are regular rods and the tendency to form club-shaped rods and slightly branched cells is not strong. This tendency is the norm in the coryneform bacteria, which include the genera *Corynebacterium* and *Arthrobacter*. The tendency to cell branching is even more strongly expressed in the mycobacteria. These are followed by the proactinomycetes, which form transient mycelia, and the sequence is completed by the actinomycetes. Many members of the above groups can be recognised easily by their cell shape, colonial morphology, and physiological properties. Others can only be identified by various biochemical characters.

Caryophanon latum can be included here also. It is a trichome-form-

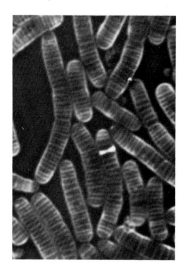

Fig. 3.4. Caryophanon latum, *a filament-forming, peritrichously flagellated bacterium.*
(Picture: M. P. Peshkoff.)

ing, flagellated bacterium that can be isolated regularly from cow dung. The gram-positive, filamentous rods are exceptionally large ($3 \times 15 \mu m$) (Fig. 3.4).

3.6   Coryneform bacteria

Corynebacterium.   The genus *Corynebacterium* (Greek *coryne*, club) was established in 1896 to comprise forms of the *Corynebacterium diphtheriae* type. Apart from their morphological variability, these organisms are characterised by a 'snapping apart' of the cells during cell division; the connecting walls on either side of the newly made cell wall appear to separate at different rates, so that the two cells seem to twist away in opposite directions. In addition, they undergo multiple fissions, so that one large cell may divide into several short rods. *C. diphtheriae* is the causative agent of diphtheria. It is, however, unrepresentative of the genus in its physiological properties, since it grows as a microaerophile or even as an anaerobe, whilst most corynebacteria are aerobic. Its pathogenicity is due to its invasion of the larynx and tonsils, and production of an exotoxin that circulates in the blood and attacks cells of the cardiac muscle, kidneys, and nerves, giving rise to post-diphtherial paralysis.

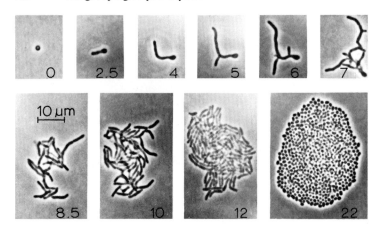

Fig. 3.5. *Development of a microcology of* Arthrobacter pyridinolis *on agar film.*

The numbers give the incubation times in hours. Phase-contrast micrograph. (From Kolenbrander, R. E., Lotong, N. & Ensign, J. C. (1976). *Arch. Microbiol.* **110**, 239.)

Only strains which have been lysogenised with phage produce the exotoxin. Thus toxin production is a consequence of a genetic alteration of the bacterium by the phage. This is known as **'phage conversion'**. In addition, the toxin is only produced if the supply of iron to the cells is sub-optimal.

The genus *Corynebacterium* also contains several other animal pathogens and many widely distributed plant pathogens (*C. michiganense, C. poinsettiae, C. fascians*). *C. mediolaneum* was the first bacterium used for biological conversion of steroids (1938).

Arthrobacter. Several coryneform bacteria that grow profusely in soil are comprised in this genus. *Arthrobacter* is characterised by a marked tendency of the cells to produce branched and coccoid forms. Some members are motile and flagellated and all are aerobic. *Arthrobacter* can be isolated easily from dry soils; together with bacilli, it can withstand several months of dry storage (in soil) whilst most non-spore-forming bacteria are killed under such conditions. *Arthrobacter* is pleomorphic, i.e. it assumes various shapes; in young colonies and liquid media it grows as irregularly shaped, long rods, whilst only coccoid forms are found in old cultures (Fig. 3.5). Another group of coryneform bacteria in soil consists of several cellulose-utilising species of the genus *Cellulomonas*.

Members of the genus *Arthrobacter* are found in various habitats, but they appear to be the quantitatively predominant representatives of the **autochthonous soil microflora**, that is, they are predominant in soils in which easily metabolisable substrates have been degraded and in which humus has remained as the major fraction of organic material. Under unfavourable conditions, *Arthrobacter* can grow slowly in its coccoid form. It can be assumed that the majority of the cocci found in soils by Winogradsky were cells of *Arthrobacter*. Other strains and species of the genus are found on plants and in the active sludge of sewage plants.

Other genera and species.   Many coryneform bacteria excrete glutamic acid and other amino acids into the medium (Ch. 10.2.2) and, because of this property, they have become important in industry. Other typical forms grow on soft cheeses; for example, *Brevibacterium linens*, which is mildly proteolytic, plays a role in the ripening of cheese. Fairly recently, the propionibacteria were also assigned to the coryneform bacteria group (Ch. 8.3).

As mentioned above, the coryneform bacteria can be regarded as an intermediate group between the lactic acid bacteria and the mycobacteria in morphological and physiological properties. The tendency for branched cell formation increases in the series propionibacteria, coryneform bacteria, mycobacteria. In this same series, there is a general transition from anaerobic to strictly aerobic metabolism. Despite many efforts, it has not yet been possible clearly to differentiate the genera belonging to the coryneform bacteria. Knowledge of GC content, murein composition, and other properties and the application of numerical taxonomy are needed for a new classification of this extremely important and ecologically differentiated group of microorganisms.

3.7   Mycobacteria

Mycobacteria are invariably aerobic. Morphologically they are intermediate between the corynebacteria and the proactinomycetes (Nocardia). They do not form mycelia but grow in the form of irregularly shaped, slightly branched cells. They are non-motile and gram-positive. One way in which they differ from corynebacteria is that they are **'acid fast'**. In 1882 Ehrlich noted that tubercle bacilli (*Mycobacterium tuberculosis*) could not be decolorised by acid treatment after staining with aniline dyes. According to the Ziehl–Neelsen method, fixed bacterial smears are heated with carbol fuchsin, rinsed, and then differentiated with HCl-alcohol. Mycobacteria and nocardia are not decolourised by this acid treatment and are designated **'acid fast'**. A few saprophytic mycobacteria can be decolorised with HCl-alcohol, but not with aqueous HCl. The resistance to acid is due to the high levels of **mycolic acid** in the cell wall, which make the cells of mycobacteria waxlike and strongly hydrophobic.

Corynebacterium, Mycobacterium, and *Nocardia* exhibit a number of similar features in their cell wall composition, as well as differences. Their murein skeleton resembles that of the gram-negative bacteria, but it is complexed with an arabinogalactan, a polysaccharide consisting of arabinose and galactose. This is bound to lipids, namely, mycolic acids. **Mycolic acids** are branched hydroxyacids (R^1–CHOH–CHR^2–COOH) carrying aliphatic chain substituents in positions 2 and 3. The aliphatic chains vary in length: in corynebacteria they have 32–36 carbon atoms, in nocardia, 45–58, and in the mycobacteria, 79–85. Only the long-chain aliphatic substituents render the cells acid fast.

Mycobacterium tuberculosis is the pathogen causing tuberculosis in man and was described by R. Koch in 1882. Infection of the lungs leads to formation of nodules (tubercles), tissue destruction and dissemination of the infective foci in the body. The disease is liable to occur or take hold under conditions of malnutrition and exhaustion. Antibiotics like streptomycin and the chemotherapeutic drug isonicotinic acid hydrazide (INH) have almost eliminated this disease in industrialised countries. INH inhibits the formation of mycolic acid, and thus causes loss of acid fastness; it is effective against *M. tuberculosis* at low concentrations.

Unfortunately, millions of inhabitants of the tropics still suffer from leprosy. The pathogen *M. leprae* grows in the skin and forms swellings leading to tissue destruction in the face and extremities. Therapy is less effective than that against tuberculosis.

3.8   True actinomycetes

True actinomycetes are bacteria that grow in the form of mycelia. Their natural occurrence is mostly restricted to soils. They are gram-positive and are related to the coryneform bacteria and mycobacteria by an almost continuous sequence of intermediate forms. They are aerobic with very few exceptions. The name of this group is derived from the first-described anaerobic species *Actinomyces bovis* which causes actino-mycosis, the 'ray-fungus disease' of cattle.

Actinomycetes can be cultivated easily on simple media and can be identified by their growth in and on the surface of agar and their forma-tion of aerial mycelia, substrate mycelia, spores, and sporangia (Figs 3.6, 3.7). The **proactinomycetes** (*Nocardia*) form substrate and aerial mycelia that disintegrate into rod-shaped cells in older cultures. They do not produce true spores (Figs 3.6, 3.8).

Members of the large genus *Streptomyces* have permanent mycelia; their aerial mycelia are often very well developed and contain aerial hyphae (sporophores), which serve to enhance the spread of the organism by budding off conidia. The structure of the sporophores (i.e. whether they are straight, wavy, spiral, bunched, etc.), colonial morphology, colour, size and odour are diagnostic characters that are used to differentiate the many species and strains. The fragrance which emanates from freshly ploughed soil in spring is due to streptomycetes. An oil called geosmin can be isolated from *Streptomyces griseus* and is responsible for this odour. It is a 1,10-dimethyl-9-decalol. Knowledge about streptomycetes has advanced considerably because of their practical importance as producers of many effective antibiotics. Streptomycin (from *S. griseus*), chloramphenicol (from *S. venezuela*), and aureomycin and tetracyclin (from *S. aureofaciens*) are the most successful therapeutics among the hundreds of antibiotics isolated.

Many streptomycetes degrade cellulose, chitin, and other recalcitrant natural substances. One cellulose-degrading organism, widely distributed in soil and in rotting aqueous sediments, is *Micromonospora*. It has flat colonies with no aerial mycelia and its spores occur singly at the ends of weakly branched sporophores. *Microbispora* is morphologically similar but produces aerial mycelia and paired conidia.

Several actinomycetes (*Actinoplanes, Streptosporangium, Ampullariella*) do not produce spores directly on the aerial mycelia, but in sporangia. *Streptosporangium* is a cellulose-degrading aerobic streptomycete. On solid media it grows at first by a substrate mycelium, but forms aerial mycelia at a later stage. The tips of the aerial mycelia enlarge and form spherical sporangia 5–8 μm in diameter; these can reach 18 μm at maturity. The supporting hypha grows into the spherical end cell, where it assumes a helical form and pinches off sporangiospores. In *Streptosporangium* these are non-motile. *Actinoplanes* grows submerged on plant remains and also produces its spores within buttonlike sporangiospores; a flagellar bundle confers motility on these spores.

Dermatophilus congolensis is another actinomycete producing motile spores. It causes dermatitis of the dorsal skin in sheep and horses and can grow on solid media as smooth or rough colonies, forming a dense substrate mycelium. The hyphae divide longitudinally and transversely, so that up to eight parallel rows of coccoid cells are produced and liberated by autolysis of the hyphal wall. These coccoid spores are also motile by means of flagella.

The spores of actinomycetes are usually not heat-resistant, but they can withstand dehydration. The only actinomycete that forms heat-resistant spores is *Thermoactinomyces vulgaris*. This is thermophilic and occurs as part of the bacterial flora of damp haystacks and piles of

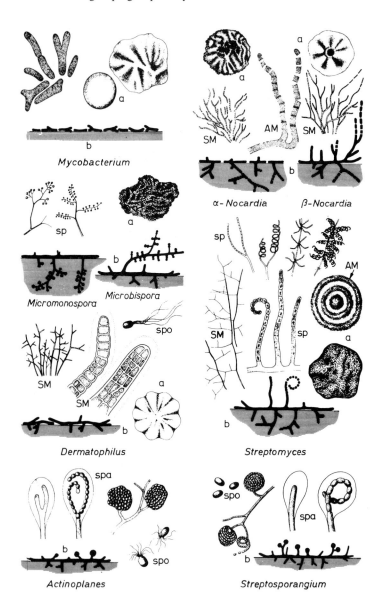

Mycobacterium

α-*Nocardia*   β-*Nocardia*

Micromonospora   *Microbispora*

Dermatophilus

Streptomyces

Actinoplanes   *Streptosporangium*

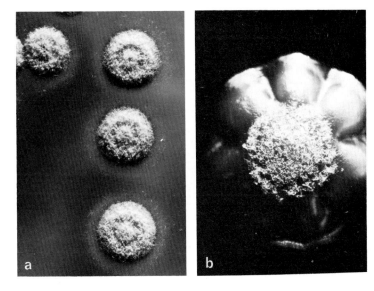

Fig. 3.7. *Colonial forms of streptomycetes.*

(a) Colonies of *Streptomyces* with aerial mycelia after growth for five weeks on glycerol-nitrate agar. (b) First appearance of aerial mycelium on a colony of a *Streptomyces* strain. (Picture: P. Hirsch.)

Fig. 3.6. *Mycobacteria, nocardia and actinomycetes.*

(a) Representative colonial forms for the different genera; (b) cross sections through growths on agar surfaces. SM, typical growth forms of the substrate mycelia; AM, typical growth forms of the aerial mycelia; sp, sporophores; spa, sporangia; spo, non-flagellated and flagellated spores.

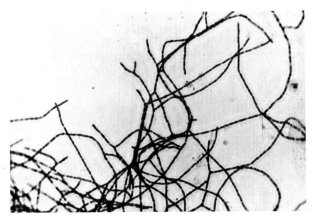

Fig. 3.8. *Substrate hyphae of* Nocardia saturnea.
Light micrograph of a smear stained   (Picture: P. Hirsch.)
with carbol fuchsin.

organic waste, where heat is generated. In their structure and dipicolinic acid content, these spores resemble the endospores of *Bacillus* and *Clostridium*.

3.9   Endospore-forming rods and cocci

The ability to produce more or less heat-resistant spores is restricted, with few exceptions, to a group of gram-positive, motile rods with peritrichous flagella. The aerobic and facultatively anaerobic rods belong to the genera *Bacillus*, *Sporolactobacillus*, and *Sporosarcina*, and the anaerobic rods belong to the genera *Clostridium* and *Desulfotomaculum*. Many spore formers are widely known because of their biochemical capacities. Only some representatives of the large genera *Clostridium* and *Bacillus* will be described here.

Aerobic spore formers.   The aerobic spore formers live in soil. Many bacilli form chains or filaments. They can be differentiated into the following groups according to the shape of their spores and vegetative cells (Fig. 3.9). (I) The spores of the majority of bacilli are oval or cylindrical in shape and no wider than the vegetative cells (*Bacillus megaterium*, *B. cereus*, *B. subtilis*, *B. licheniformis*, *B. anthracis*, *B. thuringiensis*).

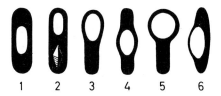

Fig. 3.9. *Typical spore-forming cells.*

(1) Central spore without distension of the mother cell (*Bacillus megaterium*). (2) Terminal spore without distension of the mother cell (*Bacillus thuringiensis* with protein inclusion body). (3) Terminal spore, mother cell distended ovally (tennis racquet shape) (*Bacillus macerans*). (4) Central spore, mother cell distended to spindle shape: clostridium form (*Bacillus polymyxa*). (5) Terminal spherical spore, mother cell distended to drumstick shape: plectridium form (*Bacillus sphaericus*). (6) Lateral spore, mother cell distended to spindle shape (*Bacillus laterosporus*).

(II) The oval spores are wider than the vegetative cells; during sporulation the cells become distended (*B. polymyxa, B. macerans, B. stearothermophilus, B. circulans*). (III) Almost spherical spores in terminally distended vegetative cells (*B. pasteurii*).

(I) *B. megaterium*, with dimensions of 2×5 µm, is a giant among the rod-shaped eubacteria. *B. cereus* is somewhat smaller. This species now also includes a variant called *B. cereus* var. *mycoides* because of its fungoid type of growth pattern on agar surfaces. There are 'right- and left-turning' strains; the colonial morphology is unmistakable (Fig. 3.10). Closely related to *B. cereus* is the anthrax bacillus, *B. anthracis*, which is non-flagellated and surrounded by a capsule containing glutamic acid. The insect pathogen *B. thuringiensis* is also related. *B. subtilis*, which is called the 'hay bacterium' because it is easily isolated from hay by enrichment culture, and *B. licheniformis*, produce polypeptide antibiotics. The latter organism can derive its energy not only from aerobic respiration but also from fermentation and nitrate respiration.

(II) *B. polymyxa* (formerly called *B. asterosporus*) takes its name from its profuse slime production and the star-shaped cross section of its barrel-shaped spores. It produces 2,3-butanediol, as does *B. licheniformis*. *B. stearothermophilus* is a decidedly thermophilic organism with an optimum growth temperature of 50–65 °C.

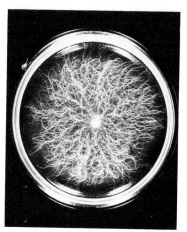

Fig. 3.10. *Filamental growth of* Bacillus cereus *var.* mycoides.

On agar medium these form a colony which resembles a fungal colony. (Picture: D. Claus.)

(III) *B. pasteurii* is known as the classic urea-degrading organism; it produces urease constitutively, hydrolyses urea to CO_2 and ammonia, and is adapted to grow at high pH values. *Sporosarcina urea* is physiologically similar; although it resembles sarcinae morphologically, it is reckoned among the bacilli because of its physiological characteristics, i.e. thermoresistance, dipicolinic acid-containing spores, and aerobic metabolism.

Anaerobic spore formers.   These organisms do not need O_2 for growth. The species in the genus *Clostridium* usually lack cytochromes and catalase. Most clostridia contain high levels of flavin enzymes and, on contact with air or oxygen, they form hydrogen peroxide, which is toxic to these cells. Spore-forming, sulphate-reducing bacteria, once included with the clostridia, have been placed in the new genus *Desulfotomaculum* (*nigrificans, orientis, ruminis*) because they contain protohaem-like pigments. Overall the spores of anaerobic spore formers are usually considerably wider than the vegetative cells and, according to the position of the spores, the mother cells assume various shapes.

The clostridia can ferment a large number of substrates, including polysaccharides, proteins, amino acids and purines (Ch. 8.5). Therefore, they can be differentiated according to their preferred substrates into (*Clostridium butyricum, C. acetobutylicum, C. cellulosae-dissolvens*), peptoclostridia (*C. histolyticum, C. sporogenes, C. tetani, C. botulinum*), and uric acid-degrading clostridia (*C. acidi-urici*). Among their fermentation products are butyrate, butanol, acetone, 2-propanol, and, in many cases, large quantities of gas (CO_2 and H_2). *C. pasteurianum*, as well as some other clostridia, can fix nitrogen; *C. aceticum* converts fructose or a mixture of CO_2 and H_2 to acetate.

Oscillospira guillermondii can be mentioned here as an addendum. It is an exceptionally large ($5 \times 100 \ \mu$m), spore-forming anaerobic bacterium that forms cell chains. It occurs in the appendix of guinea pigs and is also frequently found in the rumen of ruminants.

3.10   Pseudomonads and other gram-negative rods

It has become common to refer to all polarly flagellated, gram-negative rods as 'pseudomonads'. Frequently such physiologically highly special-ised eubacteria as *Nitrosomonas, Methylomonas*, the thiobacilli, and even phototrophic bacteria (*Rhodopseudomonas*) have been designated in this way. However, such usage has only morphological significance and in no way defines a taxonomic unit.

The family Pseudomonadaceae consists of gram-negative, polarly flagel-lated, straight and slightly curved rods that grow aerobically and are not spore formers. They obtain their energy by aerobic respiration and, in some cases, by anaerobic respiration (nitrate respiration, denitrification), but never by fermentation. The Pseudomonadaceae are chemo-organo-trophs, though some are facultative chemolithotrophs. The genus *Pseudo-monas* is the prototype of this family and is characterised by the proper-ties discussed below.

The metabolic and physiological properties of pseudomonads are characterised by the wide spectrum of substrates these organisms can use. They can even utilise a large number of heterocyclic and aromatic compounds that are not attacked by other bacteria. They generally metabolise sugars via the Entner–Doudoroff pathway (Ch. 7.2.3). Some *Pseudomonas* species oxidise sugars incompletely and excrete sugar acids (gluconate, 2-oxogluconate). Because of their simple requirements, pseudomonads are ubiquitous. They are present in soil, water, sewage and air. When media containing mineral salts and organic acids or sug-ars are exposed to air, pseudomonads are usually the first colonisers. Many can be recognised by their production of water-soluble pigments, i.e. the blue-green derivative of phenazine, pyocyanin, and the yellow-green fluorescing pigments. Some of the excreted fluorescent pigments function as siderophores (Ch. 7.7).

***Pseudomonas* species.**   *Pseudomonas aeruginosa* (formerly *P. pyocyanea*) is an aquatic bacterium that can cause opportunistic infections in man, giving rise to inflammation of the middle ear, wound infections producing greenish-blue pus, and, in compromised patients, even septicaemia. *P. fluorescens* and *P. putida* are other soil and aquatic species that can oxidise a very large number of organic compounds. Many strains showing plant pathogenicity have recently been unified in the species *P. syringae*. The aquatic bacterium *P. saccharophila* was used in the discovery of the Entner–Doudoroff pathway of sugar dissimilation.

Xanthomonas. The yellow-pigmented plant pathogens of the Pseudomonodaceae family have been unified in the genus *Xanthomonas*. The yellow pigment is a polyene compound containing bromine. Certain strains of *Xanthomonas campestris* secrete exopolysaccharides (xanthan) that are resistant to enzymic degradation. These polysaccharides are produced industrially and used to increase the viscosity of aqueous solutions such as printing ink, diet soups, and packet desserts.

Other gram-negative aerobic rods. Genera that resemble the pseudomonads metabolically are *Alcaligenes, Agrobacterium* and *Rhizobium*, the acetic acid bacteria *Acetobacter* and *Gluconobacter* (Ch. 10.1), and the free-living nitrogen fixers *Azotobacter, Beijerinckia* and *Derxia* (Ch. 13.2).

Alcaligenes, Rhizobium, Agrobacterium. These genera include bacteria that resemble the aerobic pseudomonads in their energy metabolism (respiratory system), but they are not polarly flagellated. They have either subpolar flagella or only a few (2–6) peritrichous flagella. *Alcaligenes* includes the facultative autotrophic hydrogen bacterium *A. eutrophus* (Ch. 11.4). *Rhizobium* is characterised by its ability to fix atmospheric nitrogen in endosymbiosis with leguminous plants (Ch. 13.1). *Agrobacterium tumefaciens* can produce tumours in roots, leaves, and stems of plants (Ch. 4.3; Fig. 4.15).

Chemolithotrophic bacteria. Aerobic chemolithoautotrophs (Ch. 11) are characterised by their ability to use inorganic ions or compounds as electron or hydrogen donors. They can use carbon dioxide as their carbon source and carry out CO_2 fixation via the ribulose-bisphosphate pathway. Most of these bacteria are facultative autotrophs and can also utilise organic substrates. Autotrophic bacteria belong to many genera, including *Pseudomonas, Alcaligenes, Aquaspirillum, Xanthobacter, Mycobacterium, Bacillus* and *Nocardia*.

Sheathed bacteria. The best-known filamentous bacterium is *Sphaerotilus natans*. Referred to as a 'sewage mould', it grows in contaminated streams and waters, in the drainage from sugar refineries, in weirs, and in various

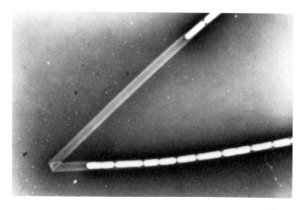

Fig. 3.11. Sphaerotilus natans *with cells in the partially emptied sheath.* (From Stokes, J. L. (1954). *J. Bacteriol.* **67**, 278.)

trickling filters. It can form threads and aggregates or, when adhering to solid substrates, it can produce long pellicles and extensive surface covers. Pipes, irrigation systems and ditches can easily become plugged. *Sphaerotilus natans* is a unicellular gram-negative bacterium with polytrichously polar flagellation. It could be regarded as a relative of the pseudomonads except for its specific growth characteristics. It grows as long chains or filaments that consist of chains of individuals held together by a thin tubular sheath (Fig. 3.11). This sheath consists of a heteropolysaccharide and can be regarded as a capsule. The bacteria multiply within the sheath by division and are able to leave the sheath as motile individual cells. On agar plates two types of colonies are often found: rough colonies that contain mainly filamentous forms, and smooth colonies consisting of single cells. Cell size, filament diameter and other secondary characters have been used to differentiate a number of species.

Filamentous bacteria that are widely distributed in iron-containing waters, ditches, wells, drainage pipes, and swamps were formerly called 'ochre bacteria' (*Leptothrix ochracea*). Their natural habitat is usually deficient in utilisable organic materials but rich in iron. Their sheaths are therefore streaked and covered by iron oxide precipitates. Ever since Winogradsky's investigations (1888), it has been assumed that these were iron-oxidising autotrophic bacteria. However, because neither physiological nor biochemical studies can support this assumption, *Leptothrix ochracea* and also *Cladothrix dichotoma*, which differs from *L. ochracea* in its growth form, are now regarded as variants of *Sphaerotilus*, distinguished only by their habitat.

3.11   Gram-negative facultative anaerobic rods

The members of this taxonomic group are characterised by their fermentation products. Under anaerobic conditions, they gain the energy for growth from fermentation and excrete several organic acids, including formic acid. Although this is not quantitatively predominant, it is the most characteristic fermentation product. Because representative members of this group, including *Escherichia coli, Salmonella, Shigella* and others, inhabit the intestinal tract (Greek *enteron*), the whole group has been called Enterobacteriaceae. These will be discussed in Ch. 8.4.

3.12   Gram-negative anaerobic bacteria

Gram-negative anaerobic rods and vibrio-like bacteria are widely distributed in anaerobic ecosystems. Until relatively recently their investigation was limited mainly by their oxygen sensitivity and carbon dioxide requirement. Their quantitative preponderance in the intestinal tract and rumen, and in sewage sludge was only recently recognised.

Species of the genus *Bacteroides* (*B. fragilis, B. succinogenes*) belong to the dominant gram-negative flora of human faeces. Up to 30% of faecal mass can consist of bacteria: 10^{10} *Bacteroides*, 10^6–10^8 coliform cells, and a similar number of both streptococci and lactobacilli have been counted in 1 g wet weight of faeces. The ratio of strict anaerobes to facultative anaerobes is about 40:1. The species of the genus *Bacteroides* have a purely fermentative metabolism. They ferment glucose to succinate, acetate, formate, lactate, and other acids.

Fusobacterium gets its name from its spindle shape; the rods are relatively long. The genus is well characterised by its chief fermentation product, butyrate. Several species occur in the oral cavity, intestinal tract, and faeces.

The genus *Leptotrichia* exists in the form of non-flagellated threads up to 200 μm long. *L. buccalis* is found in the mouth. The main product of its glucose fermentation is DL-lactate.

The vibrio-form bacteria, which should follow the three genera named above, will be discussed in Section 3.14 (*Selenomonas, Butyrivibrio, Succinivibrio*), and in connection with their ecological and metabolic properties (*Desulfovibrio*: Ch. 9.2; *Selenomonas*: Ch. 8.3; *Butyrivibrio*: Ch. 8.5).

3.13   Archaebacteria

Archaebacteria are distinguished from all other bacteria, which are collectively known as the eubacteria, by profound differences and are all found in rather extreme (special) habitats. These 'extreme' conditions seem to resemble those supposed to have prevailed in the earliest times of the earth's development, i.e. archaeic times. The archaebacteria include lithoautotrophic and heterotrophic aerobes and anaerobes. The members of this group have many properties in common that distinguish them from the eubacteria. Within the group, however, there are differences in cell shape, cell components, and metabolism, similar to the differences found among the eubacteria.

According to the present state of research, the archaebacteria can be subdivided into **three groups**: methanogenic bacteria, halophilic bacteria, and thermo-acidophilic bacteria.

Common properties.   The characters common to the archaebacteria concern their cell walls, lipids, transcription and translation apparatus, coenzymes and prosthetic groups, their mechanism of autotrophic CO_2 fixation, and energy supply. Although there are still many gaps in our knowledge, a general survey based on current research will be attempted in the following section.

The **archaebacterial cell wall** does not contain a peptidoglycan skeleton; only proteins and polysaccharides are present and, at best, a 'pseudomurein'. This explains why archaebacteria are not sensitive to antibiotics such as penicillin, cephalosporin and D-cycloserine that act on the eubacterial cell wall.

The **cytoplasmic membrane** of archaebacteria contains glycerol ethers with C_{20} (phytanyl) and C_{40} (biphytanyl) alkyl isoprenoids in place of the fatty acid glycerol esters. Neutral lipids are also found in the form of free C_{15} and C_{30} isoprenoid hydrocarbons.

Dialkylglyceroltetraether   Dialkylglyceroldiether

The DNA-dependent RNA polymerases of archaebacteria differ from those of the eubacteria in that they consist of more than four subunits and are resistant to the antibiotics rifampicin and streptolydigin. The nucleotide sequences of archaebacterial 16S and 5S RNA differ markedly from those of the eubacteria. Translation in archaebacteria is insensitive to chloramphenicol but is inhibited by diphtheria toxin, which is ineffective in eubacteria. Diphtheria toxin also inhibits translation in eukaryotes.

Some of the **prosthetic groups and coenzymes** of the archaebacteria are distinct, although they may resemble those of the eubacteria or eukaryotes. Some examples are F_{420}, a 5-deazoriboflavin derivative, the nickel-tetrapyrrol factor F_{430}, tetrahydromethanopterin, and coenzyme M. These factors were discovered in the methanogenic bacteria (Ch. 9.4). It is not yet possible to make more general statements.

Autotrophic CO_2 fixation does not occur via the ribulose bisphosphate cycle. Methanogenic bacteria fix CO_2 via the acetyl-CoA pathway (Ch. 9.4), which is also used by some eubacteria.

The process of energy conversion (regeneration of ATP) probably involves the formation of a proton potential gradient and the function of an ATP synthase, and this process could be regarded as a primitive anaerobic respiration. Carbon dioxide, sulphur, and, in a few archaebacteria, oxygen function as the electron acceptor.

The methanogenic bacteria.   Almost all the shapes known in the eubacteria can be found in the methanogens: cocci (*Methanococcus vannielii*); rods (*Methanobacterium formicicum*); short rods (*Methanobrevibacter ruminantium, M. arboriphilicus*); spirilla (*Methanospirillum hungatei*); coccal packets (*Methanosarcina barkeri*); filaments (*Methanothrix soehngenii*); and even square bacteria (*Methanoplanus limicola*). There are mesophilic and thermophilic species (*Methanobacterium thermoautotrophicum, Methanothermus fervidus*). Six families can be distinguished already, and the number of known species and genera is constantly increasing. The GC content varies between 27 and 61 mol%. The ecology and metabolism of the methanogens is discussed in Ch. 9.4.

Halobacteria.   The genera *Halobacterium, Haloferax* and *Halococcus* consist of extreme halophiles. They are aerobes and heterotrophs and are found in salterns in which seawater is evaporated for the production of salt. During the mass proliferation of the carotenoid (haloruberin) containing halobacteria, the water appears dark red. Their optimal growth range lies between 3.5 and 5 M NaCl. They also have the special property of being able to utilise light energy for their metabolism (see Ch. 12.3).

Thermo-acidophilic bacteria.   This group at present contains non-methanogenic thermophilic archaebacteria, which do not seem to have many common features. They include autotrophs and heterotrophs, extreme acidophiles and neutrophiles, and aerobes and anaerobes.

Sulfolobus acidocaldarius is found in hot acid springs and oxidises sulphur to sulphate (Ch. 11.2).

The position of *Thermoplasma acidophilus* seems quite isolated. It lacks a cell wall, as do the mycoplasmas, but grows optimally at 59 °C and pH 1–2. Its usual habitat is in heat-generating coal slag-heaps, but it has also been found in a hot spring. It has the smallest genome so far known in non-parasitic bacteria (1×10^9). It can grow heterotrophically under aerobic conditions in the presence of yeast extract. The above-named aerobic species are contrasted with a group of anaerobic species collected under the name of Thermoproteales. They were isolated from hot springs, volcanoes, and from the sea floor. They are all extremely thermophilic with temperature optima of 85–105 °C, and their metabolism is of the type described as 'sulphur respiration' (Ch. 9.3). This means they oxidise hydrogen and reduce elemental sulphur to hydrogen sulphide. The group includes facultative autotrophs (*Thermoproteus tenax*), obligate autotrophs (*Thermoproteus neutrophilus, Pyrodictium occultum*), and heterotrophs (*Desulfurococcus, Thermococcus, Thermodiscus*).

As more research is done on this group of organisms, it is becoming more apparent that the archaebacteria are early deviants from the eubacteria not only with respect to their cell components. Most of them are probably the progeny of those 'primordial' bacteria that had 'discovered' the utilisation of the inorganic hydrogen donors (H_2) and acceptors (CO_2, sulphur) which were available in the earliest era of development. They probably contributed to the deposition of reduced carbon in sedimentary rocks that occurred some 3×10^9 years ago.

3.14   Curved rods: spirilla and vibrios

Spirilla and vibrios are gram-negative aquatic bacteria, motile by means of their flagella.

Spirilla.   These are characterised by their helical form and bipolar polytrichous flagellation. They obtain their energy by respiration. There are several genera. The genus *Spirillum* contains only one species, *S. volutans*. This is a giant spirillum, found frequently in pig manure, and was characterised by its 'volutin' content, i.e. polyphosphates. In pure culture it grows only at low oxygen concentrations (about 5%) and is thus microaerotolerant. Most spirilla belong to the genus *Aquaspirillum* (*A. itersonii, A. serpens*). These also have a marked tendency not to tolerate the partial pressures of O_2 found in normal air.

Vibrios.   The vibrios are facultatively anaerobic and metabolically similar to the Enterobacteriaceae (mixed acid fermentation). the best known is *Vibrio cholerae*, the causative agent of cholera. It is transmitted by water and, hence, sewage. It grows in the intestinal tract and produces enzymes that attack the intestinal epithelium, and an exotoxin that causes very severe loss of water from the tissues, and hence dehydration of the body.

Bdellovibrio.   *Bdellovibrio bacteriovorus* is an aerobic organism that parasitises other bacteria. The cells are small and highly motile by virtue of a thick flagellum, 50 nm in diameter (Fig. 3.12); its swimming velocity is 100 μm/sec, which corresponds to about 70 body lengths/sec. When this parasite encounters a suitable host bacterium, it adheres with its unflagellated pole to the host's cell wall (Fig. 3.12) and may rotate around its longitudinal axis. Soon afterwards the host cell rounds off and assumes a spherical form, resembling a spheroplast, whilst the *Bdellovibrio* penetrates the cell wall and settles in the periplasmic space. The *Bdellovibrio* cell continues to elongate into a long cylinder until the nutrients obtained from the gradually shrinking host protoplast have been exhausted. The cylinder then undergoes multiple divisions to give rise to cells of uniform size; eventually, the host cell wall lyses and the progeny of the parasite are liberated into the medium ready to attack other host bacteria. The progressive attack and lysis of host bacteria can be seen macroscopically as the appearance of 'holes', or lytic zones, on a bacterial lawn of the host, or as a decrease in turbidity in the case of liquid cultures. In contrast to bacteriophages, which can multiply only in growing bacteria, *Bdellovibrio* can attack and lyse non-growing cultures. The several strains of *Bdellovibrio* that have been isolated from different soils are differentiated according to their host range. They lyse mainly gram-negative bacteria and seem to prefer pseudomonads and enterobacteria. Whilst the wild type is an obligate bacterial parasite dependent on host bacteria for its nutrition, a few mutants are able to grow saprophytically outside other bacterial cells on complex nutrient media. It is generally assumed that the parasitic life-style of *Bdellovibrio* represents adaptation to environments with low nutrient concentrations.

Fig. 3.12. *The bacterial parasite* Bdellovibrio bacteriovorus.

(a) Life cycle in the host bacterium; (b) bacteria attacked by *Bdellovibrio* (*Erwinia carotovora*), $\times$ 2200; (c) primary stage of attack on a host bacterium (*Pseudomonas*) by *Bdellovibrio*, $\times$ 20 000. (From Stolp, H. (1968). *Naturwissenschaften* **55**, 57.)

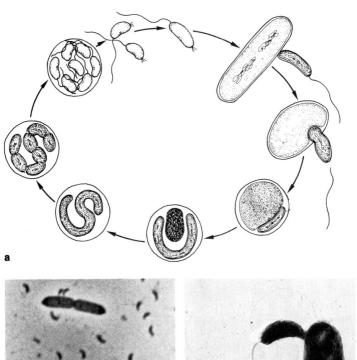

a

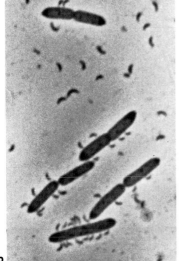

b

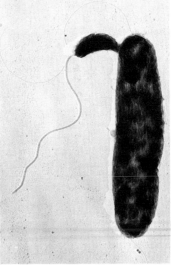

c

Strictly anaerobic vibrios.   A second group of vibrio-like bacteria is strictly anaerobic: *Desulfovibrio, Selenomonas, Butyrivibrio* and *Succinivibrio. Desulfovibrio* represents the type of metabolism known as dissimilatory sulphate reduction (Ch. 9.2). *Selenomonas sputigena* occurs in the oral cavity and dental mucus of humans, and *S. ruminantium* is a rumen bacterium. Both species are characterised by lateral flagellation and utilise the fermentation of carbohydrates to propioniate and acetate for growth.

3.15   Spirochaetes

The spirochaetes are a group of unicellular chemoheterotrophic bacteria of very characteristic shape. They are distinguished from all other bacteria by their cellular structure and the way they move. Their form is helical, like that of spirilla, but the cell body is extremely flexible, not rigid. Their diameter is extraordinarily small ($0.1–0.6 \ \mu m$) in comparison to their length ($5–500 \ \mu m$). They are able, therefore, to pass through most bacteriological filters (pore diameter $0.2–0.45 \ \mu m$) that retain other bacteria, and they can thus be selected in an enrichment procedure using filtration. Because of their small diameter they are difficult to visualise in bright-field microscopy, but they can be observed by phase-contrast or dark-field microscopy.

Cell structure.   The cells of spirochaetes can be divided into three major components: the cylindrical protoplast, the axial fibrillae, and the outer envelope membrane (Fig. 3.13). The helically wound cylinder of protoplasm is surrounded by the cytoplasmic membrane–cell-wall complex. The fibrillae wound around this are called axial fibrillae and are collectively known as the axial filament. Each fibrilla has one end attached to the cell apex and the other end is free. The number of fibrillae varies in different genera and species: *Treponema pallidum* and *Leptospira* usually have four, *Borrelia* have up to 18, and *Cristispira* have more than a hundred. About the same number of fibrillae are usually inserted at each end, and they may overlap in the middle or along the length of the cell. The outer membrane covers the fibrillae as well as the cell body.

Motility.   Although the spirochaetes lack flagella, they are able to swim, to move without solid support, or to glide over solid surfaces. The movement is produced by the action of fibrillae. The fibrillae share with flagella the nature of their protein (flagellin), the way they are inserted into the cell body, and the helical arrangement of subunits. It is assumed that rotation or contraction of the fibrillae produces the unique kind of twisting, winding or serpentine movement characteristic of spirochaetes.

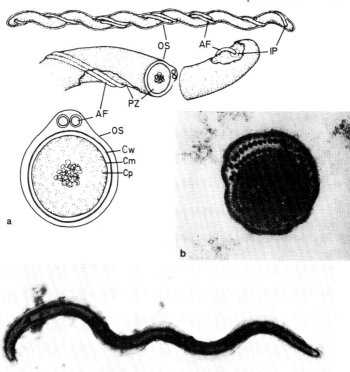

Fig. 3.13. *The cells of spirochaetes.*

(a) The protoplasmic cylinder (PZ) is surrounded by a helical axial filament, which consists in this case of two axial fibrillae (AF) which overlap. Each fibrilla is inserted in the protoplasmic cylinder at one end (IP, insertion pore). The protoplasmic cylinder with the axial filaments is surrounded by a membranous envelope, the outer sheath (OS).

Cw, cell wall; Cm, cytoplasmic membrane; Cp, cytoplasm. (From Holt, S. C. (1978). *Microbiol. Rev.* **42**, 114.) (b, c) A mouth spirochaete with several axial fibrilla. (b) Electron micrograph of transverse section, × 110 000; (c) electron micrograph of a stretch cell, × 7000 (From Listgarten, H. (1964). *J. Bacteriol.* **88**, 1087.)

Distribution, habitat and most important representatives. Free-living spirochaetes can be found in many aquatic environments: pools, lakes, even the sea. Others belong to the normal autochthonous microflora of animals. They occur in the intestinal tract of mammals, on the surface of ciliates, in the gut of wood-eating termites and cockroaches, in the stem of molluscs, in the rumen, and in various other habitats. Only a few are pathogenic, causing syphilis, relapsing fever and leptospirosis. There are five genera: *Spirochaeta, Cristispira, Treponema, Borrelia* and *Leptospira*.

Spirochaeta plicatilis is widely distributed in freshwater and seawater. It is never found in clarification sediments, but always in mesoaerobic zones of water, in village ponds, in pools, and in mud, which also contains many purple bacteria. The organism is striking because of its characteristic restless movements. It can be maintained in laboratory cultures only for limited periods. *S. zuelzerae* occurs in rotting sediments in various waters. This species is strictly anaerobic, grows in yeast-extract glucose media, and can utilise a number of sugars as well as starch. Its optimal temperature is 37–40 °C and it resembles *Treponema pallidum* in its appearance as well as in its antigenic properties; it gives a positive complement-fixation response with syphilis serum. *S. zuelzerae* and also rumen spirochaetes ferment glucose to lactate, acetate, succinate, CO_2 and molecular H_2; that is, they resemble *E. coli* in their fermentation pattern.

Cristispira lives in the 'crystal stalk' and gut of freshwater and marine mussels (*Anodonta, Pecten, Venus*, etc.). The helical pitch is steeper than in *Spirochaeta plicatilis*. The diameter of the cell is 0.5–3.0 μm. A very fine seam or band appears to wind helically around the cylindrical cell body. This seam or 'crista' corresponds in its arrangement to the axial filament, and it consists of more than 100 individual fibrillae.

The smaller types of spirochaetes belong to the Treponemataceae. *Treponema pallidum* is the causative organism of syphilis. *T. pertenue* causes yaws. Several *Treponema* species are relatively harmless parasites of the oral cavity; *T. macrodentium* can be isolated from saliva and dental plaques.

The genus *Borrelia* includes anaerobic spirochaetes that are easily stained with aniline dyes. They are parasites of various arthropods and can cause disease in man and other vertebrates (blood spirochaetes). *B. recurrentis* is the causative organism of relapsing fever. *B. anserina* was used by Ehrlich and Hata to screen the arsenicals against syphilis until they achieved their goal by developing a highly effective chemotherapeutic agent with Salvarsan. *B. burgdorferi* is the organism that causes the borreliosis Lyme disease. It is conveyed by ticks which are disseminated via red deer and birds. The infection is easily controlled by antibiotics.

The genus *Leptospira* contains the smallest aerobic spirochaetes. They have a diameter of 0.1–0.25 μm and are 4–8 μm long. They are characterised by their hook-shaped, crooked ends. *L. biflexa* can be isolated from freshwater, including tapwater, ponds and pools. It grows on the usual nutrient media and is aerobic. Among the pathogenic *Leptospira* species are *L. icterohaemorrhagiae*, the causative agent of Weil's disease, *L. pomona*, which causes Swineherd's disease, and *L. canicola*, the causative agent of icterus infectiosus. These have been well investigated. They gain entry via contaminated food and drink, pass into the blood stream, kidneys or liver, and cause dysfunction of these organs, resulting in haemorrhagic jaundice.

3.16   Gliding bacteria

Only a few groups of bacteria are able to move by gliding or creeping. They are grouped together as 'gliding bacteria' and subdivided into:

    (I) Bacteria that contain intracellular sulphur, of which there are trichome-forming (*Beggiatoa, Thiothrix*) and unicellular (*Achromatium*) representatives.

    (II) Sulphur-free bacteria existing as trichomes, such as *Vitreoscilla, Leucothrix*, and *Saprospira*, as well as the 'mouth oscillaria' *Simonsiella* and *Alysiella* (Fig. 3.14).

    (III) Unicellular, rod-shaped bacteria, including the myxobacteria, the *Cytophaga* group and the *Flexibacter* group.

    (IV) The threadlike gliding bacterium *Chloroflexus* is discussed with the phototrophic bacteria in Chapter 12.1.

    (V) Cyanobacteria, if they are motile at all, move by gliding. They are discussed in Section 3.21.

(I) *Beggiatoa* is a colourless, threadlike sulphur bacterium. It consists of trichomes of uniform thickness and is similar in construction to *Oscillatoria*. Several species are identified by their diameter (1.5–35 μm). The cells are usually filled with sulphur droplets, which makes the colourless threads appear white. The threads are motile by gliding. *Beggiatoa* is an aerobic organism and looks like masses of spider's webs either covering the black putrid mud of slow-moving waters or in the sea when water containing hydrogen sulphide is exposed to atmospheric oxygen. The sulphide is oxidised to sulphate. The intermediate production of elementary sulphur leads to its transient accumulation intracellularly. Winogradsky (1888) derived his concept of chemolithoautotrophy, i.e. energy supply by oxidation of reduced organic compounds coupled with synthesis of cellular material from CO_2, from his studies of *Beggiatoa*. Some *Beggiatoa* strains found in natural habitats require organic nutrients.

Thiothrix is not freely motile. Bunches or tufts of trichomes are attached by their bases to solid surfaces. Each trichome consists of a base and apex, and it tapers from 5 to 2 μm. Multiplication is by gonidia, which are formed by the rounding off of apical cells. Gonidia can glide

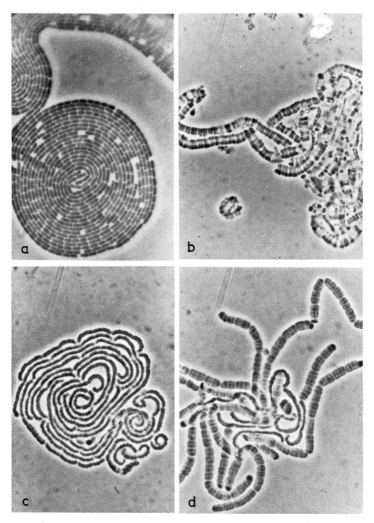

Fig. 3.14. *Filament-forming bacteria.*

(a) Colony of *Vitreoscilla* species.
(b) *Alysiella filiformis.* (c) Colony of
Simonsiella crassa before it begins to
creep. (d) *S. crassa*, flat and
perpendicular filaments, some
creeping.
(Picture: V. B. D. Skerman.)

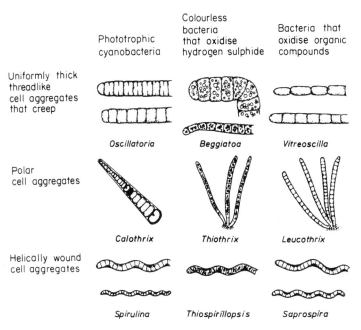

Fig. 3.15. *Comparison of some cyanobacteria and related forms of non-phototrophic bacteria.*

over solid surfaces. In most instances, several gonidia settle together and grow into the multicellular filaments. *Thiothrix* is much more widespread than *Beggiatoa* and grows in waters in which rotting organic material gives rise to hydrogen sulphide.

(II) *Vitreoscilla* is a colourless, aerobic, multicellular, filamentous bacterium which moves by gliding and multiplies by fragmentation of the filaments (Fig. 3.14). It can be isolated from cow dung.

Leucothrix grows epiphytically on marine algae, and in its manner of growth it is the organotrophic equivalent of *Thiothrix*. The filaments grow in bunches or tufts and adhere with their bases to a solid surface.

The sulphur bacterium *Thiospirillopsis floridana* and the organotrophic *Saprospira grandis* can be compared to the helically wound cyanobacterium *Spirulina*. In Fig. 3.15 the morphologically similar representatives of the three metabolic types (phototrophic cyanobacteria; colourless bacteria that oxidise hydrogen sulphide; bacteria that oxidise organic compounds)

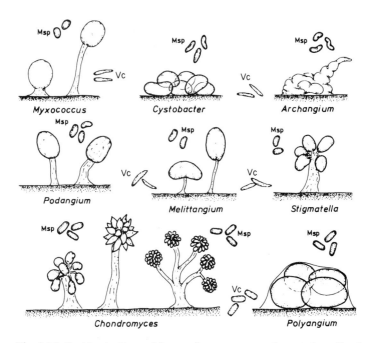

Fig. 3.16. *Fruiting bodies and forms of myxospores and vegetative cells of some myxobacteria.*

The fruiting bodies are not drawn to a uniform scale. The vegetative cells of the genera shown in the upper two rows are spindle-shaped (rods with pointed ends); those of *Chondromyces* and *Polyangium* are rods with blunt ends.
Msp, myxospores; Vc, vegetative cells.
(After Reichenbach, H. (1974). *Biologie in unserer Zeit* **4**, 33.)

are shown diagrammatically and arranged so that those with similar morphological structure are shown next to each other.

(III) Myxobacteria are strictly aerobic chemoheterotrophic organisms with gliding motility. They are soil bacteria and are characterised in their natural habitat by the formation of fruiting bodies that are very small (less than 1 mm). Such fruiting bodies are found in decaying plant material, rotting wood, tree bark, and on the faeces of herbivores. They can be isolated from the latter, after incubating the faeces for several weeks in damp soil.

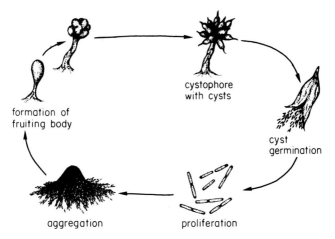

cystophore
with cysts

formation of
fruiting body

cyst
germination

aggregation   proliferation

Fig. 3.17. *Developmental cycle of* Chondromyces apiculatus *with formation of fruiting bodies.*

After aggregation of the cells, a fruiting body consisting of a mucous stem and cysts is formed. The cysts are organs of distribution and they release the myxospores on germination. These then develop into vegetative cells.

On solid media myxobacteria form very extensive flat colonies. When the vegetative cells inside the colonies aggregate, they differentiate into fruiting bodies that differ in shape, size, and pigmentation for the various genera and species of the myxobacteria (Figs 3.16, 3.17). During maturation, the cells inside the fruiting bodies become dormant, i.e. they are converted to myxospores. These can be spherical (*Myxococcus*) or rod-shaped (Fig. 3.16) and may be enclosed in cysts. Bacteriolytic and cellulolytic species can be distinguished by their mode of nutrition. Most of the myxobacteria can lyse bacteria by exoenzymes, whilst only the genus *Polyangium* contains cellulolytic species.

The *Cytophaga* group contains the genera *Cytophaga* and *Sporocytophaga*, which became known by their ability to degrade cellulose in the soil aerobically. They exhibit gliding motility like the myxobacteria, but do not form fruiting bodies. Some species are facultative anaerobes and can ferment glucose with the production of organic acids. In *Sporocytophaga*, the spindle-shaped vegetative cells can change into spherical, encapsulated lasting forms that resemble the myxospores of *Myxococcus* but are called microcysts (Fig. 3.18). *Cytophaga* and *Sporocytophaga* can be easily enriched on cellulose, i.e. filter paper (see Ch. 14.1).

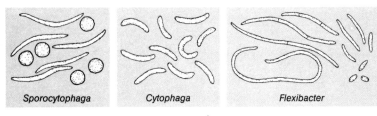

Fig. 3.18. *Cell forms of the genera* Sporocytophaga, Cytophaga *and* Flexibacter.

Flexibacter in young cultures forms many cells 100 μm long with few septa; the cells are very actively motile. With increasing periods of incubation these thread-like cells divide into shorter, and eventually coccoid, forms. (After Reichenbach, H. (1974). *Biologie in unserer Zeit* **4**, 33.)

The *Flexibacter* species are aquatic bacteria. They consist of long, very flexible cells that are not considered multicellular (Fig. 3.18). During continuous cultivation these become shorter and eventually fragment into coccoid cells. Many forms contain carotenoids and show yellow, pink, or orange pigmentation. The causative agent of the columnaris fish disease (*Chondrococcus columnaris*) is now assigned to the genus *Flexibacter* as *F. columnaris*.

3.17   Prosthecate and budding bacteria

This group contains organisms whose form differs markedly from that of typical bacteria either by the presence of protheca or buds or hypha-like protrusions, or by the formation of extracellular stalks or masses of slime (Figs 3.19, 3.20).

Budding and prosthecate bacteria.   Budding or sprouting is the term applied to the mode of multiplication that is characteristic for the 'budding' yeasts. Contrary to binary fission, it is an unequal cell division, which proceeds via localised growth. The daughter cell (bud) is usually smaller than the mother cell and reaches normal size only after it has become separated from the mother cell. Various aquatic and soil organisms belong to the budding bacteria. *Hyphomicrobium vulgare*, a denitrifying bacterium which can be obtained by enrichment culture in media containing nitrate and methanol, is a regular inhabitant of stagnant water, including water-baths in laboratories; it forms its buds at the ends of long hyphae. Another organism with similar habits is the non-

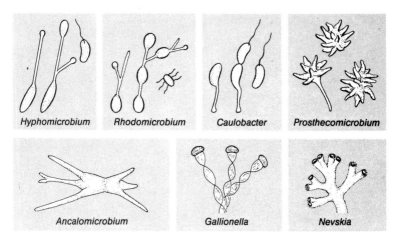

Fig. 3.19. *Prosthecate and stalked bacteria.*

sulphur purple bacterium *Rhodomicrobium vannielii*. Extracellular stalks and other protuberances are known as prosthecae. The best known are the species of the *Caulobacter* group (*Caulobacter vibrioides*, *Asticcacaulis*) that are also found as mats or pellicles on water-baths, etc. They have a characteristic form and a complex life cycle. The polarly flagellated rods adhere to solid surfaces, or even to other bacteria, with their flagellar pole, which then grows out into a stalk; the cell divides normally and the daughter cell then forms a new flagellum at the free pole.

Careful examinations of surface films and the surfaces of Crustaceae, aquatic plants, and the fauna and flora of water surfaces have yielded further unusually shaped bacteria; *Prosthecomicrobium* and *Ancalomicrobium* are examples of these.

Stalked bacteria.   Some widely distributed bacteria are sessile by means of a stalk consisting of slime. *Gallionella ferruginosa*, for example, is a bean-shaped cell which excretes a slime on its concave side. This concave side can be seen microscopically to consist of a helical band encrusted with ferrous hydroxide. *Gallionella*, the best-known iron bacterium, grows profusely, especially in the spring, in iron-containing waters such as streams, drainage pipes, etc. *Nevskia ramosa* has been isolated a number of times from the pellicles it forms on ponds, moorland ditches, and water-baths. Its characteristic polar secretion of slime apparently occurs only under conditions of nutrient deficiency.

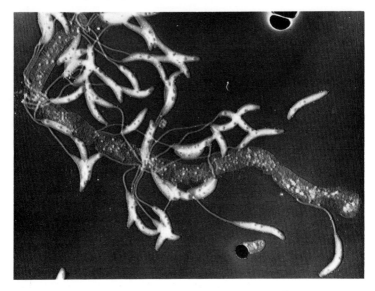

Fig. 3.20. Caulobacter *on dead cells of* Bacillus megaterium.
Electron micrograph (approximately
× 4000). (Picture: A. L. Houwink).

3.18   Obligate cellular parasites

The fact that some bacteria are absolutely dependent on living cells for their growth and multiplication was mentioned in Section 3.14 on *Bdellovibrio bacteriovorus*. It is probable that many bacteria that occur as endosymbionts in insects and ciliates are obligately restricted to these locations. The basis of such obligate cell parasitic forms of life is usually attributed to degenerative changes in metabolism. Among the best studied of the obligately intracellular bacteria are the rickettsiae and chlamydiae. Both are pathogens of animals and humans and their cell envelope structure is that of gram-negative organisms.

Rickettsiae.   The rickettsiae are named after H. T. Ricketts, who discovered American 'Rocky Mountain spotted fever'. This group is also referred to as the 'spotted fever' (typhus fever) group after the disease produced by the best-known of these pathogens (*Rickettsia prowazekii*). Their natural distribution is by host vectors such as lice, fleas, ticks, mites, etc. in which they exist as harmless parasites or even symbionts. On being transferred to other animal hosts or humans by bites, scratches, or inhalation, they produce very serious disease symptoms. Although the size of rickettsiae is of the same order of magnitude as pox viruses, they can be differentiated quite unequivocally from any viruses. They contain DNA as well as RNA in a ratio of 1:3.5. The cells are surrounded by a cell wall that contains muramic acid and is lysozyme sensitive. Nuclear regions and cell walls can also be distinguished in electron micrographs of thin sections.

Most rickettsiae have never been cultured except in living cells, but they can be grown in incubating chicken eggs or in experimental animals; about 10^9 cells can be produced in the yolk sac of a chicken egg. A few enzymes of intermediary metabolism can be demonstrated in isolated cells, but the metabolic activity of the cells declines on storage; respiration can be restored by addition of ATP, organic acids and amino acids. It appears that the rickettsiae are able to develop their own metabolism, but they are apparently unable to control uptake and excretion of metabolites because of the permeability characteristics of their cell envelope.

The best-known pathogens among the rickettsiae are those of the typhus group. *R. prowazekii* is the causative agent of typhus fever. The reservoir is humans, and the organism is transmitted by lice (head lice and clothes lice). The lice are rapidly (in a few days) killed by the organism, and infection is via their faeces. *R. typhi* is the causative organism of endemic and murine typhus, which produces a similar but less severe syndrome. The organism is spread by rats which remain symptomless and is transmitted from rat to rat and to humans by fleas.

Whilst the above rickettsiae are relatively sensitive to heat and dehydration, another organism, *Coxiella burnetii*, which causes Q-fever, can survive outside the host. It is transmitted by ticks to sheep, goats, and cattle and can infect humans not only by tick bites but also via animal dust, infected soil, and consumption of milk. The usual pasteurisation of milk (heating at 60 °C for 30 min) does not kill *Coxiella*.

Chlamydiae.   Chlamydiae are human pathogens. *Chlamydia trachomatis* causes trachoma, the Egyptian eye disease that starts as conjunctivitis and leads to blindness, and the venereal disease lymphogranuloma venereum. In both cases transmission is by contact. *C. psittaci* is the causative agent of ornithoses, the best known of which is a psittacosis, a feverish pneumonia. The main hosts of chlamydiae are birds.

On the basis of their biochemical characteristics, chlamydiae belong to the prokaryotes (bacteria) and not, as formerly thought, to the viruses. They contain RNA and DNA in a ratio characteristic of bacteria, and they synthesise substances which eukaryotic cells are unable to produce, such as muramic acid, diaminopimelic acid, D-alanine, and folic acid. These properties are in accord with their sensitivity to penicillin and sulphonamides. Their genome is very small (relative size, 0.66×10^9) and corresponds to only about one quarter of the genetic information of *E. coli*. Chlamydiae grow only in living cells and are cultured in chicken eggs and tissue cultures. Their dependence on the metabolism of host cells is apparently due to absence of an ATP-generating system of their own. They are unable to phosphorylate glucose or to metabolise it. On the other hand, they are extraordinarily permeable to ATP and CoA. They can therefore be regarded as 'energy parasites'.

The obligate cell parasites among the bacteria are apparently the result of a regressive development. Their adaptation to their host cells has been accompanied by loss of various synthetic capacities.

3.19   The mycoplasma group

The members of the Mycoplasma group (class Mollicutes) are the smallest independently replicating prokaryotes. They do not have any cell walls. Since the protoplasts are surrounded only by a cytoplasmic membrane, they are osmotically extremely labile. The genome size of several mycoplasmas (*Mycoplasma* and *Ureaplasma*) corresponds to only a fraction of that of *E. coli*. With a chromosome size of 500–900 kb, they have the smallest genome of any prokaryote capable of autoreplication. The order Mycoplasmatales has therefore been elevated to a special class of bacteria with the name **Mollicutes** (soft skinned) to express the phylogenetic differentiation of this group from all other bacteria.

The first representative of the mycoplasmas described was the causative organism of pleuropneumonia, a lung infection of cattle. This organism grows on agar media containing serum in small colonies that have a 'fried-egg' appearance. Similar growth forms have therefore been designated as *p*leuro*p*neumonia-*l*ike *o*rganisms (PPLO). Mycoplasmas have been recognised as causative organisms for a number of diseases, as contaminants in tissue cultures, and as harmless saprophytes. The colonies consist of cells and fragments of various sizes and can be described as cocci, filaments, discs and rosettes. They multiply by binary fission, by fragmentation of filaments and rings into coccoid cells, and by a kind of sprouting. In liquid media they are often found as very irregular and sometimes branched forms (Fig. 3.21) that can pass through membrane filters, rather like viruses.

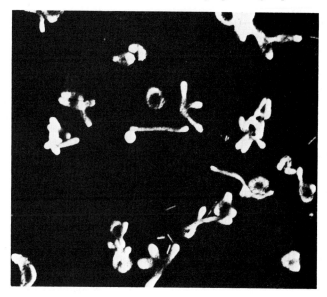

Fig. 3.21. *Mycoplasma*.

Cells of the organism causing broncho-pneumonia in the rat, grown submerged in nutrient solution. Electron micrograph, × 11200.

(From Klieneberger-Nobel, E. & Cuchow, F. W. (1955). *J. gen. Microbiol.* **12**, 95.)

Distribution and species.   The members of the Mycoplasma group (genera *Mycoplasma, Acholeplasma*, and *Spiroplasma*) are parasitic bacteria. They do not kill their hosts, but they produce predominantly chronic infections, and in this sense they are very successful parasites.

In animals they may appear as harmless parasites on the serous epithelia of the respiratory and genital tracts (in mammals and birds). They are membrane parasites in that they adhere tightly to the epithelial cells of the serous membranes. They do not excrete toxins but because of the intimate contact between the parasite, which does not have a cell wall, and the host cell, even weakly toxic metabolites like ammonium ions and hydrogen peroxide may have toxic effects on the host cells. The animal parasites of the mycoplasma group are divided into two genera. The members of the genus *Mycoplasma* require cholesterol or addition of complex steroids for growth (i.e. media containing blood serum). For the genera that do not require cholesterol or similar materials, a new genus *Acholeplasma* has been designated. Whilst infections with mycoplasmas can be symptomless in some animals, inflammation of the respiratory system, the lungs or udder occur in others. The host specificities of *Mycoplasma* species are expressed in the species designation, as in *M. canis, M. gallisepticum, M. hominis.*

In plants mycoplasmas cause yellowing diseases. They are predominantly localised in the phloem part of the vascular system, and, because of their morphological similarity to a spirillum, they have been collected in the genus *Spiroplasma. Spiroplasma citri* causes a yellowing disease in citrus trees. Similar forms have been demonstrated in other plants (maize, rice, Bermuda grass, etc.). *Spiroplasma* has also been found in bees and grasshoppers and it may be assumed that insects are not only carriers but also hosts of *Spiroplasma* species.

Biochemical properties.   The Mycoplasma group is differentiated from all other bacteria not only by the lack of a cell wall, but also by biochemical characters. The organisms grow only in isotonic or hypertonic media (with sorbitol or sucrose) and require purines and pyrimidines, as well as lipids and steroids. The lack of quinones and cytochromes suggests a very limited respiratory chain.

Relation to L-forms.   A strain of *Streptobacillus moniliformis* that grew as irregular protoplasts was isolated in 1934. These cells were called L-forms after the Lister Institute in London where they were isolated. Naked protoplasts that are able to grow can also be isolated from *Salmonella, E. coli* and *Proteus* as well as from other bacteria by cultivation on serum agar with penicillin (100 μg/ml). They produce 'fried-egg' type colonies which resemble those of the *Mycoplasma* species above. Two types of L-forms have been isolated: labile forms, which revert back to normal cells with complete cell walls on cultivation without penicillin; and stable forms, which do not form cell walls even in the absence of penicillin. It was at first assumed that the *Mycoplasma* types arose by mutation of normal bacteria to stable L-forms. However, genome size and GC content of mycoplasmas contradict their origin from eubacteria and suggest that they constitute a separate class.

3.20   Anaerobic anoxygenic phototrophic bacteria

The anaerobic phototrophic bacteria (Rhodospirillales) are characterised by their possession of photosynthetic pigments and by their dependence on light as an energy source. **Four families** are distinguished on the basis of important physiological properties: purple sulphur bacteria (Chromatiaceae), non-sulphur purple bacteria (Rhodospirillaceae), green sulphur bacteria (Chlorobiaceae), and the *Chloroflexus* group (Chloro-flexaceae). They constitute a natural phylogenetic group and will be discussed in relation to photosynthesis in Chapter 12.

3.21   Aerobic oxygenic phototrophic bacteria: cyanobacteria

Because of their mode of cell division by binary fission, the cyanobacteria were grouped with the bacteria as Schizophyta for quite a long time. But because of physiological properties that they share with green plants, they were also assigned to the plant kingdom and called the 'blue-green algae'. They were thus treated according to the taxonomic rules of the botanists. When it became possible to distinguish unequivocally between the prokaryotes and eukaryotes, the cyanobacteria were allocated to the bacteria.

The cyanobacteria share with the algae and higher plants photosynthesis accompanied by release of molecular oxygen, as well as the possession of chlorophyll *a* and other pigments. They were therefore regarded as algae and designated the blue-green algae. However, F. Cohn had already regarded them as Schizophyceae on the basis of their cell division, and hence as belonging with the Schizomycetes (today's bacteria) to the Schizophyta. In fact, their cellular structure, murein-containing cell wall, possession of 70S ribosomes, and other important properties characterise them as gram-negative prokaryotes. The cyanobacteria are the largest, most diverse, most widely distributed group of photosynthetic prokaryotes, and their abilities to grow in extreme habitats and to fix atmospheric nitrogen render them of great importance in the economy of nature. Some cyanobacteria are motile. Their movement, though, is never produced via flagella, but consists of gliding or crawling over solid surfaces. Such gliding movement is also characteristic of some other groups of bacteria.

Morphology and classification.   The cyanobacteria include unicellular and multicellular forms and can be divided into five groups on the basis of their morphology (Fig. 3.22).

> Group 1. Unicellular rods and cocci are collected in the group **chroococcal cyanobacteria**. The cells are seen either as individuals or as aggregates which are kept together by capsules or slime. Cell division occurs only by binary fission or budding. This group includes *Synechococcus* (formerly *Anacystis nidulans*), *Gloeocapsa*, *Gloeothece* and *Gloeobacter violaceus*.

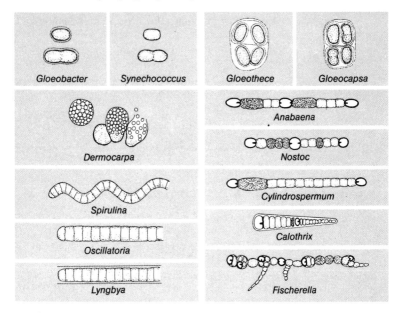

Fig. 3.22. *Cyanobacteria.*

Heavily drawn cell walls and polar granules characterise heterocyts; solid cells represent akinetes; thin lines outside trichomes characterise sheaths. (Redrawn from Rippka, R., Deruelles, J., Waterburry, J. B., Herdman, M. & Stanier, R. Y. (1979). *J. gen. Microbiol.* **III**, 1.)

Group 2. The **pleurocapsular cyanobacteria** also includes unicellular forms, but only those which can also multiply by multiple fission. During this process, many small cells, so-called baeocytes, appear within the dividing mother cell. Examples of this group are *Pleurocapsa, Dermocarpa* and *Myxosarcina.*

The following three groups are characterised by threadlike cell aggregates; they form trichomes (chains of cells). Growth is intercalatary, that is, by cell division within the trichome. The trichomes exhibit gliding motility. Multiplication also occurs through breakup of the trichomes and formation of hormogonia. For this reason, these filamentous blue-green algae have also been called 'hormogonal blue algae'. Three groups of such trichome-forming cyanobacteria are now identified.

Group 3. **Filamentous cyanobacteria without heterocysts**. Here the trichomes consist only of vegetative cells. Typical of this group are *Oscillatoria, Spirulina, Lyngbya, Phormidium* and *Plectonema.*

Group 4. **Filamentous cyanobacteria with heterocysts**. When trichomes are grown without fixed nitrogen, they differentiate into heterocysts. In some cases, akinetes (thick-walled, resting cells) may occur. This group includes the genera *Anabaena, Nostoc* and *Calothrix.*

Group 5. **Filamentous cyanobacteria with heterocysts**. The members of this group differ from those of the previous group by their cell division in more than one plane. The best-known genus in this group is *Fischerella.*

Ecology.   The cyanobacteria are distributed in lakes and other waters, in soil, and in rice fields. They can be seen with the naked eye as dark blue or black growth on rocks and in the littoral zone of freshwater lakes and in the oceans. The black lines (referred to as ink streaks) that are often seen on chalk cliffs and boulders and mark the watershed are due to chroococcal cyanobacteria. In eutrophic lakes there are often sudden blooms of blue-green (*Anabaena*) or red-tinted (*Oscillatoria rubescens*) cyanobacteria (see Ch. 17.1). Their ability to fix atmospheric nitrogen enables many cyanobacteria to occur as 'pioneers' in poor habitats such as sandy beaches and desert rocks. They can find protection and moisture in crevices and fissures and are able to grow endolithically. Nor are they discouraged by other extremes. Some unicellular cyanobacteria (*Synechococcus lividus*) are so acid-tolerant that they can grow in hot acid springs (pH 4.0, 70 °C). Other species live symbiotically: *Nostoc* lives in the lichen *Peltigera* and in the roots of *Cycas* and *Gunnera*; *Anabaena azollae* grows in the leafy cavity of the tropical aquatic fern *Azolla.*

The cell: structure and components.   The detailed architecture and cellular fine structure of the cyanobacteria conform almost completely to that of the gram-negative bacteria (Fig. 2.4). The protoplast is surrounded by a cell wall which has a peptidoglycan layer enclosed by an outer membrane containing lipopolysaccharides. Many forms excrete exopolysaccharides as soluble slime, or as **capsules** that surround individual cells, or as **sheaths** that surround the trichomes.

The **photosynthetic apparatus** is present in the form of **thylakoids**, which occur either parallel to the cytoplasmic membrane or coiled at the periphery of the protoplasmic space (Fig. 3.23). The thylakoid membrane contains chlorophyll *a*, β-carotene, and oxo-carotenoids like myxoxanthophyll, echinenon, and zeaxanthin, as well as components of the

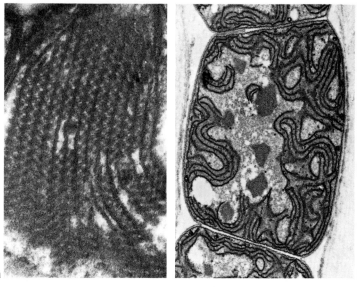

Fig. 3.23. *The photosynthetic membrane systems of cyanobacteria.*

(a) Rows of phycobilisomes on the thylakoid membranes of *Microcoleus vaginatus.* (b) In *Nostoc muscorum* the double lamellae (thylakoid membranes) appear wavy, singly, or in groups. The outer layer of the multi-layered cell wall is visible. (a) From Wildman, R. B. & Bowen, C. C. (1974). *J. Bacteriol.* **117**, 866. (b) From Menke, EW. (1961). *Z. Naturforsch.* **16b**, 543.

photosynthetic electron transport system. The special feature of the thylakoids of cyanobacteria (and red algae) are the phycobilisomes, disclike structures attached to the outer surface of the thylakoids. They consist of the phycobiliproteins phycocyanin (75%), allophycocyanin (12%) and phycoerythrin, and some colourless polypeptides. The last two components constitute about 12%. The phycobiliproteins in turn are composed of proteins and their prosthetic groups, **phycocyanobilin** and **phycoerythrobilin**. They function as 'pigment antennae' and deliver the energy that they absorb mainly to photosystem II. Chlorophyll *a* serves only photosystem I. The phycobilisomes can constitute up to 50% of the total cellular protein.

The **phycobilins** are very similar to bile pigments. During their synthesis, porphyrin is formed first; on opening of the ring, the methylene carbon atoms are released as carbon monoxide. The synthesis of phycobilin is one of the few processes where carbon monoxide is known to be formed.

Only one of the cyanobacteria, *Gloeobacter violaceus*, lacks thylakoids and phycobilisomes; it has chlorophyll *a* localised in the cytoplasmic membrane and the phycobiliproteins are attached as a continuous layer to the internal surface of the cytoplasmic membrane.

In many of the cyanobacteria the composition of incident light influences the ratio of blue and red pigments. In green and blue light, phycoerythrin is synthesised predominantly; in red light, phycocyanin is predominant. This complementary 'chromatic adaptation' ensures efficient utilisation of light in such habitats as under leaf canopies, or in the blue light of deep waters.

Cellular inclusions. All the cyanobacteria are apparently capable of accumulating polysaccharides in the form of **glycogen** granules and phosphate as **polyphosphate** granules, whilst **poly-β-hydroxybutyrate** is stored by only a few species.

Cyanophycine granules are a type of storage material that is found only in cyanobacteria. They have been identified as polypeptides by their positive reaction with protein dyes. They consist of poly-aspartate with arginine attached to all the free carboxyl groups, so that they contain aspartate and arginine in the ratio 1:1. This polymer apparently functions as a nitrogen reserve. It decreases under nitrogen starvation and increases again on addition of a nitrogen source. It is stored predominantly in the heterocysts. However, it may also function, to a lesser degree, as an energy store, since arginine can serve to regenerate ATP under anaerobic conditions, via breakdown into ornithine and carbamoyl phosphate.

Carboxysomes (see Ch. 2.2.7) are found in many cyanobacteria. **Gas vacuoles** are commonly found in aquatic forms that occur in stratified waters or as algal blooms.

Specialised cells. Cyanobacteria are able to form a number of highly specialised cell structures, which have no parallel in other groups of bacteria.

Heterocysts can be observed in the light microscope by virtue of their thick cell walls, weak pigmentation, and refractile polar granules. Electron microscopy allows observation of their detailed structure (Fig. 3.24). The polar granules are cyanophycin grains, and the compact layers that surround the gram-negative cell wall consist of polysaccharides of glucose, galactose, mannose, and xylose in β-1,3-glycosidic linkage. Heterocysts are resistant to the action of lysozyme. They are connected to the neighbouring vegetative cells of the trichome by pores.

The heterocysts function **as the sites for nitrogen fixation** under aerobic conditions. They are formed in response to a lack of fixed nitrogen

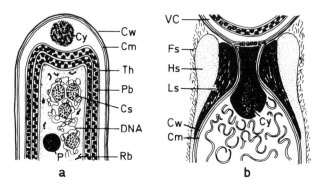

Fig. 3.24. *Longitudinal sections through cells of cyanobacteria.*

(a) Vegetative cell; (b) heterocyst.
Cm, cytoplasmic membrane; Cs,
carboxysomes;
Cy, cyanophycin bodies; Fs, fibrous
layer; Hs, homogenous layer; Ls,
lamellar layer; P, polyphosphate;

Pb, phycobilisome; Rb, ribosomes;
Th, thylakoid; VC, vegetative cell;
Cw, cell wall.
(Redrawn after Stanier, R. Y. & Cohen-
Bazire, G. (1977). *Ann. Rev. Microbiol.*
31, 225.)

(NH_4 or NO_3). The morphological differentiation is accompanied by biochemical alterations. Nitrogenase is synthesised whilst the phycobiliproteins are degraded, though chlorophyll *a* is conserved. The mature heterocysts, therefore, contain no phycobiliproteins and no functional photosystem II, and they cannot produce oxygen. They contain only photosystem I, which enables them to carry out cyclic photophosphorylation and ATP regeneration. These changes provide the appropriate conditions for the functioning of the oxygen-sensitive nitrogenase. Heterocysts are supplied with organic carbon compounds by the vegetative cells and deliver fixed nitrogen mainly in the form of glutamine.

Akinetes are 'survival' forms. They are recognised by their size, intense pigmentation and thick cell walls. They are morphologically differentiated cells, analogous to the heterocysts, and are either intercalated in (in *Anabaena*) or terminally arranged on (in *Cylindrospermum*) the trichomes (Fig. 3.22).

Hormogonia are short sections of the trichome formed by breakage of longer filaments. Their formation promotes propagation. In *Oscillatoria* their formation entails the sacrifice of at least one cell of the trichome, as the cells are connected by a common peptidoglycan layer that is not divisible. This is referred to as 'transcellular division'.

Baeocytes are small spherical reproductive cells of the pleurocapsulated cyanobacteria. They are formed by multiple fission within a considerably enlarged cell that is surrounded by a thick fibrous exopolysaccharide layer. In *Dermocarpa*, for example, rapid binary divisions lead to the formation of from 4 to 1000 baeocytes.

Gliding movements.   Many of the cyanobacteria are motile, for example, the trichome-forming varieties, all hormogonia, and many baeocytes. Movement is possible only by gliding, which requires a solid surface. The movement takes place by rotation of the trichome around its longitudinal axis, which makes the threadlike fibrils appear to swing or to oscillate (*Oscillatoria*). A spot of dye applied to the surface of *Oscillatoria princeps* was found to describe a helical line with a 60° pitch during forward motion. Studies of the fine structure showed fibrils inside the cell wall with a similar helical turn. This correlation suggests that the movement may be based on torsional waves by the fibrillae. The direction of movement can be reversed and many cyanobacteria are phototactic and accumulate in areas of suitable illumination.

Nitrogen fixation.   All cyanobacteria that can form heterocysts are capable of nitrogen fixation. The heterocysts are cells that are morphologically and physiologically specialised for nitrogen fixation (see section above on heterocysts). The discovery that the genetic information for the synthesis of nitrogenase (the *nif* gene) is present even in pleurocapsular cells and in non-heterocyst-forming cyanobacteria (*Oscillatoria* group) was surprising at first. It appears that the expression of nitrogen fixation is blocked under the usual growth conditions in the light (in these organisms) because the enzyme nitrogenase is extremely sensitive to oxygen. However, the synthesis of the enzyme can be derepressed and its presence can be demonstrated by suitable manipulation of conditions. Incubation of cells in the absence of fixed nitrogen, anaerobically in the light, but with addition of the herbicide DCMU (dichlorophenylmethylurea) to inhibit photosystem II and hence the evolution of oxygen, leads to formation of nitrogenase. With this technique it has been possible to show that more than 50% of all strains examined have the ability to produce nitrogenase. Some of the strains of chroococcal cyanobacteria are also capable of nitrogen fixation. How the nitrogenase in these is protected from the photosynthetically produced oxygen is not known.

Anaerobic metabolism.   Several cyanobacteria are found in waters that have significant concentrations of H_2S (about 5 mmol/l). Studies of *Oscillatoria limnetica* have shown that photosystem II is inactive in the presence of H_2S and that an anaerobic, anoxygenic photosynthesis takes place, similar to that known to occur in the anaerobic purple sulphur bacteria:

$$CO_2 + 2H_2S \rightarrow \langle CH_2O \rangle + H_2O + 2S$$

The ability of many cyanobacteria to function as facultative anaerobes is probably important in only a few habitats.

Obligate photoautotrophy.   Many of the cyanobacteria are apparently obligate photoautotrophs; they can grow only in the light. Only a few strains can grow chemo-organotrophically by oxidation of sugars in the dark. In these cases the growth rates are always much lower than under photo-autotrophic conditions.

Prochloral bacteria.   Phototrophic organisms, which show some characteristics of prokaryotes together with some of green algae, have been discovered recently. On the one hand they have the typical cell structure of prokaryotes (gram-negative cell wall with peptidoglycan, no organelles or true nucleus, DNA genome size of 3.6×10^9) but they contain in addition to chlorophyll a, chlorophyll b, which is found only in green algae. They are also distinguished from cyanobacteria by the absence of phycobilin protein, cyanophycin and poly-β-hydroxybutyrate. Up to now, two members of this group of bacteria, closely related to the cyanobacteria, have been found. *Prochloron* grows as an exosymbiont on several members of the Ascidia, but hardly grows on any synthetic media. *Prochlorothrix hollandica* is a thread-like organism, free-living in freshwater, and can be cultured on mineral medium, in the light.

4   The viruses: distribution and structure

The designation 'virus' (poison) was used originally for pathogenic agents about which very little was known. The term eventually came to mean the group of causative agents that could pass through bacterial filters (as discovered by Iwanovski in 1892) known as 'filterable viruses' or simply 'viruses'.

The viruses differ from microorganisms in the following properties. (1) They contain only one kind of nucleic acid, either RNA or DNA (Table 4.1). (2) Only the nucleic acid is necessary (but not sufficient) for their reproduction. (3) They are unable to reproduce outside living cells. Thus, viruses are not independent organisms but use living cells for their multiplication. Reproduction occurs within the host cell, since the virus depends on the host cell for the replication of its nucleic acid and the synthesis of its protein coat. This process usually leads to the death of the host cell. Outside the host cell the terms 'virus particle' or 'virion' are used. The virus particle consists of nucleic acid and a protein coat, known as the **'capsid'**. The virus particle is thus a **nucleocapsid**. Sometimes there is also an envelope.

Viruses become demonstrable by the consequences of their development in the host. They destroy whole cell complexes and produce tissue damage, necrotic areas, and lytic halos (Fig. 4.1). Plants, animals and microorganisms are the natural hosts for viruses.

Plant viruses.   Plant viruses gain entrance to their hosts through lesions; they do not actively penetrate into plant tissues. The quantitative determination of plant viruses is based on the development of necrotic spots around artificially produced primary lesions. In nature the viruses are spread by vectors or by direct contact. Frequently, viruses enter into leaf tissue through injuries produced by rubbing. The plant parasite *Cuscuta* can penetrate into plants by means of its haustoria and it then establishes a direct link between plants with its conducting system over which the viruses can be transported. Many viruses are spread by insects. In some cases, the virus multiplies in the alimentary tract of the insect (persistent viruses); new infections of plants can occur only after a certain incubation period in the insect. Non-persistent viruses are transmitted directly and passively by the insect sting or bite. Many plant diseases

143

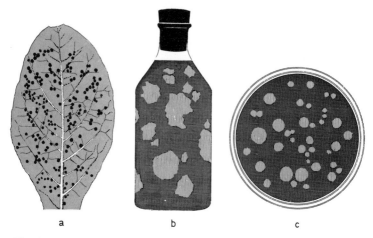

Fig. 4.1. *Demonstration of viruses by the necrotic spots or lytic zones they produce.*

(a) Necrotic spots of tobacco mosaic virus on a tobacco leaf. (b) Lytic zones of poliomyelitis virus in a tissue culture. (c) Lytic zones or plaques of bacteriophage on a confluent bacterial culture.

are caused by viruses. Potato viruses are of great economic importance. The most intensively investigated and best-known plant virus is the tobacco mosaic virus (TMV). Most plant viruses have RNA as their genetic material.

Animal (pathogenic) viruses. In humans and other animals, viruses cause many diseases; smallpox, chickenpox, measles, rabies, poliomyelits, influenza, the common cold, foot-and-mouth disease (of cattle), etc. Animal viruses are also transmitted by direct contact or via insects, and they apparently gain entry into the host cell by phagocytosis or pinocytosis. To investigate viruses in the laboratory it is necessary to use experimental animals or fertilised chicken eggs. Some viruses, however, can be cultivated in tissue cultures, and their presence can be determined quantitatively. The genetic material of animal viruses can be either DNA or RNA. Whilst DNA is usually present as a double-stranded helix, RNA is found single-stranded or double-stranded.

Bacterial viruses. Viruses that use bacterial cells as hosts are called bacteriophages. There is hardly a single species of bacteria where sufficient investigation has not found a phage. The presence of bacteriophages is recognized by the appearance of 'plaques' or lytic holes in a continuous bacterial lawn. In a bacterial suspension, phage multiplication can lead to complete lysis in a short time. Phage nucleic acid occurs either as double- or single-stranded DNA, or as a single- or double-stranded RNA. The phages of *E. coli* have served as models for bacteriophages generally. Such research on phages and their reproductive cycles has yielded important insights into the transmission of genetic material from cell to cell.

4.1   Viruses

Structure of viruses.   A **virus particle** or **virion** consists of nucleic acid. DNA or RNA, that is covered by a protein coat called a **capsid**. The combined nucleic acid and capsid, called the **nucleocapsid**, can be either naked or enclosed by a **membrane** (Figs 4.2, 4.3). TMV, papilloma viruses and adenoviruses, for example, are naked nucleocapsids. Among the enveloped viruses are influenza virus and herpes. The capsid itself consists of subunits called **capsomers**. In most cases the capsids are symmetrically constructed. Two kinds of symmetry have been recognised: helical symmetry and cubical symmetry.

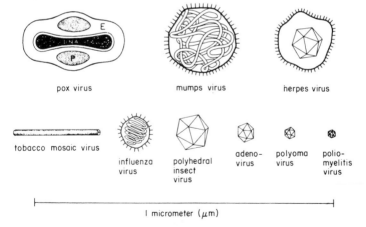

pox virus

mumps virus

herpes virus

tobacco mosaic virus

influenza virus

polyhedral insect virus

adeno-virus

polyoma virus

polio-myelitis virus

|— 1 micrometer (μm) —|

Fig. 4.2. *Form and size of various virus particles.*

DNA, virus DNA;
P, elliptical protein body;
E, envelope.

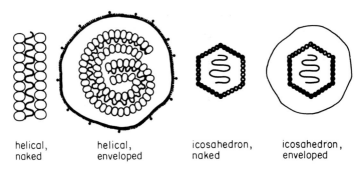

| helical, | helical, | icosahedron, | icosahedron, |
| naked | enveloped | naked | enveloped |

Fig. 4.3. *Structural types of virus particles.*

Four architectural types are represented: two with helical and two with cubical symmetry, each as a naked and an enveloped virion.

Classification of viruses. Viruses are extremely host-specific, and within a given host also tissue- and cell-specific. Among the animal pathogens, for example, those that develop in nerve cells are called neurotrophic, those that are found in lymphocytes are called lymphotrophic and those that are specialised for mucous membranes and epithelial cells are called myxotrophic viruses.

The viruses pathogenic for higher plants are named according to the host and the visible effects that they produce. Very few viruses that attack algae, fungi or protozoa have so far been examined – or discovered. There are, therefore, no attempts yet to classify these. Bacteriophages are named after the host organism where they were first discovered, and are then given letter and number identification.

The classification of animal pathogens is usually limited to family names which are commonly based on disease symptoms (pustules, swellings, tumours), nature and size of its nucleic acid (pico-RNA) or on the nucleic acid replication mechanism (retroviruses). The number of known viruses is immense and this very condensed survey can in no way do justice to their role as pathogens nor to the part they have played in research that has led to the enormous progress in molecular biology.

Structural forms of viruses. In the following sections four viruses known to cause disease will be described: two virions with helical symmetries, one with no envelope (TMV) and one with an envelope (influenza virus), and two virions with cubical symmetry, one with no envelope (poliomyelitis) and one with an envelope (herpes). Table 4.1 represents a survey of viruses according to their structural properties.

Table 4.1. *Morphological classes of viruses*

Naked capsids		Capsids with envelopes	
Helical structure			
RNA	tobacco mosaic virus and many other plant viruses	RNA	myxoviruses: influenza virus, parainfluenza virus, mumps, measles
DNA	coliphage fd		
Polyhedral structure (icosahedron)			
RNA	picornaviruses: foot and mouth, ECHO, polio, reoviruses	RNA	retroviruses[a]: sarcoma, leukaemia, carcinoma
cyclic DNA	papovaviruses[a]: papilloma, polyoma	RNA	togaviruses: SFV, encephalitis, yellow fever
	SV40	DNA	herpes simplex (shingles),
single-stranded cyclic DNA	coliphage ΦX174, M113		varicella (chicken-pox), EB virus (infectious mononucleosis)
Composite viruses (icosahedral head + helical tail)			
DNA	large bacteriophages: (T2, T4, T6)		
Complex virions			
DNA	pox viruses (Variola) cowpox (vaccinia)		

SFV, Semliki Forest Virus; EB, Epstein–Barr; SV, Simian Virus;
ECHO, Enteric Cytopathic Human Orphan virus.
[a] Oncogenic viruses.

Tobacco mosaic virus. TMV is the model example of a virion with helical symmetry. It can be easily obtained from expressed juice of TMV-infected plants.It is rod-shaped with a diameter of 18 nm (Fig. 4.4a). This rod-shaped nucleocapsid consists of about 2100 capsomers, which are helically arranged to form a hollow cylinder. Each capsomer is a polypeptide chain consisting of 158 amino acids in known sequence. The RNA is embedded in the wall of the hollow cylinder between the capsomers, the RNA strand following the helical arrangement (Fig. 4.4b).

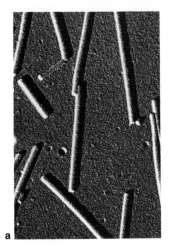
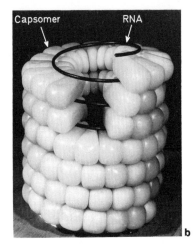

Fig. 4.4. *Tobacco mosaic virus.*

(a) Electron micrograph after carbon-platinum shadowing, × 65 000. (Picture: H. Frank.)

(b) Model (from Karlson (1980). *A Short Textbook of Biochemistry.* Stuttgart: Thieme.)

Influenza virus.   The particles of influenza virus have a diameter of 110 nm (Fig. 4.5a). The nucleocapsid is helically arranged as in TMV, though it is not rod-shaped, but multiply twisted or 'rolled up' (Fig. 4.5b). The nucleocapsid is surrounded by an envelope which is part of the membrane of the host cell from which the virion originated. The envelope has spikes on its outer surface; these serve to adsorb the virion to the host cell and contain proteins and the enzyme neuraminidase. This enzyme splits a component of the host-cell membrane (*N*-acetylneuraminic acid) and apparently renders the mucus that covers the epithelium of the nasopharyngeal tract more liquid. Multiplication of the virus takes place inside the host cell, whilst the liberation of the virions occurs by a kind of budding. Observation of this process led to the recognition that the envelope of the virus particle consists of the host-cell membrane, though the latter may be modified by virus-coded proteins (e.g. neuraminidase).

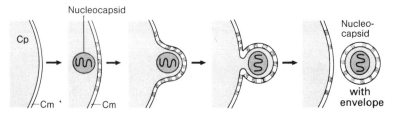

Influenza virus occurs in a great many varieties. The target tissues that are attacked depend on the host specificity of the virus and on the receptor properties of the cells. The virus attack can lead to inhibition of cellular metabolism or to the destruction of the cell. The virus is antigenic and induces formation of antibodies by the hosts. The virus strains responsible for the large influenza epidemics are characterised by their virulence and pathogenicity.

Polyhedral viruses without envelope.   Many viruses that appear spherical are actually polyhedral. The preferred polyhedral form is the icosahedron (20 faces), a body of 20 equilateral triangles and 12 vertices (Figs 4.5c, 4.6). The capsid of such viruses consists of two types of capsomers: in the vertices there are five-cornered pentons consisting of five proteins (protomers); the planes and edges are occupied by six-cornered hexons consisting of six protomers. The assembly of the capsid from the capsomers follows the laws of crystallography; according to these the smallest icosahedral capsid would consist of 12 pentons, the next larger one would have 12 pentons and 20 hexons. There are viruses that have 252, and even 812 capsomers. A large number of viruses are arranged on the icosahedral principle; the poliomyelitus virus, the virus of foot-and-mouth disease, adenoviruses and the SV40 tumour virus are examples (Fig. 4.5d).

> Construction of the virus capsid from many identical subunits may be explained by the fact that the nucleic acids of many viruses have only a small particle weight, i.e. are quite short. Their information content therefore suffices for only a few polypeptide chains. Of these the majority have to have enzymic functions for the reproduction of the virus in the host cell. The principle of constructing the capsid from a large number of identical subunits guarantees the maximal effectiveness for a minimum expenditure of genetic information.

Polyhedral viruses with envelopes.   The architectural form of an icosahedron surrounded by an envelope is found, for example, in the causative agents of chickenpox (*Varicella*), shingles (*Herpes zoster*) and vesicular stomatitis.

The icosahedral capsid of herpes viruses consists of 162 capsomers. The envelope is almost certainly derived from the inner nuclear membrane of the host cell. Herpes viruses multiply inside the nucleus of the host cell. The capsids are covered by the inner nuclear membrane of the host, liberated by budding, and guided to the outer surface by the endoplasmic reticulum. Chickenpox is a non-serious disease of children. The varicella virus infects the upper respiratory tract and is then distributed by the circulatory system; eventually the virions settle in the skin and

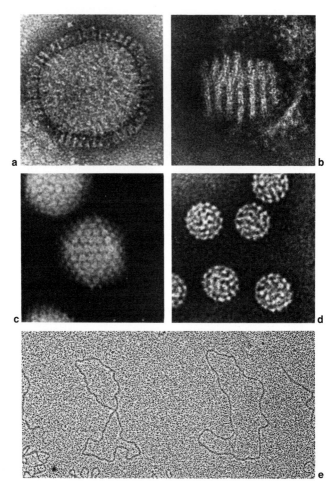

Fig. 4.5. *Some animal viruses and their nucleic acids.*

(a) Influenza virus A2. (b) Nucleocapsid of influenza virus A2; the
contrast medium, phosphotungstic
acid, has penetrated into a broken
particle as in (a), and made the
nucleocapsid visible. (c) Adenovirus;
the icosahedral form of the particle
can be recognised. (d) SV40 (Simian
virus 40); this tumour virus, much
smaller than adenovirus, appears
round although it is also constructed on the icosahedral
principle. (e) DNA of SV40; the
double-stranded circular DNA

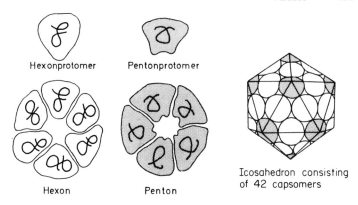

Hexonprotomer   Pentonprotomer

Hexon   Penton

Icosahedron consisting
of 42 capsomers

Fig. 4.6. *Possible capsid components of icosahedral viruses.*

Two types of capsomers are represented, a hexagonal capsomer (hexon) and a pentagonal capsomer (penton); the former consists of six protomers, and the latter consists of five protomers. Protomers, in turn, consist of one or two polypeptide chains. At the right, an icosahedron consisting of 42 capsomers: 12 pentons and 30 hexons.

cause the typical flat blisters. Shingles is found in partially immune persons; it is apparently produced by reactivation of the varicella virus. Both illnesses are thus caused by the same virus.

Pox viruses.   The pox viruses are the largest among the animal pathogens. Their construction is quite different from the four types mentioned above. They contain DNA, proteins, and several lipids. They are therefore called complex virions (Table 4.1). The virus particles of smallpox (variola) and of cowpox (vaccinia) have the shape of a rounded-off square. They consist of an inner body which contains the double-stranded DNA, a protein-containing double layer, elliptical protein bodies, and a covering membrane; all of this is covered by closely applied threads. The virus particles are very resistant to dehydration and, hence, very infectious. Smallpox is a disease to which only primates (humans and apes) are susceptible. Cattle, rabbits and sheep, on the other hand, are sensitive to vaccinia virus. Both viruses, vaccinia and variola, have common

Fig. 4.5 (*cont.*)

molecules have a contour length of about 1.7 μm; at the right and left the ends of broken circles can be seen. Magnification: (a–d) × 250 000; (e) × 65 000. Preparation: (a–d) negative contrast with phosphotungstic acid. (Pictures: (a, b, d, e) H. Frank; (c) H. Gelderblom, Max-Planck-Institute for Virus Research.)

antigens. This is the reason that protective vaccination against smallpox makes use of vaccinia virus obtained from calves, which produces only a very mild reaction in man. This active vaccination leads to the production of serum antibodies that also confer immunity against smallpox (variola virus).

4.2   Bacterial viruses (bacteriophages)

Isolation and demonstration.   Bacteriophages can be easily isolated by suspending a host bacterium in a nutrient medium and inoculating with material from a location where the bacterial strain occurs naturally. If this enrichment culture is incubated under conditions that are favourable for the bacteria in question, the phages present in the inoculum can multiply rapidly. The virus, of course, will multiply only in living cells. By filtering or centrifuging down the unaffected cells, one can obtain a supernatant 'lysate' in which the number of phage particles can be determined (titrated). This makes use of the fact that whilst solid media inoculated with a phage-free bacterial suspension and suitably incubated will produce a continuous 'lawn' of bacterial growth, inoculation with a suspension containing countable numbers of bacteriophage particles will produce 'plaques' (holes) in the bacterial lawn. In each place where a phage particle was deposited and attacked a bacterial cell, rapid lysis of increasing numbers of adjoining bacteria (attacked by progeny of the original phage particle) will lead, after a certain time, to bacteria-free spots, i.e. 'plaques'. These can be easily distinguished macroscopically from the background of confluent growth and hence can be counted (Fig. 4.1c). By using appropriate methods, one can obtain rapid multiplication of phages in bacterial suspensions, or from growth of bacteria on solid media. The bacteria are removed by centrifugation and any remaining in the supernatant can be killed with chloroform, so that a phage lysate containing 10^{10}–10^{13} phage particles/ml can be obtained.

Morphology of bacteriophages.   The shape and form of bacteriophages has been elucidated mainly for the T series of *E. coli* phages. The coliphage T2 consists of a polyhedral head, about 100 nm in length, and a tail of similar length. It is therefore called a composite virus (Table 4.1). The head consists of capsomers and contains DNA; protein and DNA each comprise about 50% of the head. The tail of coliphage T2 has a rather complicated structure consisting of at least three parts. A hollow stylus is surrounded by a contractile sheath which bears on its distal end a base plate covered with claw-like tail fibres and host-specific adsorption spikes. Electron microscopy of negatively stained preparations shows two alter-

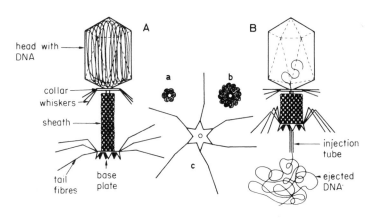

Fig. 4.7. *Model of a T2 phage.*

(A) Phage with stretched sheath before adsorption. (B) Phage with contracted sheath after adsorption and injection. (a) Transverse section through the stretched tail; 6 sheath-protein units in one plane.

(b) Transverse section through the contracted tail; 12 sheath-protein units in one plane. (c) View onto the basal plate of a phage ready for adsorption, showing free tail fibres.

Fig. 4.8. *Various shapes of bacterio-phages (a–d) and geometrical shapes of phage heads (e, f).*

(a) Threadlike form of coliphage fd; (b) head (hexagonal outline) and tail with contractile sheath (e.g., coliphage T2, T4, and T6); (c) head with long, flexible, non-contractile tail (e.g. coliphages T1 and T5); (d) head with short tail (e.g. coliphages T3 and T7, salmonellaphage P22); (e) Octahedron; (f) icosahedron. (According to Bradley, D. E. (1967). *Bacteriol. Rev.* **31**, 230.)

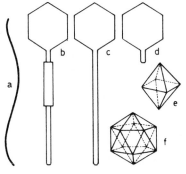

native states. In one of these the head is only weakly contrasted and the sheath appears contracted. In the other, the head is sharply contrasted from an electron-dense background and the sheath appears stretched. Fig. 4.7 is a schematic representation of these observations: (A) represents the active, DNA-containing phage; (B) shows the phage after injection of DNA into a bacterium.

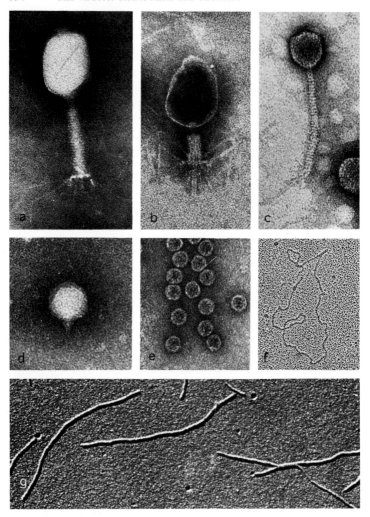

Fig. 4.9. *Several forms of bacteriophages.*

(a) Coliphage T2; (b) T2 with contracted tail protein and emptied head; (c) coliphage lambda; (d) coliphage T7 with short tail; (e) RNA-coliphage fr; (f) circular DNA molecule (replicative form) of coliphage fd; (g) coliphage fd (these have a circular DNA that is single-stranded). Magnification: (a–e) × 168 000; (f, g) × 50 000. Preparation: (a, b) negative contrast with phosphototungstic acid; (c–e) negative contrast with uranylacetate; (f) after spreading in cytochrome and conical shadowing; (g) obliquely shadowed. (Pictures: H. Frank.)

Many bacteriophages are structurally less complex. Several types can be distinguished according to the form of the mature phage (Figs 4.8, 4.9). Most bacteriophages contain double-stranded DNA. In the course of the last few years, however, several phages with single-stranded DNA and some with single-stranded RNA have been discovered. The RNA-containing phages R17 and $Q\beta$ (Fig. 4.9e) have the smallest genomes known: 3500–4500 nucleotides.

4.2.1   Multiplication of a virulent phage: the lytic cycle

The multiplication of viruses in their host cell is a very complicated process. The individual synthetic processes, from attack of the host cell to liberation of the mature phage particles, have been extensively investigated by biochemical, genetic and morphological studies on bacteriophages of the T series (T2, T4 and T6). These investigations made use of the fact that the phage DNA contained 5-hydroxymethylcytosine in place of cytosine, so that phage DNA synthesis could be followed easily. Furthermore, bacteriophage mutants that are blocked in one of the steps of the multiplication process, or able to multiply only under certain conditions, were obtained. These mutants made it possible to follow morphological development of the phage inside its host cell (morphopoeisis) and the temporal sequence in the syntheses of phage units and their assembly.

Like other viruses, bacteriophages are non-motile. When a suspension of free phage particles is mixed with a suitable bacterial suspension, accidental contact leads to attachment of a phage particle to a bacterial surface (adsorption), followed by injection of the phage DNA. Eventually, after a period of synthesis and maturation of phages, lysis of the host cells liberates newly formed phage particles into the suspending medium (Fig. 4.13).

Adsorption.   Not every phage is adsorbed by every bacterium. The specific host–phage relationship is based on the specificity of adsorption. This is determined by the receptors in the cell wall of the bacterium. The receptors for some phages are part of the lipoprotein component and the receptors for other phages are contained in the lipopolysaccharide layer. Lack of such receptors is most probably a cause of phage resistance of a bacterial cell. If phages are added in excess, multiple adsorption of up to 200–300 phages (per host cell) can occur.

Intracellular development of phages.   Following adsorption, the phage injects its DNA into the host cell. In phage T2, this injection apparently

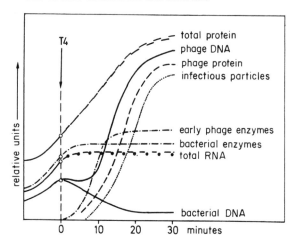

Fig. 4.10. *Time course of biosynthetic processes in* E. coli *after infection with bacteriophage T4.*

(After Luria, S. E. & Darnell, J. E. (1967). *General Virology*, 2nd edn. New York: John Wiley and Sons.)

consists of the anchoring of the base plate and contraction of the sheath which effects penetration of the hollow stylus into the bacterial cell. Experiments with ^{32}P-labelled nucleic acids and ^{35}S-labelled proteins have shown that only the nucleic acid penetrates to the inside of the host cell, the protein remaining on the outside. The protein coat can be sheared from the host cell without any effect on phage multiplication. During the so-called '**latent period**', which in *E. coli* has an average duration of about 25 minutes, no phage could be demonstrated in artificially ruptured bacteria. The injected phage DNA causes an immediate far-reaching change in the metabolism of the infected cell (Fig. 4.10). The synthesis of bacterial DNA stops abruptly. Within a few minutes after infection synthesis of bacterial RNA and proteins also ceases, but the total protein content continues to increase, and DNA synthesis is resumed at an even higher rate. At first, phage DNA is synthesised at the expense of degraded bacterial DNA. This conversion and the subsequent *de novo* synthesis of phage DNA could be followed by measuring the increase in 5-hydroxymethylcytosine, which is specific for some of the T-phages. The enzymes needed for this DNA synthesis are made shortly after injection; these are the so-called 'early proteins'. The 'late

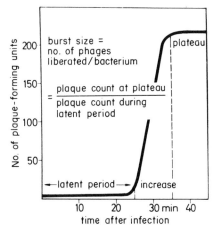

Fig. 4.11. *Determination of latent period and burst size.*

This diagrammatic representation is based on experiments on the multiplacation of phage T2 in *E. coli* B. A young bacterial culture was mixed with a phage suspension. After infection of the cells, the excess, unadsorbed phage was inactivated by addition of phage antiserum. After suitable (high) dilution, samples were removed at regular interals and plated onto agar with excess of phage-sensitive bacteria. The number of plaque-forming units remained at five for 25 minutes (latent period) and then rose to 235 (plateau). This gave an average of 47 phage particles/ infected cell (burst size).

proteins' include the coat proteins and the phage lysozymes or 'endolysins'; these are made only during the second half of the latent period.

The final **maturation** consists of the combination of the phage DNA with the coat proteins to give the mature, infectious phage particle. Maturation of the T phages is a complicated process which occurs in several steps. First, protein-filled capsids are synthesised. After lysis of the proteins in the centre of the capsid, the completed heads are filled with an amount of DNA that is specific for each phage type, and the heads are then closed. Finally, the tail components are added. The sequence of steps was worked out from study of conditionally lethal mutants that can carry out normal synthesis at 25 °C but have various steps blocked at 43 °C.

Eventually the bacterial cell wall is softened by the phage lysozyme and **liberation** of the phage particles follows. This explosive rupture of the bacterial cells can be observed with the dark-field microscope. The duration of the latent period and the burst size vary within wide limits and are dependent on the type of phage, on the bacterial host, and on the milieu (Fig. 4.11). In the case of some bacteria like *Haemophilus influenza* and *Bacillus subtilis*, it has been possible to infect them with native DNA, isolated from bacteriophages. Such treatment, which corresponds to genetic transformation, has been called 'transfection'.

4.2.2   The development of temperate phages: lysogeny

The phages that have been described so far always lyse the infected bacteria and are therefore referred to as **virulent** phages. Some bacteriophages, however, infect their host bacteria but do not multiply or produce lysis, and these are considered **temperate**. Apparently, they replicate synchronously with the host. Occasionally, in about one case in 10^2–10^5 of such **lysogenic** bacteria, a spontaneous resumption of independent phage multiplication and subsequent lysis may take place. To provide evidence for the liberation of infectious particles, another bacterial strain for which the phage is virulent must be used as an indicator. On mixing lysogenic bacteria with an excess of the sensitive indicator strain and inoculation of a nutrient agar plate with the mix-

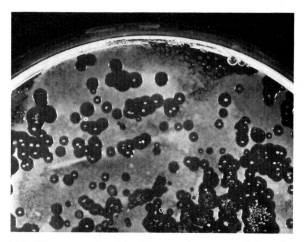

Fig. 4.12. *Plaques produced by lysogenic bacteria and free phage in a confluent growth of bacteria.*

The agar surface was inoculated with a thick suspension of non-lysogenic, sensitive bacteria (*Bacillus megaterium*) which contained a few cells of a lysogenic strain of the same species and some free phage; the central colonies are produced by growth of the lysogenic bacteria.

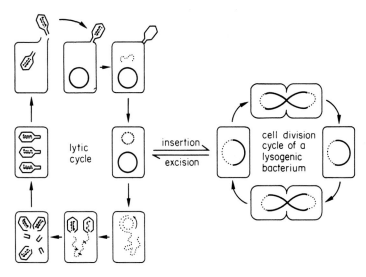

Fig. 4.13. *Life cycle of a temperate phage as seen in phage lambda.*

Infection of *E. coli* with phage lambda can result in either phage multiplication and lysis (lytic cycle) or the lysogenisation of the bacterium. The phage DNA is present in a linear double-stranded form. Inside the bacterium it is closed to give a circle. The circular DNA can remain autonomous or can be integrated into the bacterial DNA. In the former case the lytic cycle takes place. The closed circular DNA is replicated. According to the 'rolling circle' process, this produces a chain of many copies of the phage DNA. The phage genes bring about the synthesis and assembly of the head and tail proteins and the packing of one DNA copy into each phage head. Heads and tails combine spontaneously (self assembly). At lysis of the host cell, about 100 mature phages are liberated which can then infect other cells. The circular close phage DNA may, however, lose its autonomy and become integrated into the host DNA (this is also referred to as insertion of the DNA). The cell is now lysogenic for phage lambda. The latent phage or 'prophage' is replicated with the host chromosome. The lysogenised bacterium can go on dividing indefinitely without undergoing lysis. Excision of the phage DNA (from the host chromosome) can occur spontaneously or can be induced by treatment with UV light or mutagenic agents. This results in lytic multiplication of the phage DNA.

ture, the lysogenic cells can grow into colonies; however, every once in a while some phage particles will be liberated. These immediately attack the sensitive bacteria and produce plaques, in the centre of which the progeny of the lysogenised bacteria are preserved (Fig. 4.12).

Lysogenic bacteria have the potential ability to produce phage without showing any morphological or serological evidence for this. These non-infectious phages which can be passed from cell to cell of the host organism are termed **prophages**; they are hereditary in the same way as other genetic properties of the bacterial cell. The fact that all the progeny of a lysogenised cell are themselves also lysogenic must mean that the prophage has to be replicated in synchrony with the host chromosome (Fig. 4.13).

Lysogenic bacteria are immune to the particular phage that they harbour as prophage. This prophage-induced **immunity** is not due to any inhibition of phage adsorption (as has been described for virulent phages) but is caused by the production of a cytoplasmic repressor protein which inhibits the reproduction of vegetative phage. This repressor protein also represses the reconversion of prophage to vegetative phage, as well as the formation of all phage proteins. The development of the lysogenic state is thus dependent on the formation of the repressor protein. Lysogenised bacteria only very rarely undergo spontaneous lysis without any external influence. On the other hand, a variety of agents (e.g. UV light, alkylating agents, mitomycin C) can induce all cells containing prophages to liberate infectious phage particles. The success of such **induction** procedures depends on the genetic constitution of the prophage and on the physiological state of the host, as well as on the culture conditions. The induction must depend on the destruction or inactivation of the existing repressor molecules. In mutants of temperate phages that form a thermolabile repressor, a mere increase in the temperature to 44 °C is sufficient to induce lysis of the bacteria.

Integration and excision of phage lambda.   Studies on phage lambda (λ), which is lysogenic for *E. coli* K12, have shed light on how the prophage is related to the bacterial chromosome. Lysogenisation by phage lambda is used in the study of temperate phage development. The length of the lambda phage chromosome is about 2% that of the bacterial host chromosome.

In the free phage, DNA is present as a linear, double-stranded molecule (Fig. 4.14) although one of the two strands projects beyond the double strand at each end by about 12 nucleotides. These two single-stranded ends are complementary; they can hybridise by base-pairing and are referred to as 'sticky ends'. When these DNA molecules are kept in solution *in vitro* the complementarity of the single-stranded ends leads to an equilibrium mixture of linear and circular DNA. A similar ring closure apparently occurs upon infection of the cell with phage lambda. The two open ends of the strands are closed by polynucleotide ligase; this bacterial enzyme functions to repair single-strand breaks in a

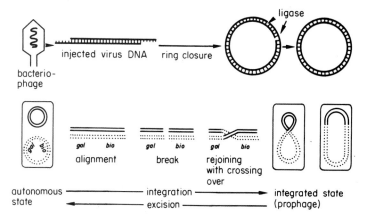

Fig. 4.14. *Integration (insertion) of phage lambda into the chromosome of* E. coli *K12, and its excision.*

DNA is present inside the phage particle in the linear double-stranded form with unpaired complementary ends. In solution or in the bacterium, the complementary 'sticky ends' associate and the gaps are closed by a ligase. The closed circular double strand now aligns with the chromosome (between the genes *gal* and *bio*). Both strands break and join with the double strand of the partner.

This process of alignment, breakage, and crosswise rejoining leads to the integration (or insertion) of the phage DNA into the host DNA. The phage has been converted to a prophage and the cell is lysogenic for phage lambda. The excision of the lambda DNA and the conversion to the autonomous form may proceed by the reverse of the process.

double-stranded polynucleotide. The integration of the linear phage DNA into the closed circular state is brought about without any phage enzymes. In the lysogenised cell the prophage is firmly attached to the host chromosome. Thus, in conjugation experiments the prophage DNA is transferred from the donor to the recipient cell together with the host chromosome. Genetic experiments show that the lambda phage DNA must be integrated at a specific locus on the host chromosome (between the galactose operon and the biotin region). At first it was thought that the phage DNA was just attached to the host chromsome at this location. The mapping of phage characters and recombination experiments, however, showed that in lysogeny the phage DNA is not just attached but must be inserted into the host chromosome.

The **insertion** of the phage DNA into the host chromsome apparently proceeds by alignment, breaking, and crosswise rejoining (Fig. 4.14). An enzyme called lambda integrase is responsible for this reaction (process). It can recognise the two non-homologous DNA sequences, one on the chromosomal DNA, and the other on the phage DNA. It brings about close alignment of the two double strands. Both double strands are broken and then rejoined crosswise. The separate steps of this site-specific recombination can be followed in Fig. 4.14. In the integrated state, the phage DNA is replicated together with the bacterial DNA and this is regulated in the same way as the replication of the bacterial chromosome. The information contained in the integrated phage DNA is not expressed. Only by transition of the prophage into the vegetative state can the autonomy of the phage DNA be re-established and lead to multiplication of the phage within the cell. This retrogression can occur spontaneously or by induction (e.g. by UV irradiation). **Excision** of the phage DNA from the bacterial DNA proceeds most probably by a reversal of the process of insertion. The excision of phage DNA is usually very precise: more than 99% of the phage particles produced by lysogenised cells are identical with the original infecting phage. This must mean that at excision the phage DNA is split at exactly the same location as at integration. In only a few instances (about one in 10^5) is the excision found to be abnormal (see Transduction, Ch. 15.2.3).

Once the prophage has reverted to the vegetative state by excision, it regains its autonomy and can multiply inside the bacterial cell like a virulent phage. The excision thus leads to the lysis of the host cell and liberation of lambda phages.

4.3   Relation of viruses and plasmids to tumour formation

Malignant tumours (cancers) can arise in a number of ways, but they are all related to DNA, the hereditary material of the cell. Whatever the origins of the oncogenic process, the eventual malignant growth is directed by the DNA of the freely proliferating tumour cells.

The conversion of a normal cell into a malignant cell, i.e. the oncogenic transformation, is due to a transformation or reorientation of DNA; the agent that stimulates the proliferation of cells is a gene product. Although there is at present no general oncogenesis theory that includes all types of malignancy, the investigations on virus- and plasmid-induced tumours have led to a number of wide-ranging conclusions.

In the following sections we shall discuss three examples of tumour formation: (1) the production of plant tumours; (2) the production of animal tumours by DNA viruses; and (3) the production of animal tumours by RNA viruses (retroviruses).

4.3.1   Formation of plant tumours

Plant tumours, the so-called crown galls, root galls, or plant cancers, can occur in many kinds of plants. These tissue proliferations reduce the nutrient flow in the plant. Such growths can also be induced experimentally in many cases. The typical tumours (Fig. 4.15) are produced by infection with *Agrobacterium tumefaciens*, a peritrichously flagellated, gram-negative soil bacterium which resembles *Rhizobium*. Infection is by entry of the bacteria through wounds and their proliferation in the intercellular spaces. There are virulent and avirulent strains of *A. tumefaciens*. The virulent strains contain a large plasmid called Ti (tumour-inducing).

The real infective agent is the plasmid DNA. This penetrates the cell and is incorporated into the plant cell genome. This process is called **oncogenic transformation**. It was demonstrated by transfer of a plug of transformed cells to healthy tissue, that after transformation, the presence of bacteria is unnecessary for infection. Only a part of the plasmid DNA, not the whole plasmid, is integrated into the host DNA. This part carries the genetic information for the production of **opines**. These are compounds derived from arginine. They are produced by the transformed plant cell, which is unable to utilise them; they are metabolisable only by *A. tumefaciens*. Thus, this *Agrobacterium* is exploiting the Ti plasmid to provide it with an exclusive supply of photosynthesis

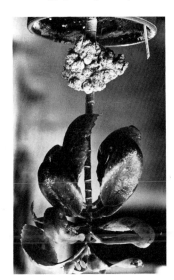

Fig. 4.15. *Plant tumour on the stem of* Kalanchoe blossfeldiana.

Tumour formation was induced by inoculation of the cortex with *Agrobacterium tumefaciens*. (Picture: U. Kaiser.)

products of its host plant. Other Ti genes are concerned with the formation of auxins and cytokinins which stimulate the division of plant cells and the growth of the tumour.

The natural ability of the Ti plasmid to transmit heterologous bacterial DNA into plant cells opens the possibility of using this plasmid as a vector for the introduction of foreign DNA into plants. Using recombinant DNA techniques (Chapter 16) it is possible to integrate foreign DNA into the Ti plasmid (in place of the virulence gene) so that, after transmission, it can undergo recombination with the plant genome, and finally be expressed. In this way recombinant tobacco plants have been produced which form a luciferase system and hence can glow. Resistance to antibiotics, herbicides and insect pests has also been transferred to various plants. The most successful such transfers, up to now, have been achieved in the Solanaceae (tobacco, potato, *Rauwolfia*, *Petunia*, *Datura* and others). The rapid progress of research in this field already suggests success in gene technology with monocotelydonous plants. Whether the ability to fix atmospheric nitrogen will one day be transferred to cultivated plants depends primarily on the extreme oxygen sensitivity of the nitrogenase system.

4.3.2   Formation of animal tumours by DNA viruses

Investigations on the origins of malignancy in animals are usually carried out on tissue cultures. When cells of animal tissues, such as chicken or hamster organs or human fibroblasts, are inoculated into a suitable nutrient medium they multiply and grow on the inner surface of the culture vessel. They normally continue to proliferate only until they make contact with each other; contact inhibition occurs and the result is a single-cell layer of confluent growth. When these normal cells are infected with a tumour virus, they lose the contact inhibition and continue to proliferate, growing into several layers. This multilayered growth is found only in cultures of cancerous cells. Individual cells can be easily isolated and propagated as 'pure cell lines', i.e. clones, from such oncogenically transformed cell cultures.

In the animal body the uncontrolled proliferation of cells produces tumours. If the body can contain and encapsulate these growths they are called **benign** tumours. However, if they go on growing without inhibition and invade other tissues to form **metastases**, they are called **malignant** tumours or **cancers**.

An example of tumour formation in animals by a double-stranded DNA virus is the Simian virus 40 (SV40). It attacks a number of hosts and tissues as suggested by the group name **polyoma** viruses (oma = tumour). This belongs to the best-researched tumour viruses and has also been examined for its suitability as a gene vector for genetic manipulation in animals.

SV40 is a simple, naked icosahedrovirus (72 capsomers) containing a closed, circular, double-stranded DNA molecule. The virus can be transferred from hosts, like hamsters or mice, to tissue culture cells and will multiply in these. In some host cell lines (permissive cells) the virus is lytic and its multiplication kills the cells. In other, non-permissive cells, the virus can establish lysogeny without reproducing. In rare cases (1 per 10^{-5}), pure DNA can be stably integrated in the host cell. The genetically altered cell may be **oncogenically transformed**, exhibiting uncontrolled growth and tumour formation. The transformed cell produces a protein (T-antigen) which initiates the replication of cellular DNA. Injecting such transformed cells into animals leads to rapid tumour formation.

The oncogenic transformation of cells by a virus such as SV40 is in many ways similar to the integration of phage lambda into the host genome of *E. coli* (establishing lysogeny). However, insertion of SV40 DNA can take place at numerous loci of host cell DNA, and is therefore not a strictly locus-specific recombination. There are also other mechanisms of tumour formation by DNA viruses.

4.3.3   Formation of animal tumours by retroviruses

Tumour formation in animals can also be caused by RNA viruses (retroviruses). These belong to the icosahedral viruses with envelopes. They have a (+)RNA genome, that is single-stranded RNA. Examples of oncogenic RNA viruses are those that produce Rous sarcoma in chickens and leukaemia in mice. The name **retroviruses** refers to the participation of reverse transcriptase in their multiplication (Ch. 2.2.2). Multiplication of these viruses can not occur by simple replication of the RNA but requires transcription into DNA, and its subsequent integration into a chromosome of the host cell. The integration is a necessary step in the multiplication of the virus; only integrated viral DNA can be transcribed (into virus RNA). Because the integration into host DNA is part of the viral life cycle, its frequency is very high. It is probable that integration can occur at any site on the host DNA. The replication of a single-stranded RNA, a (+)strand, proceeds in the following steps (Fig. 4.16): (1) reverse transcription by the virus-specific reverse transcriptase to a complementary DNA strand; (2) the DNA is copied by the cellular DNA polymerase to a linear double-stranded DNA; (3) the linear double-stranded DNA is covalently closed to the circular form (ccc); (4) integration into the host genome; (5) transcription of the viral DNA into

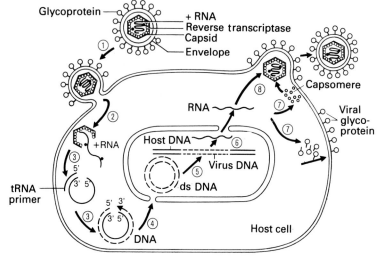

Fig. 4.16. *Developmental cycle of a retrovirus.*

The virus particle consists of a single-stranded RNA, reverse transcriptase (RNA-dependent DNA polymerase), the capsid protein and the envelope. It is adsorbed onto the specific receptors of the host cell via a glycoprotein. The nucleocapsid is admitted by a kind of pinocytosis (1) and the RNA is liberated (2). The reverse transcriptase synthesises a DNA-copy of the virus RNA (3).

Following synthesis of a DNA double-strand (4) and further replication, the DNA can be integrated into the host genome (5). The RNA then synthesised inside the nucleus serves as mRNA (6) for the synthesis of the capsid and glycoproteins, as well as the viral RNA (7). After assembly (8), the nucleocapsid is enveloped and liberated by exocytosis.

mRNA and viral RNA; (6) inclusion in the capsid; (7) envelopment of the virus particle during budding of the cytoplasmic membrane. This virus multiplication is not lytic and does not kill the cell.

The integrated DNA of the retrovirus is replicated together with the genome of the host cell (i.e. in the sarcoma), and is therefore present in all sarcoma cells. The oncogenic development, that is formation of the tumour, is due to expression of the viral gene '*src*'. This gene codes a kinase which phosphorylates proteins. The base sequence of the viral *src* gene is similar to that of a host cell gene whose product plays a role in regulation of growth in normal cells. This suggests that oncogenes of retroviruses are of cellular origin and occurred in those animals in which the retrovirus usually multiplied.

How can one explain the pathogenic effect of viral oncogenes if they are merely copies of normal cellular genes? One hypothesis proposes that the viral oncogenes differ, even if only slightly, from their cellular precursors, and, although showing similar enzyme activities, may attack different cellular targets. In contrast to this '**mutation hypothesis**', the '**dosis hypothesis**' envisages the causation of cancer by retroviruses as due merely to an overdose, rather than to any specific properties of the viral protein.

The **oncogene theory** can today be applied to all tumour viruses: each tumour viral oncogene is derived from a normal gene of animal cells. The gene products are involved in the regulation of growth and differentiation of animal cells.

Viroids.   Aetiological agents of some plant diseases have been demonstrated recently in the form of small, naked, i.e. not protein-covered, RNA molecules. These have been called viroids. Viroids are circular, closed, single-stranded RNA with a chain length of about 360 nucleotides (i.e. a relative particle mass of 12×10^4). Thus they are about 10-fold smaller than the infectious RNA of the smallest RNA virus so far known and, hence, are the smallest aetiological agent of any disease (so far known). They cause diseases of potatoes, citrus, cucumbers, chrysanthemums, hops, coconut palms and other plants.

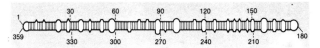

Prions.   Aetiological agents of diseases like Creutzfeld–Jakob syndrome in man and scrapie in sheep are still largely unknown, except that they appear to be nucleic acid-free small proteins, of approximately 250 amino acids. It is thought possible that these activate a latent gene of the host which codes for this protein, and that this causes the illness.

4.4   Important human viral pathogens

The common cold and influenza are about the commonest human illnesses. They are caused by RNA viruses which mainly infect the upper respiratory tract. They are transmitted between humans by droplet infection. The symptoms of the common cold (rhinitis, inflammation of the seral mucosa in the nose and throat) are caused by rhinoviruses, all small, single-stranded RNA viruses without envelope (picorna and corona viruses). They multiply in the mucosal cells which are killed. The optimal temperature for their replication is 33 °C, about the temperature of the nasal cavity. The lack of development of any persistant immunity against the common cold is most probably due to the large number of serotypes in the rhinoviruses.

The influenza viruses belong to the orthomyxovirus group, RNA viruses with envelopes. The illness at first resembles the common cold, but the inflammation is not limited to the nose and throat area: it also affects the lungs and strongly depresses general health. As the virus is very easily transmitted, it often causes widespread attack and 'flu epidemics'. The pandemic of 1957 was caused by the appearance of a highly virulent virus mutant, to which no immunity existed anywhere. Immunity against the capsid and envelope proteins of the influenza virus can last for several years. However, sometimes infection of one cell with several virus particles can lead to exchange and '**antigenic shift**', so that the virus becomes resistant to the pre-existing antibodies, leading to its uninhibited development in a previously immune individual.

Apart from the influenza and common cold viruses, the Human Immune Deficiency virus (HIV) is now one of the most widely known viruses, not because its incidence is anywhere near that of the above two, but because of the fatal disease, AIDS, that it causes. AIDS (Acquired Immune Deficiency Syndrome) was recognised as a disease of the immune system because infection with the HIV virus was accompanied by infections with typical opportunistic organisms. Such infections with opportunistic pathogens, like *Pseudomonas aeruginosa*, some protozoa, yeasts and other fungi, are very rarely found in individuals with a normally functioning immune system. They usually attack individuals weakened by some other illness or treatment, and become pathogenic when the central immune system is compromised.

HIV is a retrovirus, and therefore depends for its replication on the integration of its genome into that of the host (Ch. 4.3, Fig. 4.16). HIV is also a lymphotropic virus and specifically infects T_4 lymphocytes. These do not actually produce antibodies, but play an essential part as helper cells in the antibody production by B-lymphocytes. Practically no T_4 lymphocytes are demonstrable in AIDS patients. The HIV virus thus abolishes an important link in the chain of antibody production (immune defence) and thus renders the individual prone to all infectious diseases and to tumour formation.

Viral infections in general are currently among the most prominent infectious diseases. This is easily explained by the fact that bacteria offer a variety of targets for therapeutic agents to inhibit their growth. The multiplication of viruses, on the other hand, is intimately coupled to essential metabolic processes of the host cell, such as nucleic acid synthesis. It is, therefore, extremely difficult (up to now more or less impossible) to inhibit intracellular viral growth without serious damage to the host cell metabolism. The development of antiviral therapeutics has therefore met with little success so far, and the old-fashioned methods for dealing with the common cold, for instance, still seem the best. Cheers!

5   The fungi (Mycota)

The name of the fungi is derived from their most obvious representatives, the mushrooms (Greek, *mykes*, Latin, *fungus*). They are eukaryotes and share with plants the possession of a cell wall, liquid-filled intracellular vacuoles, microscopically visible streaming of the cytoplasm and (almost universal) lack of motility. However, they do not contain photosynthetic pigments and are chemo-organoheterotrophs. They grow aerobically and obtain their energy by oxidation of organic substances. Compared to the plants, which are organised into stems, roots and leaves, fungi show only very limited morphological differentiation and practically no functional differentiation.

The vegetative body.   The vegetative body is a **thallus**. It consists of filaments about 5 μm in diameter which are multiply branched and spread over or into the nutrient medium. The filaments or **hyphae** consist of a cell wall and cytoplasm with its inclusions. The hyphae may be without cross walls (in the lower fungi) or divided into cells by septa in the higher fungi. However, even in the septate hyphae, the cytoplasm of the cells is continuous via a central pore in the septum (Fig. 5.1). The total of the hyphal mass of a fungal **thallus** is called the **mycelium**. In certain stages, often during transition to the sexual or asexual reproduction phase, the mycelium forms tissuelike aggregates, the so-called **plectenchyma**. A typical plectenchyma is the 'flesh' of the mushroom. In the higher fungi, the mycelium may also form thick strands, **rhizomorphs**, which function to transport nutrients.

Growth and reproduction.   Fungal hyphae elongate at their apices (apical growth). In most fungi every part of the mycelium has the potential for growth (elongation); a small piece of mycelium is sufficient for inoculation to produce a new thallus. However, the forms and mechanisms involved in the reproduction of fungi are extremely diverse and are used as the basis for classification. Two kinds of reproduction are distinguished, namely sexual and asexual. Most fungi can reproduce in both ways.

Asexual reproduction of fungi is mostly by budding, fragmentation, or formation of spores. **Spore formation** is the most widely distributed

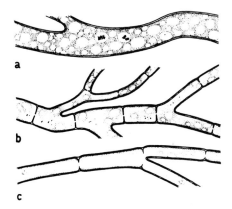

Fig. 5.1. *Somatic fungal hyphae.*

(a) The hyphae of Phycomycetes are aseptate. (b) Eumycetes are characterised by septate hyphae.

(c) In *Leptomitus lacteus* (Oomycete) the hyphae are constricted at intervals.

and most highly differentiated method. **Conidiospores** are budded off at hyphal apices (in *Penicillium, Aspergillus*). When these arise inside **sporangia** (i.e. receptacles), the fungi are grouped as **sporangiospores** (*Mucor, Rhizopus*). In the lower fungi, **sporangia** are often motile by means of flagella and are called **zoospores**. The flagella conform to the typical eukaryotic model: they originate from a **blepharoplast** in the cytoplasm and consist of eleven parallel fibrils of which nine peripheral fibrils are arranged concentrically around two central ones (9 + 2).

The asexual reproduction characteristic of yeasts (budding fungi) is budding; the mother cell forms an outgrowth which receives a daughter nucleus, whereupon the nucleated outgrowth is pinched off as a 'bud' (Fig. 5.2). Asexual reproduction can also occur by fragmentation of the hyphae into single cells, the **oidia** or **arthrospores** (e.g. in the milk mould *Endomyces lactis*). In some fungi these cells are surrounded by a thick wall and are referred to as **chlamydospores**. Finally, there are some yeasts (*Schizosaccharomyces*) which reproduce by binary fission in a manner similar to bacteria.

Sexual reproduction.   This, as in all other eukaryotes, comprises the union or conjugation of two nuclei. In different fungi, the nuclear fusion may occur at different intervals after the first parental contact. Sexual reproduction can usually be divided into three phases. The first is

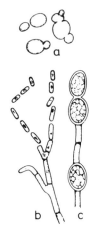

Fig. 5.2. *Asexual reproduction in some fungi.*

(a) By sprouting or budding (yeasts); (b) by fragmentation of hyphae into single cells which are called arthrospores or oidia and which behave like spores (*Collybia* sp.); (c) by formation of thick-walled chlamydospores (*Fusarium*). (From Alexopoulos, C. J. (1966). *Introduction to Mycology*. Stuttgart: Fischer.)

plasmogamy, the fusion of two protoplasts. The resulting cell has two nuclei. This nuclear pair or **dikaryon** does not need to fuse immediately, but it can persist in the dikaryotic state during the rest of the cell division, the two nuclei dividing simultaneously (conjugative division). The fusion of the two haploid nuclei (**karyogamy**) may occur later, often only after formation of a fruiting body, to give the diploid nucleus of the **zygote**. Following karyogamy, **meiosis**, the reduction division of the chromosomes to the haploid number, takes place. These three processes or stages, plasmogamy, karyogamy, and meiosis, may occur in immediate sequence in some fungi, but in others they can occur during quite different stages of development.

In the lower fungi the phase of sexual reproduction is initiated by the formation of **gametes**, i.e. sexual cells. When the gametes formed by the male and female parental cells are indistinguishable morphologically they are called **isogametes**. The gametes are often formed inside morphologically differentiated cells, which are called **gametangia**, and when these are morphologically distinct, the male gametangia are called **antheridia** and the female ones are called **oogonia**.

The ways in which the gametes are transferred and plasmogamy achieved can again be subdivided into various kinds. In lower fungi, especially in aquatic ones, both gametes are usually motile (planogametes) and fuse outside the gametangia (i.e. after liberation from the gametangia). In the **oomycetes** only the male gamete is motile; it penetrates the oogonium and fertilises the ovum. **Zygomycetes** are characterised by **gametangiogamy**, the fusion of whole, multinucleate gametangia into a **coenozygote**.

Table 5.1. *Survey of some important groups of fungi*

Myxomycetes (true slime moulds)	Phycomycetes (lower fungi)	Eumycetes (higher fungi)		
		Ascomycetes	Basidiomycetes	Deuteromycetes
Fuligo septica	Chytridiomycetes	Protoascomycetes	Heterobasidiomycetes	*Aspergillus*
Lycogala	Chytridiales	Endomycetaceae	Tremellales	*Penicillium*
epidendron	Blastocladiales	Saccharomycetaceae	Uredinales	*Phoma*
Cribraria	Monoblepharidales	Euascomycetes	Ustilaginales	*Monilia*
rufa		Plectomycetes	Homobasidiomycetes	*Candida*
Physarum	Oomycetes	(Kleistothecia)	Hymenomycetes	*Alternaria*
	Saprolegniales	*Aspergillus*	Polyporaceae	
Acrasiomycetes	Leptomitales	*Penicillium*	Agaricaceae	
(cellular slime	Peronosporales	Pyrenomycetes	Boletaceae	
moulds)		(Perithecia)	Hydnaceae	
Dictyostelium	Plasmodiophoromycetes	*Sordaria*	Clavariaceae	
		Neurospora	Corticiaceae	
	Zygomycetes	*Xylaria*		
	Mucorales	*Nectria*	Gasteromycetes	
	Entomophthorales	*Claviceps*	Lycoperdales	
		Discomycetes	Phallales	
		(Apothecia)	Nidulariales	
		Rhytisma		
		Peziza		
		Helvella		
		Morchella		
		Tuberales		

When the male and female gametangia originate from the same vegetative body (produced from a single spore), the organism is referred to as a **homothallic** or **hermaphrodite** fungus (**monozoic**). In heterothallic, or **dizoic**, fungi the thalli are either male or female, that is, they bear only male or female sex organs. Homothallic fungi can be self-fertilising (**autogamous**). However, in some homothallic fungi no self-fertilisation occurs due to some physiological inhibitory mechanism, which is referred to as **incompatibility**. This is the case in *Neurospora*, for example, which, though homothallic, needs conjugation between members of different types (+ and –) to establish fertilisation; individuals belonging to the same type are incompatible (Table 5.1).

Classification.   The classification of fungi, like that of bacteria, is designed mainly for practical application but it also bears some relation to phylogenetic considerations. The nomenclature is binomial, with a generic and a specific name (e.g. *Aspergillus niger*). Species are collected in genera, genera in families (suffix -aceae), families in orders (suffix -ales), and orders in classes (suffix -mycetes). The division of Mycota, or fungi and moulds, includes the true slime moulds (Myxomycetes), the lower fungi (Phycomycetes), and the higher fungi (Eumycetes).

A complete presentation of the taxonomy, morphology, and physiology of fungi can be obtained from a number of textbooks on mycology. In this book, only a number of representative members of the various groups, those that can be regarded as model systems or that are of particular practical importance, can be discussed.

5.1   Acrasiomycetes (cellular slime moulds)

The Acrasiomycetes are called cellular slime moulds to distinguish them from the true slime moulds, which form plasmodia. Another term, 'social amoebae', derives from the curious formation of well-formed fruiting bodies by a large number of cooperating individual cells (amoebae). In Fig. 5.3, the fruiting bodies of the Acrasiomycetes and those of the Myxomycetes are presented side by side to show their superficial resemblance. The Acrasiomycetes comprise about two dozen species which are free-living soil inhabitants. The most extensively studied are *Dictyostelium mucoroides* and *D. discoideum*. These are easily isolated from humus-containing soils. In pure culture on agar media or in nutrient solutions, the amoebae feed on bacteria; under experimental conditions these are usually *E. coli* or *Enterobacter aerogenes*.

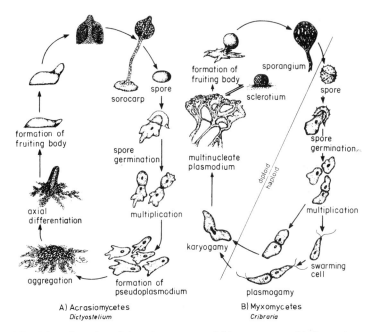

Fig. 5.3. *Life cycles of Acrasiomycetes and Myxomycetes with formation of fruiting bodies.*

(A) Life cycle of a cellular slime mould (*Dictyostelium*). The naked, single-celled amoebae form an aggregation plasmodium; from this develops a fruiting body, differentiated into stem and head.

(B) Developmental process of the true slime moulds. The myxamoebae aggregate to a multinucleate plasmodium. This gives rise to the fruiting body.

Developmental cycle. The basic units of Acrasiomycetes are naked, uninucleated, haploid amoebae (Fig. 5.3A). They move over solid media by means of pseudopodia, feed by phagocytosis of bacteria and multiply. Eventually, the amoebae migrate towards an **aggregation centre** and form an aggregation plasmodium which is called a **pseudoplasmodium** to distinguish it from the multinucleate, but unicellular, true plasmodium of the Myxomycetes. Although the individual amoebae maintain their identity, the pseudoplasmodium functions as a unit. It forms a 'slug'. A 'cap' is formed in which the axis of the fruiting body, the **sorophore**, becomes differentiated. The cells on the upper surface form a stem, which is enveloped in a cellulose coat, whilst the cells from the posterior or lower part migrate to the apex of the stem where they form a spherical head, the **sorocarp**, and develop into spores. The spores are encysted amoebae. On germination of a spore, a pore appears in the cellulose coat through which the amoeba is liberated to begin a new cycle.

The nutritional (vegetative) stage is sharply differentiated from the morphogenetic phase. Absorption of nutrients ceases some time before the beginning of aggregation, and the aggregation phase can be suppressed for a time by repeated addition of food (bacteria). The developmental cycle of the Acrasiales represents a model for the formation of an individual (unitary) body from a number of independent cells. The induction of aggregation and formation of the fruiting body by a so-called 'higher command' (or the 'god of the amoebae') is brought about by a diffusible substance that has been called 'acrasin'. In *Dictyostelium discoideum* this has been shown to be identical with cyclic AMP (adenosine-3',5'-monophosphate).

5.2   Myxomycetes (true slime moulds)

The Myxomycetes form fruiting bodies that are very similar to those of the myxobacteria and of the Acrasiomycetes, although they are larger than either of these. The developmental cycle is shown in Fig. 5.3B. The Myxomycetes occur in damp places in wood, on fallen leaves, bark, timber, and old fence-posts. Their sometimes conspicuously coloured fruiting bodies, about 0.5–1 cm in size, are easily visible. The young, cherry-sized fruiting bodies of *Lycogala epidendron* are a splendid scarlet colour, whilst the smaller, stemmed fruiting bodies of *Cribraria rufa*, for example, have sporangia with a delightful, elegantly bizzare structure. The plasmodium of the yellow *Fuligo septica* appears as hand-sized, foamlike masses on tree stumps, in tanneries, and various other habitats.

Development.   The spores liberated from fruiting bodies germinate on moist surfaces and produce flagellated swarmers, or **myxamoebae** (Fig. 5.3B). These feed on liquid nutrients or by phagocytosis of bacteria, yeasts, fungal spores, etc. The **myxoflagellates** lose their flagella after a time and enter an **amoeboid** stage. These cells are mononucleate. Eventually, they fuse in pairs (**plasmogamy** and **karyogamy**) to become **myxozygotes**. These diploid amoeba remain as such or fuse with other amoebae to form true plasmodia, which are then multinucleate. Under favourable nutritional conditions, the number of nuclei increases by repeated mitotic divisions. The plasmodia are negatively phototaxic (i.e. light avoiding) and achieve a favourable situation by means of hydrotaxis and chemotaxis. Movement of the plasmodium appears to involve a protein similar to myosin B (demonstrated in *Physarum polycephalum*).

The plasmodia give rise to the fruiting bodies or sporangia. The transition to this phase is characterised in physiological terms by an alteration in stimulus sensitivity. The plasmodia leave their dark and moist locations and migrate towards the light. A reduction division (meiosis) can be demonstrated cytologically. This is followed by the formation of a more or less complicated sporangium which has a firm envelope on its outer surface (the **peridium**). Numerous small, membrane-enveloped, mononucleate spores arise in its interior. The residues that remain between the spores form a network or 'skeleton' which is called the **capillitium**. On maturation and opening of the **peridium**, the spores are blown out of the sporangium by air currents.

5.3   Phycomycetes (lower fungi)

The Phycomycetes comprise a large group of fungi that have unseptate and multinucleate vegetative bodies, despite multiple branching of the hyphae. This type of body is referred to as a coenocytic thallus. Most of the lower fungi produce spores in sporangia. The most primitive forms are adapted to an aquatic mode of life and form motile spores and gametes. In the transition from the aquatic to the more advanced amphibian and terrestrial forms, motile stages are encountered only infrequently.

Chytridiomycetes.   The Chytridiomycetes are predominantly aquatic fungi; a few representatives are found in soil. They are of microscopic size and their cell walls appear to consist mainly of chitin. Many are parasitic on algal plankton and aquatic plants. An economically important parasite of cultivated plants is *Synchytrium endobioticum*, the causative agent of many potato diseases. *Rhizophidium pollinis* parasitises pine pollen and is a popular subject for demonstrations and teaching.

Oomycetes.   The Oomycetes are aquatic and terrestrial fungi that reproduce asexually by means of biflagellated zoospores. *Saprolegnia* and *Leptomitus* are known as 'water moulds' and live in water. The Peronosporales have advanced to a terrestrial mode of life. They are obligate parasites that undergo the whole of their life cycle inside higher plants. They also form zoospores. Some of the most devastating pathogens belong to this group: *Phytophthora infestans* causes potato blight, and *Plasmopara viticola* is the false mildew of vine.

Saprolegnia is widely distributed and can be easily isolated and cultured. It can be brought into enrichment culture by a 'baiting'

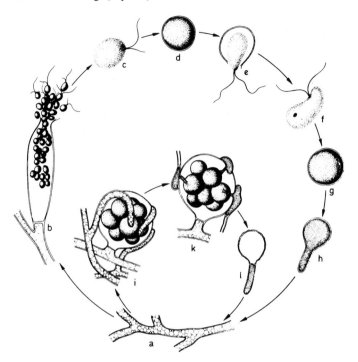

Fig. 5.4. *Life cycle of* Saprolegnia *sp.*

(a) Somatic hyphae; (b) sporangium with primary zoospores; (c) primary zoospore; (d) encapsulated zoospore; (e) germination; (f) secondary zoospore; (g) encapsulated zoospore; (h) germination; (i) oogonium with spherical oospheres and antheridia; (k) as in (i), but with fertilisation tubes of antheridia penetrating into the oogonium, in cross section; (l) germination of an oospore. (From Alexopolous, C. J. (1966). *Introduction to Mycology*. Stuttgart: Fischer.)

procedure: a dead fly with wings outspread and its legs pointing downwards is placed as bait on the water surface of a vessel filled with pond water. In a few days the fly is found to be surrounded by hyphae and sporangia. The formation of sporangia and the 'slipping' of the zoospores can be followed microscopically (Fig. 5.4).

An interesting feature of *Saprolegnia* and related genera is the occurrence of **diplany**: two swarming phases occur sequentially. The primary zoospores released from the sporangia undergo encystment following a first swarming period. These cysts release a second zoospore which becomes encapsulated after a second swarming period. Only this cyst undergoes germination with formation of a germination tube and hyphae.

Sexual reproduction occurs by direct contact between the gametangia, that is, between the antheridium and oogonium. Most of the Saprolegniaceae are hermaphrodites or homothallic; the conjugatory antheridia and oogonia arise from the same vegetative body. The oogonia are spherical, have thick walls, and contain several 'eggs' (oospheres). The antheridia are smaller, arise at the ends of the hyphae, and, when mature, attach either singly or several at a time to an oogonium. Conjugation tube arise from the antheridia, penetrate the oogonial wall, and make contact with the oosphere. A single nucleus (per germination tube) penetrates into an oosphere and fuses with its nucleus to give a diploid zygote nucleus. After fertilisation, each oosphere surrounds itself with a thick wall and becomes an oospore. After a lengthy resting period, this germinates by means of a germination tube. Meiotic nuclear division takes place. The developmental cycle is completed with the formation of new sporangia.

Zygomycetes.   The name zygomycetes is derived from the mechanisms of sexual reproduction, especially from the formation of the zygospore. The coenozygote or zygospore arises by fusion of two gametangia (gametangiogamy) which connect the parental hyphae by a kind of 'bridge' or 'yoke' (Greek, *zygos*) (Fig. 5.6). The zygomycetes are the most highly developed Phycomycetes adapted for terrestrial life. They are divided into three orders: Mucorales, Entomophthorales, and Zoopagales, of which only the first will be described here.

The **Mucorales** live on rotting organic materials; some are coprophilic, i.e. they prefer excreta as substrate; horse droppings and filtrates obtained from these have been the basis of many valuable studies. Names such as *Mucor mucedo, Rhizopus nigricans* (the common bread mould), *R. oryzae, R. arrhizus, R. rouxii, Phycomyces blakesleeanus, Choanephora cucurbitarum, Blakesleea*, etc. are well known not only to the mycologist, but also because of their industrial importance, to chemists and biotechnologists.

Fungi generally grow only sparsely and for a limited time under anaerobic conditions. On exclusion of atmospheric oxygen they can resort to fermentation, and a number form lactic acid or ethanol. At the same time, they adopt a **new growth habit**. *Mucor racemosus*, for example, forms a **sprouting mycelium** under anaerobic conditions, and the newly formed cells then multiply by budding, like yeasts.

The mucors can spread rapidly, both by the rapid growth of their hyphae and by the proliferation of numerous sporangiospores. Some, *Rhizopus stolonifer* (*R. nigricans*) for example, form stolons that can bridge distances of several centimetres.

180   The fungi (Mycota)

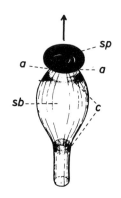

Fig. 5.5. *Sporangiophore of the Phycomycete* Pilobolus.

The arrow indicates the direction in which the sporangium (sp) will be thrown after tearing off from the subsporangial bladder (sb). (c) Carotinoid-rich areas; (a) the place where the sporangium is torn off. (From Nultsch, W. (1968). *General Botany*, 3rd edn. Stuttgart: Thieme.)

Asexual reproduction occurs by formation of sporangia and sporangio-spores. Vertical branches arise from the luxuriously growing mycelium, become delineated by a septum, and swell at their apices into spherical heads. An outer zone, rich in cytoplasm, separates from a poor inner zone; they are separated by a cell wall, the columella, which arches into the sporangium. Hundreds or even thousands of nuclei can be found in the peripheral zone, each surrounded by cytoplasm and developing into sporangiospores. Some of the mucors bear small sporangia, or sporangioles, on branched sporangial carriers, each sporangium containing only one or a few spores.

The sporangium of *Pilobolus* has a somewhat different form (Fig. 5.5). The carrier hypha enlarges into a bladder just below the sporangium, which then sits as a hemispherical black cap on the swollen tip. Extensive water uptake produces a high internal pressure, and on maturation of the sporangium the carrier is torn off at the columella, and the sporangium, including the columella, is catapulted up to 2 m high ('Pilobolus' means thrower). *Pilobolus* is also a ballistics expert and the sporangia are well aimed. The sporangial carriers are positively photo-trophic and grow towards the light with the sporangium aligned towards the light siource. The sporangia of *Pilobolus* are only formed on media containing faecal extracts. The necessary factor belongs to the siderophores and has been called coprogen.

Sexual reproduction and the developmental cycle can be exemplified by *Rhizopus nigricans* (Fig. 5.6). The liberated sporangiospores are multi-nucleate. They germinate under favourable conditions and develop a highly branched aerial mycelium. Where the branches make contact with the substrate, rhizoids are formed that can penetrate into the substrate. Immediately above these, one or several sporangial oophores are formed. Sexual reproduction in *R. nigricans* can occur only when two physiologi-

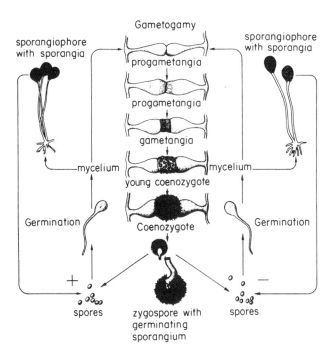

Fig. 5.6. *Life cycle of* Rhizopus nigricans.

cally differentiated, compatible (+ and –) mycelia come into contact. As these approach, copulation branches are formed that enlarge into progametangia and become enriched with cytoplasm and nuclei. They eventually separate from the carrier hyphae by means of septum formation. The cell walls in the contact zone of the gametangia disintegrate and the protoplasts fuse (gametangiogamy). Each (+) nucleus pairs with a (–) nucleus and nuclear fusion takes place. During this phase the coenozygote enlarges and forms a thick-walled zygospore. After a resting phase, the zygospore opens and germinates into a germ sporangium, the nuclei undergoing meiotic division. The vegetative body, therefore, is haploid.

Some of the mucors are homothallic and self-fertile.

5.4   Ascomycetes

The Ascomycetes, together with the Basidiomycetes, form the higher fungi (Eumycetes). They are characterised by a septated mycelium and formation of conidiospores. They do not form any flagellated cells. The name Ascomycetes is based on the possession of an **ascus**, a sac-like structure that is characteristic for this group, in which the **ascospores** are produced. Both karyogamy and meiosis take place inside the ascus. The ascus stage is the end stage of sexual reproduction and is also referred to as the **perfect** or **main fruiting** formation. Many Ascomycetes reproduce asexually by means of **conidia**. This subsidiary 'fruiting formation' is also designated the **imperfect stage**. In a number of fungi only the imperfect stage, i.e. conidium formation, is known, and these fungi are called 'fungi imperfecti' or Deuteromycetes.

Developmental cycle.   The germination tube arising from the ascospore develops into a mycelium (Fig. 5.7). In many cases, this then produces conidiophores bearing large numbers of conidia. These also germinate and form mycelia that resemble those derived from the ascospores. The asci are produced on the same mycelium as the conidia, but at a later stage.

The **sexual phase** is initiated by the formation of **ascogonia**. An ascogonium typically bears a trichogyne which receives the male nuclei, which are thus led from the antheridium via the trichogyne into the ascogonium (plasmogamy) where the nuclei pair but do not yet fuse. The ascogonium now gives rise to the so-called ascogenous hyphae, each of whose cells contains one male and one female nucleus (dikaryotic hyphae). The nuclei divide simultaneously. Fusion of the dikaryon is initiated by a specific cell division, '**hook formation**'. The hyphal apex curves in the form of a hook; the nuclear pair divides conjugatively. The upper pair of nuclei are separated by a septum both from the stem cell and from the hook. The hook then fuses with the stem cell, thus producing another dinucleate cell. The upper hook cell becomes the ascus in which the fusion of the two nuclei occurs. The resulting primary ascus nucleus then undergoes two divisions of which one is meiotic. The eight daughter nuclei then form the eight ascospores via further cell divisions. The number of divisions can be smaller (four spores) or very large (up to more than 1000 spores). Both the ascospores and the mycelium are thus haploid.

Fruiting bodies.   With few exceptions, the asci are formed in fruiting bodies (**ascocarps**). These represent the envelope or the cushion in which the sexual organs reach maturity. The hyphal network gives the charac-

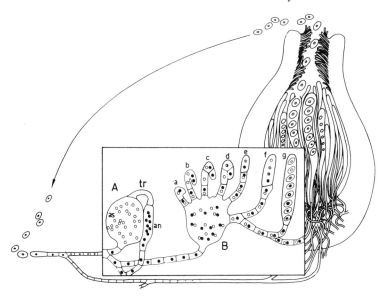

Fig. 5.7. *Life cycle of a homothallic Ascomycete.*

(A) Ascogonium before plasmogamy; (B) ascogonium with ascogenic, dikaryotic hyphae and the subsequent stages of hook and ascus formation; (a) hook formation; (b) hook after division of the paired nuclei; (c) formation of septum across hook; (d) karyogamy in the ascus cell and fusion of hook with stem cell; (e, f, g) divisions of the primary ascus nucleus; (g) formation of the eight ascospores.

as, ascogonium; an, antheridium; tr, trychogyne.

teristic shape to the fruiting body. Three different forms are distinguished (Fig. 5.8): (1) the completely closed fruiting body called the **cleistothecium** which is characteristic of plectomycetes; (2) a usually flask-shaped fruiting body called a perithecium which is typical for the pyrenomycetes; (3) an open, bowl-shaped fruiting body called an apothecium which is typical for discomycetes. In addition, there are some fungi that bear naked asci (protoascomycetes). In the truffles (Tuberales) the ascocarps remain closed.

Yeasts.   Yeasts, or budding fungi, belong to the protoascomycetes. The typical kind of asexual reproduction for yeasts is budding (Fig. 5.2). Fission occurs very rarely. The buds may continue to adhere as pseudo, or budding mycelia, or they may separate completely. The ascospores are produced in a naked ascus, derived from a zygote or from a vegetative cell.

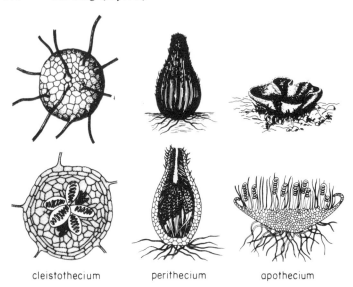

cleistothecium   perithecium   apothecium

Fig. 5.8. *Pictures of arrangements and cross-sections of fruiting bodies (ascocarps) that are characteristic for plectomycetes (cleistothecium), pyrenomycetes (perithecium) and discomycetes (apothecium).*

The members of the family Endomycetaceae form a mycelium, in addition to buds. In *Endomycopsis*, hyphae, buds, and asci with ascospores are found together. In the species *Endomyces lactis* (also known as *Geotrichum candidum* or *Oospora lactis*) arthrospores are formed by fragmentation of the hyphae.

The Saccharomycetaceae (the true yeasts) (Figs 5.9, 5.10) lack a mycelium. Brewer's and baker's yeast are physiological variants of *Saccharomyces cerevisiae*. The haploid buds can fuse (copulate). Karyogamy can be followed immediately by meiosis and the formation of a few ascospores. However, diploid cells can continue to multiply by budding; these diploid cells are larger and physiologically more active than the haploid cells. Predominantly diploid or even polyploid 'races' of yeasts are used industrially.

Thanks to its small haploid genome (only three times that of *E. coli*) and the small number of chromosomes (16 linear chromosomes of 200–2200 kb) as well as its short doubling time (90 min), *S. cerevisiae* has become the model organism for molecular genetics research in eukaryotes.

The asporogenous yeasts can be considered as even more reduced (i.e.

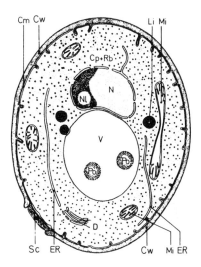

Fig. 5.9. *Cross-section through a yeast cell.*

The production of a single daughter cell by budding has left a scar. Cm, cytoplasmic membrane; Cp, cytoplasm; D, dictyosome; ER, endoplasmic reticulum; Li, lipid droplet; Mi, mitochondria; N, nucleus; Nl, nucleolus; Po, polyphosphate; Rb, ribosomes; V, vacuoles; Sc, scar; Cw, cell wall.

having a limited life cycle). Only a few form mycelial networks; most multiply entirely by budding. Some of the genera belonging to the asporogenous yeasts are *Candida, Torulopsis, Cryptococcus, Rhodotorula, Pullularia*, etc. (Fig. 5.11).

In nature, yeasts are found in all habitats where fermentable, sugar-rich liquids, extracts and secretions are available, for example in the nectar of flowers and on fruits and leaves. *Pullularia pullulans* ('soot' yeasts) form a black coating on leaves that are covered with honeydew.

Plectomycetes.   The Plectomycetes are cleistothecial fungi. The very important genera *Aspergillus* and *Penicillium* belong to this group. They are identified by their conidial stage (Fig. 5.12). These organisms will be further discussed in the context of physiological problems. Their highly branched, multinucleate mycelia bear large numbers of conidiophores which arise individually on the hyphae. A hyphal cell, the base cell, branches and forms a vertical hyphae. In *Aspergillus* this terminates in a swollen end, on the surface of which sterigmata grow out. Chains of

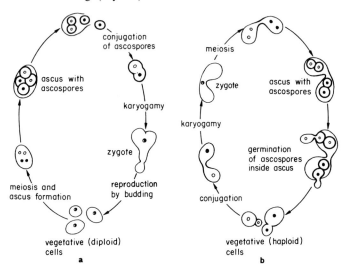

Fig. 5.10. *Life cycles of yeasts.*

(a) In *Saccharomyces cerevisiae* (mainly diploid) conjugation follows immediately on formation of the ascospores.

(b) In *Zygosaccharomyces* (haploid) haploid vegetative cells conjugate; the diploid phase is restricted to the zygote.

conidia arise on the sterigma, giving the appearance of strings of beads. These are pigmented (black, brown, ochre, green, etc.) and give the fungal colony a typical colour.

Many of the aspergilli and penicillia cause damage to organic materials, such as timber, fruit, leather, etc. *Penicillium roqueforti* and *P. camemberti* (now often replaced by the faster-growing *P. caseicolum*) bestow the characteristic flavour of Roquefort and Camembert cheeses. *Penicillium notatum* and *P. chrysogenum* are the well-known penicillin producers.

Pyrenomycetes.   The pyrenomycetes are **perithecial** fungi. A typical perithecium has its own, true wall. The asci arise in the base or in the lower part of the flask-shaped fruiting body and are accompanied by paraphyses. The inside of the **neck is covered with periphyses**.

A large number of pathogenic fungi belong to the pyrenomycetes. They include the obligately parasitic true mildews (*Erysiphe, Uncinula necator, Sphaerotheca mors-uvae*, etc.) and the saprophytic *Chaetomium* species, among them the common object of genetic studies *Neurospora. Sordaria fimicola*, among others, is coprophilic. The black *Xylaria* and

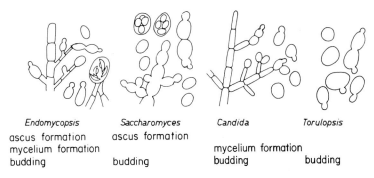

Endomycopsis
ascus formation
mycelium formation
budding

Saccharomyces
ascus formation

budding

Candida

mycelium formation
budding

Torulopsis

budding

Fig. 5.11. *Yeasts can be distinguished by their ascus formation, mycelium formation, and budding.*

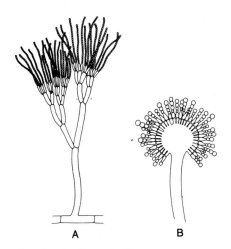

A   B

Fig. 5.12. *Secondary fruiting forms in Plectomycetes.*
(A) *Penicillium*; (B) *Aspergillus.*
(From Nultsch, W. (1968). *General Botany*, 3rd edn. Stuttgart: Thieme.)

Hypoxylon species grow on tree stumps. *Nectria galligena* and *N. cinna-barina* cause malignant growths on trees. *Claviceps purpurea* is the causative agent of ergot in rye; other species of *Claviceps* attack various grasses.

Development of a pyrenomycete. The developmental history of the pyrenomycetes can be illustrated by that of the ergot fungus *Claviceps purpurea* (Fig. 5.13). The ascospores infect the ovaries of the grain during the flowering period. The mycelium penetrates the ovary and turns it into a soft white mass. The surface is wrinkled, and in the furrows a large number of small hyaline conidia are borne on the thickly massed hyphal termini. The conidia, suspended in a sweet syrup (honeydew), are dispersed by insects. The surface eventually dries out and the fungus-infested seed vessel turns into a horny sclerotium. At harvest time the sclerotia fall off and hibernate in the soil. After stimulation by frost and in the presence of sufficient moisture and favourable temperatures in the spring, germination takes place. Perithecial heads borne on stems arise from the sclerotia. Their peripheral layers bear the perithecia with asci that contain eight threadlike (filamentous) ascospores. The sclerotia contain highly active alkaloids (lysergic acid derivatives, ergotoxins, and ergotamine) which are pharmacologically useful. Ergot may be produced on a commercial scale by cultivation of deliberately infected rye. Another species, *Claviceps paspali*, can also be grown in submerged culture.

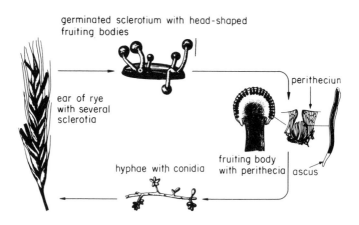

germinated sclerotium with head-shaped fruiting bodies

ear of rye with several sclerotia

peritheciun

hyphae with conidia

fruiting body with perithecia

ascus

Fig. 5.13. *Life cycle of the ergot fungus* Claviceps purpurea.

Discomycetes.   The discomycetes are apothetical fungi. Several of the more striking woodland fungi (*Peziza, Morchella, Helvella*, and truffles, i.e. Tuberales) belong to this group, as well as some pathogens like *Monilinia fructicola, Sclerotinia sclerotiorum, Rhytisma acerinum*, and *Lophoderma*, to name but a few. The apothecia are open, plate- or bowl-shaped fruiting bodies. In some of the woodland species they are pigmented bright red, yellow or orange, whilst others may be black or brown. *Pyronema omphalodes* (*P. confluens*), the model object for demonstrating the development of asci, grows on ground that has been burned.

5.5   Basidiomycetes

The Basidiomycetes are regarded as the most highly developed group of fungi. The distinguishing organ of the Basidiomycetes is the **basidium**, an upright fungal cell that corresponds to an ascus. Four **basidiospores** are usually pinched off from this. They are mononucleate and haploid. The basidiospores also resemble ascospores in being the result of plasmogamy, karyogamy and meiosis; the two latter processes occur, respectively, in the ascus and in the basidium. The mycelium of Basidiomycetes consists of septate hyphae. The white strands, which can be seen with the naked eye amongst woodland litter, consist of hyphal bundles surrounded by an envelope, and these are called rhizomorphs.

Developmental cycle of a hymenomycete.   After germination of the basidiospore, a primary mycelium develops which consists of septated hyphae with mononucleate cells. The secondary **dikaryotic** mycelium is produced when hyphae of two compatible strains meet and their mono-nucleate protoplasts fuse (somatogamy). At each cell division the nuclei divide synchronously. The cell division and the nuclear division in many Basidiomycetes involve formation of a tubular outgrowth called a **clasp** (Fig. 5.14). This mechanism ensures that the new cell contains one of each daughter nuclei. When the cell is ready for division a hook is formed between the two nuclei, a and b; this then curves backwards. The proximal nucleus b then migrates into the hook and both nuclei divide. The proximal part of the cell now contains the daughter nuclei a' and b' and becomes separated off by a septum. At the same time the hook fuses with the mother cell and allows the nucleus b to move back into the posterior part of the cell. The proximal cell is then also divided off from the hook by a septum; both daughter cells, i.e. the proximal and the posterior one, then contain one of each nuclei a and b (Fig. 5.14).

The dikaryotic mycelium can grow into highly organised fruiting bodies which are well known as mushrooms of various kinds. The basidia

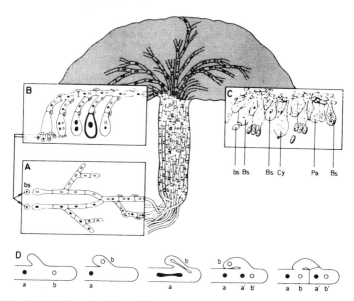

Fig. 5.14. *Life cycle of a mushroom.*

The inset areas show the hyphae and basidia at high magnification. (A) Development of septate hyphae from the basidiospores (bs) and plasmogamy with subsequent clasp formation (drawn at higher magnification in (D); see text for further explanations). (B) Formation of basidia with sequential stages of basidiospore formation. (C) Longitudinal section through a hymenium, with basidospores (bs), basidia (Bs), cysts (Cy) and paraphyses (Pa).

are formed in a certain layer of the fruiting body, the **hymenium**. This is composed of basidia and sterile hyphae, paraphyses, and cystids. The basidia are formed by enlargement of an upright cell and karyogamy takes place inside this. The zygote nucleus undergoes meiosis and produces four haploid nuclei. Meanwhile, four sterigmata have been formed containing the initial stages of basidiospores, and the nuclei migrate into these. The basidiospores are actively hurled out of the fruiting body. Accumulations of basidiospores show that they are pigmented. Their colours – brown, black, purple and ochre spores have been observed – serve as a diagnostic feature.

The above process of development, with a few modifications, also applies to the homobasidiomycetes. They have the kind of basidia described above. The hymenomycetes are distinguished from the gastero-

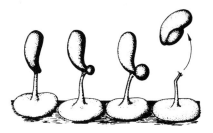

Fig. 5.15. *Spore formation in* Sporobolomyces.
The spore is projected by the
extrusion of a water droplet.

mycetes by the location of the hymenium. In the latter, the fruiting body
does not open to expose the hymenium layer; the basidiospores are only
liberated by the disintegration of the fruiting body (*Lycoperdon, Bovista,
Geastrum, Cyathus, Phallus*).

The fungi such as Tremellales, Uredinales and Ustilaginales belong to
the heterobasidiomycetes. The construction of their basidia differs from
that of the homobasidiomycetes. In several groups the pro-basidium is
covered by a rough envelope and behaves as a resting spore. Unfortunately, this is not the place to consider the attractive subject of basidial
modifications and adaptations to environmental conditions, the vegetative cycle of the host, etc. However, a small family of yeast-like fungi can
be mentioned, the Sporobolomycetaceae. They form conidia that are
borne on sterigmata. These conidia are actively hurled outwards and are
therefore often called ballistospores. *Sporobolomyces salmonicolor* repro-
duces like yeasts, by budding. Each cell, however, can produce a sterigma
which may bear a kidney-shaped spore. When these ripen, a droplet of
water is extruded at the lower end, and the spores are hurled about
0.1 mm into the air (Fig. 5.15). This seems to be the standard mechanism
for the 'shooting' of basidiospores by those forms possessing free-stand-
ing basidia (hymenomycetes).

5.6   Fungi imperfecti (Deuteromycetes)

This class contains all those fungi that do not have a sexual (perfect)
stage, as well as those where none has so far been demonstrated. The
conidial stages of these fungi are very similar to those of some well-
known Ascomycetes. It is assumed, therefore, that the fungi imperfecti
may represent conidial stages of Ascomycetes whose ascus stage has not

yet been discovered or has been lost in the course of evolution. On the other hand, even the fungi imperfecti are not completely asexual. **Parasexuality** has been demonstrated in these, as well as in Basidiomycetes and some Ascomycetes. Thus, they exhibit the processes of plasmogamy, karyogamy and meiosis, but these do not occur at defined locations of the vegetative body or in special developmental stages (i.e. they occur at random). The primary mycelium is normally homokaryotic, that is, it contains only one type of nucleus. Occasionally, fusion of protoplasts containing different kinds of nuclei gives rise to **heterokaryosis**. The alien nucleus which has been introduced into a mycelium can reproduce, and its daughter nuclei can spread through the mycelium. Eventually karyogamy and meiosis take place. The parasexual cycle can thus allow a similarly effective recombination of nuclear material as does true sexuality. The classification of the fungi imperfecti is based on the secondary fruiting forms and other external traits and serves exclusively the practical aims of naming and identification.

6 Growth of microorganisms

6.1 Nutrition of microorganisms

The growth of microorganisms is dependent on the presence of water. The substances from which microorganisms synthesise their cell material and obtain their energy, the nutrients, are dissolved in water. Different microorganisms have very different requirements for composition of nutrient media as well as for other environmental conditions. Because of this, numerous recipes for the composition of microbiological media have been devised. Basically, all nutrient media must fulfil the following minimal requirements: they must supply as utilisable compounds all elements that take part in the synthesis of the cell substance.

Elementary nutrient requirements. The elementary composition of cells is divided into the ten macroelements which are present in all cells, carbon, hydrogen, oxygen, nitrogen, sulphur, phosphorus, sodium, potassium, calcium, magnesium and iron (C, H, O, N, S, P, K, Na, Ca, Mg, Fe), and the microelements or trace elements; manganese, molybdenum, zinc, copper, cobalt, nickel, vanadium, boron, chlorine, selenium, silicon, tungsten, as well as others that are not required by all organisms. The heavy metals are mostly part of enzymes which are involved in the metabolism of inorganic elements and compounds (O_2, N_2, H_2, S, SO_4^{2-}, SO_3^{2-}, NO_3^{2-}, NO_2^{2-}, NH_4^{2+}). Most of these trace elements required at micromolar concentrations occur as impurities in the salts of the macroelements and also reach the nutrient media via contamination of glass vessels and dust particles. Special procedures are therefore necessary to demonstrate a requirement for trace elements. Many of the heavy metals (Hg, Cu, Zn, Ni, Co, Cd, Ag, Cr, Se) are toxic at millimolar concentrations. Most elements are provided as salts in nutrient media: Table 6.1 shows the composition of a simple synthetic medium plus a trace element stock solution (Table 6.2).

Carbon and energy sources. Organisms that can obtain their energy via photosynthesis or by oxidation of inorganic compounds can use carbon dioxide as their main carbon source. These carbon-autotrophs reduce

Table 6.1. *Example of a simple synthetic nutrient solution*

K_2HPO	0.5 g
NH_4Cl	1.0 g
$MgSO_4 \cdot 7H_2O$	0.2 g
$FeSO_4 \cdot 7H_2O$	0.01 g
$CaCl_2 \cdot 2H_2O$	0.01 g
Glucose	10.0 g
Water	1000 ml
Trace element stock solution	1 ml

Table 6.2. *Trace element stock solution*

$ZnCl_2$		70 mg
$MnCl_2 \cdot 4H_2O$		100 mg
$CoCl_2 \cdot 6H_2O$		200 mg
$NiCl_2 \cdot 6H_2O$		100 mg
$CuCl_2 \cdot 2H_2O$		20 mg
$NaMoO_4 \cdot 2H_2O$		50 mg
$Na_2SeO_3 \cdot 5H_2O$		26 mg
[$NaVO_3 \cdot H_2O$		10 mg]
[$Na_2WO_4 \cdot 2H_2O$		30 mg]
HCl (25%)		1.0 ml
Distilled water	to	1000 ml

[ ], required by only a few organisms.

CO_2. All other organisms obtain their cell carbon predominantly from organic compounds. These commonly serve as both carbon source and energy source; they are partially assimilated into the cell material and partially oxidised to provide energy. The quantiatively predominant organic nutrients in the biosphere are the polysaccharides cellulose and starch. The monomeric building blocks of these polymers, glucose, can be utilised by a great many microorganisms. In addition, practically all other naturally occurring organic materials can be broken down and utilised by some microorganisms.

Accessory nutrients.   Many organisms need, in addition to minerals, carbon and energy sources, some accessory nutrients, known as growth

Table 6.3. *Well-established solution of
vitamins for soil and water bacteria*

Biotin	0.2 mg
Nicotinic acid	2.0 mg
Thiamine	1.0 mg
4-Aminobenzoate	1.0 mg
Pantothenate	0.5 mg
Pyridoxamine	5.0 mg
Cyanocobalamine	2.0 mg
Distilled water	100 ml

2–3 ml of the solution are added per
1000 ml nutrient solution

factors or vitamins. These are substances that are part of the cell but cannot be synthesised from simple building blocks by the organism in question. There are three types of 'accessory' factors: amino acids, purine and pyrimidine bases, and the vitamins. The amino acids and purines plus pyrimidines are components of proteins and nucleic acids, respectively, and are therefore required in appropriate amounts; the vitamins, on the other hand, are components of coenzymes or prosthetic groups, i.e. they function catalytically and are therefore required in only minute quantities (Table 6.3). Organisms that have such accessory requirements are known as auxotrophs, in distinction to prototrophs, which are independent of accessory food factors.

Sulphur and nitrogen.   Both these elements are present in cells predominantly as reduced compounds, namely as sulphydryl and amino groups. Most microorganisms can assimilate these two elements as oxidised compounds and can reduce sulphates and nitrates. The most common sources of nitrogen for microorganisms are ammonium salts. A few prokaryotes can reduce molecular nitrogen (N_2). Other microorganisms may require amino acids as nitrogen sources in which the nitrogen is already present in an organic form. Similarly, not all microorganisms can carry out sulphate reduction; some require hydrogen sulphide or cysteine as a sulphur source.

Oxygen.   Oxygen is always present in the form of water, as well as in carbon dioxide and many organic substances. However, many organisms are additionally dependent on molecular oxygen (O_2). The main function of O_2 is to act as a terminal electron acceptor in aerobic respiration; the O_2 being reduced to water. Actual incorporation of molecular oxygen into the cell substance occurs only when methane or long-chain and aromatic hydrocarbons serve as carbon sources.

In their relation to oxygen, at least three groups of organisms can be distinguished. **Obligate aerobes** can obtain their energy only via aerobic respiration and are dependent on O_2. **Obligate anaerobes** can grow only in the absence of oxygen; for these, oxygen is toxic (see Ch. 7.4). **Facultative anaerobes** can grow either in the presence or absence of oxygen. Among these one must distinguish two types: lactic acid bacilli, for example, can grow in the presence of oxygen, i.e. they are **aerotolerant**, but they cannot utilise oxygen and they obtain their energy exclusively via fermentation. Other facultatively anaerobic bacteria (the Enterobacteriaceae) and many yeasts can switch from respiration in the presence of O_2 to fermentation in its absence for their energy supply.

Many, probably most, aerobic bacteria are actually **microaerophilic**, that is, they require oxygen for energy, but they cannot tolerate it at the partial pressure in air (0.2 bar) but only at 0.01–0.03 bar.

6.2   Nutrient media and growth conditions

Many unexacting microorganisms, such as several pseudomonads of soil and water, but also *E. coli*, can grow abundantly in nutrient solutions of the composition detailed in Table 6.1. A number of microorganisms also require one or other of the trace elements, vitamins, or other additions. When a nutrient solution can be made up entirely from defined chemical compounds it is called a **synthetic** or defined medium. It is desirable to find for each microorganism the minimal nutrient requirements and to develop a minimal medium that contains only the components actually required for growth. Exacting species may require many accessory substances; thus a minimal medium developed for *Leuconostoc mesenteroides* contains 40 components.

Complex media.   In the case of many exacting bacteria, the actual nutrient requirements are not completely known. These organisms are cultured in nutrient solutions that contain yeast extracts, yeast autolysates, peptones, or other meat extracts. For some groups of microorganisms such substances as malt extract, hay infusions, plum juice, carrot juice, coconut milk, and, for coprophilic fungi, even horse dung infusions may be used. For economic reasons, media are often made up with complex substances such as molasses, cornsteep liquor, soybean extract, whey, etc. which are cheap, industrial by-products, rather than from pure chemicals. All such nutrient media are known as **complex** or undefined media.

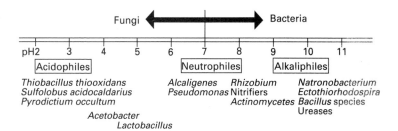

Fig. 6.1. *pH ranges that are tolerated or favoured by various bacteria and fungi.*

Solid media.   To obtain solid media, nutrient solutions have certain solidifying agents added to them, which give them a jellylike consistency. Gelatine, which was the first such solidifying agent, is only rarely used now because it melts at 26–30 °C and also because many microorganisms can liquefy it. The almost ideal solidifying agent is **agar**, introduced into bacteriological methodology in 1883 by one of R. Koch's collaborators, W. Hesse. This is a highly branched complex polysaccharide obtained from algae. It is added to aqueous nutrient solutions at a concentration of 15–20 g/l. Agar melts only at 100 °C but remains liquid down to 45 °C (or less). Very few bacteria are able to digest it. If solid media without any organic components are required, silica gel is used as the solidifying agent.

Hydrogen ion concentration.   The ions H^+ and OH^- are the most mobile of all ions; therefore even small changes in their concentrations have large effects. The attainment of the optimal initial pH and the maintenance of the pH during growth of a culture are therefore of great importance. Most organisms grow best when H^+ and OH^- ions are present in approximately equal concentrations (pH 7). Many bacteria, however, prefer higher pH values, i.e. a slightly alkaline medium. Some examples of these are the nitrifiers, rhizobia, actinomycetes, and urea-digesting bacteria (Fig. 6.1). Only a few are **acid tolerant** (lactobacilli, *Acetobacter, Sarcina ventriculi*) or even **acidophilic (*Thiobacillus*)**. Fungi prefer lower pH ranges. Inoculation of soil samples into complex media of different pH values will give predominantly fungi on the media at pH 5 and predominantly bacteria on the media at pH 8.

The maintenance of a constant pH during growth of a culture is especially important for those organisms that produce acid but are not acid tolerant (lactobacilli, Enterobacteriaceae, many pseudomonads). To avoid self-poisoning of long-term cultures by acid production, the media must be buffered or be free from fermentable substrates. A certain buffering capacity, though limited to values above pH 7.2, is given by inorganic phosphates. In the case of more pronounced acid production, addition of calcium carbonate to the medium is recommended, or sodium bicarbonate if insoluble components are undesirable; in the latter instance, though, it must be remembered that bicarbonate ions are in equilibrium with (dissolved) CO_2 and with the CO_2 content of the gas phase (i.e. air).

$$CO_2 \underset{\text{(gaseous)}}{} \rightleftharpoons CO_2 \underset{\text{(dissolved)}}{} \rightleftharpoons CO_2 + H_2O \rightleftharpoons H_2CO_3 \rightleftharpoons H^+ + HCO_3^-$$

The relationship between pH, bicarbonate concentration, and partial pressure of CO_2 in the atmosphere is given by the Henderson–Hasselbach equation: the concentration of carbonic acid equals the product of the CO_2 partial pressure and the solubility coefficient α:

$$pH = pK' + \log \frac{c(HCO_3^-)}{p(CO_2)\alpha}$$

Many bacteria, however, are fairly insensitive to small pH variations in the range 6–9. If the pH of the medium changes rapidly there may be a transient change in the intracellular pH, but this is usually readjusted to the original pH within about 30 minutes.

The damage produced by unsuitable pH is not actually due to the hydrogen and/or hydroxyl ions; these only increase the undissociated proportion of weak acids or bases which penetrate more readily into the cell than their dissociation products. The undissociated acids are the physiologically more active form. Cells take up the dibasic succinic acid and the tribasic citric acid more rapidly the lower the pH of the medium.

Carbon dioxide.   Nutrient media for CO_2-fixing, autotrophic bacteria usually contain sodium bicarbonate and are incubated in a CO_2-containing atmosphere in a closed system. Alternatively they can be bubbled with air or CO_2-enriched air. In all cases, the relationship between pH, bicarbonate concentration, and CO_2 partial pressure of the gaseous atmosphere, as described above, must be taken into consideration.

However, even heterotrophic organisms that assimilate organic carbon need CO_2. Many parasitic bacteria that occur in blood, tissues, or gastrointestinal tracts are adapted to a higher CO_2 content in their atmosphere than that in air. Such bacteria must be incubated in a gaseous atmosphere containing 10% CO_2, by volume. Furthermore, it must be kept in mind that removal of CO_2, as by absorption in KOH, will inhibit the growth of almost all bacteria (see CO_2 fixation, Ch. 11.5).

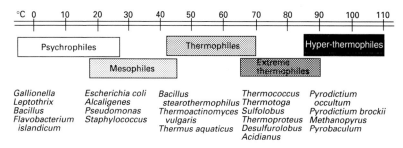

Fig. 6.2. *Growth temperature ranges of different bacteria.*

Water content and osmotic pressure. Microorganisms vary widely in their requirements with regard to water content. To compare solid materials and aqueous solutions with respect to available water, the parameters **water activity (a_w)** or relative humidity are used. These parameters are related to the vapour phase which is in equilibrium with a solid material or an aqueous solution. They give the ratio of the water concentration in the vapour phase over the material in question, and the water concentration in the gaseous phase over pure water, at a given temperature.

Microorganisms can grow over a range of water activities of 0.998–0.6 (a_w). The lowest water activity tolerated for growth has been recorded for the osmotolerant yeast *Saccharomyces rouxii* which grows at a_w of 0.6. *Aspergillus glaucus* and other moulds can grow at a_w of 0.8, but most bacteria need water activities of more than 0.98. The only exceptions are halophilic bacteria with a_w requirements to 0.75.

Temperature. Bacteria also differ with regard to the temperatures they require for growth (Fig. 6.2). Most of the soil and aquatic bacteria are **mesophilic**, i.e. they have their maximal growth rates at temperatures in the range of 20–42 °C. **Thermotolerant** organisms are those that can grow in temperatures of up to 50 °C (*Methylococcus capsulatus*). **Thermophilic bacteria** grow at maximal rates at temperatures above 40 °C and their temperature limit is in the region of 70 °C (*Bacillus stearothermophilus*, *Thermoactinomyces vulgaris*). **Extreme thermophiles** are organisms whose growth optimum is above 65 °C (*Thermus aquaticus*, *Sulfolobus*); some of these can grow above 70 °C (several species of the genera *Bacillus* and *Clostridium*) or 80 °C (*Sulfolobus acidocaldarius*) and even at 105 °C (a strictly anaerobic, sulphur-reducing bacterium). Bacteria that grow between 80 and 100 °C are called **hyper-thermophilic**. At the other end of the temperature range for growth are the **psychrophilic**

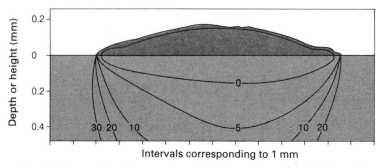

Fig. 6.3. *Oxygen distribution under and inside a colony of* Escherichia coli *after growth on complex agar.*

Partial pressures of oxygen after three days' incubation at 30 °C were determined by means of an oxygen microelectrode. Values are expressed as percentage of the partial pressures obtained in air-saturated agar.

(or **cryophilic**) organisms. Among these are predominantly some marine bacteria (photobacteria) and the iron bacteria (*Gallionella*); they reach their maximum growth rates at temperatures below 20 °C.

Aeration. All microorganisms that are obligate aerobes need oxygen as the final electron acceptor. When these bacteria grow on the surface of agar plates or in thin layers of liquid, in contact with air, the oxygen supply is usually sufficient. However, in liquid media of greater depth, aerobic bacteria can grow only in the surface layers because oxygen is continuously consumed and the deeper layers become anaerobic (Fig. 6.3). When aerobic bacteria are required to grow throughout a liquid medium, it is necessary to ensure a continuous oxygen supply by aeration. Microorganisms can utilise only dissolved oxygen. Whereas the mineral salts and organic nutrients of a medium can be supplied at concentrations sufficient for several hours' or even days' growth, the very low solubility of oxygen in aqueous solutions makes this limiting. One litre of water that is in equilibrium with air at atmospheric pressure and 20 °C contains 6.2 ml or 0.28 nmol oxygen. This amount is just enough to oxidise 0.046 mmol or 8.3 mg glucose (about one thousandth of the usual glucose concentration in nutrient media). Thus, oxygen cannot be stored in the nutrient medium but must be supplied continuously. Fortunately, most microorganisms are adapted to very low concentrations of dissolved oxygen, but a certain minimal value, the 'critical oxygen concentration' must be maintained for adequate respiration of the cells.

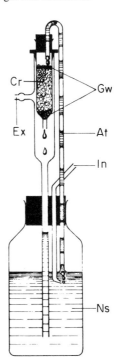

Fig. 6.4. *Apparatus for percolating a carrier material (soil, glass beads, etc.) with nutrients and air.*

The exit port (Ex) is connected to a suction device by which air is continuously and slowly removed from the vessel; fresh air is drawn in through the air inlet (In) at the same rate, forcing the nutrient medium up through the ascending tube (At) from the nutrient solution in the vessel (Ns). Nutrient solution and air are thus percolated through the carrier material (Cr). Gw, glass wool.

The rate of solution of oxygen in the liquid can be increased by providing a large area of gas–liquid interphase, and by increasing the partial pressure of oxygen in the gas phase. Liquid cultures are usually aerated by air, or by gas mixtures of O_2, N_2 and CO_2. A number of means for obtaining large surface areas have been tried: (1) thin-layer cultures; (2) agitation of the liquid by shaking (reciprocal or rotary shakers); (3) rotation of horizontally held flasks around their longitudinal axis; (4) forced aeration of a liquid column with air under pressure through a gas distributor (fritted glass); (5) percolation through columns of granular material (Fig. 6.4); (6) mechanical stirring. For submerged cultures of aerobic microorganisms a combination of forced aeration through sintered glass or spargers and mechanical stirring are often used. Some fermentors and the 'Waldhof' system utilise the vortex produced by vigorous stirring. Fig. 6.5 shows some of the culture vessels designed to give maximal surface area to liquid layers, and some of the apparatus developed for submerged culture of aerobic microorganisms.

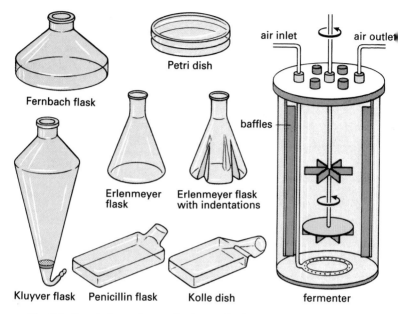

Fig. 6.5. *Vessels for surface and submerged culture of aerobic microorganisms.*

It must also be kept in mind that even in a well-aerated fermenter, or in natural waters, the distribution of oxygen is not always even. Clumping of bacteria, for example, can produce local microenvironments with lowered partial pressure of O_2. Such semi-anaerobic microenvironments can also be provoked by suspended material in natural waters. One can simulate these conditions experimentally by addition of solid particles (clay, cellulose, chitin) to bacterial suspensions. The bacteria then grow adhering to the surface of the particles and suffer oxygen lack. **Facultative anaerobes**, which switch either to fermentation (*E. coli*) or nitrate respiration (*Pseudomonas denitrificans*) under conditions of oxygen lack, are especially suited to demonstrate these effects.

Anaerobic culture.   Exclusion of oxygen from the culture milieu is essential for the growth of strictly anaerobic bacteria. Anaerobic techniques make use of de-aerated boiled nutrient media, free of air bubbles, in sealed bottles; oxygen-free gaseous atmosphere in desicators or anaerobic jars; the use of oxygen-absorbing substances (alkaline pyrogallol, dithionite) and other means. Addition of reducing agents (ascorbic acid, thioglycollate, cysteine, or sulphide, if tolerated) to nutrient media can reduce or counteract the toxic effects of aerobic oxygen. Even very oxygen-sensitive bacteria can be transferred in the open atmosphere, provided that a continuous stream of oxygen-free nitrogen through the culture vessel prevents contact of the medium with air (Hungate technique). Alternatively one can use inoculation chambers which are filled with oxygen-free nitrogen, argon or hydrogen. As an indicator for anaerobic conditions, resazurin can be added to media: in the presence of oxygen this is blue, if conditions are anaerobic it is colourless, and after reoxidation, it is red. Also, a beaker with alkaline glucose–methylene blue solution, which is decolorised under anaerobic conditions, can be added to the incubation jar.

6.3   Nutritional types

The concepts 'heterotrophic' and 'autotrophic', which were established to distinguish the modes of nutrition of plants and animals, are insufficient to characterise the much more diverse types of nutrition among microorganisms. Newer, summary designations of nutritional types refer to the **energy source**, the **hydrogen donors**, and the **carbon source**.

Energy source.   According to the mechanism of **energy conversion** into the biochemically useful form of ATP, organisms can be divided into two principal metabolic types: **phototrophic** and **chemotrophic**. Those organisms that can use electromagnetic radiation (light) as the energy source for growth are called **phototrophs** (photosynthesisers). The phototrophic organisms comprise two large groups: the anaerobic phototrophic bacteria, which do not evolve oxygen, and the aerobic phototrophs, i.e. cyanobacteria, algae and green plants, which produce oxygen in light. The term **chemotroph** (or chemosynthetic) indicates energy gain by oxidation–reduction reactions of nutrient substrates, irrespective of the way in which the biochemical energy is obtained, whether by respiration or fermentation.

Hydrogen donors and carbon sources.   All organisms that use organic compounds as **hydrogen donors** are called **organotrophs**. This term is used as an antonym to **lithotroph**, which is used to designate the ability to use inorganic hydrogen donors such as NH_3, H_2S, S, CO_2, Fe^{2+} and others. The concepts 'autotroph' and 'heterotroph' have been narrowed down in meaning and refer only to the **source of cellular carbon**. Microorganisms are **autotrophs** if they can obtain the major part of their cellular carbon by carbon dioxide fixation. They are **heterotrophs** if they obtain their cell carbon by assimilation of organic compounds.

In general, classification by the basic processes of energy conversion and the hydrogen donor is sufficient. Green plants, cyanobacteria, and purple sulphur bacteria are **photolithotrophs**, nitrifying bacteria are **chemolithotrophs**, and animals and the vast majority of microorganisms are **chemo-organotrophs** (the source of cellular carbon is included in the designation only in special cases). Since in most microorganisms lithotrophy is linked to autotrophy, one may also speak of **photoautotrophs**, **chemoautotrophs**, and **chemoheterotrophs**.

6.4   Selective culture methods

Our knowledge of the diversity of microorganisms is based on two kinds of procedures. Some microorganisms became recognisable by their colonial characteristics, accumulation of substances, or changes in their environment. By producing visible evidence of their presence many of these microorganisms are suitable for **direct isolation**. Appropriate growth media and conditions for such organisms could be readily determined. Many different types of microorganisms, however, could be investigated only after S. N. Winogradsky and M. W. Beijerinck had developed the techniques of enrichment culture.

Enrichment culture.   The principle and the practice of this technique are really very simple. Enrichment conditions for a given organism are those that enable it to compete successfully and outgrow other organisms that may be present in the inoculum. Thus, one can impose environmental conditions by choice of a number of factors (nature of carbon, energy and nitrogen sources, gaseous atmosphere, hydrogen acceptors, temperature, light, pH, etc.). On inoculation of such a medium with a mixed population of microorganisms such as a sample of soil or mud, the organisms that are most highly adapted to the particular growth conditions provided will outgrow the others and gain dominance (in numbers). By repeated subculturing in the same medium and under the same conditions and finally plating out on solid medium of the same composition, the enriched strain or species can then be isolated. Frequent subculture at short intervals in liquid medium prevents the growth of accompanying organisms that might utilise excretion products or even autolysates of the cells that are primarily favoured. Suitable starting materials, i.e. inocula, are samples from locations where natural selection and enrichment has already taken place; carbon monoxide-utilising organisms from gas work effluents; haemoglobin-utilising strains from abattoir wastes, and hydrocarbon-oxidising organisms from oilfields and refineries.

The enrichment culture technique makes it possible to isolate microorganisms with all possible combinations of nutrient requirements, provided that the desired type does exist in nature. For very specialised microorganisms the enrichment conditions can be highly selective. A mineral medium, free of fixed nitrogen and exposed to light, is extremely selective for nitrogen-fixing cyanobacteria. If such a nutrient solution is supplemented with an organic carbon and energy source and incubated aerobically in the dark, it will become enriched with *Azotobacter*, whilst anaerobically *Clostridium* will flourish. The success of an enrichment culture depends on satisfying only the **minimal nutritional requirements** of the metabolic type that one desires to isolate. Thus, for instance, if bacteria are sought that can oxidise methane or hydrogen, with nitrate or sulphate as hydrogen acceptor, it is imperative to exclude oxygen from the growth milieu; otherwise aerobic bacteria that can oxidise methane or hydrogen would predominate. Selection methods can also be based on the resistance or tolerance of an organisms with respect to acid or alkali, heat, or radiation. Quite often selective techniques can include 'counter selection' of accompanying organisms by including selective inhibitors in the media. Thus, an azide-containing medium allows, under aerobic conditions, the growth of lactic acid bacteria, whilst the growth of other aerobes is inhibited. Azide, cyanide and H_2S select against aerobic organisms that have cytochromes involved in their respiratory processes. Selective inhibition is used in medical diagnosis for identification of *Corynebacterium diphtheriae* (tellurite-containing media) and of pathogenic Enterobacteriaceae (bismuth agar). The technique of counter selection with penicillin for the purpose of enriching auxotropic mutants is described in Ch. 15.1.5. Addition of penicillin to media is also used to suppress gram-positive bacteria. Growth of fungi, yeasts, protozoa and other eukaryotic microorganisms can be suppressed by addition of cycloheximide.

Sometimes inocula used for enrichment culture may contain several variants of a similar metabolic type; these variants may differ only slightly, in pH optima or growth rates, for example. In this case only the best adapted or most rapidly growing strain will prevail and overgrow the others, so that they cannot be isolated. If **the aim** is to **obtain the largest possible number of strains** that can grow under the selective conditions, the '**direct plate**' method can be used. If the inoculum is distributed at a suitable dilution over a solidified selective medium (an agar plate), the favoured metabolic types will give rise to individual colonies, and if the distance between the colonies is adequate, there will be no competition for nutrients. The more slowly growing strains are therefore not overgrown by the faster growing ones and can be isolated. Table 6.4 gives the important selective conditions for a number of representative

Table 6.4. *Conditions for enrichment culture of certain bacteria*

Phototrophic microorganisms: main carbon source CO_2

Under illumination	anaerobic	H_2		
		organic acids	photo-assimilated	$\lambda > 800$ nm
				Rhodospirillaceae
		H_2S	as H-donor	Chromatiaceae
		H_2S	as H-donor	$\lambda > 715$ nm Chlorobiaceae
	aerobic	NH_4Cl orKNO_3	as N-source	green algae
		N_2	as N-source	cyanobacteria

Chemolithotrophic (autotrophic) bacteria: main carbon source CO_2

		H-donor	H-acceptor	
In the dark, no organic compounds	aerobic	NH_4^+	O_2	*Nitrosomonas*
		NO_2^-	O_2	*Nitrobacter*
		H_2	O_2	H_2 bacteria
		$H_2S, S, S_2O_3^{2-}$	O_2	*Thiobacillus*
		Fe^{2+}	O_2	*Thiobacillus ferrooxidans*
	anaerobic	$S, S_2O_3^{2-}$	NO_3^-	*Thiobacillus denitrificans*
		H_2	NO_3^-	*Paracoccus denitrificans*
		H_2	CO_2	methanogens

Chemo-organotrophic (heterotrophic) bacteria

Anaerobes	*With external H-acceptor:*	
	KNO_3, 2% plus organic acids	pseudomonads } denitrifying
	KNO_3, 10% plus YE	spore formers }
	Without external H-acceptor:	
	glutamate, histidine	*Clostridium tetanomorphum*
	lactate plus YE	*Veillonella*
	starch plus NH_4^{+a}	*Clostridium*
	starch plus N_2^a	*C. pasteurianum*
	glucose plus NH_4^+	*Enterobacter* and fermenters
	glucose plus 1% YE, pH 5	lactic acid bacteria
	lactate plus 1% YE	propionic acid bacteria
Aerobes	lactate plus NH_4^+	*Pseudomonas fluorescens*
	mannitol, benzoate plus N_2	*Azotobacter*
	starch plus NH_4^{+a}	*Bacillus polymyxa* and similar
	4% ethanol plus 1% YE, pH 6.0	*Acetobacter, Gluconobacter*
	5% urea plus 1% YE	*Sporosarcina ureae*
	petroleum plus NH_4^+	*Mycobacterium, Nocardia*
	cellulose plus NH_4^+	*Sporocytophaga*

YE, yeast extract.   [a] Pasteurised inoculum.

Fig. 6.6 *'Streaking out' method for isolation of a pure culture of an aerobic bacterium.*

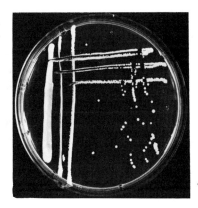

A suitable dilution of a bacterial suspension is 'streaked out' on an agar medium with a platinum loop. Successive streaks transfer decreasing concentrations of the inoculum. The final, well-separated colonies have originated most probably from single cells. The single colony in the upper part of the plate is due to an air contaminant.
(Picture: B. Lehmann.)

metabolic types. It summarises the data presented in the discussion of enrichments for individual metabolic types.

Pure culture.   A pure culture is defined as the progeny (clone) of a single cell. To establish a pure culture, demonstrate its purity beyond doubt, and maintain it free from contaminants is one of the most important tasks for microbiologists. The isolation of pure cultures (i.e. of a given organism) is carried out, with very few exceptions, on or in solid media. First of all, a single cell must be separated from a cell population, and the colony that results from its multiplication must remain separate from other cells and other colonies. Aerobic bacteria are isolated by Koch's pour-plate method, or, less laboriously, by streaking with a platinum wire loop over the surface of a suitable agar plate (Fig. 6.6). Anaerobic bacteria are suspended in liquefied agar medium at 45 °C and incubated under exclusion of oxygen (Fig. 6.7). By careful separation of single colonies, their suspension in suitable liquid, and repeated streaking out or 'plating' on nutrient agar of the same composition, it is possible to obtain pure cultures of the majority of microorganisms.

The isolation of a pure culture can also be carried out in liquid media, provided that the particular organism is quantitatively predominant in the starting material. By serial dilution of the suspension in medium, a stage can be reached where only one cell is present in the medium; a clone arising from this must then represent a pure culture.

Mixed culture.   Natural populations normally consist of a mixture of different microorganisms. A variety of interrelationships can exist among these. They can be classified as competitive for common substrates, as **commensalism** or **mutualism** (see Ch. 17.2). To study such relationships

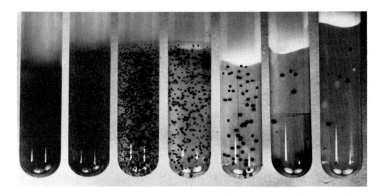

Fig. 6.7. *Serial dilution of purple sulphur bacteria in soft agar (0.8%) after incubation for one week with illumination.*

This demonstrates the isolation of a pure culture of anaerobic bacteria according to the dilution technique in shaken cultures. The agar column is covered with a layer of paraffin and oil to prevent access of atmospheric oxygen. (Picture: B. Lehmann.)

and others, the employment of mixed cultures is coming increasingly into use. In batch cultures as well as in continuous culture systems, defined conditions can be employed, and successions of different microorganisms and their metabolic products can be monitored. These provide evidence for antagonistic or synergistic relationships among the organisms. A desired mixed culture can be constructed by mixing inocula from pure culture. Experiments with defined mixed cultures can lead to insights into the complex interrelationships among the microorganisms in their natural habitat.

For use in home and industry, pure cultures are by no means universal; many processes employ mixed cultures, which are sometimes called 'natural pure cultures'. Examples of this are sourdough, 'kefir', tea, fungus and yeast. Mixed cultures also play a considerable role in sewage and effluent treatments, especially in the degradation of xenobiotics in industrial effluents.

6.5   The physiology of growth

Growth can be considered as the increase in living substance; usually the number of cells or the total mass of cells. The **growth** rate measures change in either cell number or cell mass per unit time. In unicellular organisms growth involves increase of cell numbers. Bacterial cells multiply by **binary fission**. At first cell size doubles, and the cell then divides into two daughter cells which have approximately the same size as the original 'mother' cell. The time required for a doubling of cell numbers is known as the **generation time**, whilst the time required for doubling of the cell mass is referred to as the **doubling time**. Under conditions where cell mass and numbers double in the same time interval, the generation time (g) and doubling time (t_d) are of course equal. The reciprocal value $1/g$ = number of doublings per hour is called the growth rate, v and has the dimension of h^{-1}.

6.5.1   Methods of determining bacterial numbers and bacterial mass

During growth of a population in batch culture, for example a suspension of bacteria in an Erlenmeyer flask, there is not necessarily a constant or unique relationship between increase in bacterial mass and cell numbers.

After inoculation of the nutrient medium, for example, some bacteria may divide more rapidly than the rate of increase in mass; in this case the cells become smaller. At a later stage the rate of increase in cell mass may exceed the increase in cell numbers, so that the cells become larger. It is necessary, therefore, to distinguish between increase in cell mass and cell numbers. On the other hand, when dealing with those growth phases where the **increase** in cell mass and numbers is **is known to be equal**, these two parameters do not need to be considered separately. Under such conditions of **balanced growth**, with so-called 'standard cells', a parameter **proportional to total cell mass**, such as photometric extinction or optical density, can be determined instead of cell numbers. (The proportionality between extinction and cell mass has to be ascertained, however, for each set of conditions, i.e. for a given organism in a given medium.) The cell mass per unit volume (litre or ml) is then referred to as the **cell concentration** or **cell density** (g/l or mg/ml).

Determination of bacterial numbers.   Not all the cells in a bacterial population are necessarily viable. Only those cells are regarded as living, or viable, that can grow on or in nutrient agar to produce colonies, or that can grow to suspensions in liquid nutrient media. The method of viable counting determines the number of such viable cells in a population, whilst 'total cell counts' include all visible or otherwise demonstrable cells, including those that are 'non-viable' or damaged.

Total cell count.   (1) The most widely used method for determining total counts involves enumeration, using a microscope, of the number of cells suspended in a thin layer of agar and placed in a counting chamber of known volume (according to Neubauer or Thoma). With a layer 0.02 mm deep and an area 0.05 mm square (i.e. a volume of 5×10^{-8} cm^3), the number of cells counted under the microscope must be multiplied by 2×10^7 to give the total cell number/ml. (2) Counts relative to known numbers of small particles, for example, those of erythrocytes in blood (approximately 5×10^6/ml), is one of the oldest methods. (3) An electronic instrument, the Coulter counter, has greatly facilitated total counting, it utilises the loss of conductance of an electrolyte solution that occurs when a bacteriuma (or small particle) passes through a narrow orifice. (4) With cell numbers below 10^6/ml, a membrane filtration method can be used. A known volume of marine, pond, or drinking water is passed through a membrane filter that is then dried, stained, and made transparent for microscopic enumeration of the cells on the filter (or a known area thereof).

Viable counts.   Usually this involves counting the colonies produced by the viable cells under favourable growth conditions. According to Koch's pour-plate method, an aliquot of a suitably diluted suspension of the culture is mixed with nutrient agar at a temperature where it is liquid (40–45 °C), poured into petri dishes, and allowed to set. The suspensions can also be spread over the agar surface of a petri dish using a sterile spreader or triangular spatula. Alternatively, the cells can be deposited on a suitable filter (membrane filter) that can then be placed onto nutrient agar or nutrient-coated cards. In all cases, the number of colonies produced after suitable incubation of the nutrient media is counted. The application of Koch's pour-plate method, as well as the other methods derived from it, is suitable only for homogeneous suspenions of a given strain or species, but not for counting individuals cells of different species in a mixed population.

Determination of bacterial mass.   The choice of method for determinations of bacterial mass depends on the context, i.e. what the determined mass is related to. Thus, for determinations of growth yields, wet or dry weight estimations are commonly used. To evaluate metabolic and enzymic activites, however, protein or nitrogen content of a given bacterial suspension is more pertinent. Quite often, the choice of method is dictated mainly by speed and simplicity, and indirect methods, which have to be calibrated, are therefore often preferred over the direct methods.

Direct methods.   (1) Determination of the wet weight after centrifugation. After drying the centrifuged cells to constant weight, one can determine the dry weight. Both these procedures are subject to considerable systematic errors. (2) Total nitrogen content (by micro-Kjeldahl with microdiffusion of ammonia) and total carbon (according to van Slyke–Folch) can be more accurately determined. (3) In routine determinations, bacterial protein can be readily quantified. Modifications of the biuret reaction and other colorimetrically accessible colour reactions are very serviceable. Micromethods are based on estimations of representative protein constituents (such as tyrosine or tryptophan in the Lowry or Folin–Ciocalteu methods).

Indirect methods.   Methods that are based on measuring the turbidity of cell suspensions are very useful for determining bacterial mass. Usually the optical density or turbidity of a suspension is measured as extinction, though for some purposes nephelometry may be more accurate. The linearity between the measurements and bacterial mass (concentration) extends over only a very limited range of cell concentrations. Since the light scattering of the cells is influenced by size (diameter), shape, refractive index, as well as composition and turgor of the cells, it is necessary to calibrate the optical measurements against more direct parameters (i.e. dry weight, nitrogen or carbon concentration) for any particular conditions. (2) Metabolic functions that are directly related to growth, such as oxygen uptake, production of carbon dioxide, or production of acid, can also give an adequate measure of microbial mass. Such determinations are useful in cases where other methods are unsuitable, for example, when dealing with very low concentrations of cells. Measurements of metabolic functions can be made by a variety of methods: titrimetric, manometric, electrochemical, etc. For actual and not just relative measurements of microbial mass, measurements using these methods also need to be calibrated to direct measurements of dry weight, etc.

6.5.2   Exponential growth and generation time

Bacteria reproduce by binary fission. Their multiplication therefore corresponds to a geometric progression: $2^0 \rightarrow 2^1 \rightarrow 2^2 \rightarrow 2^3 \dots 2^n$. The number of cells increases during each time interval by a constant factor. This is referred to as **exponential growth**. Taking a unit volume of a growing batch culture containing N_0 cells, then the number of cells, N, after n divisions will be $N_0 \times 2^n$ Applying logarithms, this becomes $\log N = \log N_0 + n\log 2$ and for the number of cell divisions

$$n = \frac{\log N - \log N_0}{\log 2}$$

For the number of divisions per hour, also known as the division rate (v) this gives

$$v = \frac{n}{t} = \frac{\log N - \log N_0}{\log 2(t - t_0)}$$

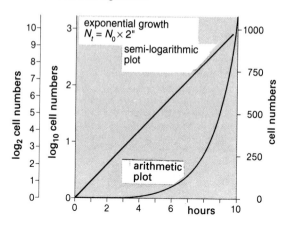

Fig. 6.8. *Exponential growth of unicellular organisms.*
Arithmetic and semi-logarithmic
plots of cell numbers versus time.

The time interval for one division is called the generation time

$$g = \frac{t}{n} = \frac{1}{v}$$

Thus if a cell suspension (culture) increases in ten hours from 10^3 to 10^9 cells (per unit volume), the division rate will be

$$v = \frac{\log 10^9 - \log 10^3}{0.3010 \times 10} \approx \frac{6}{3} = 2 \text{ (divisions / hour)}$$

and the generation time is 30 minutes.

A plot of the number (or mass) of cells on the ordinate against the time on the abscissa (both arimetrically) gives an exponential curve (Fig. 6.8). Such an arithmetic representation of a growth curve is, however, unsuitable for dealing with a large number of cell divisions since only the early or late divisions (depending on the chosen range of measurements) will be recognisable. It is preferable, therefore, to use a semi-logarithmic plot (Fig. 6.8), i.e. with the logarithms of the cell concentrations on the ordinate. Such a logarithmic plot shows **exponential growth** as a straight line, the slope of the line corresponding to the division rate; the steeper the slope, the greater the division rate. Because exponential growth is characterised by a linear relationship between time and logarithm of cell numbers (or mass), it is also referred to as **logarithmic growth**.

In studies of bacterial growth kinetics, individual cells can be ignored and the growing population is considered as an **autocatalytically multi-**

plying syustem. Calculations are based on bacterial mass (x) or a measurement that is strictly proportional to it (i.e. optical extinction under defined conditions). The rate of change in the value of x during any time interval is then proportional to the initial value of x, and thus follows the kinetics of a first order reaction. Thus, during exponental growth:

$$\frac{dx}{dt} = \mu x$$

where μ is the growth rate constant. Integration then leads to :

$$x = x_0 \cdot e^{\mu t}$$

and for a doubling of x

$$2x_0 = x_0 \cdot e^{\mu t} d$$

From this follows:

$$2 = e^{\mu t} d \text{ or } \ln 2 = \mu t_d$$

Hence

$$\mu = \frac{\ln_2}{t_d} = \frac{0.693}{t_d}$$

The growth constant, μ, is therefore related to the reciprocal of the doubling or generation time, i.e. the growth rate v by:

$$v = \frac{1}{t_d} = \frac{\mu}{0.693}$$

The two parameters, μ and v are functions of the same growth process, i.e. of an exponential growing bacterial population.

6.5.3   Bacterial growth in batch culture

If bacteria are inoculated into a nutrient solution and incubated under suitable conditions, they will usually continue to multiply until one necessary factor approaches exhaustion and becomes growth limiting. If during this period no nutrients are added or waste products removed, the growth in such a closed system is called a batch culture and it obeys the same laws as does the growth of multicellular organisms. A batch culture thus behaves like a multicellular organisms with genetically determined limitations of growth.

Growth of a bacterial culture can be depicted graphically by plotting the logarithms of cell numbers or viable counts against time. A typical **growth curve** of this kind (Fig. 6.9) is sigmoidal in shape and can be divided into a **number of growth phases**, which are regularly present but

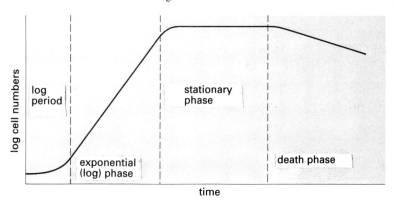

Fig. 6.9. *Growth curve of a bacterial culture.*

may appear more or less strongly expressed (or vary somewhat in extent). These are the lag phase, exponential or logarithmic phase, stationary phase, and death phase. Growth on solid media proceeds basically in the same way but much higher cell concentrations are involved.

The lag phase.   This occupies the time interval between inoculation and establishment of the maximum division rate. The actual duration of the lag phase depends on the previous cultural history, the age of the culture, and the composition and suitability of the nutrient medium. If the inoculum is derived from an 'old' culture, i.e. one in the stationary phase, the cells will need to synthesise RNA, ribosomes, enzymes, etc. to adapt to the new growth conditions. Again, if the carbon and energy sources in the new medium differ from those in the old, adaptation to these novel conditions will often involve synthesis of new enzymes that were not required for growth in the previous culture and were therefore not synthesised. The synthesis of such new enzymes is induced by the presence of the new substrate(s).

A good example of this effect of substrate on enzyme synthesis is the phenomenon called **diauxie** (Fig. 6.10). The appearance of biphasic growth or a double growth cycle is found in media that contain mixtures of substrates. In a mixture of glucose and sorbitol, for example, *E. coli* will utilise only the glucose at first. Glucose will induce the synthesis of those enzymes required for its utilisation and at the same time will repress the synthesis of enzymes required for sorbitol utilisation. These latter are only produced when all the glucose has been metabolised. Hence the two lag phases in such cultures can be explained by these regulatory mechanisms.

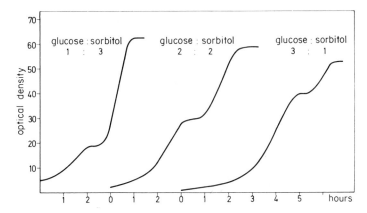

Fig. 6.10. *Biphasic growth (diauxie) of* E. coli *in nutrient media containing glucose and sorbitol in the proportions shown.*

(After Monod, J. (1958). *Recherches sur la croissance des cultures bactériennes.* Paris: Hermann.)

Changes in the quantitative composition of bacteria during the lag phase are most clearly seen in their RNA content. The RNA concentration increases 8-fold to 12-fold, and this increase indicates the participation of RNA and ribosomes in the synthesis of enzymes and protein.

The exponential phase.   The exponential or logarithmic growth phase (the log phase) is characterised by a constant minimal division or doubling rate. The actual logarithmic division rate is dependent on the particular organism and the growth conditions. Enterobacteria can grow with a doubling time of 15–30 minutes. *E. coli* can grow at 37 °C with a doubling time of 20 minutes. For other bacteria the generation time may be much longer, many soil bacteria grow with generation times of 60–150 minutes and *Nitrosomonas* and *Nitrobacter* have doubling times of 5–10 hours.

In many bacteria, cell size and protein content are constant during the log phase; the culture can be said to consist of 'standard cells'. When this can be established and cell numbers, dry weight and cellular protein all increase at the same rate, any one of these can be used for measuring growth rate. In many cases, however, the cells undergo changes in size and/or composition in batch culture even during logarithmic growth because the milieu is also undergoing continuous changes. The substrate concentration decreases, the cell concentration rises, and metabolic end products may accumulate. However, since the generation time remains relatively constant during the log phase, it is the most suitable phase for measurements of growth rates. The influence of environmental factors such as pH, temperature, redox potential, aeration, and the utilisation of different substrates is studied by following the increases in cell numbers or turbidity (extinction) during exponential growth.

The stationary phase. This phase begins when the cells can no longer reproduce. As the growth rate depends on, among other factors, the concentration of substrate, and because this decreases during growth, the growth rate of a culture usually begins to decline even before all substrate has been consumed. The transition from the exponential to the stationary phase is therefore usually gradual. Apart from substrate limitation, other factors such as very high cell concentrations, low partial pressure of oxygen, and accumulation of toxic metabolic end products can also lead to decrease in growth rate and initiation of the stationary phase. During the stationary phase, storage material may be consumed, a proportion of ribosomes may be degraded, and enzymes may still be synthesised. These various processes are dependent on the nature of the growth-limiting factor. Only very sensitive cells die off rapidly. As long as the energy necessary for cell maintenance can be supplied by utilisation of reserve materials or protein, the bacteria may remain viable for a considerable time.

In many microbial processes that are aimed at the formation of secondary metabolites (for example production of penicillin) the stationary phase is the real production phase. In biotechnology, therefore, a **trophophase** of growth is distinguished from an **idiophase**, i.e. a production phase. Although the cells no longer grow in the idiophase, they still utilise added substrates and incorporate precursor substances into the final product.

The bacterial mass that is synthesised when the stationary phase is reached is known as the yield, and it is dependent on the amounts and nature of the nutrients and the culture conditions.

The death phase. The death phase and the causes of bacterial death in normal nutrient media have not been thoroughly investigated. The situation is clearer in cases where acids are accumulated (*Escherichia, Lactobacillus*). The viable count can decrease exponentially. In some cases cell lysis occurs due to cellular enzymes (autolysins).

6.5.4   Growth curve parameters

When the growth of a batch culture is followed by means of dry weight determinations, the growth parameters of primary interest are the yield, the exponential growth rate, and the duration of the lag phase (Fig. 6.11).

Yield. The yield is the difference between the initial and the maximum bacterial mass: $X = X_{max} - X_o$. It is expressed in grams of dry weight. Of special significance is the relationship of the yield to substrate

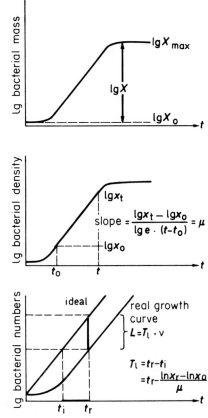

Fig. 6.11. *Growth parameters: yield, growth rate and lag phase.*

consumption (X/S). When both of these values are expressed in weight units, the ratio is called the yield coefficient or growth yield, Y. The yield is also frequently related to the concentration of the substrate and calculated as the molar growth yield Y_m (g cells/mol substrate). This molar growth yield enables one to relate the yield to the amount of ATP available from metabolism of a given energy source (substrate). This leads to an energy yield coefficient (g cells/mol ATP) that can be calculated when the catabolic pathway and its energy yield for a substrate is known.

For anaerobic cultures of E. coli and Klebsiella pneumoniae whose growth rate was limited by glucose supply, respective Y_{ATP} values of 12.4 and 14 g cells/mol ATP have been determined. In the anaerobic bacteria, which obtain all their energy by fermentation, Y_{ATP} is a largely constant value. Significantly higher values of Y_{ATP}, for a new bacterium for example, suggest the existence of additional energy-yielding metabolic reactions. Values of Y_{ATP} have also been determined for aerobically growing bacteria. They seem to depend on the growth conditions and the necessary synthetic activities of the cells, i.e. whether the nitrogen source for cell synthesis is in the form of ammonium ions, nitrate ions, or organic nitrogen compounds.

Exponential growth rate.   The exponential growth rate is a measure of the speed of cellular growth in the exponential phase. It is calculated from the bacterial concentrations x_0 and x_t at the times t_0 and t, according to the equation

$$\mu = \frac{\log x_t - \log x_0}{\log e(t - t_0)} = \frac{\ln x_t - \ln x_0}{(t - t_0)}$$

where $\log e = 0.43429$. The doubling time is

$$t_d = \frac{\ln 2}{\mu}$$

The lag phase like the exponential growth rate is an important parameter for judging the properties of an organism and the suitability of a medium. The lag period T_1 is the time interval between the time t_r at which the culture has reached a certain density x_r and the time t_i at which it would have reached the same density if it had been growing exponentially from the time of inoculation (l = lag phase; r = real growth; i = ideal growth).

$$T_1 = t_r - t_i = t_r - \frac{\ln x_r - \ln x_0}{\mu}$$

As the parameter T_1 can be used when two cultures with the same exponential growth rates are compared, the lag period is usually expressed in terms of generation time (g) rather than in absolute time. The difference between the observed, real growth and the ideal growth, expressed in multiples of generation time is $L = T_1 \cdot v$. The L value therefore states by how many doublings the real culture lags behind the ideal culture that would have grown at the exponential rate throughout. These L values are used in comparisons of data on the influence of different nutrients, inhibitors and environmental conditions on growth.

6.5.5 Bacterial growth in continuous culture

In a batch culture the cultural conditions undergo continual change; the bacterial concentration rises and the substrate concentration diminishes. For many physiological investigations, however, it is desirable to keep the cells over extended periods during which substrate concentrations and other cultural conditions are constant and the cells grow at a constant exponential rate. Such a situation can be approximated by frequent transfer of the cell population to fresh nutrient medium. The aim is reached more simply and more completely by constant addition of new growth medium to a growing cell population and concomitant withdrawal of equal volumes of the bacterial culture. This is the basis of continuous culture carried out in a **chemostat** or a **turbidostat**.

Growth in the chemostat.   The chemostat (Fig. 6.12) consists of a culture vessel and a reservoir that supplies nutrient medium at a constant rate. Forced aeration and mechanical stirring of the culture are used to ensure optimal oxygen supply and almost instantaneous equal distribution of the nutrients throughout the culture vessel. New medium is continuously added to the culture vessel at a constant rate, and bacterial culture is withdrawn at the same rate. If the volume of the culture vessel is V litres and the medium is supplied at a **rate** of $f = (l/h)$, then the **dilution rate** is $D = f/V$, so that D gives the **volume change per hour**. If the bacteria initially present in the culture vessel ($X = g/l$) were unable to grow, they would be washed out of the culture vessel with a **wash-out rate**.

$$D \cdot x = \frac{dx}{dt}$$

The bacterial concentration in the culture would thus decrease exponentially as $x = x_o \cdot e^{-Dt}$. Growth of bacteria in the culture vessel is also exponential, and the **rate of increase** is given by the expression

220 Growth of microorganisms

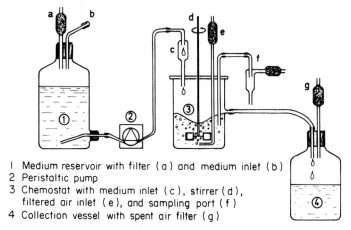

1 Medium reservoir with filter (a) and medium inlet (b)
2 Peristaltic pump
3 Chemostat with medium inlet (c), stirrer (d),
  filtered air inlet (e), and sampling port (f)
4 Collection vessel with spent air filter (g)

Fig. 6.12. *Principle of continuous culture in a chemostat.*

$\mu x = \mathrm{d}x/\mathrm{d}t$, so that the bacterial concentration increases exponentially as $x = x_0 \cdot \mathrm{e}^{-\mu t}$. The rate of change in bacterial concentration, $\mathrm{d}x/\mathrm{d}t$, inside the culture vessel is thus composed of the two above rates, i.e. $\mathrm{d}x/\mathrm{d}t = \mu x - Dx$. Thus, if the **growth rate** μ and the **dilution rate** D are equal, the loss through wash-out and gain by bacterial growth are in balance, hence the change in bacterial mass is zero and bacterial concentration remains constant. Under these conditions the culture is in **steady state**: the exponential increase in cell mass is balanced by a negative exponential process of the same magnitude.

The culture in a chemostat is controlled by substrate concentration; the stability of the system rests on this limitation of growth rate by the concentration of a growth-limiting substrate (hydrogen donor, N, S, or P source). If this substrate limitation is used to keep the actual growth constant μ smaller than the maximal growth constant possible at that substrate concentration, μ_{max}, the dilution rate D can be varied over a fairly wide range without risk of wash-out. Of course, the dilution rate must not exceed μ_{max}.

The dependence of the growth constant μ on the substrate concentration c_s follows a saturation curve (Fig. 6.13). In general, bacteria can grow at low substrate concentrations (for example 10 mg glucose/l medium) at maximal rate; μ becomes proportional to substrate concentration only at very low values. K_s is the substrate concentration at which μ is half the maximal rate constant ($\mu = \frac{1}{2}\mu_{max}$). K_s is one of the fundamental growth parameters of a chemostat culture, together with Y (yield) and μ_{max}.

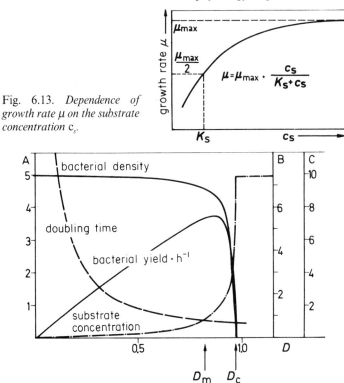

Fig. 6.13. *Dependence of growth rate μ on the substrate concentration c_s.*

Fig. 6.14. *Relationships between bacterial concentration, substrate concentration, doubling time, and bacterial yield in the steady state, at different dilution rates (D) in a chemostat.*

The values are calculated for a bacterial culture with the following parameters: $\mu_{max} = 1.0$ h⁻¹, $Y = 0.5$, and $K_s = 0.2$ g/l with a substrate concentration in the incoming nutrient solution of $S_r = 10$ g/l. Ordinates: (A) bacterial yield Dx (g/l·h); (B) doubling time t_d (h);

(C) substrate concentration in the culture vessel c_s (g/l). Abscissa: dilution rate D (h⁻¹); D_m, dilution rate for maximal yield; D_c, wash-out point. (After Herbert, D., Elsworth, R. & Telling, R. C. (1956). *J. gen. Microbiol.* **14**, 601.)

Figure 6.14 shows the bacterial concentration, the substrate concentration, the doubling time, and the bacterial yield all plotted against the dilution rate D. When the dilution rate D is varied between zero and the wash-out rate D_c, there is little variation in the bacterial concentration.

In this range the bacteria respond to an increase in dilution rate with a decrease in doubling time (increase in growth rate). The increasing dilution rate and the similarly increasing medium flow rate with the decreasing doubling time, however, produce an increasing expulsion of bacteria. This reaches a maximum at the dilution rate D_m. Above D_m it decreases rapidly.

The substrate concentration in the culture vessel and hence in the culture leaving it (i.e. the outflow) is close to zero for a wide range of low dilution rates. Only when the dilution rate approaches the maximum growth rate does some of the substrate reach the outflow, i.e. is washed out. With further increase in dilution rate, the substrate concentration in the outflow eventually equals that in the inflow of nutrient solution.

The stability of the flow balance in a chemostat is based on the limitation of the growth constant by substrate concentration (see above). The growth rate μ is kept at a low value. If the flow rate is kept constant over considerable periods, the chemostat can be easily run as a self-regulatory system.

Growth in the turbidostat. Continuous culture in a chemostat can be contrasted to that in a turbidostat. As the name suggests, this is based on keeping a bacterial concentration or turbidity constant. A turbidity probe controls the nutrient flow by means of a switch. The culture vessel contains all nutrients in excess, and the bacteria grow at almost maximal growth rate. The running of a turbidostat is technically more complicated and demanding than that of a chemostat.

Fundamental differences. There are some fundamental differences between growth of a classical batch culture and growth in continuous culture in a chemostat. These differences should be emphasised once more.

Batch culture must be viewed as a closed system (in a way, as a multicellular organism) whose development consists of a lag phase, exponential phase and 'death' phase (i.e. like youth, maturity, age and death). The culture conditions are different at each moment. Automation is hardly possible in such a culture.

Continuous culture represents an open system that approaches a '**steady state**'. The time factor is more or less eliminated, and the environmental conditions for the organism are constant. Such a system can be easily automated.

6.5.6   Synchronisation of cell division

To study metabolic processes in relation to the cell division cycle, it is necessary to have a population of cells that divide at the same time, i.e.

synchronously. The equal phasing of the various processes in different cells can be achieved by 'synchronisation' of a culture. This can be brought about by a number of manipulations, i.e. temperature changes, light stimuli, nutrient limitation, and collecting cells of uniform size by filtration. A cell population that has been treated by one of these techniques will divide simultaneously for a small number of divisions but will then revert to asynchronous division, so that the increase in cell numbers (following synchronisation) changes from a stepwise to a continuous progression.

6.6   Growth inhibition and 'death' in microorganisms

A number of chemical substances slow the growth of microorganisms or inhibit it altogether. If the growth is halted in the presence of a chemical but can resume once the chemical has been removed, the effect is called **bacteriostatic**. **Bactericidal agents** are those that lead to loss of viability. Both effects are concentration dependent. It is noteworthy, however, that among bacteria there are types of organisms that can tolerate what are considered to be general metabolic poisons (H_2S, CO, phenol, etc.) and can even use these as energy sources. For quite a large number of antimicrobial agents, the target area in the cell and the mode of action are more or less understood.

Damage to structural components and the cell envelope.   At relatively high concentrations (70%) ethanol causes coagulation of proteins and acts bactericidally. Phenols, cresols, neutral soaps and surface-active agents (detergents) attack the cell envelope and destroy the semi-permeability of the cytoplasmic membrane. The membranes consist predominantly of lipids and proteins. Detergents have a polar structure and consist of lipophilic groups (long-chain hydrocarbons or aromatic rings) and hydrophilic ionising groups. They accumulate in the lipoprotein membranes, which are similarly polar in structure, and interfere with their functions. Because of their wide spectrum of antimicrobial effects, detergents are used as general disinfectants on surfaces, clothing, etc. Some polypeptide antibiotics (polymyxin, colistin, bacitracin, subtilin) and some antimicrobial agents from plant sources resemble detergents in their effects.

Damage to enzymes and important metabolic processes.   Some heavy metals (copper, silver, mercury, among others) act as potent poisons of enzymes and they function even at very low concentrations (oligodynamic action). In the form of salts ($HgCl_2$, CuCl, $AgNO_3$) and in organic combinations (e.g. 4-hydroxymercuribenzoate), they bind to SH groups of enzymes and cause alterations in the tertiary and quaternary structure of these proteins. The functional mercapto group of coenzyme A can be blocked in this way. Cyanide is a respiratory poison which binds to the iron group and blocks the function of the terminal enzyme of aerobic respiration, i.e. cytochrome oxidase. Carbon monoxide inhibits respiration by competing with molecular oxygen at the cytochrome oxidase step; it acts as a competitive inhibitor. Antimycin A inhibits electron transport in the respiratory chain by blocking cytochrome c reductase. The compound 2,4-dinitrophenol uncouples respiratory chain phosphorylation. Fluoroacetate blocks the tricarboxylic acid cycle because it is at first 'activated' like acetate and converted to fluorocitrate (lethal synthesis) which then blocks the enzyme aconitase and hence any further metabolism of citrate.

Competitive inhibition.   Inhibition of the conversion of succinate to fumarate by malonate can be taken as a model of competitive inhibition. The effect is highly specific and occurs at low concentrations of malonate. However, increasing the concentration of succinate will partially or completely reverse the inhibition of the enzyme succinate dehydrogenase by malonate. This is in contrast to the inhibition of respiration by cyanide, for example, which cannot be relieved by increasing the substrate concentration, i.e. the partial pressure of oxygen. It is thought that in the inhibition of succinic dehydrogenase by malonate, the normal substrate, succinate, competes with the **structural analogue** or **antimetabolite**, malonate, for the catalytic centre of the enzyme. Competitive inhibition is based on structural similarities of the inhibitors to the normal cellular components. The uptake of an antimetabolite into the cell, therefore, can have various effects, especially on biosynthetic processes (see below). In the following diagram three metabolites, succinate, 4-aminobenzoate and arginine, are shown with their respective antimetabolites, malonate, sulfanilamide and canavanine.

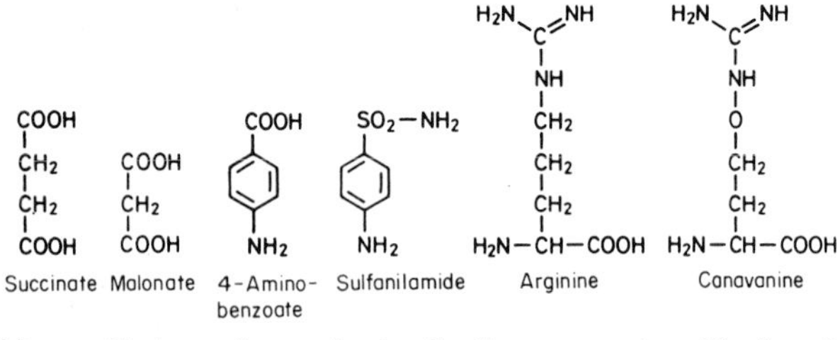

Succinate   Malonate   4-Amino-   Sulfanilamide   Arginine   Canavanine
                                  benzoate

Inhibitory effects on the synthesis of cell components.   The best-known example of growth inhibition by assimilation of a structural analogue to a cell component is the effect of sulfanilic acid derivatives. The antibacterial action of sulfanilamides was discovered empirically by Domagk; it became clear only later that the structural similarity to 4-aminobenzoic acid (see above) was the key for understanding its mode of action. 4-Aminobenzoic acid is part of a coenzyme, namely tetrahydrofolate. Most bacteria can synthesise this from simple building blocks. However, when 4-aminobenzoate or sulfanilamides are added to nutrient media, they are taken up by the cells and assimilated into folate; in the case of sulfanilamides, this results in the synthesis of a non-functional coenzyme and thus eventually leads to cessation of growth. The effect of sulfanilamides can be counteracted by increasing doses of 4-aminobenzoic acid; the inhibition (of growth) is thus based on a competitive mechanism. In animals, folate can neither be synthesised *de novo*, nor from intermediates and must be supplied as the complete coenzyme. Sulfonamides can therefore not be incorporated into the coenzyme and are not injurious. The selective toxicity of sulfonamides and their usefulness as chemotherapeutic agents is the result of the high synthetic capacity of bacteria and the much more limited synthetic abilities of animals.

The inhibition of succinic dehydrogenase by malonate and the growth inhibition produced by derivatives of sulfanilic acid are examples of antagonistic relations between normal metabolites of the cell and structurally similar compounds. This **antagonism** between metabolites and antimetabolites (structural analogues) can be effective at different levels. Antimetabolites can prevent the incorporation of the normal metabolite and thus inhibit synthesis of important cell components; they may themselves be incorporated into polymers and result in a loss or diminution of activity of an enzyme or nucleic acid.

Inhibition of protein synthesis by antibiotics.   Protein synthesis in prokaryotes is specifically inhibited by a number of antibiotics. The target is the function of the 70S ribosome. Streptomycin and neomycin inhibit the correct incorporation of amino acids into polypeptides. Erythromycin inhibits the functioning of the 50S subunit. Tetracycline inhibits the combination of aminoacyl-tRNA with the ribosome. Chloramphenicol apparently inhibits the formation of the peptide bond by peptidyltransferase. It is used chemotherapeutically as a highly effective bacteriostatic agent, and it is also useful in biochemical research as a selective inhibitor of protein synthesis without effecting other metabolic activities. The above-named antibiotics can, of course, have similar effects on mitochondrial or chloroplast ribosomes. However, since the mitochondrial membrane is almost impermeable to streptomycin, this antibiotic has little effect on eukaryotic organisms at the low concentrations at which it acts on prokaryotes. The division of organelles in eukaryotes is inhibited only at thousandfold higher concentrations. If streptomycin at high concentrations is applied to growing eukaryotic organisms (yeasts, *Euglena*, growth points of higher plants), it leads to a diluting out of mitochondria and chloroplasts and results in cells and tissues with considerably lower content of these organelles.

Inhibition of nucleic acids by antibiotics.   The synthesis of nucleic acids is also inhibited by a number of antibiotics. Mitomycin C selectively prevents DNA synthesis without inhibiting RNA and protein synthesis. The effect is thought to be due to cross-linking of the double-stranded DNA and strand breakage. Actinomycin D forms a complex with double-stranded DNA by combining with guanine; it prevents the synthesis of all three types of RNA, but not the replication of DNA. Rifampicin acts on the DNA-dependent RNA polymerase and thus inhibits the synthesis of RNA.

Inhibition of cell wall synthesis.   The inhibition of peptidoglycan synthesis by penicillin, cephalosporin, and other cell wall effective agents has already been discussed (Ch. 2.2.4).

Death and 'killing' of microorganisms.   So-called cell death in microorganisms is defined as the irreversible loss of the ability to grow and reproduce or, as it relates to experimental practice, the loss of 'colony-forming ability'. Many cell injuries that lead to 'death' can be repaired under certain conditions, i.e. they can be overcome. Well known is the reactivation after UV irradiation or heat effects (see Ch. 15.1.4). Quantitative estimations of '**death**', i.e. 'loss of viability', in microorganisms are only possible **for populations**, not for individual cells. In many cases the rate of loss of viable cells at any one time has been found to be proportional to the number of viable cells; it thus seems to follow first order reaction kinetics: $N = N_0 \cdot e^{-kt}$ (k, exponential 'death' rate). This applies to sterilisation by irradiation, for example.

6.6.1   Sterilisation methods

The 'killing'', of microorganisms that is, irreversible loss of the ability to grow, is a fundamental part of microbiological methods and of food conservation; it therefore needs some consideration. **Sterilisation** is the process of freeing any material of **living** microorganisms **or their dormant forms**. One must differentiate sterilsiation from partial sterilisation (i.e. **pasteurisation**) and **conservation**, i.e. keeping sterile. When a sterile material, or one that has been inoculated with a certain type of microorganism, becomes infected with other, not deliberately added organisms, it is said to be contaminated (or subject to contamination). The concepts of **disinfection** (killing of all pathogenic microorganisms), **asepsis**, **antisepsis** and **infection** are used less in microbiology than in the field of hygiene.

Table 6.5. D_{10} *values (decimal reduction times) of spore suspensions from three aerobic spore-forming bacteria*

Spores from	Decimal reduction times in seconds at					
	105 °C	120 °C	130 °C	140 °C	150 °C	160 °C
Bacillus cereus	12.1	4.2	2.6	1.3	1.0	0.7
B. subtilis	27.8	4.5	3.1	2.1	1.1	0.5
B. stearothermophilus	2857.0	38.6	8.8	3.9	2.4	1.4

(Modified after Miller, I. & Kandler, O. (1967). *Milchwissensch.* **22**, 686).

Microorganisms vary in their susceptibility to methods of sterilisation. Differences occur from species to species, but they also depend on water content, pH of the medium, age of cells, spores, etc. The killing rates are thus dependent on a number of factors in the environment as well as on the type of microorganisms. Instead of 'killing rates', the extent of killing of a given population under given conditions is often expressed as the D value, the time needed to kill 90% of the cells, also called the decimal reduction time (D_{10}) (Table 6.5).

Sterilisation or partial sterilisation can be achieved by moist heat, dry heat, filtration, irradiation, or chemical methods.

Moist heat.   The vegetative cells of most bacteria and fungi are killed at temperatures around 60 °C within 5–10 minutes; yeasts and fungal spores are killed only above 80 °C, whilst bacterial spores need about 15 minutes at 120 °C. The decimal reduction times given in Table 6.5 allow calculation of the necessary exposure to moist heat of some spore-forming, very heat-resistant bacteria. It should be remembered, though, that the sterilisation programme also depends on the extent of contamination; larger numbers of thermoresistant spores require longer periods of sterilisation.

To reach temperatures above the boiling point of water, an **autoclave**, a vessel that allows heating under pressure, must be used. The actual temperature of the steam (produced from water) in the autoclave is dependent on the pressure (Fig. 6.15), but the temperature at a given pressure is considerably lower if any air is present in the chamber. Because the effectiveness of sterilisation depends on the temperature and not the pressure, it is necessary to ensure the elimination of air from the sterilisation vessel. This can be done by allowing the valve to be open during the initial heating of the steam so that steam and air can be

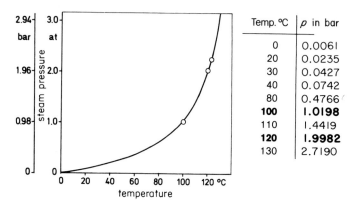

Fig. 6.15. *Pressures of water-saturated steam.*

expelled, or by evacuation. It would be more appropriate to monitor the temperature in the autoclave, rather than the pressure, but because of its simplicity and for reasons of safety, it is more common to register the pressure. The necessary duration of the sterilisation process also depends on the size (i.e. the heat capacity) of the apparatus and vessels to be sterilised; this can be derived from the data in Table 6.6.

A similar effect of sterilisation can also be achieved by **fractional sterilisation** (tyndallisation). This consists of heating media and solutions on three successive days to 100 °C for 30 minutes and leaving them at incubator temperatures during the intervening times, during which spores can germinate so that the resulting vegetative cells will be killed by the following period of heating to 100 °C.

For many purposes the destruction of vegetative microorganisms, i.e. partial sterilisation, may be sufficient. This can be achieved by the process of **pasteurisation**, heating to 75–80 °C for 5–10 minutes. Milk, for example, is usually pasteurised, but for even shorter periods so that its palatability is not affected. Two pasteurisation methods are in use (for milk). A short-term one (20 sec at 71.5–74 °C) and a 'high-heat' method (2–5 sec at 85–87 °C). Sterilisation of milk can also be obtained by an 'ultra-heating' method. In this method superheated steam is injected into the milk, producing a temperature of 135–150 °C to which the milk is exposed for 1–2 seconds. Subsequently the milk is allowed to expand through a jet and simultaneously cooled so that the water added by the steam injection is driven off.

Partial sterilisation is also involved in the **preserving** of fruit. The usual heating of preserving vessels for 20 minutes at 80 °C kills off vegetative

Table 6.6. *Sterilisation times for liquids in different vessels in the autoclave at 121–123 °C*

Vessels	Volume	Exposure time (min)
Test tubes	20 ml	12–14
Erlenmeyer flasks	50 ml	12–14
Erlenmeyer flasks	200 ml	12–15
Erlenmeyer flasks	1000 ml	20–25
Erlenmeyer flasks	2000 ml	30–35
Bottle	9000 ml	50–55

cells and fungal spores, though bacterial spores remain viable. However, the low pH associated with the acidity of such fruits inhibits germination of bacterial spores. Thus, conserved fruit often keeps for years in spite of the presence of viable bacterial spores. There are apparently no heat-resistant bacterial spores which can germinate below pH 4.5. Less acid fruits and vegetables (beans, peas, carrots, mushrooms) can also be preserved by pasteurisation if a tablespoon or two of vinegar is added to ensure a sufficiently low pH. The strawberry mould *Byssochlamys nivea* is often found in pasteurised strawberries. The ascospores of this fungus are resistant to 86 °C; at this temperature its D_{10} value is 14 minutes.

Dry heat.   The sterilisation of bacterial spores by dry heat requires higher temperatures and longer exposure times than sterilisation by moist heat (Table 6.7). Materials that are relatively insensitive to high temperatures, such as glass vessels, powders, oils, etc. can be sterilised by heating for 2 hours at 160 °C in a dry steriliser or sterilising oven. For materials that have a high heat capacity or thermal insulation properties, the time taken to reach the sterilising temperature must be taken into account. In each case it is advisable to run temperature controls with indicators or sterilisation controls with spore-bearing soil. Heating for 30 min at 180 °C can be used if the material to be sterilised can tolerate it; experience shows that all spores are killed by such treatment. The lethal effect of heat is due to the coagulation of cellular proteins.

Filtration.   Solutions containing temperature-sensitive substances (vitamins, amino acids, sugars, etc.) are most conveniently sterilised by filtration. Unglazed porcelain (Chamberland candles) were already in use in Pasteur's laboratory. Now Berkfield filters (sintered silica) are used in laboratories and for sterilising drinking water. In addition Seitz filters, sintered glass and membrane filters are suitable. Some filter materials are

Table 6.7. *Sterilisation of bacterial spores by dry heat: required exposure times*

Spores of	Exposure times in minutes at						
	120 °C	130 °C	140 °C	150 °C	160 °C	170 °C	180 °C
Bacillus anthracis				60–120	9–90		3
Clostridium botulinum	120	60	15–60	25		10–15	5–10
Clostridium tetani		20–40	5–15	30	12	5	1
Soil bacteria				180	30–90	15–60	15

obtainable with different pore sizes so that organisms of different sizes and shapes can be separated by differential filtration. Unidirectional filters can be attached to syringes and are used routinely for sterilisation of substances which are sensitive to heat. Virus particles, however, pass through filter membranes.

It should be noted that sugars like glucose and fructose may be hydrolysed or interconverted on autoclaving or even boiling. Glucose has maximal stability in the pH range of 3–5, at which it can be autoclaved in aqueous solution. However, at pH 8, even boiling for 30 minutes changes 40% of glucose to fructose. Metal salts (Fe, Mn, Mo, etc.) accelerate this conversion. As fructose is converted to humic acid under these conditions, any nutrient media that have been subjected to such treatment often appear brown or black.

Irradiation. Among the different kinds of radiation (UV, X-rays, and gamma rays) that are sometimes used for complete or partial sterilisation, UV irradiation is the most important for use in the laboratory. The radiation of most UV lamps is rich in rays of the wavelength region around 260 nm which is preferentially absorbed by nucleic acids, and exposure for any considerable time is lethal for bacteria (Ch. 15.1.4; Fig. 15.3). UV irradiation is suitable for partial sterilisation of rooms; bacteria are quickly killed off, whilst fungal spores which are less UV-sensitive are killed much more slowly.

Ionising radiation. X-rays, UV and gamma-rays (e.g. ^{60}Co) work by forming hydroxyl radicals which attack macromolecules. Even very small radiation doses are sufficient to destroy cells. This is explained by the fact that only one complete copy of DNA is present in most cells, whereas there are many copies of most proteins and polysaccharide molecules. Thus a single hit on a DNA molecule leads to 'cell death', without any changes being demonstrable in other molecules. Ionising radiation can therefore be employed for sterilisation of foods and other solid materials.

Chemical methods.   Sterilisation by ethylene oxide has been found very useful for the sterilisation of food, pharmaceuticals, instruments, and apparatus. It will kill vegetative cells as well as spores, but is effective only in the presence of water (i.e. 5–15% water content). It is used in a mixture with nitrogen or carbon dioxide as a gas containing 2–50% ethylene oxide. Another chemical, β-propiolactone (propane-3-olide) has been introduced for the preservation of thermolabile materials in nutrient solutions. This compound is much more active than ethylene oxide but is thought to have considerable carcinogenic and other side effects. It is added at 0.2% to the complete nutrient solution which is then incubated at 37 °C for 2 hours. On standing overnight the propiolactone is completely degraded. Carbohydrates are not attacked.

β-Propiolactone   Diethyldicarbonate   Ethylene oxide

Drinks can also be sterilised with diethylcarbonate (0.003–0.020%). The traditional microbicidal agents, bromine water (1%), sublimate, i.e. $HgCl_2$ (1% in alcohol), silver nitrate (0.5%), or calcium hypochlorite (1% Cl_2) are suitable for the external **sterilisation of seeds** from which sterile plants are to be grown. Treatment is for 5–30 minutes. However, before treatment with these reagents, it is essential to ensure that the seed surface is completely wettable. This can be achieved by prior washing with soap or surface-active agents.

To clean glassware and render it free of viable microorganisms, it is usually enough to use a suitable detergent dissolved in hot water, such as SDS (sodium dodecyl sulphate) or even ordinary domestic washing-up preparations. Depending on the further use of the glassware, however, these have to be removed by copious rinses in clean (preferably distilled) water.

6.6.2   Conservation procedures

Organic materials are subject to microbial degradation unless they are protected from the actions and the multiplication of microorganisms by various methods and conditions. A number of procedures are suitable for the preservation and conservation of organic materials. The most important are the methods for the protection of food and food products.

The special field of **food microbiology** deals with the relevant problems.

Foodstuffs are spoiled for human consumption not only because of degradation by microorganisms (aerobic decomposition and anaerobic putre-
faction) but also through contamination with toxin-producing bacteria or
fungi. The most important toxin producers in foods are *Clostridium
botulinum* and several *Staphylococcus* species. The former produces a highly
lethal exotoxin that attacks the nervous system, i.e. a neurotoxin.
Staphylococci produce an enterotoxin that is responsible for food poisoning and acts largely on the intestinal tract. Some fungi produce mycotoxins,
of which **aflatoxin**, produced by *Aspergillus flavus*, has become the most
widely known.

Conservation procedures for the prevention of microbial food spoilage
make use of a number of possibilities. Physical and chemical methods
can be utilised.

Physical methods.   Sterilisation by heat has already been discussed. Tinned
foods are usually autoclaved. Acid fruit juices are stable, even if only
pasteurised so that vegetative cells have been killed, but spores are still
viable; endospores of bacteria cannot germinate in acid media. **Sterile
filtration** through small pore, pressed filter discs of asbestos or cellulose is
used for sterilisation of fruit juices, mineral water and therapeutica. **Centrifugation and filtration** are also used to interrupt fermentation at the
appropriate stage in wine making so that a residual sweetness remains.

The ancient and widely practised methods of **drying** certain foods utilises the fact that growth of microorganisms requires a certain water content (usually above 10%). Rolled oats, dried fruits, hay and silage owe
their durability to their dry state and are rapidly attacked by moulds and
bacteria when exposed to moist air, with consequent absorption of water.

Treating food products by **irradiation** has so far only been in limited
use. UV irradiation is used predominantly for the sterilisation of air and
rooms in dairies, refrigerated storage, large bakeries, and similar institu-
tions. So far, little use has been made of the possibility of treating foods
with ionising radiation. The safety of irradiation by gamma-rays has been
tested and established on several occasions. It is also evident that the low
radiation doses required for sterilisation will not cause significant alterations in the sterilised goods.

A safe method, which is also used more and more in the home, sur-
planting the preserving process, is **storage at low temperatures**. Deep freez-
ers and deep-freeze food stores kept the frozen goods at temperatures
below $-20\,°C$. The storage of food at these temperatures does not significantly decrease the viability of microorganisms or destroy toxins, but it
completely inhibits microbial growth. Even psychrophilic bacteria are unable
to grow below $-12\,°C$.

Chemical methods.   Conservation **by acidity** utilises the fact that only a
few microorganisms can grow at low pH and under anaerobic conditions.
Pasteurisation is usually sufficient to get rid of these; heat resistant spores

do no germinate below pH 4.0. A natural way of conservation by acidity is involved in the production of sauerkraut, pickled gherkins, and sausages like salami or cervelat. In many cases acetic acid, lactic acid, citric acid or tartaric acid added. Acidified but non-pasteurised foodstuffs are subject to spoilage by yeast and other fungi under aerobic conditions.

Meat and fish products are preserved by **smoking**. This process consists of lowering the water content of the food and penetrating the food with antimicrobial substances such as phenols, cresols, aldehydes, acetic and formic acids.

Salting is carried out by immersing the food in 14–25% NaCl; this treatment leads to loss of water and suppresses the growth of spoilage-producing microorganisms; only a few halophilic bacteria can multiply under these conditions.

Sugar at high concentrations (about 50%) is growth inhibitory. The preservation of marmalade, jams, and syrups is primarily due to their acid and sugar content.

The use of **chemical preservatives** is necessary for the conservation of several food products. Wine owes its preservation, until now, to the addition of sulphite. Wine and fruit juices can also be preserved by addition of diethylcarbonate.

Further methods for the **preservation of food products** utilise the addition of sorbic acid, benzoic and formic acids. Citrus fruit is surface treated with biphenyl or o-phenylphenolate. Finally, the inhibition of microbial growth by antibiotics has also been attempted.

7 Basic mechanisms of metabolism and energy conversion

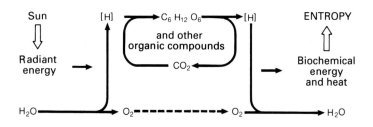

| O₂-producing phototrophic organisms | organotrophic aerobically respiring organisms |

Two processes were contrasted in the discussion of the carbon cycle (Chapter 1), namely, **photosynthesis** with accompanying fixation of carbon dioxide and evolution of oxygen; and the consumption of oxygen and liberation of carbon dioxide which occurs in the **mineralisation** of organic compounds. With regard to the **transformation of mass**, the two processes are complementary; the transition of carbon from a gaseous, inorganic form to a solid or semi-solid organic compound and the reciprocal process of mineralisation are the most obvious. However, if one views both these processes from the point of view of **energy transformation**, carbon appears of lesser importance than hydrogen. As early as 1848, J. R. Meyer expressed this as 'Plants take up a force, light, and produce a force, the chemical potential' (force is used in the sense of energy). The light energy of the sun is transformed to chemical energy in photosynthesis by splitting water into hydrogen and oxygen, and then converting this hydrogen in combination with carbon (from carbon dioxide) into a metastable state (see above diagram). The major part of this stabilised hydrogen is transiently fixed in the form of carbohydrates. This potential difference between hydrogen and oxygen produced by plants serves as the energy source for all aerobically respiring, organotrophic organisms. These organisms remove the hydrogen from its combination with carbon and oxidise it with oxygen in the biochemical oxyhydrogen reaction that yields energy. This oxidation of hydrogen proceeds in a stepwise fashion in such a way that the available energy can be converted to chemical energy in discrete portions. Globally, the 'phototrophic plants – organotrophic organisms' system is integrated into the processes of converting radiant energy to heat and results in the slowing down of the entropy increase.

7.1   Basic considerations

Metabolism and metabolic pathways.   Vegetative cells are dependent on a continuous supply of energy, not only during growth, but also in a resting state. The living cell represents the most highly ordered state of matter. Energy is required both for the formation of this ordered state and for its maintenance. This energy that is required for the maintenance of life and for the synthesis of cell components is obtained by metabolism, i.e. by the ordered transformation of substances in the cell. The energy sources are the nutrients which are acquired from the environment. They are transformed in the cell by a series of successive enzymic reactions via specific metabolic pathways. The metabolic pathways have two functions: to provide **precursors** for cell components and to provide **energy** for synthetic and other energy-requiring processes.

The transformation of substances in the cell (i.e. **cell metabolism**) that leads from simple nutrients like glucose, long-chain fatty acids, or even aromatic compounds to *de novo* synthesis of cell material can be simplified by division into three major phases. The nutrients are first broken down into smaller fragments (breakdown or **catabolism**) and then converted in the reactions of **intermediary metabolism** or amphibolism to a series of organic acids and phosphate esters. Both these pathways are completely integrated. The many low molecular weight compounds represent the **substrate** from which the **building blocks** of the cell are synthesised. These building blocks are the amino acids, purine and pyrimidine bases, sugar phosphates, organic acids, and other **metabolites**. They are the end products of sometimes long synthetic reaction chains. The polymeric **macromolecules** (nucleic acids, proteins, reserve materials, cell wall constituents) which make up the composition of the cell, are synthesised from these building blocks. These two phases of the biosynthesis of cell material, the synthesis of the building blocks and the synthesis of polymers from these, are collected in the terms **synthetic metabolism** or **anabolism** (Fig. 7.1).

Unity in biochemistry.   The principle of 'unity in biochemistry' (unitary biochemistry) is one of the few enduring dogmas of the century. It expresses the assumption that the biochemistry of all life forms on this planet is basically the same. This principle is exemplified by the

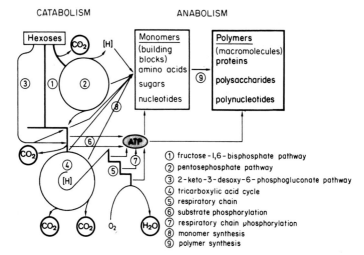

Fig. 7.1. *Metabolic map of aerobically respiring cells catabolising hexoses.*

uniformity of cellular building blocks, including their optical rotation; the universality of adenosine triphosphate (ATP) as the elementary quantum of biological energy; the universality of the genetic code; and the universality of the pathways of sugar degradation and of the respiratory chain. The major metabolic pathways are also almost identical in all living organisms. There are a few groups of bacteria in which the basic schemes are modified, with a few routes predominating and others abridged or atrophied. The metabolic strategies of microorganisms can be easily traced back to a common plan. It can be assumed that the metabolic pathways developed in the course of evolution, and the biochemical apparatus typical for aerobic organisms developed fairly late, when oxygen became available. It is at present difficult to decide whether abbreviated metabolic pathways are primitive traits or the result of a loss of metabolic steps.

Breakdown of carbohydrates.   Carbohydrates are the quantitatively predominant products of plant photosynthesis, as has been mentioned already in the description of the carbon cycle. They are also the most general nutrients for most microorganisms; for this reason the following considerations will be based primarily on glucose as nutrient and substrate of cellular metabolism. The entry into metabolism of other natural materials that can be used as nutrients will be dealt with in other contexts (Chapter 14).

Macromolecules are usually broken down to mono- or dimeric building blocks outside the cell by exoenzymes and are absorbed as such.

Hexoses are usually split in half after various preparatory reactions. The products of the cleavage are then converted to pyruvate. This occupies a key position in intermediary metabolism and is the starting point for synthetic and further catabolic reactions. Pyruvate is decarboxylated to a two-carbon compound, which combines at first with a suitable acceptor molecule (oxaloacetate) and enters the **tricarboxylic acid cycle** (TCA; also called the citric acid cycle), where it is oxidised via a series of reactions to carbon dioxide. Oxaloacetate is regenerated in this cyclical process. The hydrogen atoms (or reducing equivalents) which are obtained in the dehydrogenation reactions enter the respiratory chain system which leads to the regeneration of ATP (oxidative phosphorylation). With each turn of the tricarboxylic acid cycle, the two-carbon compound (acetyl-CoA) yields 2 molecules of CO_2 and four times 2 [H]. This series of reactions constitutes the balance of the tricarboxylic acid cycle.

The intermediary compounds of the tricarboxylic acid cycle, however, comprise several organic acids that are also the starting material for biosynthetic processes (2-oxoglutarate, succinate, oxaloacetate). The tricarboxylic acid cycle, therefore, functions not only as the terminal oxidation pathway of nutrients, but also as a large distributor of starting materials for the synthesis of building blocks. If such intermediates were to be continuously withdrawn from the cycle, it would come to a halt because the acceptor molecule would not be regenerated. This is avoided by anaplerotic (**replenishing**) sequences that provide additional intermediary compounds to the tricarboxylic acid cycle to compensate for the losses caused by biosynthetic processes. The anaplerotic pathways are of special importance for organisms that grow on simple carbon compounds (C_1 and C_2 compounds) or on other substrates that are metabolised via these simple compounds.

The function of enzymes. The conversion of chemical substances in the cell is carried out by enzymes. Each transformation of a metabolite into another is due to a specific enzyme. Enzymes are proteins and function as catalysts. The most important functional properties of an enzyme are the recognition of the specific metabolite (substrate), its catalytic action, and the potential for regulation of its activity.

Enzyme-catalysed reactions are initiated by the binding of the metabolite (substrate of the enzyme) to the enzyme protein. Usually, an enzyme deals only with one metabolite, its substrate, and catalyses its transformation into a second metabolite until equilibrium is reached. Each enzyme is therefore characterised by a substrate specificity (it deals only with one metabolite and its conversion product) and by a reaction specificity (it catalyses only one of several possible conversion reactions that a metabolite could undergo). The **recognition of the substrate** by the enzyme is part of the enzyme-substrate binding process. The substrate is bound to a very specific site on the enzyme, its catalytic centre. Steric and ionic properties of the substrate are the characteristics that are recognised by the enzyme. It is thought to 'fit' the enzyme (catalytic) site in a 'lock and key' analogy.

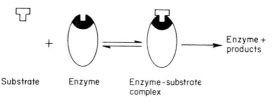

| Substrate | Enzyme | Enzyme-substrate complex |

Enzyme proteins function as **biological catalysts** and lower the **activation energy** (for a reaction). The chemical transformation of a metabolite occurs on the enzyme at normal temperatures. Thus enzymes allow reactions to take place that would otherwise occur only at high temperatures or under non-physiological conditions that cells cannot tolerate.

The velocity of an enzyme-catalysed reaction is greater by about ten orders of magnitude than that of the same non-enzymic reaction; increase in velocity by a factor of 10^{10} shortens a half-time of 300 years to one second. A very important property of enzymes, which has been fully recognised by biochemists only during the last decade or so, is the **regulatory alterability** of their **catalytic activity**. These regulations of catalytic activities offer at least one explanation for the harmony of metabolic processes in the cell. The activities of at least some enzymes, usually one in any specific synthetic pathway, can be regulated. These enzymes recognise not only the substrate at the catalytic centre, but also recognise, at another centre, the relevant end product of the synthetic reaction chain or other low molecular weight compounds whose influence on the enzyme activity is advantageous. Thus these enzymes have a second binding site, the regulatory centre. It is envisaged that the binding of end products or other metabolite(s), called effectors, is transmitted to the catalytic centre and produces an alteration in the catalytic activity. End products of synthetic reactions function as negative effectors. Positive effectors cause an increase in enzyme activity. Thus, the concentrations of metabolites that function as effectors regulate the activity of the enzyme and thereby the velocity of the metabolic flux that it catalyses. The effectors are structurally unrelated to the enzyme substrate, i.e. they are sterically different; they are therefore called allosteric effectors, and their regulatory binding sites on the enzyme are called allosteric centres.

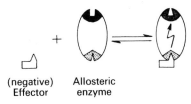

Coenzymes and prosthetic groups.   For the uptake and transfer of substrate fragments, for example, hydrogen, methyl groups, or amino groups, enzyme proteins make use of low molecular weight compounds known as coenzymes and prosthetic groups (Table 7.1; Fig. 7.2). They are more or less tightly bound to the enzyme. Substances which accept a substrate group while bound to one enzyme protein are coenzymes (but more appropriately, co-substrates or transfer metabolites). If the low molecular weight substances are tightly bound to one enzyme protein and transfer the substrate group without being dissociated from the enzyme, they are referred to as prosthetic groups of the enzyme protein.

Coenzymes are of special importance in so far as they cannot be synthesised by many organisms and must be supplied as nutrients in the form of vitamins. Many lactic acid bacteria, soil and aquatic bacteria, as well as other unicellular organisms require one or the other of the vitamins listed in Table 6.3, or their precursors, as supplements for growth.

Interconversions of energy.   The metabolic pathways sketched above (hexose catabolism, the tricarboxylic acid cycle, and respiratory chain) result in the oxidation of sugar to carbon dioxide and water. The energy liberated in these reactions amounts to the same value as that liberated by the complete combustion of sugar. The subdivision of glucose oxidation into many enzyme-catalysed and theoretically fully reversible reactions offers the opportunity to convert some of the released energy into a biochemically utilisable form without the occurrence of high reaction temperatures.

Many metabolic reactions release only small amounts of energy. These are of use to the cell only because the equilibrium of the reaction lies to the product side. The metabolism of some intermediary compounds, however, is accompanied by the release of larger amounts of free energy ($-\Delta G = 40$–60 kJ/mol or 10–15 kcal/mol); this energy is conserved via **substrate-level phosphorylation** in the form of ATP and can then be made available for other, energy-requiring, metabolic reactions. This type of ATP regeneration involves substrates (intermediary compounds) and enzymes.

Table 7.1. *Coenzymes and prosthetic groups, their functions as hydrogen, group, or electron carriers, and their relation to vitamins*

Coenzyme or prosthetic group[a]	Function: transfer of	Vitamin
NAD(P) (Section 7.1 of this chapter)	hydrogen, e^-	nicotinic acid
FMN (Fig. 7.9)	hydrogen, e^-	riboflavine
FAD (Fig. 7.2)	hydrogen, e^-	riboflavine
Ubiquinone (Fig. 7.9)	hydrogen, e^-	–
PQQ (Fig. 7.2)	hydrogen, e^-	PQQ
F_{420} (fig. 9.7)	hydrogen, e^-	–
F_{430} (Fig. 9.7)	hydrogen, e^-	–
Cytochrome (Fig. 7.9)	e^-	
Biotin (Chapter 8.3)	carboxy groups	biotin
Pyridoxal phosphate (Fig. 14.15)	amino groups	pyridoxin
Tetrahydrofolate (Chapter 8.6)	formyl group	folate, 4-aminobenzoate
Coenzyme A (Fig. 7.2)	acyl groups	pantothenate
Coenzyme M (fig. 9.7)	methyl group	–
Lipoate (Fig. 7.2)	acyl groups and hydrogen	lipoate
Thiamine pyrophosphate (Fig. 7.2)	aldehyde groups	thiamine
B_{12} coenzyme (Fig. 7.2)	carboxy and methyl group transfer	cobalamin
Methanopterin (Fig. 9.7)	formyl, methenyl, methyl group	–
HTPT (Fig. 9.7)	methyl group	–
Methanofuran (Fig. 9.7)	carboxy, formyl group	–

[a] Chemical formulae located in this book as indicated.

The major part of the energy obtainable by oxidation of substrates, however, is converted to the biochemically utilisable form of ATP by a special energy-transducing machinery: **respiratory chain phosphorylation**, an oxidative phosphorylation in the respiratory chain.

Metabolites. Even a superficial knowledge of the compounds that take part in cellular metabolism shows that many of these substances are present in the phosphorylated form, i.e. as esters of phosphoric acid. The non-phosphorylated intermediates contain carboxyl groups or ionisable basic groups. It would appear that many enzymes can only deal with

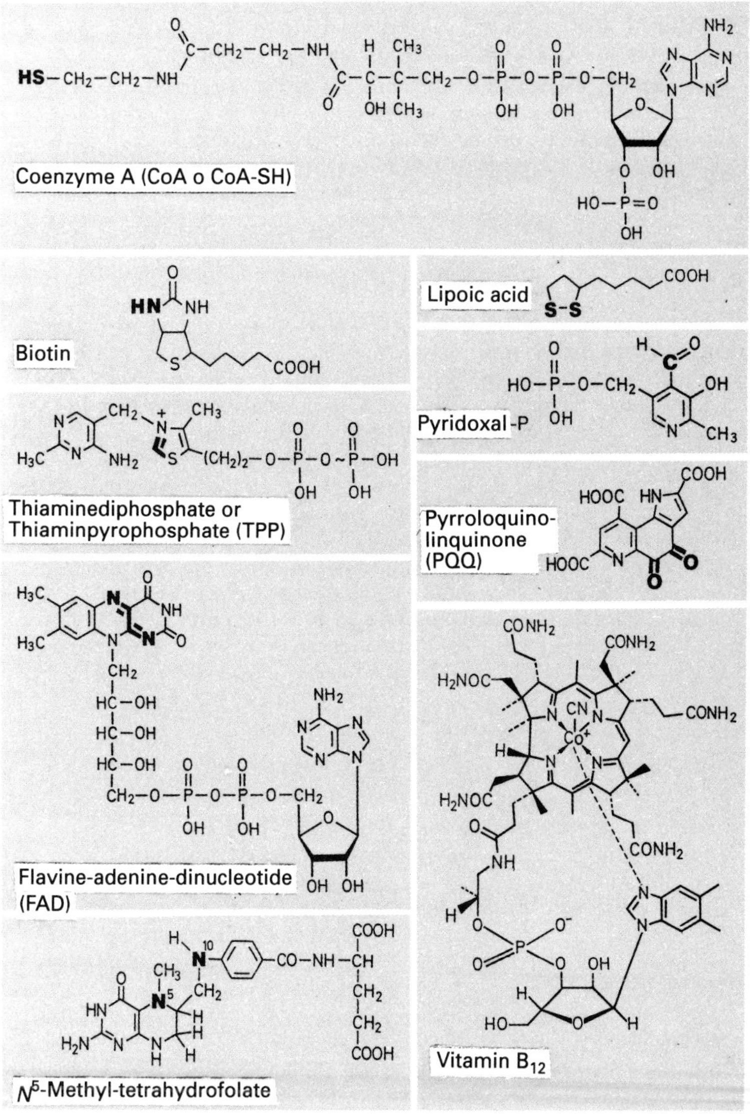

Fig. 7.2. *Structural formulae of some coenzymes and prosthetic groups.*
Reactive groups are shown bold.

metabolites that have ionised or charged groups. Uncharged molecules or groups are always bound to coenzymes or prosthetic groups; some form Schiff's bases with the diamino acid lysine contained in the active centre of the enzyme. Only compounds at the beginning and end of metabolic pathways are unionised, i.e. many initial substrates and several end products (glucose, fructose, ethanol, acetone, 2-propanol, glycerol and many others). Quite apart from the generalisations that can be drawn, there is the question of whether the occurrence of ionised intermediary compounds is related to enzyme functions or to specially effective mechanisms for retention of the metabolites inside the cell.

Dehydrogenation and pyridine nucleotides.   The oxidation of organic compounds involves the transfer of electrons. The electrons are transferred from the **electron donor** to the **electron acceptor**. In biological substrate oxidations two electrons are usually transferred simultaneously with the release of two protons (H^+) from the substrate. This oxidation of a substrate, formally equivalent to the loss of two hydrogen atoms, is called dehydrogenation. The following terms are used synonymously: **hydrogen donor** and **electron donor**; **hydrogen acceptor** and **electron acceptor**; **oxidation** and **dehydrogenation**; **reduction** and **hydrogenation**. The enzymes that remove hydrogen atoms from a substrate are called dehydrogenases and their names are related to the **hydrogen donor** (lactate dehydrogenase, malate dehydrogenase, etc.). Many dehydrogenases transfer the hydrogen to one of two coenzymes, nicotinamide adenine dinucleotide (NAD) or nicotinamide adenine dinucleotide phosphate (NADP).

R = H : NAD
R = PO$_3$H$_2$: NADP

The functional, active group of these coenzymes is the nicotinic acid amide. One hydrogen atom with its electron pair is transferred (as hydride ion) from the substrate to the pyridine ring, whilst the second hydrogen becomes a proton in solution. The transfer of the hydrogen is stereospecific: some enzymes (alcohol dehydrogenase, lactate dehydrogenase) transfer to one (the A) side of the pyridine ring, whilst other dehydrogenases (glyceraldehyde phosphate dehydrogenase) use the other (B) side of the pyridine ring.

$$NAD^+ + Ethanol \longrightarrow Acetaldehyde + NADH + H^+$$

For brevity, such reversible dehydrogenations are also written in the following way:

$$CH_3-CH_2OH + NAD \rightleftharpoons CH_3-CHO + NADH_2$$

The reduced forms of both coenzymes, in contrast to the oxidised forms, have an absorption maximum in the spectrophotometer at 340 nm. The reduction and oxidation of the coenzymes can therefore be followed by changes in absorption at this wavelength. This is the basis of many optical methods for determining the activities of dehydrogenases.

The two coenzymes are freely dissociable: that is, they dissociate from the dehydrogenase protein after having combined with the hydrogen which they then transfer, after binding to another dehydrogenase, to the hydrogen acceptor. Their function as such 'hydrogen transporters' has earned them the name of 'transport metabolites'. $NADH_2$ transfers its hydrogen preferentially to precursors of fermentation products or channels it into the respiratory chain, whilst $NADPH_2$ is mostly involved in reductive steps of biosynthetic processes.

ATP and other energy-rich compounds.   Energy-requiring processes in the cell are made possible by the participation of adenosine triphosphate (ATP). ATP is the chemical form in which energy, obtained by photosynthesis, respiration, or fermentation, can be utilised by the cell. **ATP is the universal transfer agent of chemical energy between energy-yielding and energy-requiring reactions**. It is the international currency, so to speak, in the energy market of the cell. ATP services such diverse processes as synthesis of building blocks and macromolecules, osmotic regulation, and cell movement. The pyrophosphate bonds between the phosphate groups are 'energy rich', that is, they have a **high group-transfer potential**. In other words, they need more energy for their formation than a normal esterification, and reciprocally, their cleavage liberates a large amount of energy (with water as the hydrolysing agent, $\Delta G_0' \approx -30$ kJ) or conserves it in the reaction products (Table 7.2).

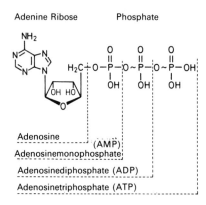

Adenine Ribose   Phosphate

Adenosine ------- (AMP)
Adenosinemonophosphate
Adenosinediphosphate (ADP)
Adenosinetriphosphate (ATP)

Table 7.2. 'Energy-rich' and 'energy-poor' compounds of biochemical importance. The 'free energy' – $\Delta G_0'$ of hydrolysis at pH 7.0 under standard conditions is shown

Substrate	$-\Delta G_0'$ (kJ)	(kcal)	Substrate	$-\Delta G_0'$ (kJ)	(kcal)
Acetylphosphate	44.0	10.5	glycoside	12.6	3.0
Acetoacetyl-CoA	44.0	10.5	sucrose	27.6	6.6
Acyl-AMP	55.7	13.3	UDP-glucose	31.8	7.6
Phosphocreatine	37.7	9.0	aldose-1-phosphate	20.9	5.0
Phosphoenolpyruvate	54.4	13.0	ATP $\rightarrow$ (ADP + P_i)	31.0	7.4
Simple phosphate esters	12.6	3.0	ATP $\rightarrow$ (AMP + P_i)	31.8	7.6

ATP as a coenzyme of metabolite activation.   Many intermediary compounds require activation by group transfer to convert them to a reactive state. The following three types of ATP hydrolysis are utilised for this.

Sugars are activated by being converted to sugar-phosphates:

glucose + ATP $\rightarrow$ glucose-6-phosphate + ADP

Ribose-5-phosphate is activated by the transfer of the diphosphate residue (pyrophosphate group):

ribose-5-phosphate + ATP $\rightarrow$ phosphoribosyl-diphosphate + ADP

Some organic acids, all amino acids, and inorganic sulphate are activated by transfer of the AMP group with hydrolysis to a diphosphate:

fatty acid + ATP → fatty acyl-AMP + diphosphate

amino acid + ATP → aminoacyl-AMP + diphosphate

Sulphate + ATP → sulphate-AMP + diphosphate

The reactions can be brought to completion so that complete substrate transformation is assured, via hydrolysis of the diphosphate (by a pyrophosphatase), thus removing it from the equilibrium.

These remarks should suffice to point out the universal significance of ATP and to lead to an appreciation of the metabolic diversity among bacteria. The metabolic strategies of different organisms can be considered from the viewpoint of the maximum yield of ATP to be gained from the available nutrients under the given environmental conditions.

Regeneration of ATP.   Three processes exist for the regeneration of ATP, namely **photosynthetic phosphorylation** (see Ch. 12.2, 12.2.2), **oxidative** or **respiratory chain phosphorylation** (Section 7.4 of this chapter), and **substrate level phosphorylation** (see Section 7.2.1 of this chapter). The first two processes have in common the formation of ATP by ATP synthase. Substrate-level phosphorylation can occur at several reactions in intermediary metabolism. The ATP-regenerating reactions of most importance in carbohydrate metabolism are catalysed by phosphoglycerate kinase, pyruvate kinase and acetate kinase. In the fermentation of sugars by bacteria and yeasts, ATP regeneration depends entirely on these enzymes. In all the phosphorylation processes, ADP serves as the phosphate acceptor (with few exceptions). Adenosine monophosphate (AMP) must first be converted to ADP, with the participation of ATP, by adenylate kinase (AMP + ATP $\rightleftharpoons$ 2 ADP) before it can be phosphorylated to ATP.

In the following sections, the four most important reaction sequences of glucose catabolism will be briefly presented: the initial cleavage to C_3 compounds, the oxidation of pyruvate, the tricarboxylic acid cycle, and the respiratory chain and its function. Some details that are important for understanding special metabolic processes will also be mentioned. In general, though, and for a more penetrating view of metabolism and biochemistry of microorganisms, a textbook of biochemistry should be consulted.

7.2   Pathways of hexose breakdown

There are several ways of converting glucose to three-carbon (C_3) compounds, including pyruvate which is one of the most important intermediary compounds of metabolism. The most widely distributed catabolic pathway proceeds via *f*ructose-1,6-*bis*phosphate (FBP) and is called the FBP pathway, glycolytic breakdown, glycolysis, or, after the chief research workers who elucidated it, the **Embden–Meyerhof–Parnas** pathway (Fig. 7.3). Another sequence of reactions that can be carried out by most living organisms can be combined into a cycle that is known as the oxidative **pentose-phosphate pathway**, the **hexosemonophosphate pathway**, or the **Warburg–Dickens–Horecker** scheme (Fig. 7.4). The reverse reaction sequence comprises the most important way for the regeneration of CO_2 acceptors in autotrophic CO_2 fixation. The **Entner–Doudoroff breakdown** mechanism, also known as the **KDPG pathway** because of the characteristic intermediate 2-*k*eto-3-*d*eoxy-6-*p*hosphogluconate, is apparently confined to bacteria. (Fig. 7.5). Other, related breakdown mechanisms have more specialised significance.

| β-D-Glucose | Glucose-6-phosphate | Fructose-6-phosphate | Fructose-1,6-bisphosphate |

In the cell, glucose is first phosphorylated on carbon 6 (C-6) by the enzyme hexokinase, with ATP functioning as the phosphate donor. **Glucose-6-phosphate** (G-6-P) is the metabolically active form of cellular glucose, and the starting point for all three breakdown mechanisms.

| Glyceraldehyde-3-phosphate | 1,3-Bisphosphoglycerate | 3-Phosphoglycerate | 2-Phosphoglycerate |

| Phosphoenolpyruvate | Pyruvate | Dihydroxyacetone-phosphate | Glycerol-3-phosphate |

7.2.1   Fructose-1,6-bisphosphate pathway (glycolysis)

In the fructose-1,6-bisphosphate pathway (Fig. 7.3), glucose-6-phosphate is converted to the form in which it can be split, by first being isomerised to fructose-6-phosphate by glucose phosphate isomerase and then being phosphorylated on C-1 by 6-phosphofructokinase from ATP. The resulting fructose-1,6-bisphosphate is cleaved by fructose-bisphosphate aldolase into two triose-phosphates, dihydroxyacetone-phosphate and glyceraldehyde-3-phosphate. These two triose-phosphates are held in equilibrium by the enzyme triose-phosphate isomerase. Dihydroxyacetone-phosphate can be reduced to glycerol-phosphate by glycerol-phosphate dehydrogenase, and the glycerol-phosphate can then be hydrolysed to glycerol and orthophosphate by glycerol-1-phosphatease. However, in the normal course of events, the dihydroxyacetone-phosphate produced by the aldolase reaction is converted to glyceraldehyde-3-phosphate which is then oxidised.

This dehydrogenation is one of the most important steps with respect to the energy yield of the glycolytic pathway, as well as for other reactions that result in the production of glyceraldehyde-3-phosphate. A portion of the energy obtainable from the oxidation of glyceraldehyde-3-phosphate to 3-phosphoglycerate ($\Delta G_0 = -67$ kJ) is conserved in the form of an **energy-rich phosphate bond**. The aldehyde group is first attached to an SH-group of the enzyme glyceraldehyde-phosphate dehydrogenase and the hydrogen is transferred to NAD. The resulting **acyl-S-enzyme** complex is an **energy-rich thioester**. By exchange of the S-enzyme group with orthophosphate (a phosphorolysis) the energy is conserved

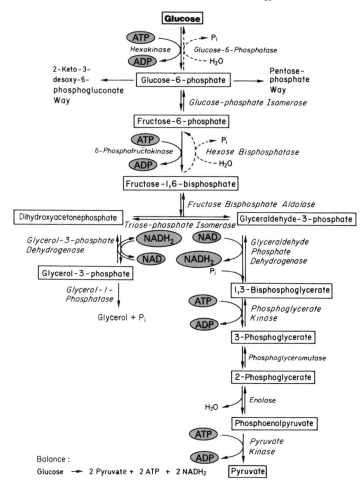

Fig. 7.3. *The fructose-1,6-bisphosphate pathway of glucose catabolism (glycolysis).*

in the **1,3-bisphosphate glyceric acid**, namely in the 1-phosphate. The enzyme phosphoglycerate kinase then transfers this energy-rich phosphate to ADP, yielding ATP and 3-phosphoglycerate. Because the energy-rich phosphate is formed on the substrate, this kind of phosphorylation is termed **substrate-level phosphorylation**. This oxidation of glyceraldehyde-3-phosphate is dependent on the enzyme protein and the presence of orthophosphate and ADP. Lack or exhaustion of any of these components results in the termination of glycolysis. This fact is important for the regulation of glucose catabolism (the Pasteur effect).

3-phosphoglycerate is next converted to 2-phosphoglycerate by phosphoglyceromutase and then hydrolysed to **phosphoenolpyruvate** by the enzyme enolase. This is again an enol ester, whose energy-rich **phosphate group** is transferred to ADP by pyruvate kinase and thus conserved. The resulting pyruvate is the precursor of a number of further catabolic, synthetic, and interconversion processes.

The reactions of the fructose-1,6-bisphosphate pathway are completely reversible, with the three exceptions of the hexokinase, the 6-phospho-fructokinase, and the pyruvate kinase reaction. If all the triose-phosphate produced by the cleavage of fructose-1,6-bisphosphate is converted to pyruvate, then the net balance of glucose breakdown via this pathway is the formation of 2 molecules of pyruvate, 2 molecules of ATP (i.e. 4 minus 2), and 2 molecules of $NADH_2$.

The two energy-conserving reactions in the conversion of glyceraldehyde-3-phosphate to pyruvate are the **most important energy-yielding reactions for anaerobic organisms**. All microorganisms that ferment carbohydrates, with only a few exceptions, are entirely dependent on the energy they obtain from the oxidation of glyceraldehyde-3-phosphate to pyruvate.

7.2.2   The pentose-phosphate pathway

In the pentose-phosphate pathway (Fig. 7.4), glucose-6-phosphate is dehydrogenated by glucose-6-phosphate dehydrogenase to 6-phospho-gluconolactone, with transfer of the hydrogen to NADP. The 6-phospho-gluconolactone is hydrolysed, either spontaneously or enzymically (gluconolactonase), to 6-phosphogluconate. The latter is then dehydrogenated to 3-keto-6-phosphogluconate by 6-phosphogluconate dehydrogenase and decarboxylated to **ribulose-5-phosphate**. This constitutes the end of the actual oxidation process.

The following reactions can be regarded as merely interconversions of pentose-phosphates into hexose-phosphates and vice versa. Furthermore, the addition of these reactions to the initial oxidation reactions yields a metabolic cycle. Ribulose-5-phosphate is in equilibrium with ribose-5-phosphate and xylulose-5-phosphate. Ribose-phosphate is an important building block for the synthesis of nucleotides and nucleic acids. The pentose-phosphates can be converted to two fructose-6-phosphates and

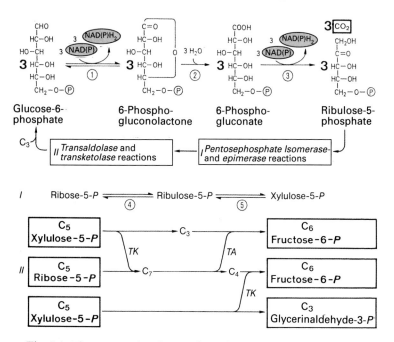

Fig. 7.4. *The pentose-phosphate pathway for the oxidative catabolism of glucose-6-phosphate.*

The oxidative steps culminate in the formation of ribulose-5-phosphate. The ribulose-5-phosphate exists in an enzyme-catalysed equilibrium with ribose-5-phosphate and xylulose-5-phosphate. The pentose-phosphates are converted to two fructose-phosphates and one glyceraldehyde-3-phosphate by the actions of transketolase and transaldolase. These reactions are completely reversible; in the reverse direction, they participate in the ribulose-monophosphate cycle of formaldehyde fixation and in the ribulose-bisphosphate cycle of carbon dioxide fixation, as well as in other cyclical processes. The enzymes involved are: (1) glucose-6-phosphate dehydrogenase; (2) lactonase; (3) 6-phosphogluconate dehydrogenase; (4) phosphoribose isomerase; (5) ribulose-5-phosphate-3-epimerase; TK, transketolase; TA, transaldolase.

only one glyceraldehyde-3-phosphate by transketolase and transaldolase. Isomerisation of the fructose-6-phosphate to glucose-6-phosphate and condensation of two triose-phosphates to hexose phosphate then closes the cycle. One revolution of the cycle thus converts three molecules of glucose-6-phosphate into two molecules of fructose-6-phosphate plus one molecule of glyceraldehyde-3-phosphate, yielding three molecules of CO_2 and three times 2 $NADPH_2$. The enzymes glucose-6-phosphate dehydrogenase and phosphogluconate dehydrogenase of most, if not all, bacteria can transfer the hydrogen from their substrates to NAD as well as to NADP.

The pentose-phosphate cycle is probably a subsidiary pathway whose importance lies in its provision of essential precursors (pentose-phosphates, erythrose-phosphate, glyceraldehyde-3-phosphate) and reducing equivalents for synthetic processes. Pentose-phosphate as precursor for nucleotide and nucleic acid synthesis is thus obtainable via dehydrogenation and decarboxylation of glucose-6-phosphate, as well as by the transaldolase and transketolase reactions from fructose-6-phosphate.

7.2.3   2-keto-3-deoxy-6-phosphogluconate pathway

Glucose-6-phosphate is at first dehydrogenated to 6-phosphogluconate, as described for the pentose-phosphate pathway. Removal of water from 6-phosphogluconate by a phosphogluconate dehydrase then yields **2-keto-3-deoxy-6-phosphogluconate** (Fig. 7.5). The keto-deoxy-phosphogluconate is then cleaved by a specific aldolase into pyruvate and glyceraldehyde-3-phosphate, which can be further oxidised to pyruvate via the glycolytic pathway.

The different degradative pathways show considerable differences in their yields of ATP, $NADH_2$, and $NADPH_2$. The fructose-bisphosphate pathway yields 2 mol ATP and 2 mol $NADH_2$ per mol glucose converted to pyruvate, whereas the 2-keto-3-deoxy-6-phosphogluconate pathway yields only one mol ATP and one of $NADPH_2$. The formation of one mol $NADPH_2$, therefore, seems to be equivalent in terms of energy balance to one mole of ATP plus one mole $NADH_2$. This is in agreement with the observation that the transfer of hydrogen from $NADH_2$ to $NADPH_2$ by transhydrogenase is in many cases energy dependent and involves the consumption of one mol ATP.

Microorganisms differ considerably in the extent to which they utilise the different pathways (Table 7.3). The enzymes of the **fructose-bisphosphate pathway** seem to be part of the basic cellular equipment, though the pathway may be utilised only in the reverse direction (bridging the irreversible steps with other enzymes) in many bacteria. The **pentose-phosphate pathway** also appears to be of universal importance. The **2-keto-3-deoxy-6-phosphogluconate pathway** is widely distributed among bacteria, its principal importance being the utilisation of gluconate. Thus, whilst *E. coli* and *Clostridium* species, for example, utilise glucose via the fructose-bisphosphate pathway, gluconate can enter their intermediary metabolism via the 2-keto-3-deoxy-6-phosphogluconate reaction.

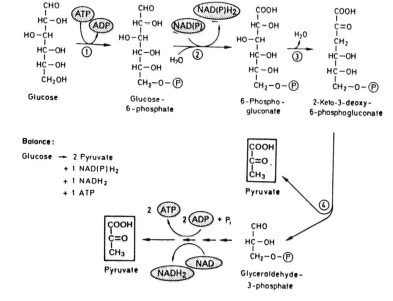

Fig. 7.5. *The 2-keto-3-deoxy-6-phosphogluconate (Entner–Doudoroff) pathway for the oxidative catabolism of glucose.*

The enzymes involved are: (1) hexokinase; (2) glucose-6-phosphate dehydrogenase; (3) phosphogluconate dehydrase; (4) phospho-2-keto-3-deoxy-gluconate aldolase. The 6-phosphogluconolactone produced as an intermediate between glucose-6-phosphate and 6-phosphogluconate has not been included.

Clostridia and some aerobic bacteria can catabolise gluconate via a variant of the 2-keto-3-deoxy-6-phosphogluconate pathway: gluconate is first converted to 2-keto-3-deoxygluconate by a gluconate dehydratase, and is phosphorylated from ATP only at this step by a keto-deoxy-gluconate kinase; the 2-keto-3-deoxy-6-phosphogluconate is cleaved by phospho-2-keto-3-deoxygluconate aldolase.

Table 7.3. *The participation of different pathways in the catabolism of hexose (%)*

Species	Fructose-1,6-bisphosphate pathway (%)	Pentose-phosphate pathway (%)	2-keto-3-deoxy-6-phosphogluconate pathway (%)
Candida utilis	70–80	30–20	
Streptomyces griseus	97	3	
Penicillium chrysogenum	77	23	
Escherichia coli	72	28	
Bacillus subtilis	74	26	
Pseudomonas aeruginosa		29	71
Gluconobacter oxydans		100	
Pseudomonas saccharophila			100
Atcaligenes eutrophus			100

7.2.4 Oxidation of pyruvate

Pyruvate stands in the centre of intermediary metabolism and can be converted to many anabolic products. In many organisms the pyruvate produced by catabolic reactions is mainly oxidised to acetyl-CoA. In bacteria, three reactions play the predominant part in this:

(1) pyruvate + CoA + NAD $\rightarrow$ acetl-CoA + $NADH_2$ + CO_2

(2) pyruvate + CoA + 2 Fd $\rightarrow$ acetyl-CoA + 2 FdH + CO_2

(3) pyruvate + CoA $\rightarrow$ acetyl-CoA + formate

Reaction (1) is catalysed by the multienzyme complex pyruvate dehydrogenase. This enzyme is present in all aerobic organisms and serves predominantly for the formation of acetyl-CoA to enter the tricarboxylic acid cycle. This will be discussed in detail in the following paragraphs (Fig. 7.6). Reaction (2) is catalysed by pyruvate: ferrodoxin oxidoreductase which plays an eminent role in many anaerobic bacteria, such as clostridia. Reaction (3) is catalysed by pyruvate: formate lyase. This enzyme is found in many anaerobic bacteria that excrete formate (formate fermentation, Ch. 8.4), especially Enterobacteriaceae, but also phototrophic organisms.

Yeasts, and some bacteria which excrete ethanol have a fourth enzyme for the oxidation of pyruvate:

(4) pyruvate $\rightarrow$ acetaldehyde + CO_2

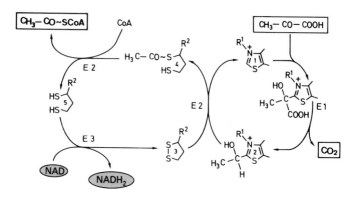

Fig. 7.6. *The steps involved in the dehydrogenation of pyruvate.*
See text for explanations.

This enzyme, pyruvate decarboxylase, splits pyruvate to acetaldehyde and CO_2, the acetaldehyde being subsequently reduced to ethanol.

Pyruvate dehydrogenation by pyruvate dehydrogenase.   Pyruvate is converted to acetyl-CoA and CO_2 by the multienzyme complex pyruvate dehydrogenase with the participation of several cofactors (Fig. 7.6).

> The multienzyme complex can be resolved into three proteins: pyruvate dehydrogenase (E1), dihydrolipoamide transacetylase (E2), and dihydrolipoamide dehydrogenase (E3).
>
> $$\text{pyruvate} + \text{TPP} \xrightarrow{\text{E1}} \text{hydroxyethyl-TPP} + CO_2$$
>
> $$\text{hydroxyethyl-TPP} + \text{lipoate} \xrightarrow{\text{E2}} \text{6-S-acetyl-dihydrolipoate} + \text{TPP}$$
>
> $$\text{acetyl-dihydrolipoate} + \text{CoA} \xrightarrow{\text{E3}} \text{acetyl-CoA} + \text{dihydrolipoate}$$
>
> $$\text{dihydrolipoate} + \text{NAD} \xrightarrow{\text{E4}} \text{lipoate} + \text{NADH}_2$$
>
> In the first reaction, on E1, the pyruvate is bound to the 2-position on the thiazole ring (1) of the thiamine pyrophosphate (TPP) and CO_2 is split off. The resulting hydroxyethyl-TPP (2) then reacts with the lipoate (3) bound to E2, which is thereby reduced and has the acetyl residue (4) bound to the secondary SH-group. E2 further catalyses the transfer of the acetyl group to CoA, leaving dihydrolipoate (5). This is then reoxidised by E3 with reduction of NAD (3).

This pyruvate dehydrogenase multienzyme complex does not occur in strictly anaerobic bacteria.

7.3   The tricarboxylic acid cycle

The tricarboxylic acid cycle serves to oxidise the two-carbon compound acetate to carbon dioxide by the removal of hydrogen (Fig. 7.7). Three of the participating dehydrogenases transfer the hydrogen to NAD(P), whilst succinic dehydrogenase transfers it directly to a quinone. The coenzymes usually transfer the hydrogen to the respiratory chain.

At first acetyl-CoA is condensed with oxaloacetate to citrate by the enzyme citrate synthase, with the liberation of CoA. Although citrate is a symmetrical molecule, it is metabolised asymmetrically. Aconitate hydratase catalyses the reversible interconversion of the three tricarboxylic acids:

$$\text{citrate} \rightleftharpoons \textit{cis}\text{-aconitate} \rightleftharpoons \text{isocitrate}$$

Isocitrate dehydrogenase then catalyses the reaction that leads from isocitrate to 2-oxoglutarate. This enzyme occurs in an NAD- and an NADP-specific form. The intermediate oxalosuccinate apparently remains bound to the enzyme. The next enzyme, 2-oxoglutarate dehydrogenase, catalyses a reaction that is analogous to the pyruvate dehydrogenase reaction; in addition to the enzyme protein, it involves the participation of thiamine pyrophosphate, lipoate, CoA, NAD, and Mg^{2+}. Succinate can then be liberated directly from the resulting succinyl-CoA by a CoA-acylase, or by a coupled reaction with phosphorylation of ADP:

$$\text{succinyl-CoA} + \text{ADP} + P_i \rightleftharpoons \text{succinate} + \text{CoA} + \text{ATP}$$

In the next reaction, succinate dehydrogenase oxidises the succinate to fumarate and transfers the electrons to ubiquinone and cytochrome b. Fumarase (fumarate hydratase) catalyses the hydroxylation of fumarate. This reaction is stereospecific and yields 2-malate. This is then dehydrogenated to oxaloacetate by malate dehydrogenase so that the acetate acceptor is regenerated. Apart from the formation of succinyl-CoA, all reactions of the tricarboxylic acid cycle are reversible.

The balance of acetate metabolism via the tricarboxylic acid cycle yields 2 molecules of CO_2 and 8 [H], 6 at the level of pyridine nucleotide and 2 at the flavoprotein level. In addition, one energy-rich bond is formed (in the 2-oxoglutarate dehydrogenase reaction).

The tricarboxylic acid cycle serves not only for the **terminal oxidation** of nutrients, but also for the **generation of biosynthetic precursors** (2-oxoglutarate, oxaloacetate, succinate). The removal of these intermediates, however, would lead to a lack of oxaloacetate to function as the acetate acceptor, and thus to a cessation of the tricarboxylic acid cycle. To compensate for such losses of tricarboxylic acid cycle intermediates,

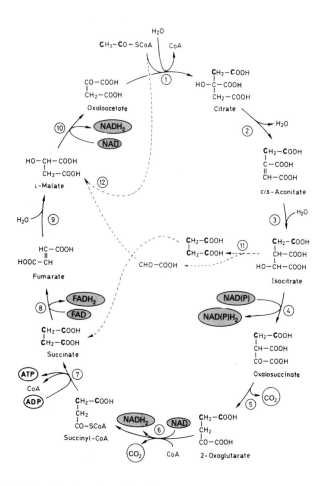

Fig. 7.7. *The tricarboxylic acid cycle.*

Up to reaction 8, the carbon atoms derived from acetate are indicated by bold letters to illustrate the asymmetrical catabolism of citrate. The glyoxylate cycle is indicated by dashed arrows. The enzymes are: (1) citrate synthase; (2,3) aconitate hydratase; (4,5) isocitrate dehydrogenase; (6) oxoglutarate dehydrogenase; (7) succinate thiokinase; (8) succinate dehydrogenase; (9) fumarase; (10) malate dehydrogenase; (11) isocitrate lyase; (12) malate synthase.

so-called replenishing reactions, or **anaplerotic sequences**, come into play. Among the most important mechanisms for the replenishment of the tricarboxylic acid cycle with four-carbon dicarboxylic acids are the carboxylation of pyruvate and phosphoenolpyruvate ($C_3 + C_1 \rightarrow C_4$). These reactions will be discussed in detail under the heading of accessory cycles (Section 7.5 of this chapter).

7.4   The respiratory chain and electron transport phosphorylation

Whilst most anaerobic organisms can regenerate ATP only by substrate-level phosphorylation, respiring organisms have a far more efficient mechanism at their disposal for the regeneration of ATP. This is a special apparatus, the **respiratory chain** or **electron-transport chain** and the enzyme ATP synthase. Both systems are located in the cytoplasmic membrane of prokaryotes and in the inner mitochondrial membrane of eukaryotes. The reducing equivalents ([H] or electrons) derived from substrates enter the respiratory chain inside the membrane and the electrons are finally transferred to oxygen (or other terminal electron acceptors). The reactions of the respiratory chain can be considered as a biochemical oxyhydrogen reaction. It differs energetically from the purely chemical oxidation of hydrogen by the fact that a considerable part of the free energy is conserved in the form of ATP as biologically utilisable energy, and only a small part is lost as heat.

Mechanisms of electron-transport phosphorylation.   The reducing equivalents (protons and electrons) obtained from substrates are transported to the inner mitochondrial or cytoplasmic membrane. They are transferred across the membrane in such a manner that an electrochemical gradient is generated, with a **positive potential** at the **outer surface** and a **negative potential** at the **inner surface** of the membrane (Fig. 7.8). This potential gradient is a function of the precise arrangement of the respiratory chain components in the membrane. Some of the components transfer electrons and others transfer hydrogen. The arrangement of the transfer components in the membrane results in the uptake of protons at the inner surface and their release at the outer surface during the transport of electrons from substrates to oxygen. This can be visualised as a looped pathway of electrons through the membrane during which protons are transported from the inner to the outer surface. This system of electron and proton transport is known as the **respiratory chain** or **electron-transport chain** and, with respect to its function, is also loosely referred to as a **proton pump**. This is the major function of the system.

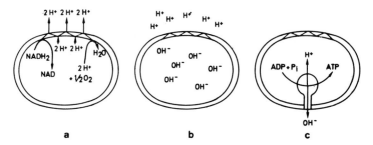

Fig. 7.8. *The respiratory chain and electron-transport phosphorylation in and at the cytoplasmic membrane of protocytes and the inner membrane of mitochondria.*

(a) NADH$_2$ oxidation and proton extrusion; (b) electrochemical gradient between inner and outer surfaces; (c) regeneration of ATP as a consequence of the backflow of protons.

The proton-motive force, or the **electrochemical gradient** of the membrane, is the driving force for the generation of ATP (and other energy-consuming processes). The membrane contains a special enzyme, ATP synthase, which synthesises ATP from ADP and P$_i$. This enzyme, localised in the membrane, protrudes from its inner surface. During the synthesis of ATP, protons migrate from the outer to the inner surface of the membrane. This synthesis of ATP during electron transport across the membrane is called **respiratory chain** or **electron-transport phosphorylation**.

To understand the respiratory process it is necessary to know: (1) the components of the respiratory chain; (2) their redox potentials; and (3) their arrangement in the membrane.

> **Membranes as sites of respiration.** The components of the respiratory chain are enzyme proteins that contain low molecular weight groups (prosthetic groups) relatively tightly bound. The earlier conclusion that respiration is catalysis of iron on surfaces (O. Warburg) has turned out to be true; the enzymes of the respiratory chain are structurally bound. The actual localisation of the respiratory chain components in the respective membranes of eukaryotes and prokaryotes is remarkably similar. The respiratory chains of *Alcaligenes eutrophus* and of *Paracoccus denitrificans* are almost exactly the same as that of mitochondria.

The components of the respiratory chain. The components of the respiratory chain are localised in the lipid bilayer of the membrane. They comprise a large number of electron- and hydrogen-transferring enzymes, coenzymes and prosthetic groups, and several dehydrogenases and transport systems. The proteins can be isolated from the membrane. The

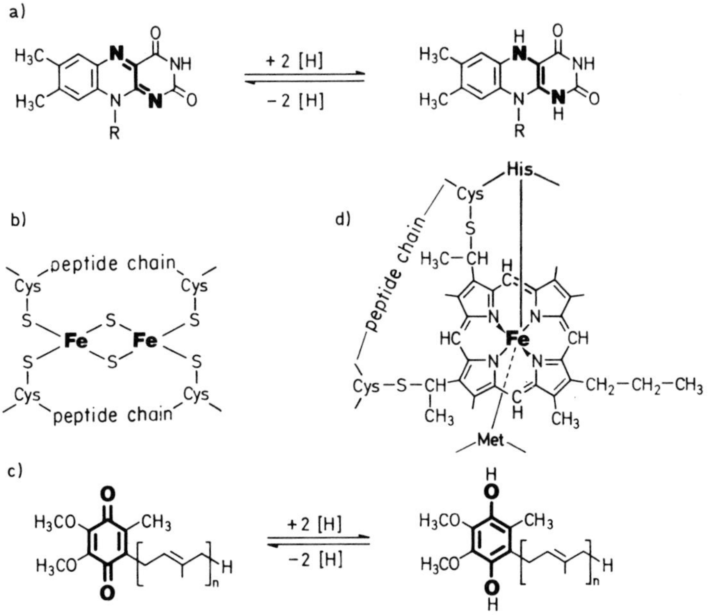

Fig. 7.9. *Formulae of the most important components of the respiratory chain.*

(a) The isoalloxazine ring system of FMN and FAD in its oxidised and reduced form; (b) the [2Fe + 2 S] centre of an iron–sulphur protein; (c) the reduction of ubiquinone to ubihydroquinone; (d) cytochrome *c*.

most important components involved in the oxidation of hydrogen are flavoproteins, iron–sulphur proteins, quinones, and cytochromes.

The flavoproteins are enzymes that contain FMN or FAD as prosthetic groups. They transfer hydrogen. The active group is the isoalloxazine system (Fig. 7.9a); it acts as a reversible redox system. The reactive centres are two nitrogen atoms, each of which can take up a hydrogen atom. The hydrogenation can occur in two steps via a semiquinone. The ability to transfer either one or two hydrogen atoms enables the flavoproteins to mediate between the two types of hydrogen transfer processes.

The **iron–sulphur proteins** are redox systems that transfer electrons. They contain iron atoms that are bound on one side to the sulphur of the amino acid cysteine and on the other side to inorganic sulphide

(Fig. 7.9b). The latter can be easily liberated as hydrogen sulphide by acidification. The cysteine residues are part of the polypeptide chain and the Fe–S centres can be considered as prosthetic groups of the polypeptide chain. The [2 Fe + 2 S] centres involved in the respiratory chain can transfer only one electron. Iron–sulphide proteins of this type, i.e. which contain two labile iron and sulphur groups, occur in several enzyme complexes of the respiratory chain. Of the total iron contained in the respiratory chain, about 80% is present in these Fe–S proteins and only about 20% is present in cytochromes.

> Apart from their participation in electron transport in membranes, Fe–S proteins are also involved in nitrogen fixation, sulphite reduction, nitrite reduction, photosynthesis, activation and liberation of molecular hydrogen, and in alkane oxidation. The Fe–S proteins are characterised by low molecular weights and strongly negative redox potentials; their E_0' values are in the region of -0.2 to -0.6 mV. Apart from the Fe–S proteins with [2 Fe + 2 S] centres (in chloroplasts and aerobic bacteria), others are known with one [4 Fe + 4 S] centre (*Clostridium, Chromatium*) and some with two [4 Fe + 4 S] centres (*Clostridium, Azotobacter*). Some of the iron–sulphur proteins are named according to their function or occurrence, as ferredoxin, putida redoxin, rubredoxin, or adrenodoxin.

Further redox systems that participate in the respiratory chain are the **quinones**. Ubiquinone (coenzyme Q: Fig. 7.9c) is found in the inner mitochondrial membrane and in gram-negative bacteria. Gram-positive and gram-negative bacteria contain naphthoquinone, and chloroplasts have plastoquinone. The quinones, and especially ubiquinone, are lipophylic and are therefore localised in the lipid phase of the membrane. They can transfer hydrogen or electrons and the transfer can occur in two stages with a semiquinone as an intermediate step. Relative to the other members of the respiratory chain, quinones are present in 10-fold to 15-fold excess. They serve as 'pools' for the hydrogens delivered by the various coenzymes and prosthetic groups of the respiratory chain; these hydrogens are then passed on to the cytochromes.

The **cytochromes** are redox systems which transfer electrons; they cannot transfer hydrogen. They accept electrons from the pool of the quinones, and with this transfer a number of protons, equivalent to the number of electrons transferred, go into solution. The cytochromes contain haem as their prosthetic group (Fig. 7.9d). The central iron atom of the haem ring participates in the electron transport by valency changes. The cytochromes are coloured and can be distinguished by their absorption spectra and their redox potentials. Cytochromes a, a_3, b, c, o and several others can be differentiated. In cytochrome c the haem group is covalently bound to cysteine residues of the apoprotein. It is water soluble (by virtue of this tight binding) and can be extracted from the membrane by aqueous solutions of salts and buffers. Cytochrome c has been found up to now in almost all organisms that possess a respiratory chain. The distribution and occurrence of the other cytochromes show considerable differences. Cytochromes are also involved in the transfer of electrons to oxygen. Cytochrome oxidase (cytochrome a_3) is the terminal oxidase (in many organisms) which reacts with oxygen and reduces it with four electrons:

$$O_2 + 4Fe^{2+} \rightarrow 2O^{2-} + 4Fe^{3+}$$

Cytochrome o, which is widely distributed in bacteria, can also react with molecular oxygen. These terminal oxidases are inhibited by cyanide and carbon monoxide.

> For a long time cytochromes were considered to be restricted to aerobic and phototrophic organisms. The discovery of cytochrome c_3 in *Desulfovibrio* therefore came as a surprise. However, the discovery that sulphate reduction by sulphate-reducing bacteria involves electron-transport phosphorylation under anaerobic conditions led to the realisation that this is formally analogous to respiration. More recently, it has been found that even the aerotolerant lactic acid bacteria *Streptococcus lactis* and *Leuconostoc mesenteroides*, as well as the anaerobic *Bifidobacterium*, produce cytochrome if they are grown on nutrient media containing haemin or blood. Cytochromes have been found even in strains of *Selenomonas ruminantium, Veillonella alcalescens, Vibrio succinogenes, Clostridium formicoaceticum* and *C. thermoaceticum*. It seems quite possible, therefore, that cytochromes and even a modest electron transport chain phosphorylation mechanism may eventually be found in other strict anaerobes.

The redox potential.   Hydrogen and electron transport are equivalent processes. The respiratory chain can be viewed as an electron-transport chain where the components oscillate between their reduced and oxidised states; that is, they behave as typical **redox catalysts**. They can therefore be assigned a redox potential, either by direct measurement (for cytochromes) or by an indirect method (for NAD, FAD).

The redox potential is a measure of the tendency of compounds or elements to deliver electrons. The redox potential is defined as the electrode potential on the hydrogen scale (E_h). Values are related to the **standard hydrogen electrode**; this is a half-cell with a solution of HCl of pH 0 and a platinum foil electrode covered by platinum black and saturated with H_2 at standard atmospheric pressure.

$$H_2 \rightleftharpoons 2H^+ + 2e^- \quad (pH\,0;\ p_{H_2}\ 1.013\ bar)$$

The **electron potential** of this **standard hydrogen electrode** is **zero**. Biological substances can be arranged in a sequence according to their redox potentials, in a manner analogous to the redox potential series of elements. The redox potential for the half-reaction (oxidised and reduced forms at equal concentrations) is designated E_0. In biochemistry, the redox potentials related to that at pH 7.0 are used and designated E_0'. At this pH the hydrogen electrode has an E_0' of $- 0.42$ V. Figure 7.10 shows the relationship between the redox potentials relative to that of the hydrogen half-cell and the pH.

As derived from the Nernst equation:

$$E = E_0 + \frac{R \cdot T}{n \cdot F} \ln \frac{c_1}{c_2}$$

The true potential of a redox system E depends on the concentration of the oxidised and reduced components:

$$E' = E_0' + \frac{0.06}{n} \log \frac{c_{ox}}{c_{red}} \quad \text{(for 30 °C)}$$

so that it becomes more negative as the concentration ratio of oxidised to reduced substance diminishes (Fig. 7.10). The redox potential is also a measure of the **maximum work**, or the **free energy** ΔG_0 that can be obtained from a reaction. The free energy of a reaction, **ΔG_0** between two redox systems, can be **calculated** from the **difference** between **their redox potentials ΔE_0**:

$$\Delta G_0 = -n \cdot F \cdot \Delta E_0 = -n \cdot 96.5 \cdot E \ (kJ / mol)$$

The E_0' values of the components of the respiratory chain extend from $- 0.32$ V for $NADH_2/NAD$ to $- 0.08$ V for flavoproteins ($FADH_2/FAD$); $- 0.04$ V for cytochrome b (Fe^{2+}/Fe^{3+}) to $+ 0.81$ V for $O^{2-}/\frac{1}{2}O_2$. Some substrates can also be assigned an E_0' value: lactate/pyruvate, $- 0.186$ V; malate/oxaloacetate, $- 0.166$ V; succinate/fumarate, $- 0.03$ V.

The free energy of the oxyhydrogen reaction derived from the difference of E_0' values of H_2 and O_2 ($- 0.42$ and $+ 0.81 = 1.23$ V) is $\Delta G_0' = - 2 \times 96.5 \times 1.23 = - 237.4$ kJ/ml. The cellular hydrogen at the level of $NADH_2$ gives a redox potential difference for final reduction of O_2 to H_2O of only 1.13 V ($+ 0.81 - (- 0.32\ V) = 1.13$ V) which is equivalent to a free energy yield of $- 218$ kJ/mol. The differences between the free

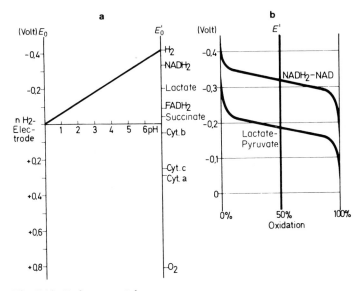

Fig. 7.10. *Redox potentials.*

(a) Dependence of the potentials, relative to the potential of the hydrogen half-cell (n-H$_2$ electrode), on pH. The normal potential E_0' is shown for some compounds. (b)

The dependence of the true potential E' of two redox systems on the concentrations of the reduced and oxidised forms.

energy yields $\Delta G_0'$ in the electron-transport steps of the respiratory chain can thus be calculated from the differences between their redox potentials (Table 7.4).

Sequence and function of the redox systems in the respiratory chain. The components of the respiratory chain can be arranged in a sequence according to their redox potentials; this sequence starts with NAD (negative redox potential) and ends in cytochrome oxidase and oxygen (Fig. 7.11A).

The electrons are transferred from NADH to oxygen via a sequence of large protein complexes – NADH-quinone reductase (also called NADH dehydrogenase), cytochrome reductase and cytochrome oxidase. These complexes traverse the cytoplasmic membrane and keep prosthetic groups – flavins, cytochromes, FeS–centres – firmly bound and fixed in a certain configuration. The electrons are transferred by NADH-

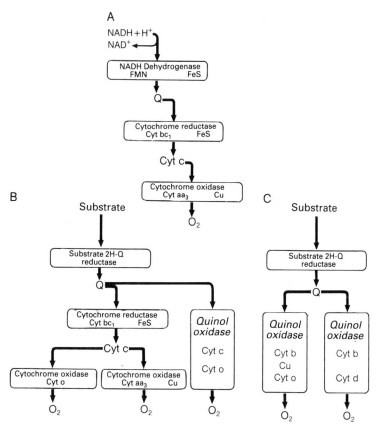

Fig. 7.11. *Diagrammatic representation of electron transport chains in the membranes of mitochondria and many bacteria.*

(A) In mitochondria and many bacteria, the respiratory chain electron transport involves three protein complexes with characteristic prosthetic groups. In many bacteria the respiratory chain may be modified and branched. In *Paracoccus denitrificans* (B) the electrons can be transported either via cytochrome reductase-cytochrome *c* and cytochrome oxidase or directly form ubiquinone via cytochrome *o* as terminal oxidase, to oxygen. In *Escherichia coli* (C) the electrons are transported either via cytochrome *b* and cytochrome *o* (low affinity for O_2) or via cytochrome *d* (high affinity for O_2) to oxygen. In oxygen deficiency, cytochrome *d* is preferentially synthesised.

Table 7.4. *Redox potentials of the components of the respiratory chain and their potential differences and energy equivalents*

Respiratory chain component	E_0' (V)	Difference (V)	$-\Delta G_0'$ (kJ/mol)	(kcal/mol)
Hydrogen	− 0.42			
		0.10	19.3	4.61
NAD	− 0.32			
		0.24	46.4	11.1
Flavoprotein	− 0.08			
		0.04	7.7	1.84
Cytochrome *b*	− 0.04			
		0.31	59.8	14.30
Cytochrome *c*	+ 0.27			
		0.02	3.8	0.92
Cytochrome *a*	+ 0.29			
		0.52	100.4	24.0
Oxygen	+ 0.81			

The underlined figures indicate where enough energy is available for respiratory chain phosphorylation.

quinone reductase – via the reduced form of ubiquinone ($UQ \cdot H_2$) – to the cytochrome reductase. This protein, also known as bc_1 complex, consists of a *b*-type cytochrome and FeS centre and cytochrome c_1. It accepts two hydrogens from $UQ \cdot H_2$ and transfers an electron to cytochrome *c*. UQ is present in large excess and transports hydrogen within the lipid bilayer. Cytochrome *c* is a peripheral membrane protein. Cytochrome oxidase, which is a protein complex containing one cytochrome *a* plus one cytochrome a_3 and Cu, transfers the electrons from cytochrome *c* to oxygen. Thus, the substrate hydrogen is ionised within the respiratory chain; the protons are then removed from the membrane by the protein complexes and the electrons delivered to oxygen. The sequence deduced from the redox potentials of the components has been confirmed by spectrophotometric and inhibitor studies.

The system, which applies to mitochondria, is found relatively rarely in aerobic prokaryotes. The bc_1 complex is found in almost all known respiratory chains, but some bacteria have branched electron transport systems and a multiplicity of endo-oxidases (Fig. 7.11B, C). Thus, there are cytochromes of the *b*-type which are called cytochrome *o* (for oxidase). These are constituted analogously to the cytochrome *a*–a_3 complex and function in a similar manner as proton pumps. Another alternative oxidase is cytochrome *d*. The branching can originate from the quinone pool or from the bc_1 complex. Which branch of the respiratory chain is actually produced may depend largely on environmental conditions, primarily on the partial pressure of oxygen.

Respiratory chain inhibitors.   The respiratory chain is inhibited or blocked by a number of cell poisons. Amytal, rotenone, and piericidin A inhibit NADH dehydrogenase. Antimycin A blocks the transfer between cytochromes b and c. Cyanide and carbon monoxide inhibit only cytochrome oxidase; the iron of cytochrome c is apparently embedded so deeply in the protein that it is unable to react with CN^- or CO. The specific effects of these inhibitors and consequent changes in the characteristic absorption spectra of the respiratory chain components have been the clues for the elucidation of respiratory chain function.

P/O ratio and energy balance.   It can be seen by inspection of the redox potentials (Table 7.4) that there are only three oxidation steps in the respiratory chain that could yield sufficient energy for the synthesis of an 'energy-rich' bond. Thus in the transfer of 2[H] from $NADH_2$ to oxygen, only three electron transfers can be coupled to phosphorylation of ADP to ATP, so that only three molecules of phosphate can be incorporated into organic compounds. This relationship is expressed as the P/O ratio (mol ATP/mol oxygen). A P/O ratio of 3 can be established experimentally in animal mitochondria with isocitrate or malate as substrates, which donate 2[H] to NAD; with succinate as substrate, the P/O ratio is only 2 because the hydrogen from succinate enters the respiratory chain only at the level of flavoprotein.

The realisation that the transfer of two hydrogen equivalents via the respiratory chain leads to the formation of three molecules of ATP allows the formulation of an **energy balance of glucose oxidation**. Assuming that one molecule of glucose is completely catabolised via the fructose-bisphosphate pathway and the tricarboxylic acid cycle and that all the hydrogen is oxidised to water by the respiratory chain, the total energy yield in terms of ATP is as follows: (a) from the fructose-bisphosphate pathway: $2 NADH_2$; (b) from the pyruvate dehydrogenase reaction: $2 NADH_2$; (c) from the tricarboxylic acid cycle: $2 \times 3 NADH_2$ and $2 FADH_2$. There is a total, therefore, of $10 NADH_2$ plus $2 FADH_2$. With P/O ratios of 3 and 2, respectively, for the respiratory chain, this gives $(10 \times 3) + (2 \times 2) = 34$ molecules of ATP. To these are added the 2 moles of ATP obtained in the fructose-bisphosphate pathway and the ATP formed from succinyl-CoA in the tricarboxylic acid cycle (2) to give an overall total of 38 molecules of ATP from each molecule of glucose metabolised to CO_2 and water by these pathways.

This calculation applies to mitochondria and to many bacteria. In a number of bacteria, however, there are only two phosphorylation points for the transfer of hydrogen from $NADH_2$ to oxygen, i.e. the P/O ratio is only 2. This is the case, for example, in aerobically growing *E. coli*; their aerobic glucose respiration yields only 26 ATP.

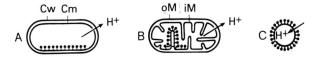

Fig. 7.12. Protein extrusion in the course of electron transport via the respiratory chain.

In bacterial cells (A) or mitochondrion (B). Protons are extruded into the suspension medium. In inside-out vesicles proton transport is inward (C). Cm, Cytoplasmic membrane; Cw, cell wall; oM and iM, outer and inner mitochondrial membranes.

Respiratory chain phosphorylation. The generation of ATP in respiratory chain phosphorylation and in photosynthetic phosphorylation takes place in membranes. ATP synthase, similar to other components of the respiratory chain, is a membrane constituent. The actual mechanism by which the respiratory chain hydrogen and electron transfer processes are coupled to the generation of ATP is still not fully understood. It has, however, been shown experimentally on a number of occasions that only vesicles or other completely membrane-enclosed structures are able to generate ATP. The electron and hydrogen transfer processes are intimately associated with a proton translocation, and this seems to be a necessary condition for the generation of ATP.

Proton transport. When oxygen is admitted to an anaerobic suspension of mitochondria or bacteria, it is found that the pH of the suspending medium declines. This leads to the conclusion that during respiration in bacteria or mitochondria, protons are extruded into the medium (Fig. 7.12A,B). In preparations of 'inside-out' vesicles (in which the originally inner surface of the membrane faces outward) from bacteria or mitochondria, respiration with reverse proton transport can be observed, leading to alkalinisation of the suspending medium (Fig. 7.12C). The proton translocation produces an electrochemical gradient. The inside of respiring mitochondria or bacteria is electrically negative and alkaline relative to the suspending medium. Both the pH gradient and the electrical membrane potential gradient exert a pull in the direction of the cell interior on the extruded protons. This proton potential, or 'proton-motive force' (ΔP), consists of the electrical membrane potential ($\Delta\psi$) and the pH difference (ΔpH) between the inner and the outer surface:

$$\Delta p = \frac{\Delta\tilde{\mu}_{H^+}}{F} = \Delta\psi - Z \cdot \Delta pH \ (mV)$$

where $Z = 2.3 \cdot R \cdot T/F$, namely 59 mV at 25 °C. The proton potential can be based entirely on the pH difference or on the membrane potential or on both.

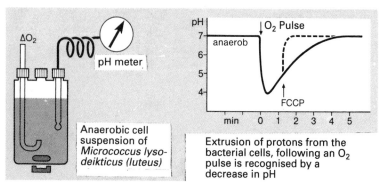

Anaerobic cell suspension of *Micrococcus lyso-deikticus (luteus)*

Extrusion of protons from the bacterial cells, following an O_2 pulse is recognised by a decrease in pH

Experimental data are consistent with the following picture: the cytoplasmic membrane of bacteria and the inner mitochondrial membrane are impermeable to ions, including protons and OH^- ions; the electrical conductivity of the membrane is low. The membranes are constructed asymmetrically; although the lipid bilayer appears symmetrical, the topography of the functional membrane proteins (electron transport chain components, ATP synthase, permeases, etc.) imparts an asymmetric character to the membrane. The spatial orientation of the enzyme molecules results in a **vectorial** metabolic function. According to the suggestion of P. Mitchell it is assumed that the respiratory chain consists of an alternating sequence of hydrogen and electron-transfer compounds arranged in loops within the membrane (Fig. 7.13). Substrate oxidation consumes protons on the inside of the membrane and releases them on the outside. Assuming three such loops, the oxidation of $NADH_2$ would involve the transport of six protons to the outside. This respiration-driven proton transport produces an electrochemical gradient between the inner and the outer membrane surface, and the proton potential is the force which powers phosphorylation, i.e. the regeneration of ATP. The biochemical energy conservation by generation of ATP is thus the consequence of the proton gradient and is accompanied by equalisation of the membrane potential. This is the content of the **chemiosmotic theory**.

Regeneration of ATP from ADP and P_i.   The synthesis of ATP from ADP and P_i is catalysed by ATP synthase. This enzyme converts the energy obtained from the electron flow into the 'energy-rich' phosphate ester bond of ATP. The enzyme has been found in all membranes which participate in energy conversion, namely in those of mitochondria, bacteria, and chloroplasts. It is rather large (relative molecular mass, 350×10^3) and complex (Fig. 7.13). It consists of a 'head' formed from a number of

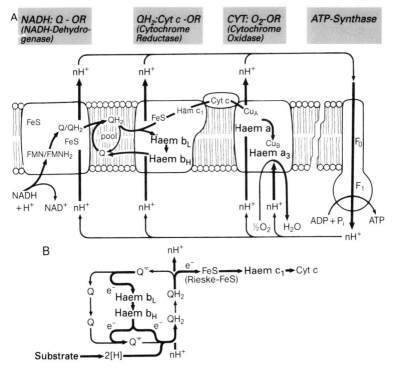

Fig. 7.13. *Diagrammatic representation showing the arrangement of large protein complexes in the respiratory chain of the inner mitochondrial membrane and the cytoplasmic membrane of bacteria.*

The electron flow from NADH via the NADH:O oxidoreductase, quinone:cytochrome c oxidoreductase and cytochrome c:O_2 oxidoreductase (cytochrome oxidase) is emphasised. Proton translocation to the outside (extrusion) is symbolised by fat black arrows. On the right-hand side ATP synthase with its F_0 and F_1-complex is indicated. The stoichimetric relations between transported protons and electrons have not been detailed. (A) The central function of the Q/QH_2 pool in connection with the quinone:cytochrome c oxidoreductase complex is shown enlarged in (B). In this reaction sequence, known as the Q-cycle, one electron is transported from ubiquinone (QH_2) via the ('Rieske') FeS-centre and haem c_1 to cytochrome c. The residual semiquinone (Q^-) is oxidised to ubiquinone (Q) by transport of an electron to haem b_1 (low potential). Haem b_1 then passes the electron to haem b_2 (high potential) which alternatively reduces Q^- and Q. OR, Oxidoreductase; Q, ubiquinone.

subunits, a stem, and a base; the latter is embedded in the lipid middle layer of the cytoplasmic membrane. ATP synthase functions by removing a water molecule from ADP and phosphate with the formation of ATP. It is at present still unclear *how* the proton flow or the proton gradient enable this phosphorylation to take place; one possibility envisages a backflow of protons to the inside through a channel or pore in the enzyme molecule, so that the energy thus liberated drives the phosphorylation reaction.

The ATP synthase is identical with F_1-ATPase; the enzyme can be demonstrated by the hydrolysis of ATP.

$$ATP + H_2O \rightarrow ADP + P_i + H^+$$

The reversibility of the reaction catalysed by ATP synthase is very important for the cell. The ATP-synthase can function in the generation of a proton potential, for example, when ATP is available by substrate phosphorylation. Thus the enzyme can function as a 'proton pump' or an 'electrogenic pump'. The reversibility of the process taking place inside the cytoplasmic membrane makes it possible to interconvert the proton potential and ATP. This convertibility is of essential importance for the coupled processes of substrate transport, flagellar movements, and biosyntheses, as shown diagrammatically in the scheme below.

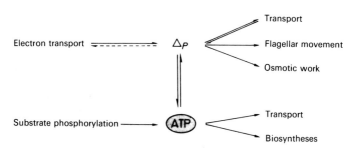

Reverse electron transport.   Some special problems are posed by bacteria that utilise hydrogen donors with redox potentials that are more positive than that of the pyridine nucleotides. Reduced pyridine nucleotides are necessary for synthetic processes, and especially for the reduction of 3-phosphoglycerate during autotrophic CO_2 fixation. Thus, pyridine nucleotides must be reduced even when sulphides, thiosulphate, sulphur, nitrite or Fe^{2+} serve as hydrogen donors. Since a direct reduction of NAD by these hydrogen donors is thermodynamically impossible, it must be assumed that in these cases, NAD (NADP) reduction is produced by a reverse, energy-dependent electron transport, driven either by ATP or the proton potential, and that ATP generation can take place only in the terminal, oxygen-reducing stages of the respiratory chain. Such reverse electron transport, accompanied by NAD reduction, has been demonstrated in *Nitrobacter, Thiobacillus* and *Comamonas carboxydovorans*.

Toxic effects of oxygen on aerobes and anaerobes.   Oxygen is the terminal electron acceptor of aerobic respiration and thus is essential for all aerobic organisms. The fact that oxygen is toxic for strict anaerobes has been known since Pasteur's experiments on butyric acid fermentation by bacteria. It was surprising, however, that oxygen also has toxic effects on aerobic organisms and that most of these contain enzymes that act to protect against the toxic products of oxygen.

In the biological sphere, three kinds of oxygen activation can be distinguished by the number of electrons that are transferred to the oxygen molecule.

$$(1) \quad O_2 + 4\,e^- \rightarrow O^{2-} + O^{2-}$$

$$(2) \quad O_2 + 2\,e^- \rightarrow O_2^{2-}$$

$$(3) \quad O_2 + 1\,e^- \rightarrow O_2^{-}$$

Reaction (1) is catalysed by cytochrome oxidase, the terminal enzyme of the electron transport chain. Four electrons are transferred simultaneously to give two O^{2-} ions, each of which then reacts with two protons to form water. Cytochrome oxidase and a few copper-containing enzymes (tyrosinase, laccase) are the only enzymes that catalyse a four-electron transfer to O^2.

Reaction (2) is characteristic for some flavin-containing enzymes (glucose oxidase, amino acid oxidase, xanthine oxidase). These enzymes transfer two electrons simultaneously and reduce oxygen to the peroxide ion O_2^{2-} which reacts with protons to give hydrogen peroxide, H_2O_2. Hydrogen peroxide is toxic to cells; it oxidises SH-groups, for example. The enzymes catalase and peroxidase have a protective function in this respect:

$$2\,H_2O_2 \xrightarrow{\text{catalase}} 2\,H_2O + O_2$$

$$H_2O_2 + 2\,GSH \xrightarrow{\text{glutathione peroxidase}} GSSG + 2\,H_2O$$

Since flavoprotein enzymes occur in many anaerobic and aerobic bacteria, the fact that almost all aerobic organisms contain catalase seems logical.

Reaction (3) is catalysed by a large number of oxidases (xanthine oxidase, aldehyde oxidase, NADPH oxidase, etc.). Only one electron is transferred with the formation of a superoxide ion O_2^-, which is a highly reactive radical. Although this is only a side reaction of the above enzymes, the superoxide radical and its reaction product with H_2O_2 ($O_2^- + H_2O_2 + H^+ \rightarrow O_2 + H_2O + OH\cdot$), the hydroxyl radical, are extremely reactive and form further reactive compounds in the cell. The enzyme superoxide dismutase exerts a protective effect against the superoxide radicals.

$$2O_2^- + 2H^+ \xrightarrow{\text{superoxide dismutase}} H_2O_2 + O_2$$

Together with catalase, the superoxide dismutase thus leads to the conversion of the superoxide radical to the harmless oxygen (the ground state). It is assumed that only organisms and cells that have superoxide dismutase are able to tolerate oxygen. The enzyme has been found in (almost) all **aerotolerant** bacteria so far examined. However, this is still a very active field of research and it is therefore advisable to refrain from over generalising.

Electron-transport processes in anaerobic bacteria.   Chemo-organotrophic organisms have two ways of regenerating biochemically useful energy (ATP) under anaerobic conditions, i.e. in the absence of oxygen: fermentation and anaerobic electron-transport phosphorylation. Fermenting organisms have at their disposal only a limited number of reactions for ATP generation, which are described as **substrate level phosphorylation** in Section 7.2.1 of this chapter and in Chapter 8.

Many bacteria, on the other hand, can carry out **electron-transport phosphorylation** even under anaerobic conditions, by transferring electrons derived from substrate via a shortened electron-transport chain to an external electron acceptor supplied in the nutrient medium, or to an internal electron acceptor derived from substrate degradation. Nitrate, sulphate, carbonate, and fumarate ions, as well as sulphur can function as electron acceptors. The respective bacteria are grouped accordingly as **nitrate reducers**, **denitrifiers**, **sulphate reducers**, **methanogens**, **acetogenic bacteria**, and **sulphur reducers**. These bacteria play an eminent part in the elemental cycles of nature (see Chapter 1). Because electron-transport phosphorylation was considered for a long time as the specific energy conservation process for respiration, tne energy conservation by electron-transport phosphorylation under anaerobic conditions is also referred to as '**anaerobic respiration**' (see Chapter 9). Electron-transport phosphorylation with fumarate as the terminal electron acceptor is not restricted to bacteria but is found in worms and even mammals. The functioning of this reaction, catalysed by fumarate reductase is indicated by the accumulation or excretion of succinate.

7.5   Accessory cycles and gluconeogenesis

Any loss of intermediary components from the tricarboxylic acid cycle for biosynthetic reactions during cellular growth is (or must be) compensated by **anaplerotic reactions** (replenishing reactions). Their specific function is to replenish oxaloacetate as the acceptor for acetyl-CoA. During growth on glucose, the glucose can serve as the precursor for all synthetic building blocks that contain glucose, ribose, deoxyribose, or other sugar derivatives. In this case the anaplerotic reactions serve predominantly for the replenishment of the tricarboxylic acid cycle. During growth on lactate, pyruvate, acetate, glyoxalate and other carbon compounds, additional metabolic pathways are necessary to maintain not only the functioning of the tricarboxylic acid cycle, but also to furnish intermediary products for the biosynthesis of sugar units (**gluconeogenesis**).

Glucose as substrate. The most important anaplerotic reactions for the replenishment of the tricarboxylic acid cycle are carboxylations of C_3 acids (pyruvate and phosphoenolpyruvate) to oxaloacetate (Fig. 7.14). These are widely distributed in animal, plant, and microbial cells. In animal tissues (liver and kidney) and in some pseudomonads, pyruvate is carboxylated by pyruvate carboxylase:

$$\text{pyruvate} + CO_2 + \text{ATP} \rightarrow \text{oxaloacetate} + \text{ADP} + P_i$$

The most widely represented carboxylation reaction is that of phosphoenolpyruvate by phosphoenolpyruvate carboxylase:

$$\text{phosphoenolpyruvate} + CO_2 + H_2O \rightarrow \text{oxaloacetate} + P_i$$

Both these reactions are practically irreversible.

Lactate, pyruvate, and other C_3 compounds as substrates. Growth of cells on pyruvate and other related compounds necessitates not only replenishment of the TCA cycle but also the net synthesis of glucose and its derivatives. The synthesis of sugars (**gluconeogenesis**) involves the same intermediary compounds that participate in glycolysis. However, the steps catalysed by hexokinase, 6-phosphofructokinase, and pyruvate kinase in the catabolic pathway are replaced by enzyme reactions that are exergonic in the direction of glucose synthesis (Fig. 7.3). In animal tissues (liver, kidney) the practically irreversible pyruvate kinase reaction is circumvented by the carboxylation of pyruvate to oxaloacetate by pyruvate carboxylase, followed immediately by a reaction catalysed by phosphoenolpyruvate carboxykinase:

$$\text{oxaloacetate} + \text{GTP} \rightarrow \text{phosphoenolpyruvate} + CO_2 + \text{GDP}$$

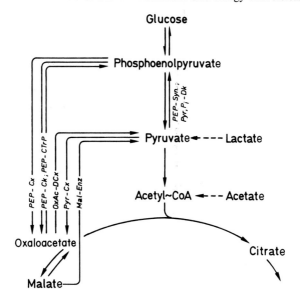

Fig. 7.14. *The most important reaction pathways connecting the C_3 compounds pyruvate and phsophoenolpyruvate with the C_4 compounds malate and oxaloacetate.*

Enzymes: Mal-Enz, malate enzyme; OxAc-DCx, oxaloacetate decarboxylase; PEP-Ck, phosphoenolpyruvate carboxykinase; PEP-Cx, phosphoenolpyruvate carboxylase; PEP-Syn, phosphoenolpyruvate synthetase; PEP-CTrP, phosphoenolpyruvate carboxytransphosphorylase; Pry-Cx, pyruvate carboxylase; Pyr, P_i-Dk, pyruvate orthophosphate dikinase.

This synthesis of phosphoenolpyruvate from pyruvate via oxaloacetate thus consumes two energy-rich phosphate bonds, one for the carboxylation of pyruvate and a second for the synthesis of phosphoenolpyruvate from oxaloacetate.

> It has become clear in recent investigations that the reverse reaction catalysed by phosphoenolpyruvate carboxykinase is the only one by which C_3 compounds can give rise to oxaloacetate in strictly anaerobic bacteria (and worms). In the presence of high concentrations of carbon dioxide in the environment, the reaction goes predominantly in the direction of oxaloacetate formation.

In *E. coli* and some other bacteria, pyruvate can be directly phosphorylated by phosphoenolpyruvate synthase (Fig. 7.14).

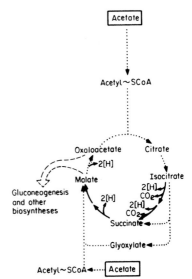

Fig. 7.15. *Metabolic pathways to supply the cell with energy and carbon building blocks during growth on acetate.*

The catabolic pathway (tricarboxylic acid cycle) is drawn with full lines and the anaplerotic pathway (glyoxylate cycle) with broken lines.
(After H. L. Kornberg.)

$$\text{pyruvate} + \text{ATP} + H_2O \rightarrow \text{phosphoenolpyruvate} + \text{AMP} + P_i$$

This reaction also consumes two energy-rich phosphate bonds (i.e. in going from ATP to AMP). The synthesis of oxaloacetate is then catalysed by phosphoenolpyruvate carboxylase. *E. coli* does not contain pyruvate carboxylase.

Propionibacteria, *Acetobacter aceti, Entamoeba histolytica* and *Fusobacterium symbiosus* contain a further enzyme that can form phosphoenolpyruvate from pyruvate, namely pyruvate orthophosphate dikinase. This catalyses the reversible reaction:

$$\text{pyruvate} + \text{ATP} + P_i \rightleftharpoons \text{phosphoenolpyruvate} + \text{AMP} + PP_i$$

It should be noted that here the energy-rich bond of the diphosphate is preserved. In the C_4-dicarboxylic acid plants, such as sugar cane and maize, this enzyme is also responsible for the synthesis of phosphoenolpyruvate, which is then converted to oxaloacetate by phosphoenolpyruvate carboxylase.

Acetate as substrate. Microorganisms are able to grow on acetate and compounds that are catabolised to acetate (fatty acids, hydrocarbons) by virtue of the glyoxylate cycle (Krebs–Kornberg cycle) (Fig. 7.15).

This anaplerotic sequence is based on the function of two enzymes, isocitrate lyase and malate synthase. Isocitrate lyase cleaves isocitrate to succinate and glyoxylate:

$$
\begin{array}{ccc}
\text{CH}_2-\text{COOH} & & \text{CH}_2-\text{COOH} \\
| & \xrightarrow{\textit{Isocitrate Lyase}} & | \\
\text{CH}-\text{COOH} & & \text{CH}_2-\text{COOH} \quad + \quad \text{CHO}-\text{COOH} \\
| & & \\
\text{HO}-\text{CH}-\text{COOH} & &
\end{array}
$$

| Isocitrate | Succinate | Glyoxylate |

Malate synthase then catalyses the condensation of a molecule of acetyl-CoA with glyoxylate to give malate:

$$
\begin{array}{ccc}
\text{CH}_2-\text{COOH} & & \text{CH}_2-\text{COOH} \\
| & \xrightarrow{\textit{Isocitrate Lyase}} & | \\
\text{CH}-\text{COOH} & & \text{CH}_2-\text{COOH} \quad + \quad \text{CHO}-\text{COOH} \\
| & & \\
\text{HO}-\text{CH}-\text{COOH} & &
\end{array}
$$

| Isocitrate | Succinate | Glyoxylate |

The combination of isocitrate lyase and malate synthase thus converts one molecule of isocitrate and one molecule of acetyl-CoA to two molecules of C_4-dicarboxylic acids. The latter can then be converted to pyruvate by the malate enzyme or to phosphoenolpyruvate by phosphoenolpyruvate carboxykinase and are thus recruited for gluconeogenesis. On the other hand they can furnish oxaloacetate for the citrate synthase reaction and thus furnish building blocks for biosynthesis. The glyoxylate cycle seems to be of little importance for the replenishment of the tricarboxylic acid cycle during the metabolism of glucose, pyruvate, or other C_3 compounds.

Glyoxylate as substrate.   When glyoxylate or its precursors (glycollate, urea) function as the carbon source, they induce the enzymes of the D-**glycerate pathway**. Two molecules of glyoxylate are converted to tartronate semialdehyde by tartronate semialdehyde synthase (also called glyoxylate carboligase) with the release of carbon dioxide. The aldehyde group is reduced to the CH_2OH group of the D-glycerate by a specific reductase, and the glycerate is then phosphorylated to 3-phosphoglycerate. The acetyl-CoA, derived from this in the usual way then enters the tricarboxylic acid cycle and is oxidised (Fig. 7.16). The presence of malate synthase ensures the replenishment of intermediates; it catalyses the conversion of a further molecule of glyoxylate with acetyl-CoA to malate.

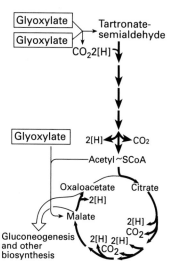

Fig. 7.16. *Metabolic pathways to supply the cell with energy and carbon building blocks during growth on glycollate, glyoxylate, or urea.*

Glyoxylate is converted to acetyl-CoA via the D-glycerate pathway and then oxidised via the tricarboxylic acid cycle (thick arrows). The anaplerotic pathway is shown with thin lines
(After L. N. Ornston and
M. K. Ornston.)

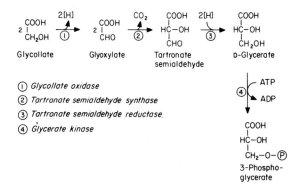

① Glycollate oxidase
② Tartronate semialdehyde synthase
③ Tartronate semialdehyde reductase.
④ Glycerate kinase

Whereas the main metabolic enzymes are always present, i.e. when cells are growing on glucose, those enzymes participating in the accessory cycles are inducible. During growth on glucose these enzymes are present only in very small amounts, referred to as the basal level of enzyme activity, and are barely demonstrable. The enzymes are only induced when the cells are placed in a nutrient medium in which acetate or glyoxylate are the sole source of carbon and energy. The enzyme content of fully induced cells can reach 100-fold, or more, the basal level. This substrate-induced enzyme level can be demonstrated by measuring enzyme activity before and after the change of substrate. Such substrate-induced production of an enzyme is convincing evidence for its role in the metabolism of the new substrate. However, final proof can only be obtained by supplying radioactively labelled precursors and identifying the labelled atoms in the appropriate intermediates and end products of the metabolic sequence.

The idea that all enzymes that participate in sugar metabolism belong to a constant enzyme equipment of cells, i.e. are **constitutive**, should also be avoided. Bacteria that grow on acetate, for example, produce only those enzymes of glucose metabolism that are necessary for gluconeogenesis; the enzymes involved only in the degradation of glucose are barely, or not at all, demonstrable in 'acetate cells'.

When cells are exposed simultaneously to two substrates, they often utilise only one at a time. During growth of *E. coli* or pseudomonads in the presence of glucose and acetate, glucose is utilised first. The enzymes necessary for the utilisation of acetate are not produced; **induction** of these enzymes does not occur while glucose is present. This is referred to as **catabolite repression** of the enzymes needed for acetate utilisation. Further details of the regulation of enzyme synthesis will be discussed in Chapter 16, 'Regulation of Metabolism'.

7.6   Biosynthesis of some low molecular weight building blocks

Biosynthesis of amino acids.   Most microorganisms as well as green plants are able to synthesis *de novo* all 20 amino acids that are required for protein synthesis. The carbon skeletons of the amino acids are derived from the intermediary compounds of metabolism. The amino groups are introduced by direct **amination** or by **transamination**. Inorganic nitrogen can be incorporated into organic compounds only via ammonia. Assimilation of molecular nitrogen, as well as of nitrate and nitrite, first involves its reduction to ammonia, before it is incorporated into organic compounds (Fig. 7.17, 1–3).

Only a few amino acids can be directly aminated by free ammonium ions. This primary assimilation of ammonia involves L-glutamate dehydrogenase (Fig. 7.17, 6) and L-alanine dehydrogenase (Fig. 7.17, 7). These enzymes catalyse the reductive amination of the corresponding 2-oxoacids without the participation of ATP. The formation of glutamine from glutamate is catalysed by glutamine synthetase. This enzyme has a much

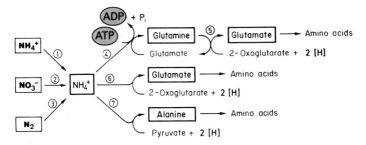

Fig. 7.17. *The most important pathways for the assimilation of nitrogen.*

Ammonium ions present in the nutrient medium are taken up directly into the cell (1). Nitrate ions are converted to ammonium ions by assimilatory nitrate reduction (2), and molecular nitrogen is converted to ammonium ions by nitrogen fixation (3). The ammonia nitrogen is incorporated into organic compounds either with participation of ATP via glutamine (4) formation, or without consumption of ATP by direct reductive amination of 2-oxoglutarate or pyruvate (6), (7).

higher affinity (lower K_m) for ammonium ions than the above-named dehydrogenases and is therefore active at very low NH_4^{2+} concentrations; the formation of glutamine requires ATP. The amide group of glutamine can be transferred to 2-oxoglutarate by glutamate synthase (Fig. 7.17, 5). This system for the assimilation of ammonia nitrogen into organic compounds is apparently always formed and utilised by bacteria and plants when the concentration of available ammonium ions is very low (less than 1 mmol/l) and especially during nitrogen fixation.

Most of the other amino acids obtain their amino groups by **transamination** with a primary amino acid. Glutamate represents the largest component (more than 50%) of the cytoplasmic, free amino acid pool.

The synthetic pathways of the 20 amino acids in microorganisms have been well researched. They start from simple compounds of intermediary metabolism (pyruvate, 2-oxoglutarate, oxaloacetate or fumarate, erythrose-4-phosphate, ribose-5-phosphate, and ATP). In most amino acids the incorporation of the amino group by **transamination** is the last step in the synthetic pathway. Some amino acids are formed by several interconversions of precursor amino acids, without transamination. The amino acids can be classified into groups by common synthetic pathways (Fig. 7.18). The synthesis of different amino acids comprise different numbers of enzymatic steps; it should be noted that the amino acids that are essential for humans are produced in other organisms only by especially lengthy synthetic routes.

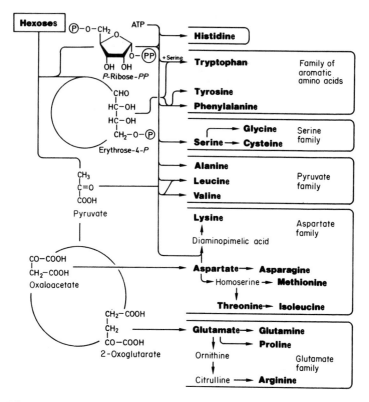

Fig. 7.18. *The 20 amino acids required for protein synthesis are synthesised from simple components of intermediary metabolism.*

The relatively rapid elucidation of these and other biosynthetic pathways is due to the use of **auxotrophic** mutants of fungi and bacteria. In many mutants **auxotrophy** is due to loss of the ability to produce a biosynthetic enzyme, so that they require the end product of the blocked pathway for growth. Such mutants have another advantageous property: they can grow not only on the end product of the blocked pathway, but also on intermediates between the blocked step and the end product. On the other hand, the substrate of the missing (or inactive) enzyme is often excreted, i.e. when enzyme b is deficient, the intermediate product B may be excreted:

$$A \xrightarrow{\text{enzyme a}} B \xrightarrow{\text{enzyme b}} C \xrightarrow{\text{enzyme c}} D \xrightarrow{\text{enzyme d}} E$$

Thus, some mutants can 'feed' other mutants that have a block at a different step of the same synthetic pathway; a mutant with a later block (enzyme d) can supply a mutant with an earlier block (enzyme b) with the necessary intermediate. The mutants in a given synthetic pathway can be placed in a sequence where one supplies the requirements of the next by such **cross-feeding experiments**. Many biosynthetic pathways have been worked out in this way, by isolation of excreted intermediary products, purification of biosynthetic enzymes, and a variety of other methods.

Biosynthesis of nucleotides.   Purine and pyrimidine nucleotides are the building blocks of nucleic acids; in addition they are contained in several coenzymes and function in the activation and transfer of amino groups, sugars, cell wall components and lipids. The synthesis of purine nucleotides follows a common path which diverges only at the level of inosine monophosphate into adenylate and guanylate. Pyrimidine nucleotides are also synthesised via a single pathway which branches out from uridylic acid.

The pentose moiety of the nucleotide is derived from ribose-5-phosphate. This can be formed in two ways: oxidatively from glucose-6-phosphate via the pentose-phosphate pathway, and non-oxidatively from fructose-6-phosphate and glyceraldehyde-3-phosphate via the transaldolase-transketolase reaction (Section 7.2.2). Ribose-5-phosphate is used in the energy-rich form of **phosphoribosyldiphosphate** for the synthesis of purine and pyrimidine nucleotides. The reduction of ribose to deoxyribose occurs at the level of the ribonucleotide and there are several reaction mechanisms.

The biosynthesis of lipids.   Fats and lipids are important components of the cytoplasmic membrane and the cell wall, and they also serve as energy reserves. In bacterial lipids, the long-chain (C_{14}–C_{18}) saturated and mono-unsaturated fatty acids predominate; multi-unsaturated fatty acids and steroids do not seem to occur, and triglycerides are rare. Complex lipids are of great importance; they consist of glycerol, which has two hydroxy groups esterified with fatty acids and the third hydroxy group is esterified with phosphate or sugar. The phosphate residue is in turn esterified with serine, ethanolamine, or glycerol. Phosphatidylglycerol, phosphatidylethanolamine, and (rarely) phosphatidylinositol, which are found in most bacteria, belong to this group of lipids. The biosynthesis of long-chain fatty acids consists of reduction and oxidation of acetyl groups. At first, the methyl group of acetyl-CoA is made more reactive in a biotin-dependent carboxylation to form malonyl-CoA.

$$CH_3\text{–}CO\text{~}SCoA + CO_2 + ATP + H_2O \rightarrow$$
$$HOOC\text{–}CH_2\text{–}CO\text{~}SCoA + ADP + P_i$$

The carboxyl group is then liberated again (as carbon dioxide) in the subsequent condensation reactions. Fatty acid synthesis takes place on a multienzyme complex, according to the overall equation:

$$CH_3-CO\sim CoA + 7\,malonyl\text{-}CoA + 14\,NADPH_2 \rightarrow$$
$$palmityl\text{-}CoA + 14\,NADP + 7\,CO_2 + 7\,CoA + 7\,H_2O$$

7.7   The uptake of solutes into the cell

Nutrients and other substances needed by the cell must penetrate the cell boundary layers before they can be metabolised. The cell wall does not present much of a barrier to small molecules and ions, but it excludes large molecules with a relative molecular mass above 600. The cell boundary component that governs the uptake of most substances into the cell is the cytoplasmic membrane.

Transport of nutrients through the cytoplasmic membrane is usually specific; only those nutrients are taken up by the cell for which transport systems are available (Figs 2.21, 7.19); transport is dependent, with few exceptions, on specific permeases and translocases. These are membrane proteins, and the names indicate that they exhibit some of the properties of enzymes. They are substrate-specific, may be substrate **inducible**, and are produced only under conditions that permit protein synthesis.

The term transport can have several quite different meanings in Cell Biology. In considering only those transport processes which occur in or through the cytoplasmic membrane, two main types are to be distinguished: **primary** and **secondary** transport. Primary transport consists of those processes that lead to the transfer of ions like H^+, Na^+, K^+, and hence to alterations in the electrochemical potential. The forces driving primary transport are either respiratory or photosynthetic electron transport, ATP-driven ion pumps (ATPases) or ion pumps driven by decarboxylation of metabolites (oxaloacetate, methylmalonyl-CoA, glutaconyl-CoA). The term **secondary transport** is applied to all processes resulting in the uptake (influx) or outflow (efflux) of cellular metabolites, which are driven by **electrochemical potential gradients**. The processes discussed here in Section 7.7 (all driven by electrochemical potential gradients) belong to this group of secondary transport.

Several types of mechanisms for the uptake of substances into the cell can be distinguished. Two of these permit only transport, but not accumulation of the material transported to the cell. On the other hand, several processes of 'active transport' lead to intracellular accumulation of the material transported (Figs 7.19, 7.20).

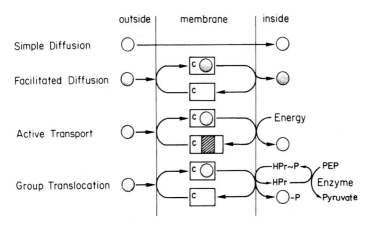

Fig. 7.19. *Schematic representation of the four mechanisms for transport of materials into the cell.*

Circle, substrate to be transported;
C, permease(carrier)-protein;
C with grey hatching, energised carrier;

PEP, phosphoenolpyruvate;
HPr, heat stable protein.
See text for details.

The non-specific penetration of substances into the cell is called simple or **passive diffusion**. It is governed by the molecular size and lipophilic properties of the material. The rates of such transport are low. Uptake of sugars by passive diffusion has never been demonstrated. Apparently water, non-polar toxins, inhibitors and other substances that are not part of the normal intracellular milieu are taken up by passive diffusion.

Facilitated diffusion.   In facilitated diffusion a substance is transported into the cell along its concentration gradient, i.e. towards equilibrium between the external and internal concentrations. The process is mediated (in most cases) by a **substrate-specific** permease, and the rate of transport is governed, over a wide range, by the substrate concentration in the medium (Fig. 7.20). Facilitated diffusion is independent of metabolic energy and the nutrient cannot accumulate inside the cell against a concentration gradient.

Active transport.   **Active transport** and **group translocation** share with facilitated diffusion the participation of substrate-specific proteins. They differ from facilitated diffusion, however, by their dependence on energy. When metabolic energy is available, the substrate can be

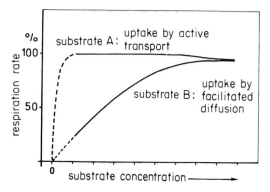

Fig. 7.20. *Substrate saturation curves for the uptake of two substrates by intact bacterial cells measured by oxygen consumption (respiration rate).*

The active and passive uptake of substrate can be recognised by the shape of the curve. Substrate A is taken up by active transport and accumulated in the cell; respiration therefore reaches its maximum rate at very low substrate concentrations. Substrate B is taken up passively and the respiration rate reaches its maximum only at relatively high substrate concentrations (10–20 mmol/l).

accumulated inside the cell **against a concentration gradient**. The basic difference between **active transport** and **group translocation** is the nature of the product that is released inside the cell. In active transport, the molecule released into the cytoplasm is identical with that taken up from the medium. In group translocation, the molecule is modified during the transport process, for example, by phosphorylation.

Various models proposed for **active transport** all include specific transport proteins in the membrane. These have been given names that indicate their presumed functions: permeases, translocases, translocator proteins, and carriers. Different transport processes are distinguished mainly by the way in which the energy necessary to drive the transport process is made available: by a proton potential, Δp (Fig. 7.21), by ATP or by phosphoenolpyruvate (Fig. 7.19). The transport of many substances, including inorganic and organic ions, as well as sugars, is driven by the proton potential Δp (Section 7.4 of this chapter). The bacterial cell maintains a proton potential by constantly pumping out protons and other ions (Na^+). This is mediated by **transport proteins** located in the membrane. Each of these proteins has a specific function. One protein is known, for example, to catalyse the simultaneous transport of a sugar molecule (lactose, melibiose, or glucose) and a proton in the same direction. This is referred to as a **symport** of two (or more) substances. Other

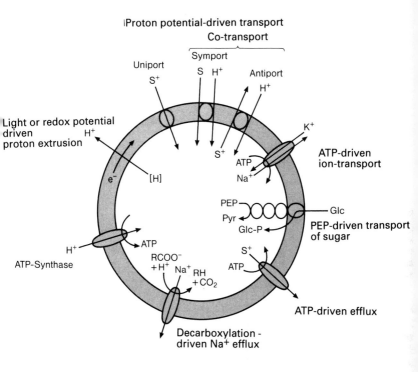

Fig. 7.21. *Summary of systems that transport ions and other metabolites through the cytoplasmic membrane.*

transport proteins catalyse the simultaneous transport of two substances in opposite directions, for example, a proton and another ion (Na^+ or an organic acid); this is called **antiport**. The ions that drive the entry of sugars into the cell are probably always H^+ or Na^+. In prokaryotes, the H^+-coupled symport seems to predominate, whereas in eukaryotes, Na^+-coupled symport is the rule.

The actual presence of such transport proteins in bacterial cells has been demonstrated (a) by isolation and insertion of the purified carrier protein in protoplasts or so-called liposomes, and (b) by isolation of defective mutants that lack a given protein and its specific function. Active transport driven by a proton potential is probably the most common mechanism for the active uptake of metabolic substrates.

The idea that specific transport proteins participate in the transport of ions has been supported by observations on some antibiotics and synthetic substances, so-called **ionophores**. **Ionophores** are low molecular weight (500–2000) compounds with a hydrophobic surface and a hydrophilic centre. They enter the lipid membrane by virtue of their hydrophobicity. The best-known ionophore-antibiotic is valinomycin. It diffuses in the membrane and mediates the transport (uniport) of K^+, Cs^+, Rb^+, or NH_4^+. In the presence of these ions, therefore, the action of valinomycin leads to an equilibration of charges, and hence to a collapse of the proton potential. Other ionophores form channels through which ions can penetrate. There are also some synthetic compounds that enhance the proton conductivity of the membrane; the best-known 'proton carrier' is FCCP (7-carbonyl-cyanide-p-trifluoromethoxy-phenylhydrazone). It acts as an uncoupler, i.e. it uncouples ATP synthesis from electron transport because it can transport protons into the cell without the participation of ATP synthase. Research on membrane transport has yielded important data that are consistent with and support the chemiosmotic theory of energy conversion.

In addition to transport systems that depend on a proton potential there are others that depend on ATP. In these the periplasmic binding proteins play a part (see Fig. 2.29).

In animal cells, the cytoplasmic membrane does not transport protons and does not produce a pH gradient. The membrane potential is probably generated by ATP-dependent pumping mechanisms, such as the sodium–potassium pump, and the Na^+ potential then drives the Na^+ nutrient symport.

Group translocation.   In group translocation the transported molecule is chemically modified; a sugar, for instance, is taken up as such and is delivered inside the cell as sugar-phosphate. Glucose, fructose, mannose, and other carbohydrates are taken up by the phosphoenolpyruvate-dependent phosphotransferase system (PTS). Four proteins are known to take part in group translocation (Fig. 7.22 I, II, III). Of these, enzyme II is an integral membrane protein; it forms the channel and it catalyses the phosphorylation of the sugar. The phosphate group, however, is not directly transferred from PEP, but is first donated by enzyme I to a small, heat-stable protein, called HPr. The phosphorylated form of HPr (HPr-P) reacts with enzyme III, which is a peripheral membrane protein. The phosphate group is then transferred to the sugar by the channel protein, enzyme II. The membrane enzymes II and III are specific for each sugar, whereas enzyme I and HPr take part in all PTS-mediated sugar transport (translocation). A few sugar transport (PTS) systems do not seem to involve enzyme III.

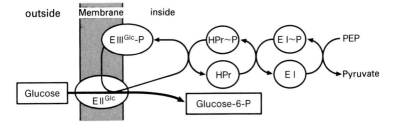

Fig. 7.22. *Transport of glucose by the phosphoenolpyruvate: glucose phospho-transferase system (PTS).*

EI, EII and EIII, enzyme I, enzyme II and enzyme III; HPr, Heat-stable protein. For further explanation see text.

The complexity of the PTS system indicates that it may function not only in the transport of sugars, but may also have a regulatory role. Thus, sugars that are transported by the PTS system inhibit the uptake and utilisation of simultaneously present other sugars (catabolite repression: Ch. 16.13).

Efflux of substances.   Even less is known about the excretion of metabolites into the medium than about uptake mechanisms. Both transport systems and uncontrolled diffusion appear to be involved. Excretion of substances takes place when these are over produced and accumulate in the cell at high concentrations. Such accumulation can be due to incomplete oxidations, defective regulation of metabolism, or fermentative processes.

The transport of iron.   Studies on a number of microorganisms have shown that they possess specific mechanisms for the uptake of iron. Under anaerobic conditions, iron is present as the ferrous (Fe(II)) ion and its concentration can be as high as 10^{-1} mol/l; it is therefore not growth limiting. In an aerobic environment at pH 7.0, however, iron is present as ferric (Fe(III)) hydroxide, which is practically insoluble; its concentration is maximally 10^{-18} mol/l. Not surprisingly, it was found that microorganisms can excrete substances that render the iron soluble by binding the Fe(III) ions in a complex which can be transported. Such substances are collectively designated as **siderophores**. They are, almost without exception, low molecular weight, water-soluble compounds (relative molecular mass less than 1500) that bind iron coordinately with very high specificity and affinity (stability constant about 10^{30}). Chemically, these iron-binding ligands can be assigned to phenolic compounds and hydroxamates. The first of these groups includes enterobactin, which has

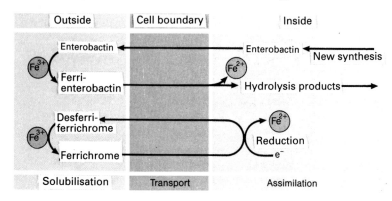

Fig. 7.23. *Examples of the mechanisms for the transport of iron into cells by siderophores.*

The upper part shows the system of the many bacteria, exemplified in enterochelin. The lower part shows the ferrichrome system of many fungi.

six phenolic hydroxy groups and is excreted by enterobacteria. The iron-free form of enterobactin is excreted into the medium and binds iron, and the ferri-enterobactin is then taken up by the cell. The iron is released inside the cell by enzymatic hydrolysis of the ferri-enterobactin complex (Fig. 7.23).

The yellow-green fluorescent pigments that are excreted by *Pseudomonas putida* and *P. aeruginosa*, also function as siderophores.

Many fungi produce ferrichromes for the same purpose. These belong to the hydroxamate siderophores; they are cyclical hexapeptides that bind ferric iron via three hydroxamate groups. These, too, are excreted into the medium in the iron-free form, combine with iron, and are transported into the cell as ferrichromes. Inside the cell the iron is reduced to the Fe(II) form, for which the ferrichromes have only low affinity so that the ferrous ions are liberated. Ferrioxamine (in actinomycetes), myco-bactine (in mycobacteria), and exocheline (also in mycobacteria) have similar functions.

Microorganisms generally excrete siderophores only when the supply of iron is growth limiting. The excretion is a result of derepression of siderophore synthesis. In the presence of soluble complexed iron, sidero-phores are synthesised in only small amounts and are retained in the cell wall where they function to transport iron into the cell.

It is of interest, in this context, that the natural defence mechanisms of higher organisms include ways of keeping the environment free of available iron. They produce iron-binding proteins that bind the iron so tightly that it is unavailable to microorganisms whose growth is therefore inhibited. Examples of these iron-binding proteins are in egg albumin (conalbumin), in milk, in tear-duct and salivary gland secretions (lactotransferrin), and in serum (serotransferrin). Thus, bacteria inoculated into chicken eggs will only grow if iron in the form of ferrous ammonium citrate is also injected simultaneously. It seems that iron may play an important role in the struggle between higher organisms and bacteria. The winner is the organism that can produce an iron-chelating substance with the highest affinity constant.

8 Special fermentations

Wherever in nature organic compounds are present, whilst oxygen is lacking, fermenting microorganisms are likely to establish themselves. Bacteria with fermentative ability initiate the degradation of biopolymers which have been deposited in conditions which oxygen cannot reach. In such oxygen-free (anoxic) environments rapidly fermenting bacteria will come to dominate (providing other conditions are suitable).

The quantitatively predominant biopolymer that is fermented in sediments of lakes and ponds, etc. is **cellulose**. The greater part of the cellulose that is eaten by herbivorous animals is excreted unchanged. If such cellulose reaches anoxic zones it is fermented by clostridia and other strictly anaerobic organisms. The fermentation products, such as alcohols, organic acids, carbon dioxide and hydrogen are then at the disposal of other bacteria. These can produce methane and, in the presence of sulphate, sulphur dioxide, by means of other specific fermentations or anaerobic respiration. These fermentations thus initiate the **anaerobic food chain**. In the sediments of freshwater lakes and in the rumen of ruminants, hydrogen and acetate are fermented to methane by methanogenic bacteria. In marine anoxigenic ecosystems hydrogen and sulphate are converted to hydrogen sulphide by sulphidogenic bacteria.

Fermenting organisms have been used in food processing and preserving for thousands of years. Representative examples are: brewing, wine production, lactic acid and yoghurt, sauerkraut, silage, cheeses and baker's yeast. Many fermentative organisms are obligate anaerobes. Others are facultatively anaerobic and can grow in the presence as well as in the absence of oxygen. **Oxygen plays no part in fermentation** processes, and the expression, coined by Louis Pasteur: 'La fermentation c'est la vie sans l'air' is still undisputed in basic science. On the other hand, the term 'fermentation' has also acquired a wider meaning in industrial microbiology (also called microbial biotechnology, these days). Because the stirred vessels employed in large-scale aerobic cultivation – for the production of biomass or metabolites – are the same as those used in the classical anaerobic fermentations (which are called fermentors), these processes are also called 'fermentations'.

Fermentation   Fermentation is an ATP-regenerating metabolic process in which degradation products of organic substrates serve as hydrogen donors as well as hydrogen acceptors. The reactions that lead to phosphorylation of ADP are oxidations. The oxidised carbon compounds are finally released from the cell as carbon dioxide. The oxidising steps are dehydrogenations in which the hydrogens are transferred to a cofactor like NAD. Intermediary products of substrate degradation then serve as acceptors for the hydrogen from $NADH_2$. The reduced products formed by the regeneration of NAD are excreted by the cell.

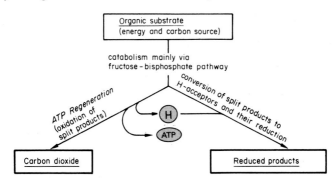

During the fermentation of carbohydrates and some other compounds, the following products are formed, either singly or in various combinations: ethanol, lactate, propionate, formate, butyrate, succinate, caproate, acetate, *n*-butanol, 2,3-butanediol, acetone, 2-propanol, carbon dioxide and molecular hydrogen. According to the quantitatively predominant or highly characteristic end products, fermentations are classified as alcoholic fermentations, lactic acid fermentations, propionic acid fermentations, formic acid fermentations, butyric acid fermentations and acetic acid fermentations.

ATP regeneration by fermentation.   One to four molecules of ATP can be produced during fermentation of glucose by microorganisms.

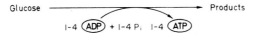

In view of the large number of possible fermentation products, it is surprising that there seem to be only a few reactions concerned in the energy conversion of substrate-level phosphorylation; only the three most important reactions are presented here:

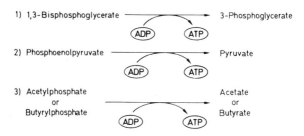

1) 1,3-Bisphosphoglycerate ⟶ 3-Phosphoglycerate
   ADP ⟶ ATP

2) Phosphoenolpyruvate ⟶ Pyruvate
   ADP ⟶ ATP

3) Acetylphosphate   Acetate
   or   or
   Butyrylphosphate   Butyrate
   ADP ⟶ ATP

Most fermenting organisms use only reaction (1) catalysed by phosphoglycerate kinase and reaction (2) catalysed by pyruvate kinase, and use pyruvate and compounds synthesised from acetyl-CoA as the necessary hydrogen acceptors. During the fermentation of 1 mol glucose only 2 (up to 4) mol ATP are generated, and the following products may be formed: lactate, ethanol, acetone, butyrate, *n*-butanol, 2-propanol, 2,3-butanediol, caproate, acetate, carbon dioxide, and molecular hydrogen.

The use of acetate kinase (reaction 3) offers the advantage of additional ATP regeneration. Acetylphosphate is produced from acetyl-CoA by phosphotransacetylase.

$$\text{acetyl-CoA} + P_i \rightarrow \text{acetylphosphate} + CoA$$

Acetylphosphate can also arise from sugar phosphates (xylulose-5-phosphate, fructose-6-phosphate) via reactions catalysed by phosphoketolase.

Whether a bacterium can utilise acetate kinase seems to depend on its ability to evolve molecular hydrogen. No hydrogen acceptors need to be synthesised for reducing equivalents (electrons) that can (after transfer to protons) be liberated as molecular hydrogen. To understand these relationships, the mechanisms for the liberation of H_2 must be discussed.

Anaerobic bacteria can oxidise pyruvate to acetyl-CoA in two ways (see oxidation of pyruvate, reactions (2) and (3), Ch. 7.2.4). In the clostridial type of reaction catalysed by pyruvate:ferredoxin oxidoreductase, ferredoxin is reduced. Its redox potential is so low E_0', -420 mV) that hydrogen can be evolved by the action of a special hydrogenase, ferredoxin:H_2 oxidoreductase:

$$2FdH \rightarrow 2Fd + H_2$$

In the reaction catalysed by pyrvate:formate lyase (enterobacterial type), formate is produced in addition to acetyl-CoA. The formate can then be cleaved by a hydrogenlyase system:

$$\text{formate} \rightarrow H_2 + CO_2$$

Both these mechanisms for the liberation of H_2 involve intermediates

(FdH and formate) with very low redox potentials, so that the reducing equivalents derived from the oxidation of pyruvate to acetyl-CoA can be released by the cell without difficulty.

This is in contrast to the hydrogen originating from the dehydrogenation of glyceraldehyde-3-phosphate in the form of $NADH_2$ which must be transferred to organic·hydrogen acceptors by most anaerobic bacteria. However, many bacteria have the ability to release even these reducing equivalents as hydrogen by virtue of an enzyme that can mediate between $NADH_2$ and ferredoxin. This enzyme, $NADH_2$: ferredoxin oxidoreductase, catalyses the reaction:

$$NADH_2 + 2Fd \rightarrow NAD + 2FdH$$

so that H_2 can be released from FdH by a hydrogenase. Since the above reaction involves a change to a more negative redox potential of hydrogen (from E_0', − 320 mV for $NADH_2$ to E_0', − 420 mV for ferredoxin), the equilibrium is unfavourable for the evolution of hydrogen, so the reaction can only continue if the evolved hydrogen can be continuously removed. Thus, organisms that have the potential ability to produce H_2 from $NADH_2$ can utilise this elegant way of releasing $NADH_2$-hydrogen as molecular hydrogen only when they grow in mixed cultures with organisms that utilise the molecular hydrogen. This does occur in nature and is referred to as **interspecies hydrogen transfer** and as a special type of symbiosis in microbial associations. The bacteria that can release the hydrogen from $NADH_2$ as H_2, in the way described above, can therefore dispense with the utilisation of acetyl-CoA for the supply of hydrogen acceptors from $NADH_2$. They can then convert their acetyl-CoA to acetylphosphate and obtain ATP from this in the acetate kinase reaction. In this way therefore, they obtain up to four molecules of ATP from the fermentation of one molecule of glucose (*Ruminococcus albus*; Section 8.5 of this chapter) and they excrete acetate as the main end-product.

The role of fermentations in the economy of nature.   Fermenting organisms play a considerable part in the metabolic cycles of nature. Cellulose found in the anerobic zones of soil sediments is fermented to the end products mentioned above, almost always including hydrogen. Hydrogen is therefore in the centre of the anaerobic food chain, with the main products being methane and/or hydrogen sulphide.

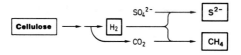

In freshwater sediments and in the rumen of ruminants, hydrogen is metabolised to methane by methanogenic bacteria, and in marine anaerobic ecosystems, hydrogen and sulphate are converted to hydrogen sulphide by sulphate-reducing bacteria.

8.1   Alcoholic fermentations by yeasts and bacteria

Fermentation of sugars with the production of ethanol is widely distributed among microorganisms. Accumulation of ethanol can occur even in plants and in many fungi under anaerobic conditions. The chief ethanol producers are yeasts, especially strains of *Saccharomyces cerevisiae*. The yeasts, like most fungi, respire aerobically, but in the absence of air they ferment carbohydrates to ethanol and carbon dioxide. A number of anaerobic or facultatively aerobic bacteria can also produce ethanol as the main or subsidiary product during fermentation of hexoses and pentoses.

8.1.1   Ethanol formation by yeasts

Yeasts have been a favourite experimental subject in the research on basic metabolic pathways discussed above. The conversion of glucose to ethanol was formulated in 1815 by Guy-Lussac in its present form:

$$C_6H_{12}O_6 \rightarrow 2\,CO_2 + 2\,C_2H_5OH$$

The normal fermentation of glucose by yeast.   The fermentation of glucose to ethanol and carbon dioxide by yeast (*Saccharomyces cerevisiae*) proceeds via the fructose-bisphosphate pathway. The conversion of pyruvate to ethanol then comprises two steps. In the first, pyruvate is decarboxylated by pyruvate decarboxylase (1), with the participation of thiamine pyrophosphate, to acetaldehyde; this is then reduced to ethanol by alcohol dehydrogenase with $NADH_2$ as the hydrogen donor (2).

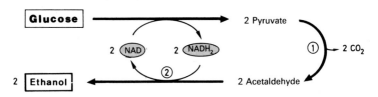

In this hydrogen transfer, the hydrogen obtained during the dehydrogenation of triose-phosphate is utilised; the oxidation–reduction balance is therefore maintained.

History of the elucidation of yeast fermentation.   The early dispute over whether alcohol formation from sugar is due to chemical contact catalysis or requires the activities of living organisms, which seems strange now, will not be discussed here. The argument about the causation of fermentation was finally settled by Louis Pasteur. He also showed that yeast can produce 20 times more cell material from a given amount of sugar under aerobic conditions than under anaerobiosis. The demonstration that in the presence of oxygen, fermentation is inhibited, the **Pasteur effect**, has become a model example of **metabolic regulation**.

In 1896–7, Buchner and Hahn observed that an extract, obtained from pressed brewer's yeast by grinding with kieselguhr and sand, frothed after the addition of sugar. This was, in fact, the first example of a complex biochemical process occurring *in vitro* i.e. in the absence of whole cells. Harden and Young (1906) made the discovery that inorganic phosphate is a requirement for the fermentation of glucose by yeast extract and is incorporated in fructose-1,6-bisphosphate. Yeast extract ferments glucose according to the Harden–Young equation:

$$2\,C_6H_{12}O_6 + 2\,P_i \rightarrow 2\,CO_2 + 2\,C_2H_5OH + H_2O$$
$$+ \text{fructose-1,6-bisphosphate}$$

Neuberg's fermentation formulae.   The methods and discoveries of C. Neuberg are of both historical and general importance. He demonstrated that pyruvate as well as glucose could be fermented by yeast. The intermediary formation of acetaldehyde could be demonstrated by trapping the acetaldehyde with hydrogen sulphite, which is practically non-toxic for yeast. On addition of hydrogen sulphite to glucose-fermenting yeast, acetaldehyde is precipitated as the addition product:

$$CH_3CHO + NaHSO_3 \rightarrow CH_2\text{–}CHOH\text{–}SO_3Na$$

Under these conditions, glycerol is formed as a new fermentation product, whilst the yield of ethanol and carbon dioxide is diminished. Fermentation in the presence of hydrogen sulphite has been exploited industrially for the production of glycerol. By trapping the acetaldehyde in this way, it cannot function as a hydrogen acceptor. In place of acetaldehyde, dihydroxyacetone phosphate becomes the hydrogen acceptor and is thus reduced to glycerol-3-phosphate, which is dephosphorylated to glycerol. The equation for this fermentation is as follows:

glucose + hydrogen sulphite $\rightarrow$ glycerol

+ acetaldehyde–sulphite + CO_2

This modified yeast fermentation has become known as **Neuberg's second fermentation**. The principle of trapping a metabolite in a pathway has become known as 'the trapping method' and became more generally used in biochemistry.

The addition of alkali ($NaHCO_3$, Na_2HPO_4) to fermenting yeast extracts also leads to the formation of glycerol because acetaldehyde undergoes dismutation to ethanol and acetate and hence does not function as a hydrogen acceptor. The equation for this fermentation is known as Neuberg's third fermentation:

2 glucose + H_2O $\rightarrow$ ethanol + acetate + 2 glycerol + 2 CO_2

The normal yeast fermentation has been designated as **Neuberg's first fermentation**. He assumed that the 2-oxopropanol (methylglyoxal, CH_3–CO–CHO) produced by the non-biological splitting of glucose was also an intermediary product of glucose fermentation.

The relationship of yeast to oxygen.   Glucose fermentation by yeast is an anaerobic process, but yeasts are aerobes. Under anaerobic conditions, yeast ferments very actively, but hardly grows. On admission of air, fermentation decreases in favour of respiration. In some yeasts, fermentation can be completely suppressed by vigorous aeration (**Pasteur effect**). Pasteur discovered this effect more than 100 years ago during investigations on fermentation processes in wine making. This effect, however, is not restricted to yeasts but is a general property of all facultatively anaerobic cells, including those of higher animals.

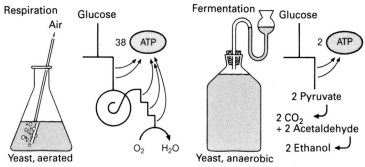

The balance sheet for glucose catabolism in a representative experiment with yeast is shown in Table 8.1. While supporting growth, aeration causes a decline in glucose consumption and in the production of

Table 8.1. *Balance of glucose consumption during anaerobic and aerobic incubation of yeast (at 25 °C) ± 0.4 mmol 2,4-dinitrophenol (DNP)/l*[a]

Incubation	Anaerobic	Aerobic	Aerobic + DNP
Glucose consumption	– 3.085	– 1.950	– 3.020
by fermentation	– 1.945	– 0.343	– 1.387
by respiration	–	– 0.356	– 0.556
Glucose catabolism	– 1.945	– 0.699	– 1.943
Assimilation	– 1.145	– 1.251	– 1.077

[a] The figures give the glucose consumption per unit time.

ethanol and carbon dioxide. These observations make sense from an energetic point of view and suggest an extraordinarily ingenious regulatory mechanism: anaerobically, one mol glucose yields only 2 mol ATP, in contrast to 38 mol ATP obtainable per mol glucose from respiration. The cell thus adapts, by regulation of substrate consumption, to the energy gain obtainable under the two conditions. The third column of Table 8.1 shows the results of an experiment in which the yeast was incubated aerobically in the presence of 0.4 mM of 2,4-dinitrophenol (DNP). DNP is an 'uncoupler' of respiratory chain phosphorylation; it abolishes the tight coupling of electron transport to oxidative phosphorylation and allows respiration to proceed without control by phosphorylation. Since the addition of DNP practically abolishes respiratory chain phosphorylation, the hydrogens obtained in the tricarboxylic acid cycle remain energetically unused. Only the energy-rich phosphate obtained from the cleavage of succinyl-CoA can be utilised. The result of this experiment, namely the increase in glucose consumption to the amount obtained under anaerobic conditions, is consistent with the uncoupling action of DNP.

The Pasteur effect seems to involve several **regulatory mechanisms** working together. One of these applies at the level of phosphorylation and can be explained by competition for ADP and P_i. The dehydrogenation step in the catabolism of glyceraldehyde phosphate requires phosphate and ADP:

$$glyceraldehyde\text{-}3\text{-}phosphate + NAD + ADP + P_i \rightarrow$$

$$3\text{-}phosphoglycerate + NADH_2 + ATP$$

Degradation of the substrate (glucose) via the FBP pathway is thus dependent on ADP and phosphate; without these, no dehydrogenation of glyceraldehyde-3-phosphate can take place. Under aerobic conditions, the ADP and phosphate are competed for by respiratory chain phosphorylations, which also leads to the synthesis of ATP. It seems plausible that the consumption of glucose, as well as the production of ethanol, is reduced by decreases in the intracellular concentrations of ADP and P_i. When respiratory chain phosphorylation is uncoupled by DNP, ADP and phosphate become available for the dehydrogenation of glyceraldehyde-3-phosphate, the aerobic glucose consumption increases to the level of the anaerobic (Table 8.1).

A second regulatory mechanism is also responsible for the Pasteur effect: the enzyme phosphofructokinase is allosterically inhibited by ATP. This inhibition by adenylate will be further discussed in the section on 'phosphofructokinase and the Pasteur effect' (Ch. 16.2.2).

Explanation of the fermentation balance according to Harden and Young. Glucose is metabolised by yeast extracts according to the Harden–Young fermentation balance. The accumulation of fructose-1,6-bisphosphate is due to lack of ATP utilisation for energy-requiring reactions in the cell-free system (in contrast to living systems), so that an excess of ATP is maintained. The yeast extract contains no phosphatase activity, so that ADP must be constantly regenerated by phosphorylation of excess glucose and/or fructose-6-phosphate.

Uses of yeast. Yeasts serve many purposes. The selection of the most appropriate species, strains, and varieties for specific purposes, from the multiplicity available, has been going on for a long time. Weakly respiring, largely fermenting yeast, so-called '**bottom yeasts**' are used in the brewing of beer. The yeasts used for ethanol production and wine-making, as well as baker's yeasts, are largely '**top yeasts**'.

Baker's yeast (*Saccharomyces cerevisiae*) is used to produce carbon dioxide to 'raise' the dough, and it must therefore be a good fermenter. It is grown in tanks with good aeration. Ethanol is always produced as a by-product, but the relative yields of yeast to alcohol can be varied by variation in aeration and glucose concentrations. In one process, sugar is supplied continuously at a rate that limits the growth rate. In this way, the appearance of fermentation products is avoided and all the sugar is used for growth. Additional nutrients (e.g. nitrogen sources) for the growing yeast are supplied by wheat-mash.

Brewer's yeasts are mostly 'bottom yeasts' (Munich, Pilsner) and are more rarely 'top yeasts' (ale, light ale, Berliner). In central Europe, beer is mostly brewed from barley; the starting material is selected from brewing barleys with a low protein content and high starch concentration. Since yeast does not contain amylase and cannot ferment starch, but only sugar, the barley starch must first be convered to sugar. This amylosis is carried out by the barley-specific amylase which is formed during seed germination. The barley grains are therefore first allowed to swell and start germinating. The 'green malt' resulting from this is dried at a certain temperature which inhibits only the germination process but does not inactivate the enzymes. The dried malt is ground and suspended in water. At medium temperatures, the starch is hydrolysed to maltose, producing wort. This is freed of spelt, hops are added, and the brew is boiled, cooled, and finally fermented by precultivated yeast in brewing casks.

For the production of **industrial alcohol** the residue of cane-sugar refining (molasses) or potatoes are used. Much alcohol can be obtained from hydrolysed wood chips or sulphite lyes from paper mills. Among the sugars found in wood, only hexoses can be fermented to ethanol; the pentoses are used in a subsequent process as the carbon source for other yeasts (*Endomyces lactis* and *Torula* species), which are then used as protein-rich cattle feed.

Many German wines are produced by spontaneous fermentation of grape juice by the yeast *Kloeckera*. To suppress the uncontrolled fermentation of wild yeasts, pure cultures of yeasts or mixtures of *Kloeckera* and *Saccharomyces* from specific vineyards are often added. The aroma and flavour of wine, however, is more dependent on the kind of grape (Riesling, Sylvaner, etc.) and the climatic and edaphic (soil) factors under which the grapes were grown, than on the kind of yeast used.

All yeast fermentation liquids contain fusel oils; propanol, 2-butanediol, 2-methylpropanol, amyl alcohol (pentanol), isoamyl alcohol (3-methylbutanol). These are products of the normal fermentative metabolism of yeasts, and their occurrence is not restricted to complex, amino acid-containing nutrient media. The main components of fusel oil are subsidary products of the metabolism of isoleucine, leucine, and valine.

8.1.2   Ethanol formation by bacteria

The pathway of ethanol formation known in yeasts (fructose-bisophosphate pathway and pyruvate decarboxylase) is utilised only by *Sarcina ventriculi* among all the bacteria so far examined. A rod-shaped, polarly flagellated, motile bacterium that produces ethanol has been isolated from 'pulque', the fermenting juice of the agave (*Agave americana*), in Mexico. This bacterium, *Zymomonas mobilis*, metabolises glucose via the 2-keto-3-deoxy-6-phosphogluconate pathway and splits pyruvate by pyruvate decarboxylase to acetaldehyde and carbon dioxide. Acetaldehyde is then reduced to ethanol. Ethanol, carbon dioxide, and small amounts of lactic acid are the only fermentation products. It is noteworthy that carbon atoms 2, 3, 5 and 6 of the glucose end up in the agave spirit, whereas yeast alcohol contains the carbon atoms 1, 2, 5 and 6 of glucose (Fig. 8.1).

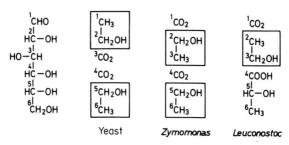

Fig. 8.1. *Origin of the carbon atoms of ethanol from the carbon skeleton of glucose in fermentation.*

Ethanol occurs as a subsidiary fermentation product in the fermentations of some Enterobacteriaceae and clostridia. The precursor of ethanol, i.e. acetaldehyde, however, is not produced by pyruvate decarboxylase directly from pyruvate, but arises via reduction of acetyl-CoA.

The heterofermentative lactic acid bacteria (e.g. *Leuconostoc mesenteroides*) produce alcohol by a completely different pathway. Glucose is first metabolised by the initial steps in the pentose-phosphate cycle to pentose-phosphate. The xylulose-5-phosphate is then attacked by phosphoketolase:

xylulose-5-phosphate + P_i → acetylphosphate

+ glyceraldehyde-3-phosphate

The acetylphosphate thus formed is reduced to ethanol by acetaldehyde dehydrogenase and alcohol dehydrogenase. The other cleavage product, glyceraldehyde-3-phosphate, is converted to pyruvate and reduced to lactate.

8.2   Lactic acid fermentation and Lactobacteriaceae

The lactic acid bacteria are collectively assigned to the family Lactobacteriaceae. Whilst this group appears rather heterogeneous morphologically and includes long and short rods as well as cocci of the stretpococcus type, it is very well characterised physiologically. All its members are gram-positive, do not form spores (with the exception of *Sporolactobacillus inulinus*), and are (with some exceptions) non-motile. They are all dependent on carbohydrates for their energy supply and excrete lactic acid. In contrast to the Enterobacteriaceae, which also produce lactic acid, they are obligate fermenters. They do not contain haemins (cytochromes, catalase). In spite of this, the Lactobacteriaceae, especially the streptococci, are able to grow in the presence of air or oxygen. They are anaerobic but **aerotolerant**; an aerobically growing bacterium that lacks catalase is in all probability a lactic acid bacterium.

Accessory factor requirements for growth.   A further characteristic of lactobacteria is their requirement for accessory factors. No member of this group can grow on a purely mineral salts medium with glucose and ammonium salts. Most require a number of vitamins (lactoflavin, thiamine, pantothenic acid, nicotinic acid, folic acid, biotin), amino acids, purines, and pyrimidines. They are therefore mostly cultivated on complex media that contain relatively large amounts of yeast extract, tomato extract, whey, or even blood. Quite surprisingly, it was recently discovered that some lactic acid bacteria (and other fermenters) can form cytochromes during growth on blood-containing media and may even be able to carry out respiratory chain phosphorylation. The lactic acid bacteria evidently lack the ability to synthesise porphyrins; when these are included in the nutrient medium, some lactic acid bacteria can form the appropriate haem pigments. The Lactobacteriaceae may thus be regarded as metabolic cripples that have lost the capacity to synthesise a number of metabolites, probably as a consequence of their specialisation for growth on milk and other media that are rich in nutrients and accessory factors. On the other hand, they have an ability that most microorganisms lack; the can utilise lactose. This ability is shared by a number of intestinal bacteria of the coliform type, as part of the Enterobacteriaceae. Lactose apparently does not occur in the plant kingdom; it is produced by mammals and is excreted and ingested in milk. The utilisation of lactose by microorganisms can be regarded therefore as an adaptation to the ecological conditions in the mammalian digestive tract. Lactose is a disaccharide that must be hydrolysed before it can enter the catabolic pathway for hexoses.

$$\text{lactose} + H_2O \xrightarrow{\ \beta\text{-galactosidase}\ } \text{D-glucose} + \text{D-galactose}$$

The enzyme β-galactosidase occurs in only a few bacteria. The hydrolysis product, galactose, after phosphorylation by a specific galactokinase is isomerised to glucose-l-phosphate. Galactose is also a component, as a galactolipid, of the thylakoid membrane in chloroplasts.

Because of the large amounts of lactate produced, the media must be well buffered. Usually calcium carbonate is added. On nutrient agar to which a suspension of calcium carbonate has been added (chalk agar), the production of lactic acid can be visualised as transparent zones around the colonies.

Occurrence and habitat.   The distribution of the lactic acid bacteria in nature is related to their high demand for nutrients and their type of energy generation (purely by fermentation). They are hardly ever found in soil or water. Their natural habits are:

(1) milk and the places where milk is produced and processed (*Lactobacillus lactis, L. bulgaricus, L. helveticus, L. casei, L. fermentum, L. brevis, Lactococcus lactis, L. diacetilactis*);

(2) intact and rotting plants (*Lactobacillus plantarum, L. delbruäckii, L. fermentum, L. brevis, Lactococcus lactis, Leuconostoc mesenteroides*);

(3) intestinal tracts and mucous membranes of animals and humans (*Lactobacillus acidophilus, Bifidobacterium, Enterococcus faecalis, Streptococcus salivarius, S. bovis, S. pyogenes, S. pneumoniae*).

Enterococcus faecalis is a normal inhabitant of human intestines, *S. bovis* occurs in ruminants, and many streptococci are harmless commensals on mucous membranes of the oral cavity and the respiratory, urinary, and genital organs. They belong to the so-called skin flora. Their presence prevents the colonisation of the skin by other, possibly pathogenic, microorganisms. When the growth of the skin flora is inhibited, for example by intensive antibiotic treatment, epithelial membranes often become infected with pathogenic dermatophites, such as *Candida albicans*. There is some reason therefore, to avoid excessive bathing with detergent-containing preparations.

Because of their production of large amounts of lactic acid and their acid tolerance, the lactic acid bacteria can easily become dominant under appropriate environmental conditions. They are therefore easy to isolate by enrichment culture in selective media. 'Natural pure cultures' occur in sour milk, certain milk products, sourdough, sauerkraut, silage, and a number of similar locations.

Carbohydrate metabolism and fermentation products.   The Lactobacteriaceae are classified according to their ability to ferment glucose solely to lactate or to additional products, i.e. as homofermentative or heterofermentative (Table 8.2). This long-standing division is consistent with the basically different catabolic pathways for sugars.

Homofermentative lactate fermentation.   Homofermentative lactobacteria produce pure or almost pure (90%) lactate. They metabolise glucose via the fructose-bisphosphate pathway, since they have all the necessary enzymes, including aldolase, and use the hydrogen obtained from the dehydrogenation of glyceraldehyde-3-phosphate (to 1,3-bisphosphoglycerate) to reduce pyruvate to lactate.

Table 8.2. *Lactic acid bacteria arranged according to shape (rods or cocci) and type of fermentation*

Cocci	Rods
Homofermentative: $C_6H_{12}O_6 \rightarrow 2CH_3\text{–CHOH–COOH}$	
Streptococci	*Lactobacilli*
Lactococcus lactis subsp. *lactis*	Thermobacteria (temp. opt. 40 °C,
Lactococcus lactis subsp. *lactis*	do not grow at 15 °C)
var. *diacetilactis*	*Lactobacillus delbrueckii*
Lactococcus lactis	subsp. *delbrueckii*
subsp. *cremoris*	*Lactobacillus delbrueckii*
Enterococcus faecalis	subsp. *lactis*
Streptococcus salivarius	*Lactobacillus delbrueckii*
subsp. *salivarius*	subsp. *bulgaricus*
Streptococcus salivarius	*Lactobacillus helveticus*
subsp. *thermophilus*	*Lactobacillus acidophilus*
Streptococcus pyogenes	*Lactobacillus salivarius*
	Streptobacteria (temp. opt. 30–37 °C,
	always grow at 15 °C)
	Lactobacillus casei
	Lactobacillus alimentaris
	Lactobacillus coryniformis
	Lactobacillus plantarum
Heterofermentative: $C_6H12O_6 \rightarrow CH_3\text{–CHOH–COOH} + CH_3\text{–CH}_2OH$ $+ CO_2$ (or $CH_3\text{–COOH}$)	
Streptococci	Lactobacilli
Leuconostoc mesenteroides	*Lactobacillus bifermentans*
subsp. *mesenteroides*	*Lactobacillus brevis*
Leuconostoc mesenteroides	*Lactobacillus fermentum*
subsp. *dextranicum*	*Lactobacillus kandleri*
Leuconostoc mesenteroides	*Lactobacillus viredescens*
subsp. *cremoris*	
Leuconostoc lactis	

This table shows the presently valid names of the lactic acid bacteria. The more common, shortened names have been used in the text.

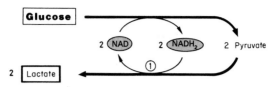

The stereospecificity of the lactate dehydrogenase and the presence or absence of a lactate racemase determines whether D(−)-, L(+)-, or DL-lactate is formed. Only a small proportion of the pyruvate is decarboxylated and converted to acetate, ethanol, carbon dioxide, or perhaps acetoin. The extent to which subsidary products are formed is dependent on the supply of oxygen.

Heterofermentative lactate fermentation.   The heterofermentative lactic acid bacteria lack the important enzymes of the fructose-bisphosphate pathway, aldolase and triose-phosphate isomerase. The initial degradation of glucose, therefore, is entirely by the pentose-phosphate pathway, that is via glucose-6-phosphate, 6-phosphogluconate, and ribulose-5-phosphate (Figs 7.4, 8.2). The latter is converted to xylulose-5-phosphate by an epimerase. This is followed by cleavage in a thiamine pyrophosphate-dependent reaction catalysed by phosphoketolase with the formation of glyceraldehyde-3-phosphate and acetylphosphate.

Washed suspensions of non-growing *Leuconostoc mesenteroides* ferment glucose almost stoichiometrically according to the equation:

$$C_6H_{12}O_6 \rightarrow CH_3–CHOH–COOH + CH_3–CH_2OH + CO_2$$

to yield lactate, ethanol, and carbon dioxide. They thus reduce the acetylphosphate via acetyl-CoA and acetaldehyde to ethanol (Fig. 8.2).

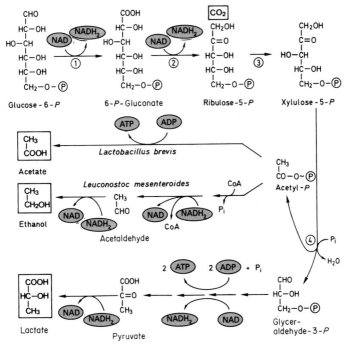

Fig. 8.2. *The heterofermentative lactic acid fermentation by* Lactobacillus brevis *and* Leuconostoc mesenteroides.

Enzymes:(!) glucose-6-phosphate dehydrogenase; (2) phosphogluconate dehydrogenase; (3) epimerase; (4) phosphoketolase. Acetylphosphate is either converted to acetate by acetate kinase with phosphorylation of ADP (*L. brevis*) or reduced to ethanol (*L. mesenteroides*). Oxidation of glyceraldehyde phosphate is by the usual fructose-bisphosphate pathway.

Other heterofermentative bacteria convert the acetylphosphate, either partially or completely, to acetate, transferring the energy-rich phosphate bond to ADP and thus gaining utilisable energy as ATP. In this case, the excess of hydrogen is transferred to glucose to give mannitol. The glyceraldehyde-3-phosphate is converted to lactate via pyruvate. *Leuconostoc mesenteroides* ferments ribose to lactate and acetate.

The heterofermentative bacteria ferment fructose with the formation of lactate, acetate, carbon dioxide and mannitol:

$$3 \text{ fructose} \rightarrow \text{lactate} + \text{acetate} + CO_2 + 2 \text{ mannitol}$$

The fructose here functions as the acceptor for excess reducing equivalents:

$$fructose + NADH_2 \rightarrow mannitol + NAD$$

Lactobacillus plantarum (synonyms: *pentosus* or *arabinosus*) metabolises glucose homofermentatively but splits pentoses by phosphoketolase to lactate and acetate. It should be pointed out here that even such a profoundly homofermentative bacterium as *Lactobacillus casei*, whilst homofermentative on glucose, metabolises ribose heterofermentatively to acetate and lactate. The presence of the ribose induces the formation of phosphoketolase. Cells that have been grown on ribose and then tested in washed suspensions actually degrade glucose heterofermentatively.

Fermentation by *Bifidobacterium*. The heterofermentative lactic acid bacterium *Bifidobacterium bifidum* takes its name from the V- or Y-shape of its cells (Latin *bifidus*, divided into two). It has become very well known because it is dominant in the intestinal tract of babies, especially those that are breast fed. This dependence of their distribution on the nutrition of babies could be traced to the high requirement of this bacterium for sugars that contain *N*-acetylglucosamine, which is found only in human milk and not in cow's milk. The members of the genus *Bifidobacterium* are strict anaerobes; they are not aerotolerant and require an atmosphere containing 10% carbon dioxide for growth. Since this requirement, which is unusual for lactic acid bacteria, was discovered, *Bifidobacterium* has also been found in the intestinal flora of adults, in several other locations, and even in putrefying mud. Several species are now distinguished.

Bifidobacterium metabolises glucose according to the equation:

$$2 C_6H_{12}O_6 \rightarrow 2 CH_3-CHOH-COOH + 3 CH_3COOH$$

The glucose is fermented via the phosphoketolase bypass. The organism possesses neither aldolase nor glucose-6-phosphate dehydrogenase but contains active phosphoketolases that split fructose-6-phosphate and xylulose-5-phosphate to acetylphosphate and erythrose-4-phosphate or glyceraldehyde-3-phosphate, respectively. Hexose is metabolised according to the following diagram.

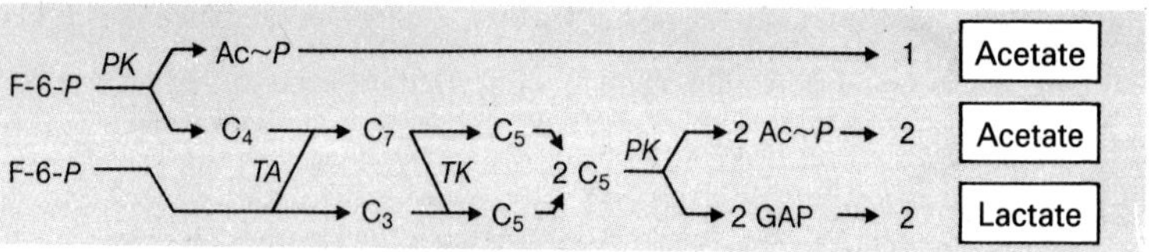

PK, phosphoketolase; TA, transaldolase; TK, transketolase; Ac~P, acetylphosphate; GAP, glyceraldehyde-3-phosphate.

Use of lactic acid bacteria in domestic and agricultural processes and in food production.   If non-sterile solutions containing sugars, complex nitrogen sources, and accessory factors are left under anaerobic conditions (or in solutions of such depth that the deeper layers are virtually anaerobic), they will soon become overgrown with lactic acid bacteria. These lower the pH to below 5 and thereby suppress the growth of other anaerobic bacteria, which are less acid tolerant. The actual type(s) of lactic acid bacteria that become dominant in such enrichment cultures depends on specific conditions. This sterilising and preserving effect of the lactic acid bacteria, due to their acid production, has led to their use in agriculture, dairying, milk-utilising industries, and domestic practice.

Silage production.   The lactic acid bacteria found on plant materials play a large part in the conservation of cattle foods. The leaves of sugar beet, potatoes, maize, grass, or lucerne are compacted in silos. Molasses is added to increase the carbon/nitrogen ratio, and formic or mineral acid is added to favour the initial growth of the acid-tolerant lactobacilli and streptococci. This leads to a controlled lactic fermentation.

> Sauerkraut is also produced by a lactic acid fermentation. Cut-up cabbage, compacted with the addition of 2–3% NaCl to produce anaerobic conditions, develops spontaneous lactic acid fermentation, at first by *Leuconostoc*, with evolution of carbon dioxide, and later, by *Lactobacillus plantarum* also.

Milk products.   Lactic acid bacteria are of decisive importance as acid and flavour producers in the dairy industry. The starting material usually consists of sterilised, or partially sterilised, milk or cream to which pure cultures are added as 'starter cultures'. A 'sour cream' butter is made from cream that is acidified by addition of *Lactococcus lactis, L. cremoris* and *Leuconostoc cremoris* and gains it special aroma from the formation of diacetyl (see Section 8.4).

Starter cultures containing *Lactococcus lactis* or *Lactobacillus bulgaricus* and *S. thermophilus* are used for the coagulation of casein in the production of curd cheeses and for certain German cheeses (Harzer, Mainzer). In contrast to these 'sour milk' cheeses, the production of hard cheeses involves precipitation of the casein by rennin; the lactic acid bacteria (*Lactobacillus casei, Lactococcus lactis*) and propionibacteria are only involved in their maturation.

> A specially aromatic buttermilk is made by the addition of the same organisms described above for the production of 'sour cream' butter. It contains, besides lactic acid and acetic acid, acetoin and diacetyl. Yoghurt consists of pasteurised, homogenised whole milk that is inoculated with *Streptococcus thermophilus* and *Lactobacillus bulgaricus* and incubated for

a short time (2–3 hours) at 43–45 °C. The name Bioghurt refers to a commercial sour milk product made by acidification with *Lactobacillus acidophilus* and *Streptococcus thermophilus*. Kefir is a milk that contains acid and ethanol. The milk (from cows, sheep or goats) is inoculated with 'kefir grains' which are partially characterised symbiotic associations of lactobacilli, streptococci, micrococci and yeasts. Acidification occurs at 15–22 °C and takes 24–36 hours. Kumiss is made from donkey milk that is inoculated with a culture containing *Lactobacillus bulgaricus* and a *Torula* yeast.

Pure lactic acid, which is used for various industrial purposes and as a food additive, is also produced by fermentation. Milk or whey is fermented by *Lactobacillus casei* and *L. bulgaricus*. For the fermentation of glucose or maltose, *Lactobacillus delbrueckii, L. leichmanii* or *Sporolactobacillus imulinus* are used. Molasses or malt are added to furnish the necessary accessory nutrients.

The acidification in sourdough, which is used for the production of some European and other types of ryebread, is also caused by lactic acid bacteria, especially *Lactobacillus plantarum* and *L. coryniformis*.

Starter cultures of lactobacilli and micrococci are also used in the production of certain sausages (salami, cervelat, etc.). The production of lactic acid and lowering of the pH by the bacteria contribute to the preservation of these types of sausages, which remain uncooked.

8.3   Propionic acid fermentation and propionibacteria

Occurrence, distribution, isolation, and systematic classification.   Propionibacteria are rumen and intestinal bacteria of ruminants (cattle, sheep), where they play a part in the formation of fatty acids, especially propionic and acetic acids, in the rumen. They are responsible for the conversion of lactate, which arises from various fermentations in the rumen, to predominantly propionate. They rarely occur in milk, nor can they be isolated from soil or water. Propionibacteria can be isolated by enrichment culture under anaerobic conditions in a lactate–yeast extract medium, inoculated with Swiss cheese. They occur in Swiss cheese, where they play an important part in maturation and flavour formation by virtue of the addition of rennin used in the early stages of the process to coagulate the milk. Rennin is an aqueous extract of calves' stomach and contains numerous viable propionibacteria. Several species are distinguished, of which *Propionibacterium freudenreichii* and its subspecies *shermanii*, as well as *P. acidi-propionici* (formerly called *P. pentosaceum*), are the best known. Another propionibacterium, *P. acnes*, is the causative organism of acne, an inflammation of the hair follicles in human skin. Apart from the genus *Propionibacterium*, the propionate forming bacteria also include *Veillonella alcalescens* (*Micrococcus lactilyticus*), *Clostridium propionicum*,

Selenomonas, and *Micromonospora*. Many other bacteria also excrete some propionate as end product of fermentation.

Growth and metabolism of the genus *Propionibacterium*.   The genus *Propionibacterium* is assigned to the coryneform bacteria (see Chapter 3). The species of this genus are gram-positive, non-motile rods that do not form spores. Club-shaped forms are often found under unfavourable conditions. Propionibacteria do not grow on solid media exposed to air. Because of this intolerance to atmospheric oxygen and their ability to grow and regenerate ATP by anaerobic fermentation, the propionibacteria were long regarded as obligatory fermenters. It has been known for some time, however, that they possess haem enzymes like cytochromes and catalase. In fact, all members of the genus *Propionibacterium* that have been examined for this were actually able to grow aerobically as well as anaerobically. Under conditions of controlled aeration, the cell yield was actually higher than anaerobically. However, during such aerobic growth, the diffusion rate of oxygen from the gas phase into the bacterial suspension must not exceed the respiration rate; measurable partial pressures of oxygen in the culture are toxic. *Propionibacterium* species should therefore be regarded as **microaerotolerant**. Under anaerobic conditions, members of the genus *Propionibacterium* ferment glucose, sucrose, lactose, and pentoses, as well as lactate, malate, glycerol, and other substrates to propionic acid. The catabolism of hexoses proceeds via the fructose-bisphosphate pathway.

In 1936, Wood and Werkman, in a study of glycerol fermentation by *Propionibacterium acidi-propionici*, discovered that this involved the net fixation of carbon dioxide. The fixed CO_2 was found in the excreted succinate; carboxylation of pyruvate with the formation of dicarboxylic acid had taken place. This carboxylation was called the Wood–Werkman reaction. It is not restricted to propionibacteria, but occurs in animals and plants and in all heterotrophic organisms. The biochemical reactions involved have already been discussed in the section on gluconeogenesis (Ch. 7.5).

Biochemistry of propionic acid formation (the methylmalonyl-CoA pathway).   The formation of propionate from lactate occurs according to the overall equation:

$$3\,CH_3\text{–}CHOH\text{–}COOH \rightarrow 2\,CH_3\text{–}CH_2\text{–}COOH$$
$$+ \, CH_3\text{–}COOH + CO_2 + H_2O$$

reduction of lactate or pyruvate to propionate follows a route called the methylmalonyl-CoA pathway because of its characteristic intermediary

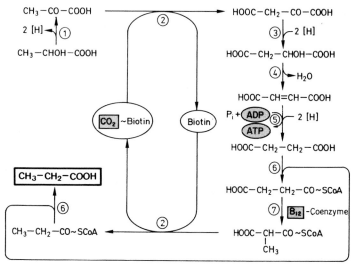

CoA-Transferase

Fig. 8.3. *Methylmalonyl-CoA pathway of propionate formation.*

Enzymes: (1) lactate dehydrogenase; (2) methylmalonyl-CoA carboxytransferase; (3) malate dehydrogenase; (4) fumarase; (5) fumarate reductase (leading to regeneration of ATP by proton translocation); (6) CoA transferase; (7) methylmalonyl-CoA mutase.

product (Fig. 8.3). Pyruvate is carboxylated to oxalocetate by methylmalonyl-CoA carboxytransferase with the participation of a biotin–carbon dioxide complex, and the oxaloacetate is then reduced via malate and fumarate to succinate. The latter step is coupled to an electron transport phosphorylation (see fumarate respiration, Ch. 9.6). The succinate is first activated by the formation of succinyl-CoA by a CoA transferase (succinyl-CoA:propionate-CoA transferase) and the succinyl-CoA is then converted to methylmalonyl-CoA by methyl-malonyl-CoA mutase with the participation of coenzyme B_{12} (cyanocobalamin). It is this intermediate which loses carbon dioxide to yield propionyl-CoA, whilst the methylmalonyl-CoA carboxytransferase mentioned above acquires the CO_2. Propionate is liberated from propionyl-CoA by the CoA transferase, which transfers the CoA to succinate. It should be noted that in this process of propionate formation, two groups (CO_2 and CoA) are transferred back from product to precursor without occurring in the free form. Another noteworthy feature is the participation of three cofactors (biotin, coenzyme A, and coenzyme B_{12}). Most of the propionibacteria form propionate by this methylmalonyl-CoA pathway, which is also used by *Veillonella alcalescens* and *Selenomonas ruminantium*.

The methylmalonyl-CoA pathway is reversible and is also used in the opposite direction, for instance during metabolism of isoleucine, valine, and odd-numbered long-chain fatty acids. The fatty acids and isoleucine yield popionyl-CoA, which is then carboxylated to methylmalonyl-CoA. The conversion of this to succinyl-CoA by methylmalonyl-CoA mutase is dependent on vitamin B_{12} (coenzyme B_{12}), even in root nodules, in rhizobia, and in animal tissues.

The acryloyl-CoA pathway. The formation of propionic acid by *Clostridium propionicum, Bacteroides ruminicola* and *Megasphaera elsdenii* occurs by a simpler route. The CoA derivative of acrylic acid, acryloyl-CoA, is the intermediate:

$$CH_3-CHOH-CO\sim SCoA \xrightarrow[H_2O]{} CH_2{=}CH-CO\sim SCoA \xrightarrow[2\,[H]]{} CH_3-CH_2-CO\sim SCoA$$

Lactyl-CoA   Acryloyl-CoA   Propionyl-CoA

8.4 Formic acid fermentation and Enterobacteriaceae

Some acid-producing fermentative organisms are collected in a physiological grouping for which formic acid is a characteristic fermentation product, though not necessarily the main one. Several other acids also occur as fermentation end products. This type of fermentation is therefore known as '**formic acid fermentation**' or as '**mixed acid fermentation**'. Since several representatives of this group are inhabitants of the intestinal tract (Greek *enteron*, intestine), the family has been named **Enterobacteriaceae**. The following familial characteristics can be enumerated: gram-negative, peritrichously flagellated, highly motile, nonsporing rods. They are facultatively aerobic, possess haemins (cytochromes and catalase), and can obtain their energy aerobically (by respiration) and anaerobically (by fermentation). They are nutritionally non-demanding and can grow on simple synthetic media containing mineral salts, carbohydrate and ammonium salts. They all ferment glucose with the formation of acids. The importance of the Enterobacteriaceae for sanitation and hygiene and for experimental research calls for a detailed account of some representatives.

Table 8.3. *Diagnostic characters for genera within the Enterobacteriaceae*

Genus	Moti-lity	Urea utili-sation	Glucose fermen-tation	Lactose fermen-tation	H_2 for-mation	Indole forma-tion	Acetoin forma-tion	Proteo-lysis
Escherichia	+	−	+	+	+	+	−	−
Klebsiella	−	+	+	+	+	−	+	−
Enterobacter	+	(+)	+	+	+	−	+	(+)
Serratia	+	−	+	−	+	−	+	+
Proteus	+	+	+	−	+	+	−	+
Citrobacter	+	(+)	+	+	(+)	+	−	−
Salmonella	+	−	+	−	+	−	−	−
Shigella	−	−	+	−	−	+	−	−
Erwinia	+	−	+	(+)	−	−	(+)	(+)

+ indicates that most of the species are positive.

Table 8.4. *The IMViC reactions for distinguishing* Escherichia coli *and* Enterobacter aerogenes

	Indole formation	Methyl red test	Acetoin formation	Citrate utilisation
Escherichia coli	+	+	−	−
Enterobacter aerogenes	−	−	+	+

Important species.   *Escherichia coli* is an intestinal inhabitant. It is not by any means the most important numerically, being exceeded in numbers by *Bacteroides* and *Bifidobacterium*. *E. coli*, however, can survive for a time outside the intestinal tract and is easily demonstrated. It is therefore very suitable for tracing faecal contamination of drinking water.

Proteus vulgaris also belongs to the normal intestinal flora but is also widely distributed in soils and water. This organism is known for its tendency to change shape (hence its name), its pronounced motility, and the tendency to swarm on agar plates so as to cover the whole surface (see Chapter 2).

Enterobacter aerogenes is in some ways a 'twin' of *E. coli* (both are designated as 'coliforms') and it is widely distributed in soils. As the name suggests, this organism produces much gas. It is differentiated from *E. coli* by only a few biochemical properties (Tables 8.3 and 8.4).

Serratia marcescens (formerly *Bacterium prodigiosum*) can be considered a pigment-forming variant of *Enterobacter*.

The genus *Erwinia* comprises plant-pathogenic species that attack leaves, stems, and roots and cause soft-rot by virtue of pectinase excretion.

Klebsiella pneumoniae is distinguished from *Enterobacter* only by formation of a thicker capsule and its lack of motility. It occurs in very virulent (highly lethal) forms of pneumonia.

Salmonella typhimurium is the most widely distributed of the bacteria that cause gastroenteritis, designated as 'food poisoning'. The toxic effect is due to mucous membrane inflammation produced by liberation of lipopolysaccharides; there is no invasion of the circulatory system. *S. typhi* is the causative agent of epidemic abdominal typhoid.

Shigella dysenteriae and related strains cause dysentery and diarrhoea.

Vibrio cholerae is the causative organism of cholera, an epidemic disease. It does not actually belong to the taxonomic group of Enterobacteriaceae but resembles it metabolically. *V. cholerae* proliferates in the intestinal tract. It adheres to the intestinal epithelium without penetrating into the cells. The cholera enterotoxin is a protein that is bound to specific receptors on the epithelial cells and causes the excretion of ions (sodium, bicarbonate and chloride) and water into the intestinal lumen.

Yersinia pestis is the causative agent of plague. *Yersinia* does not belong to the family Enterobacteriaceae but resembles it in its facultatively anaerobic modes of growth and its type of fermentation. The natural reservoir for this epidemic producer are wild rodents, mainly rats. The bacteria are transmitted to humans via infected fleas or other exoparasites and cause bubonic plague or pneumonic plague. These infections are rapidly lethal because of the organism's fast growth rate and intensive toxin production in the body.

Analysis of drinking water. Analysis of drinking water aims largely at the demonstration of *E. coli* and will be described in some detail as a simple example of a bacteriological differential diagnosis. *E. coli* is a normal inhabitant of human intestine and, as such, is completely harmless. Its presence in drinking water is not dangerous, though some strains are enteropathogens and cause diarrhoea. However, a number of causative agents of epidemics are also inhabitants of the human gut; these may be excreted in faeces (together with *E. coli*) by patients with acute disease or convalescents or carriers and could thus contaminate the water supply. The normal intestinal inhabitant *E. coli* is therefore used as an indicator for faecal contamination generally, to obviate needing to use special procedures for each epidemic. Demonstration of *E. coli* in water samples indicates contamination with intestinal content and bacteria, among which could be pathogens, so that protective measures should be taken. The total bacteria count in drinking water should be less than 100 cells per ml, and there should be no *E. coli* cell demonstrable in 100 ml.

E. coli grows well on glucose or lactose-peptone media. To achieve one-step selective conditions that support the growth of the least possible number of other bacteria, lactose is used. Utilisation of lactose requires the ability to hydrolyse this by β-galactosidase. Coliform bacteria and lactic acid bacteria have the ability to produce this enzyme, but most soil and water bacteria do not. The first indication of the presence of gas-producing bacteria is given by the evolution of gas during incubation of a sample on lactose-peptone medium in a fermentation tube (Einhorn tube). On separate inoculation of two such fermentation tubes, one with *E. coli* and the other with *Enterobacter aerogenes*, differences in gas production become apparent after a 24 hour incubation at 37 °C. *E. aerogenes* lives up to its name and produces about double the amount of gas produced by *E. coli*. The latter yields hydrogen and carbon dioxide in a ratio of approximately 1:1, whereas *E. aerogenes* produces more carbon dioxide than hydrogen.

Further methods of differentiation are necessary because some lactic acid bacteria can also hydrolyse lactose and produce gas, which could falsify the test results. On streaking a suitable culture onto eosin-methylene blue agar (lactose-peptone agar with eosine and methylene blue), the production of deep blue colonies with a metallic sheen signifies *E. coli*, whilst *E. aerogenes* forms only pink colonies that are mucoid but lack a metallic sheen. The two organisms can be more definitely differentiated by a complete fermentation analysis; this would undoubtedly be the most exact, but also laborious, method. A routine method for the differentiation of the two species has become established; it is based on the following qualitative differences: (1) indole formation from tryptophan; (2) the amount of acid produced from sugar (methyl red test); (3) production of acetoin during fermentation of glucose (Voges–Proskauer reaction); and (4) ability to grow on citrate as carbon source. These tests, known by the mnemonic 'IMViC' are presented in Table 8.4.

(1) Indole formation. Indole production from tryptophan is demonstrated with Ehrlich's reagent (*p*-dimethylaminobenzaldehyde), which gives a cherry-red coloration.
(2) Methyl red test. Acid formation changes the colour of the indicator from red to yellow (above) < pH 4.5.
(3) Acetoin formation (Voges–Proskauer reaction). Acetoin formed in the glucose-peptone medium reacts with the creatine in peptone under strongly alkaline conditions (by addition of 1 ml of 10% KOH to 5 ml medium) to give a red pigment. The sensitivity can be increased by addition of creatine and α-naphthol.
(4) Citrate utilisation. In a synthetic medium containing citrate (as sole carbon source), its utilisation can be monitored by appearance of turbidity and increase in pH (using bromothymol blue as indicator).

Fermentation products and metabolic pathways. Fermentations by facultatively aerobic bacteria, including the Enterobacteriaceae, many *Bacillus* species, and others, involve the formation of a large number of

Table 8.5. *Products of glucose fermentation by* Escherichia coli *and* Enterobacter aerogenes

		mol/100 mol glucose	
Products		*E. coli*	*E. aerogenes*
2,3-Butanediol	CH_3–CHOH–CHOH–CH_3	0	66.5
Ethanol	CH_3–CH_2OH	42	70
Succinate	COOH–CH_2CH_2–COOH	29	0
Lactate	CH_3–CHOH–COOH	84	3
Acetate	CH_3–COOH	44	0.5
Formate	HCOOH	2	18
Hydrogen	H_2	43	36
Carbon dioxide	CO_2	44	172

compounds among which organic acids predominate; the most important among these fermentation products are acetate, formate, succinate, lactate, ethanol, glycerol, acetoin, 2,3-butanediol, carbon dioxide and hydrogen. Hexoses are metabolised largely via the fructose-bisphosphate pathway, and to a minor extent by the pentose-phosphate route. Utilisation of gluconate is by the 2-keto-3-deoxy-6-phosphogluconate pathway.

Two types of fermentation have been characterised by the end products excreted under anaerobic conditions: (1) *E. coli* type; acids predominate and there is no formation of butanediol, and (2) *Enterobacter* type; production of acids is much less than that of the main product, butanediol. Table 8.5 shows the results of a representative fermentation analysis. The two types of fermentation differ especially in the reactions starting from pyruvate.

Characteristics of fermentation by *E. coli*. Fermentation of glucose by *E. coli* is characterised by the following reactions:

(1) conversion of pyruvate to acetyl-CoA and formate;
(2) cleavage of formate to carbon dioxide and hydrogen;
(3) reduction of acetyl-CoA to ethanol;
(4) lack of ability to produce acetoin and 2,3-butanediol from pyruvate.

The cleavage of pyruvate to acetyl-CoA and formate occurs only under anaerobic conditions. It is caused by the enzyme pyruvate:formate lyase (see oxidation of pyruvate, Ch. 7.2.4). This enzyme is very sensitive to

oxygen; it is maintained in the reduced state by flavodoxin and requires
S-adenosyl-L-methionine for activation.

Formate is split into carbon dioxide and hydrogen by most strains of
E. coli, as well as by other gas-forming species of Enterobacteriaceae.
The reaction is catalysed by an enzyme system called formate:hydrogen
lyase:

$$\text{HCOOH} \xrightarrow{\text{formate:hydrogen lyase}} H_2 + CO_2$$

This most probably involves the combined effects of a formate
dehydrogenase (HCOOH + X → CO_2 + XH_2) and a hydrogenase
(XH_2 → X + H_2). *E. coli* produces the two gaseous end products (H_2
and CO_2) in almost equal amounts and this stoichiometric ratio of 1:1 is
consistent with the formation of both gases by the splitting of formate.
However, variations in pH can alter the quantitative relationships.

Ethanol is formed by the reduction of acetyl-CoA in Enterobacteriaceae;
they do not contain pyruvate decarboxylase, which decarboxylates
pyruvate to acetaldehyde. A part of the acetyl-CoA is excreted as acetate; the energy-rich bond can be conserved by the reactions of
phosphotransacetylase and acetate kinase.

Lactate is formed by the reduction of pyruvate.

Succinate is produced by a process that is coupled to electron-transport phosphorylation, namely '**fumarate respiration**' (see Ch. 9.6). In the
first place, phosphoenolpyruvate is carboxylated to oxaloacetate, which
is then converted via malate to fumarate. The fumarate is reduced to
succinate by a membrane-bound fumarate reductase and the succinate is
excreted. The excretion of considerable amounts of succinate (see Table
8.5), whose synthesis comprises a CO_2 fixation steps, helps to explain the
fact that *E. coli* can obtain up to 20% of its cell carbon from carbon
dioxide.

Characteristics of the fermentations by *Enterobacter aerogenes*. *Enterobacter aerogenes* also produces a number of acids anaerobically. Quantitatively, however, these are eclipsed by the amounts of **acetoin** and
2,3-butanediol.

Acetoin formation starts with two molecules of pyruvate and includes
two decarboxylations. Thus, formation of the neutral fermentation product, butanediol, competes for the intermediate pyruvate, leading to a
decrease in acid formation. On the other hand, the formation of butanediol
involves additional liberation of carbon dioxide. The amount of additional CO_2 produced is stoichiometrically related to the amount of
butanediol formed. Table 8.5 shows that a part of the carbon dioxide is
derived from the splitting of formate, but by far the major part is derived from the formation of butanediol. This notably intensive gas pro-

duction has given *Enterobacter aerogenes* its name. These differences in fermentation products from those of *E. coli* form the bases for the methyl red test and the Voges–Proskauer test for acetoin.

The formation of **acetoin** by *Enterobacter* occurs via 2-acetyl-lactate. Active acetaldehyde (hydroxyethyl-thiamine pyrophosphate; see Fig. 7.6) combines with pyruvate in a reaction catalysed by acetyl-lactate synthase(enzyme I) to give 2-acetyl-lactate. A second enzyme (enzyme II) 2-acetyl-lactate decarboxylase removes carbon dioxide stereospecifically to yield acetoin.

2,3-Butanediol is produced by reduction of acetoin catalysed by the enzyme butanediol dehydrogenase:

$$CH_3-CHOH-CO-CH_3 + NADH_2 \rightarrow CH_3-CHOH-CHOH-CH_3 + NAD$$

Butanediol production via 2-acetyl-lactate is carried out not only by *Enterobacter aerogenes* but also by *Bacillus subtilis, B. polymyxa, Serratia, Aeromonas hydrophila* and some other bacteria. Butanediol fermentations have also found industrial applications.

Diacetyl, a compound related to acetoin, is easily produced by oxidation of the latter on exposure to air. It is also produced by some lactic acid bacteria (*Leuconostoc mesenteroides* subsp. *cremoris, Lactobacillus plantarum, Lactococcus lactis* var. *diacetylactis*, and to a lesser extent *Streptococcus salivarius* subsp. *thermophilus*), which are added to milk in the production of butter, yoghurt, and similar sour milk-derived foods because diacetyl is an aromatic agent, responsible for the flavour of butter, for example. These bacteria produce diacetyl from hydroxethyl-thiamine pyrophosphate and acetyl-CoA rather than via 2-acetyl-lactate.

Bioluminescence and luminous bacteria.   Bioluminescence, the ability to emit light, is widely distributed. In Europe, including Germany, the best-known is the luminous beetle, *Lampyris noctiluca*, whereas in North America *Photinus pyralis*, the firefly, is most commonly seen. In addition some beetles, crabs, worms, fungi (*Armillaria mellea, Panus stipticus*), Protozoa (dinoflagellates), and the luminous organs of some fish are able to emit light.

The luminous bacteria discussed here are marine microorganisms. They are chemo-organotrophs, and in their morphological and physiological characters they resemble the Enterobacteria. (They are therefore sometimes referred to as marine Enterobacteria). Some of them live a symbionts in the luminous organs of inkfish and other deep-sea fish. Whereas the selective advantage of an ability to produce luminescence is obvious in these animals, the importance of bioluminescence for unicellular organisms is still obscure.

Luminous bacteria can be easily isolated from seawater or brackish water. They develop on meat and fish as natural enrichment media, usually at low temperature. Thus, saltwater fish kept for a few days in the refrigerator (4–6 °C) and partially immersed in salt solution will develop colonies of luminous bacteria on its surface; these colonies can be easily isolated and brought into pure culture. They are not usually putrefactive: although they liberate amines, they do not produce toxic substances. To quote Robert Boyle (1667), 'A piece of meat may have been glowing in the evening, before being transformed into a palatable and wholesome meal the next day'.

All **luminous bacteria** so far isolated are gram-negative, facultative anaerobes, motile by means of flagella. They are assigned to the genera *Photobacterium* and *Vibrio* on the basis of their type of flagellation: polar or peritrichous, one to eight naked or sheathed flagella. Among the best-known and most extensively examined species are *Photobacterium phosphoreum, Vibrio fischeri, V. harveyi*, and *V. logei*. Under anaerobic conditions most luminous bacteria carry out formate or mixed acid fermentations, similar to those known in enterobacteria, and they produce formate, acetate, lactate, succinate, alcohol, carbon dioxide, and acetoin. They are halophiles like many other marine bacteria; on transfer to hypotonic solutions (distilled water), they lyse instantaneously.

Growth and bioluminescence are strongly influenced by the composition of the medium. Luminescence occurs only in the presence of oxygen. Luminous bacteria have therefore been used since the beginning of this century as very sensitive indicators for the demonstration of photosynthetic oxygen evolution by red and green algae at different wavelengths.

The luminescence process.   This can be viewed as aerobic oxidation, a branchway of respiration that does not yield ATP, but leads to the activation of an intermediate that emits light. The process of luminescence was first formulated (in 1885 by Dubois) as a result of experiments with hot-water extracts (luciferin) and cold-water extracts (luciferase) from the light organ of the rock borer *Pholas dactylus*;

$$\text{luciferin} \xrightarrow[\text{O}_2]{\text{luciferase}} \text{light}$$

Luminescence in animals. The substrates involved in bioluminescence vary in different systems. The most extensive elucidation has been achieved in the case of the American firefly, *Photinus pyralis*. The luciferin of this system has been identified as a benzothiazole derivative. Luciferase (E) catalyses the conversion of the reduced luciferin (LH_2) with ATP to an adenylate, which emits light on oxidation.

$$LH_2 + ATP + E \rightleftharpoons E \cdot LH_2 - AMP + PP_i$$

$$E \cdot LH_2 - AMP + O_2 \rightarrow light + products$$

The stoichiometric relationship between ATP and light intensity has made the 'firefly-luminescence' test a favourite for the quantitative demonstration of ATP.

Bacterial luminescence also involves several components: reduced FMN, oxgen, and a long-chain aldehyde (tetradecanal). The luciferase is a monooxygenase (see Ch. 14.11.1). The reaction can be presented as follows:

$$FMNH_2 + O_2 + R-CHO \rightarrow FMN + H_2O + R-COOH + h\nu$$

The oxidation of $FMNH_2$ most probably produces at first an excited FMN, i.e. $[FMN \cdot H_2O]^*$, which then returns to the ground state with the emission of light:

$$[FMN \cdot H_2O]^* \xrightarrow{\ h\nu\ } FMN \cdot H_2O \rightarrow FMN + H_2O$$

Bacterial luciferase is commercially available. It can be used for quantitation of ultra-micro amounts of NAD(P)H in a coupled reaction.

Autoinduction of luminscence. *Vibrio fischeri* can be isolated from seawater as well as the luminous organs of some marine fish, which the bacterium inhabits as an ectosymbiont. Whilst cultures below a certain cell density show only weak luminescence, highly concentrated suspensions produce a disproportionately strong luminescence. This phenomenon is due to the inducibility of luminescence. The inducer is formed by the cells during growth. It is therefore called an **autoinducer** and is a low molecular weight substance of known structure. It is present in almost equal concentrations in the cytoplasm and in the suspension media. At high **cellular concentrations**, therefore, the concentration of the autoinducer is also high. It is the chemical signal for the expression of the luminscence gene and the formation of luciferase. The detailed elucidation of this regulatory system explains why luminous bacteria generally do not show luminescence in the sea, but produce strong luminescence in the luminous organs of fish, where they are present at concentrations of 10^{10} cells per ml.

The genes coding for bioluminescence can be transferred as hybrid plasmids to other bacteria and even to tobacco plants, where they can be expressed. The luminescence system is also used as a marker and indicator in recombinant genetics.

8.5   Butyric acid–butanol fermentation and clostridia

Butyrate, as well as butanol, acetone, 2-propanol, and other organic acids and alcohols are typical products of carbohydrate fermentations by anaerobic spore formers (clostridia). The group clostridia, even including some specialists that only ferment ethanol, amino acids or other substances, will be discussed together in the context of butyrate formation.

Characters.   The genus *Clostridium* belongs to the family Bacillaceae. They are gram-positive, as are the other members of this family (*Bacillus, Sporolactobacillus, Desulfotomaculum* and *Sporosarcina*). Clostridia are very motile by virtue of peritrichous flagella. The vegetative cells are rods, but their shape is variable and influenced by environmental factors. The endospores are oval or spherical and deform the rod-shaped mother cell because the spore diameter is usually larger than that of the vegetative cell. The spores are heat resistant.

The clostridia are characterised physiologically by their **intensely fermentative metabolism** and by their relation to oxygen. They grow only under **anaerobic conditions**. However, they represent a complete spectrum from strict anaerobes (*Clostridium pasteurianum, C. kluyveri*) to almost aerotolerant species (*C. histolyticum, C. acetobutylicum*) (Table 8.6). Clostridia usually contain no haem derivatives (cytochromes, catalase). A few species, though, can produce cytochromes if the medium supplies precursors. Clostridia contain mostly starchlike polysaccharides as storage products.

The optimum temperature for growth of most known clostridia is in the region of 30–40 °C. In addition to these mesophiles, there are also many thermophilic species that have temperature optima between 60 and 75 °C (*Clostridium thermoaceticum, C. thermohydrosulfuricum*). In common with other Bacillaceae, clostridia can grow only at neutral or alkaline pH. Their often unwelcome growth can therefore be completely inhibited by acidification (sauerkraut, silage, tinned fruits, salami, etc.).

Substrates of clostridia.   The clostridia vary widely in the substances that they can utilise and ferment. Some clostridia are relatively non-selective and have a wide range of substrates, whilst others are known as specialists and can utilise only a few. Taken together, the clostridia can utilise a wide range of natural materials as substrates. They can metabo-

Table 8.6. *Survey of the clostridia, arranged according to fermentative properties*

Clostridium species	Substrates	Fermentation products
(1) Butyric acid formation		
C. butyricum	glucose, starch, dextrin	butyrate, acetate, CO_2, H_2
C. tyrobutyricum	glucose or lactate, glycerol + acetate	butyrate, acetate, CO_2, H_2
C. pasteurianum	glucose, starch, mannose, inulin	butyrate, acetate, CO_2
C. pectinovorum	pectin, starch glycogen, dextrin	butyrate, acetate
(2) Butanol formation		
C. butylicum	glucose	butyrate, acetate, butanol, 2-propanol, CO_2, H_2
C. acetobutylicum	glucose, glycerol, pyruvate	butyrate, acetate, butanol, acetone, acetoin, ethanol, CO_2, H_2
(3) Propionic acid formation		
C. propionicum	alanine, threonine	acetate, propionate, CO_2
(4) Caproic acid formation		
C. kluyveri	ethanol + acetate + CO_2	caproate, butyrate, H_2
(5) Stickland reaction		
C. botulinum		
C. histolyticum	proteins, amino acids	acetate, lactate
C. sporogenes		NH_3, H_2
C. sticklandii		
(6) Presence of special metabolic pathways		
C. aceticum	$(CO_2 + H_2)$ fructose	acetate
C. tetanomorphum	glutamate, histidine	butyrate, acetate, NH_3, CO_2, H_2
C. acidi-urici	urea, xanthine	acetate, formate, CO_2, NH_3

lise polysaccharides (starch, glycogen, cellulose, hemicellulose and pectins), nucleic acids, proteins, amino acids, purines and pyrimidines. Some clostridia require complex media or supplements, whilst others do not. Some can utilise molecular nitrogen as their sole nitrogen source and can fix it at a high rate (*C. pasteurianum*).

Table 8.7. *Special fermentations*

Species	Substrate	Fermentation products
Eubacterium limosum (*Butyribacterium rettgeri*)	glucose, lactate, pyruvate	butyrate, acetate, CO_2, H_2, lactate (with glucose)
Peptococcus anaerobius (*Diplococcus glycinophilus*)	glycine	acetate, CO_2, H_2, NH_3
Fusobacterium nucleatum	amino acids	acetate, lactate, ethanol, CO_2, NH_3
Clostridium oroticum	orotic acid	acetate, succinate, CO_2, NH_3

The clostridia can be grouped according to their substrate utilisation. **Saccharolytic** clostridia metabolise predominantly polysaccharides and sugars. The **peptolytic** clostridia metabolise proteins, peptones, and amino acids. In addition, they are grouped according to their fermentative properties and fermentation products (Tables 8.6, 8.7).

Enrichment and isolation.   The heat resistance of clostridial spores offers a convenient way of obtaining enrichment cultures of clostridia: namely, by using pasteurised inocula. The provision of strictly anaerobic conditions also excludes all aerobic organisms. The saccharolytic clostridia are often adsorbed onto the surface of starch grains or cellulose particles, just like many other bacteria that can metabolise polysaccharides. By washing these particles before using them in inocula (e.g. rumen contents), many bacteria are removed whilst the clostridia remain attached.

Biochemistry of fermentation and fermentation products.   Varying amounts of acids (butyrate, acetate, lactate) and alcohols (butanol, ethanol, 2-propanol), as well as acetone and gas (carbon dioxide, hydrogen), are produced during clostridial fermentations. Clostridia metabolise glucose via the fructose-bisophosphate pathway. The hydrogen removed by the dehydrogenation of glyceraldehyde-3-phosphate is usually transferred to organic acids or ketones that are synthesised from pyruvate and acetyl-CoA, respectively. The fermentations of glucose by *Clostridium butyricum* and *C. acetobutylicum* can be regarded as prototypes of clostridial fermentations. Their end products are butyrate, acetate, butanol, ethanol, acetone, 2-propanol, carbon dioxide and hydrogen. Their yields are variable and depend on conditions.

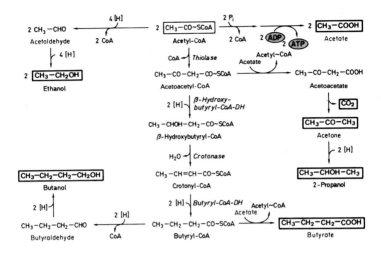

Fig. 8.4. *The formation of acetate, ethanol, n-butanol, butyrate, acetone, and 2-propanol during clostridial fermentations.*

The initiating glucose catabolism is by the fructose-bisphosphate pathway. Pyruvate is converted to acetyl-CoA by pyruvate:ferredoxin oxidoreductase. Only the reactions from acetyl-CoA are shown here.

Butyrate is the product of condensation of two molecules of acetyl-CoA to acetoacetyl-CoA, catalysed by the enzyme thiolase and subsequent reduction. Acetoacetyl-CoA is reduced by β–hydroxybutyryl-CoA dehydrogenase and $NADH_2$ to β-hydroxybutyryl-CoA. The enzyme crotonase removes water from this to give crotonyl-CoA which is then reduced by butyryl-CoA dehydrogenase, a flavin enzyme, to butyryl-CoA (Fig. 8.4). The CoA can be transferred to acetate by CoA transferase, and the liberated butyrate is excreted. The acetyl-CoA can be used for the generation of ATP by phosphotransacetylase and acetate kinase with the generation of acetate (see section on ATP regeneration by fermentation at beginning of this chapter).

$$CH_3-CO \sim SCoA \xrightarrow[CoA]{P_i} CH_3-CO-O \sim \circledP \xrightarrow[ADP \quad ATP]{} CH_3-COOH$$

In the purely butyric acid fermentation, the hydrogen derived from the oxidation of pyruvate is liberated in gaseous form. When glucose is fermented to butyrate, carbon dioxide and H_2 according to the equation

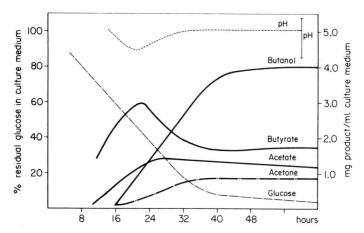

Fig. 8.5. *Time course of glucose fermentation by* Clostridium acetobutylicum.

(From Davies, R. & Stephenson, M. (1941). *Biochem. J.* **35**, 1320.)

$$glucose \rightarrow butyrate + 2CO_2 + 2H$$

a hydrogen balance is established and 3 mol ATP are regenerated per mol glucose (Fig. 8.4).

Butanol, butyrate, acetone, and **2-propanol** are the end products of glucose fermentation by *Clostridium acetobutylicum* (Fig. 8.5). This fermentation also leads to initial excretion of butyrate. With the increasing acidity, however, enzymes are induced, among them aceto-acetate decarboxylase, whose function gives rise to the accumulation of **acetone** and **butanol**. There is a close connection between the formation of acetone and butanol. The decarboxylation of a part of the aceto-acetate results in the loss of a potential hydrogen acceptor, which could have taken up two times 2[H] in the reduction to butyrate. This hydrogen, therefore, must be transferred to other hydrogen acceptors, including the excreted butyrate already formed. For its reduction to butanol, butyrate must first be activated by conversion to butyryl-CoA. The reactions involved in the conversion of butyrate and acetone to butanol are shown in Fig. 8.4. When fermentation is carried out under alkaline conditions (as, for example, in the presence of $CaCO_3$; see Table 8.8), *C. acetobutylicum* behaves like *C. butyricum*. Some strains reduce acetone and excrete 2-propanol.

Table 8.8. *Acetone-butanol fermentation by* C. acetobutylicum *in presence and absence of CaCO₃*

Fermentation products	Without CaCO$_3^a$	With CaCO$_3^a$
Butyrate	32.4	630
Butanol	411.5	45.7
Acetate	102.1	230.7
Ethanol	44.5	22.4
Acetone	222.3	13.2

^{a} As mg product/50 ml of the fermented 6% corn mash.
(From Bernhauer et al. (1936). *Biochem. Z.* **287**, 61.)

Ethanol is produced by the reduction of acetyl-CoA.

Molecular hydrogen can be derived from the cleavage of pyruvate or from the NADH$_2$ produced during dehydrogenation of glyceraldehyde-3-phosphate (see beginning of this chapter). The greater the evolution of molecular hydrogen, the less is the need for organic hydrogen acceptors (acetyl-CoA), so that the energy-rich thioester bond of acetyl-CoA can then be conserved in the formation of ATP. Thus the energy yield from the fermentation of glucose by *C. butyricum* may exceed 3 mol ATP if more than 2 mol hydrogen are liberated and correspondingly less butyrate is formed and more acetate (see *Ruminococcus* later in this section).

The production of acetone, 2-propanol, and butanol is of industrial importance. These fermentation products are used as organic solvents. Clostridial fermentation was the first process that faced industry with the task of carrying out a microbial conversion under the complete exclusion of any contaminants.

Fermentation of ethanol and acetate.   During enrichment culture for *Methanobacterium omelianskii* on media containing ethanol as substrate, an anaerobic spore former was isolated that required acetate in addition to ethanol. This bacterium, *Clostridium kluyveri*, metabolises ethanol and acetate to butyrate, caproate and hydrogen (Fig. 8.6). Acetate serves as an additional hydrogen acceptor, though it is also formed during fermentation. ATP is only regenerated by the acetate kinase reaction.

Fermentation of lactate and acetate.   *C. tyrobutyricum* was isolated from an enrichment culture containing lactate as substrate. It is also dependent on acetate as an additional hydrogen acceptor when lactate or glycerol are the main substrates:

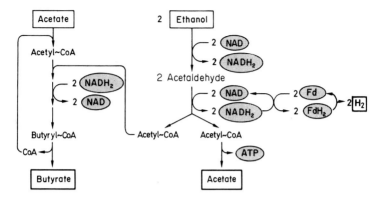

Fig. 8.6. *Fermentation of ethanol and acetate to butyrate and hydrogen by* Clostridium kluyveri.

$$CH_3-CHOH-COOH + CH_3-COOH \rightarrow CH_3-CH_2-COOH$$
$$+ H_2O + CO_2$$

The fermentation of glucose by *C. tyrobutyricum* follows the same scheme as that known for *C. butyricum* and does not need any additional hydrogen acceptors.

Fermentation of glutamic acid.   There are a multiple of fermentation processes in which amino acids are converted to fatty acids, carbon dioxide and ammonia under anaerobic conditions. Of these, only the metabolism of glutamate by *C. tetanomorphum* will be discussed here. This fermentation excited attention because it led to the discovery of the biochemical function of vitamin B_{12}, up to then only known as a vitamin. *C. tetanomorphum* was isolated from an enrichment culture which had histidine as substrate. This was metabolised via glutamate. Among the products of glutamate fermentation are butyrate, acetate, ammonia, carbon dioxide and molecular hydrogen. This catabolism of glutamate includes a number of unusual reactions (Fig. 8.7). It starts with the cleavage of the bond between carbon atoms 2 and 3 and the joining of carbon atoms 2 and 4, to give the branched amino acid methylaspartate. This reaction involves the participation of vitamin B_{12} as coenzyme. Deamination takes palce at this stage. The unsaturated mesaconate (methylfumarate) is hydroxylated, and the resulting citramalate (2-methylmalate) is then split to acetate and pyruvate. Acetate is excreted, and the pyruvate is converted to butyrate and CO_2 by the well-known pathway.

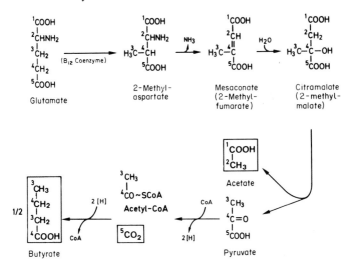

Fig. 8.7. *Fermentation of glutamate by* Clostridium tetanomorphum *via the mesaconate pathway.*

Fermentation of pairs of amino acids: the Stickland reaction. The peptolytic clostridia (Table 8.6, section 5) hydrolyse proteins and ferment the amino acids. Many of the amino acids cannot be fermented singly, however. In 1934, Stickland discovered that *Clostridium sporogenes* can readily ferment a mixture of alanine and glycine but cannot metabolise the single amino acids. According to the following overall balance equation,

$$\text{alanine} + 2\,\text{glycine} + 2\,H_2O \rightarrow 3\,\text{acetate} + 3\,NH_3 + CO_2$$

alanine must function as the hydrogen donor and glycine must function as the hydrogen acceptor:

$$CH_3\text{–}CHNH_2\text{–}COOH + 2\,H_2O \rightarrow CH_3\text{–}COOH + NH_3 + CO_2 + 4[H]$$

$$2\,NH_2CH_2\text{–}COOH + 4[H] \rightarrow 2\,CH_3\text{–}COOH + 2\,NH_3$$

The energy gain must obviously come from a **coupled oxidation–reduction** reaction. The amino acids alanine, leucine, isoleucine, valine, and methionine can function as **hydrogen donors**, and glycine, proline, arginine, tryptophane, etc. can serve as **hydrogen acceptors**. The donor amino acid is deaminated to an oxo-acid, which is then oxidatively decarboxylated to a fatty acid. This step involves a phosphorylation and therefore

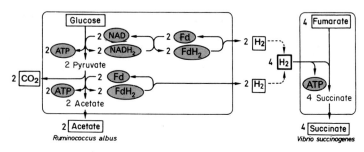

Fig. 8.8. *Fermentation of glucose by* Ruminococcus albus *and utilisation of the hydrogen produced by* Vibrio succinogenes *in a mixed culture.*

This symbiosis is an example of substrate transfer between cells (interspecies hydrogen transfer).

represents the energy-yielding reaction. The hydrogen that is first transferred to ferredoxin is then re-bound during the reductive deamination of the acceptor amino acid. Not all amino acids can be utilised by all peptolytic clostridia.

Butyrate and acetate fermentations by non-sporing organisms. Several genera of anaerobic bacteria are related to the clostridia by their type of fermentation, although they are non-sporogenous, and a number of them are gram-negative.

Most of the non-sporing butyrate- and acetate-producing organisms have been isolated from the rumen where they participate in the degradation of starch, cellulose, and other carbohydrates. They produce much hydrogen and carbon dioxide, and thus promote the formation of methane by the methanogens that are also present. *Butyrivibrio fibrisolvens* is especially noteworthy as a butyrate-forming organism in the rumen.

Ruminococcus albus, found in the rumen, is an acetate-forming coccus that utilises cellulose, xylan and many sugars. It can convert one mol glucose to 2 mol acetate plus 4 mol hydrogen and carbon dioxide, but only if the concentration of hydrogen can be kept low. This is possible in a mixed culture with hydrogen-utilising bacteria, such as *Vibrio succinogenes* (Fig. 8.8). The fermentation diagram shows that in a purely acetate fermentation, 4 mol ATP can be produced per mol glucose. Such a high efficiency of ATP regeneration, however, depends on the ability to liberate all the reducing equivalents of glucose metabolism in the form of gaseous hydrogen (see above sections on fermentations of acetate).

Clostridia as pathogens and toxin producers. Some peptolytic clostridia are pathogens that cause wound infections (gas gangrene and tetanus) and food poisoning. Their spores are widely distributed in soils. When spores of *Clostridium histolyticum* and *C. septicum* get into wounds that are not accesssible to air, or where the presence of aerobic bacteria causes anaerobic conditions by their oxygen consumption, they can germinate and grow. These organisms possess proteinases that digest collagen and other proteins with the evolution of foul-smelling and often toxic fermentation products and gas. This kind of wound infection and gas gangrene could be controlled formerly only by amputation of the affected limb(s). Another wound infection, still feared to the present day, is tetanus, caused by *C. tetani*. During growth, this bacterium excretes a highly potent nerve toxin that causes rigid paralysis of muscle (tetany).

The most dangerous food poisoning, **botulism**, is caused by *C. botulinum*. This is a widely distributed soil bacterium and develops in incompletely sterilised meat products and tinned beans, etc. It takes its name from its occurrence in sauages (Latin *botulus*, sausage). It produces a toxin that, on ingestion of the food, causes paralysis of the nervous system and is lethal by virtue of respiratory paralysis. Botulinus toxin A, which is excreted by *C. botulinum*, is a heat-labile protein. It has a 50% lethal dose (LD_{50} of 1 nanogram/kg body weight). This neurotoxin is therefore the most effective of all lethal poisons for man.

8.6   Homoacetate fermentation: carbon dioxide as hydrogen acceptor

Some clostridia (*Clostridium formicoaceticum, C. thermoaceticum, C. acidiurici, C. cylindrosporum*) can transfer the hydrogen equivalents liberated in the initial oxidation of substrate only to carbon dioxide, so as to produce acetate:

$$8[H] + 2CO_2 \rightarrow CH_3\text{–}COOH + 2H_2O$$

The thermophilic *C. thermoaceticum* and the mesophilic *C. formicoaceticum* ferment glucose predominantly to acetate. They metabolise hexose by the fructose-bisphosphate pathway and generate almost 3 mol acetate per mol glucose. In this, the major portion of the carbon dioxide produced by pyruvate decarboxylation must be re-fixed and serve as hydrogen acceptor. The formation of acetate from CO_2 and the reducing equivalents (electrons) obtained in the initial oxidation reactions proceeds according to the pathway shown in Fig. 8.9. Hexose is converted to pyruvate by the fructose-bisphosphate pathway (as in clostridia, generally). Pyruvate

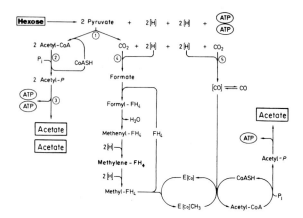

Fig. 8.9. *Biosynthetic pathway for acetate formation from hexose by* Clostridium thermoaceticum *via the acetyl-CoA pathway.*

See text for explanations
E(Co), corrinoid protein; FH_4, tetrahydrofolate; [H], hydrogen

equivalents, either as $NADH_2$ or FdH_2; CO, exogenous carbon monoxide; (CO), bound CO.

then gives rise to acetate, CO_2, FdH_2 and ATP by the enzymes pyruvate: ferredoxin oxidoreductase (1), phosphotransacetylase (2), and acetate kinase (3) (see Fig. 8.9). Carbon dioxide serves as the anaerobic hydrogen acceptor. In part it is reduced by formate dehydrogenase (4) to formate, which furnishes the methyl group of a third molecule of acetate, and in part it is reduced by CO dehydrogenase (5) to CO, which furnishes the carboxyl group of the acetate. The reduction of the formyl to the methyl group involves the participation of tetrahydrofolate (FH_4) as a coenzyme. The methyl group is subsequently transferred to a corrinoid protein (coenzyme B_{12} protein) and carboxylated by incorporation of the bound CO. The product of these reactions is acetyl-CoA, from which acetate is generated in the usual way with regeneration of ATP (Fig. 8.9).

This reductive mechanism for the synthesis of acetyl-CoA from CO_2 and hydrogen equivalents, the **acetyl-CoA pathway**, is generally identical with that used by methanogenic and acetogene bacteria with anaerobic respiration (see Ch. 9.4, 9.5).

Both *C. formicoaceticum* and *C. thermoaceticum* have been found to contain cytochrome *b*. Whether these organisms, as well as *C. aceticum* and other clostridia, can obtain energy by electron-transport phosphorylation remains to be studied (see Ch. 9.5).

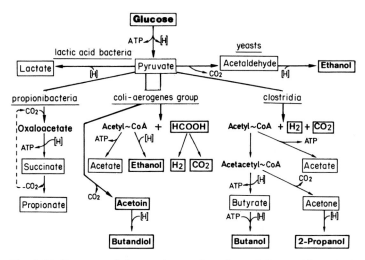

Fig. 8.10. *Summary of the reactions and products of the most important fermentations.*

8.7   Fermentable and non-fermentable natural products

Most natural products that consist of carbon, oxygen, hydrogen, and/or nitrogen can be fermented under anaerobic conditions. Fermentation is conditional on the possibility of a partial oxidation of the substrate by an exerogenic, intramolecular cleavage reaction. Thus, polysaccharides, hexoses, pentoses, tetroses and polyols are fermentable, as are organic acids, (including sugar acids, gluconate, malate, tartrate, etc.), amino acids (with the exception of the aromatic amino acids which can only be fermented under certain conditions), and purines and pyrimidines.

In contrast to these fermentable compounds are those that have been found to be non-biodegradable under anaerobic conditions: aliphatic and aromatic hydrocarbons, steroids, carotenoids, terpens, saturated fatty acids and porphyrins. Although these compounds can be oxidised and degraded under aerobic conditions, they are very stable anaerobically. Two reasons can be adduced to account for this stability: (1) Most of the compounds mentioned consist of only carbon and hydrogen atoms. No energy can be gained by their intramolecular cleavage. (2) The saturated hydrocarbons and the polyisoprenoids are oxidisable only by molecular oxygen; the first step must be catalysed by an oxygenase. The great stability of hydrocarbons under anaerobic conditions can be demonstrated in any laboratory experiment, and this stability is probably the reason why hydrocarbons survived in oil deposits. The microorganisms present at the time when oil deposits were formed probably lacked the ability to ferment paraffins, and they have not acquired it to this day (Fig. 8.10).

9 Electron transport under anaerobic conditions

In the sediments of lakes and ponds and in waterlogged soils, that is, in anoxic (oxygen-deficient) ecosystems, bacteria which gain their metabolic energy by **anaerobic respiration** can become established. Such bacteria utilise the compounds and residues produced by fermentative organisms as carbon sources and hydrogen donors. They are at the end of the anaerobic food chain (Chapter 8). These anaerobically respiring organisms can use nitrate, sulphate, sulphur, carbonate, ferric iron and several other compounds as H-acceptors. They reduce **nitrate** to **molecular nitrogen** and **NO_2, sulphate** and **elementary sulphur** to **hydrogen sulphide, CO_2** and **carbonates** to **acetic acid** or **methane**, and **ferric** to **ferrous iron**.

Figure 9.1 summarises the reducing reactions, their brief metabolic designation and the types of bacteria involved. Transfer of the electrons derived from the organic substrates to the above-mentioned inorganic ions and compounds allows electron transport phosphorylation and the appropriate gain in energy. The energetic relationships have already been discussed in Ch. 7.4. The anaerobically respiring organisms are of great importance for the understanding of the various elementary cycles in nature, and the maintenance of equilibria in the biosphere. They are all prokaryotes. Anaerobic respiration undoubtedly belongs to the kinds of metabolism that predominated in the early evolution of organisms and led to the accumulation of organic carbon found in archaeic sediments. The **products of anaerobic respiration** are very noticeable: as the release of gas bubbles (N_2, NO_2, CH_4), by their odour (H_2S), the formation of flammable gas (CH_4), and the production of diamagnetic iron oxide from non-magnetic ionic iron. Finally, it should be mentioned that these anaerobically respiring bacteria are also of considerable economic importance.

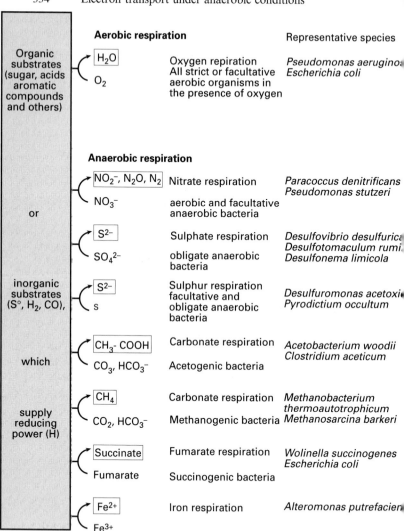

Fig. 9.1. *Processes that yield energy by electron transport phosphorylation under aerobic and anaerobic conditions.*

(Also called aerobic and anaerobic respiration.)

9.1   Nitrate respiration: denitrification and nitrate ammonification

The physiological group that can carry out nitrate respiration can transfer substrate hydrogen, respectively electrons, to nitrate which becomes reduced, with the free energy being used for electron transport phosphorylation. This process is called **nitrate respiration** or **dissimilatory nitrate reduction**. There are two types of metabolism and two groups of bacteria which have to be distinguished with respect to their ecological and biochemical roles.

(1) **Denitrifiers** are aerobic, strictly respiratory bacteria. They cannot grow anaerobically in the absence of nitrate. Under anaerobic conditions, and in the presence of nitrate as the only hydrogen acceptor, this is reduced to gaseous nitrogen dioxide (NO_2) and molecular nitrogen, which are released. Thus denitrification means the conversion of bound nitrogen (nitrate) to free N_2. This denitrification is the only biological process by which organically or inorganically bound nitrogen can be released and recycled. The denitrifiers include – to name some representative species – *Pseudomonas denitrificans, Paracoccus denitrificans, Thiobacillus denitrificans, Pseudomonas aeruginosa* and *Bacillus licheniformis*.

(2) **Nitrate ammonification** is carried out by several groups of microorganisms, especially the important group of the Enterbacteriaceae (*Escherichia coli, Enterobacter aerogenes*). These are all facultative anaerobes which are able to ferment under anaerobic conditions. However, if nitrate is available it will be used as external H-acceptor and is first reduced to nitrite. This can also be reduced, though not to nitrogen, but via the **assimilatory nitrate reduction** pathway to ammonia (NH_3) in the form of ammonium (NH_4^+). This nitrate ammonification, therefore, does not lead to the liberation of molecular nitrogen.

9.1.1   Nitrate respiration: denitrification

The conversion of nitrate to N_2 with the substrate- (organic compounds or hydrogen-) derived reducing equivalents proceeds with the following stoichimetry:

$$10[H] + 2H^+ + 2NO_3^- \rightarrow N_2 + 6H_2O$$

This proceeds in the steps depicted by the scheme below.

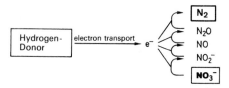

Each step is catalysed by a specific enzyme. Nitrate reductase A is a molybdenum-containing enzyme and is membrane-bound. The resulting nitrite is reduced by another membrane-bound enzyme, nitrite reductase to nitrogen oxide (NO). This is then further reduced by NO-reductase to dinitrogen oxide (N_2O), which in turn is then reduced by N_2O-reductase to molecular nitrogen (N_2). Depending on environmental conditions, the reduction of nitrate may proceed, without accumulation of intermediates, straight to the release of N_2, or intermediates like NO_2, NO, or N_2O may be accumulated and excreted. Nitrite, NO or N_2O is excreted when there is an excess of nitrate and the concentration of hydrogen donors becomes limiting. Thus, nitrogen oxides reach the atmosphere not only because of incomplete combustion of oil and coal, but also as a product of biological processes in soil and water sediments.

Apparently, there are no denitrifiers which are obligate anaerobes. All have a complete respiratory system. The enzymes required for nitrate respiration are only induced – or de-repressed – under conditions of oxygen deficiency or oxygen lack (Fig. 9.2). In many cases the presence of nitrate is necessary for induction of the enzymes, but in some anaerobiosis is sufficient. Many denitrifiers can not only grow with nitrate, but can also grow with nitrite or N_2O as H-acceptors. This shows that not only nitrate reductase A, but also the dissimilatory nitrite-, NO- and N_2O-reducing enzymes must be coupled to the electron transport chain.

Enrichment culture of denitrifying bacteria. If a nutrient medium containing various hydrogen donors, building blocks for cell synthesis, and nitrate is inoculated with soil or mud and incubated anaerobically (see Table 6.2), a number of bacterial species can be grown: (a) with a trace of peptone and ethanol or propionate: *Pseudomonas aeruginosa*; (b) with glucose: *P. fluorescens*; (c) with tartrate, succinate, or malate: *P. stutzeri*; (d) with organic acids, alcohol, and meat extract, or with high nitrate concentrations (5–12% KNO_3): *Bacillus licheniformis*; (e) with a trace of yeast extract and with molecular hydrogen as hydrogen donor: *Paracoccus denitrificans*; (f) with sulphur or thiosulphate: *Thiobacillus denitrificans*. Since some denitrifiers utilise nitrogen only or predominantly, as a hydrogen acceptor but cannot reduce it to ammonium, a nitrogen source (peptone or ammonium) must be added.

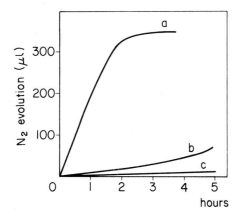

Fig. 9.2.*Rate of nitrogen production by cell suspensions of* Paracoccus denitrificans.

The evolution of N_2 is due to denitrification of nitrate with acetate as substrate under anaerobic conditions. The bacteria were grown under different conditions: (a) anaerobic with nitrate; (b) aerobic with nitrate; (c) aerobic without nitrate. (From van Olden, E. (1956.) In *The Microbe's Contribution to Biology*, ed. A. J. C. Kluyver & B. van Niel. Cambridge, MA: Harvard Univ. Press.)

Nitrogen loss in soil by denitrification.   Localised and transient denitrification in soils can be ascribed with certainty to bacterial denitrification. Denitrification is common in anaerobic locations and readily occurs under conditions of stagnant moisture, especially when organic fertilisers and nitrate are applied together. In rice fields, for example, fertilisation with nitrate may produce damage through accumulation of nitrite. Nitrite also accumulates in nitrate-containing, insufficiently ventilated drainage systems and may enter the drinking water. The dependence of nitrogen loss on the aeration in soils is a consequence of the regulation of nitrate-reducing enzyme systems in bacteria; these enzymes are induced by nitrate only under anaerobic conditions (Fig. 9.2). Oxygen represses the formation of nitrate and nitrite reductases. If the enzymes have already been induced and the cells are subsequently exposed to aerobic conditions, oxygen will compete with nitrate for electrons delivered by the respiratory chain and will inhibit the function of the nitrate reducing system.

The importance of denitrification in nature. Denitrification is the only biological process that converts fixed nitrogen to molecular nitrogen. Globally this process is of decisive importance for the maintenance of terrestrial life. In normally ventilated soils and waters, nitrate is the end product of mineralisation. The nitrate ions, because they are highly water-soluble and poorly adsorbed on soil, would tend to be washed out and accumulate in the oceans. In this way molecular nitrogen would be lost continuously from the atmosphere (by nitrogen fixation), and terrestrial plant growth and production of biomass would eventually cease.

9.1.2   Nitrate respiration: nitrate ammonification

Several facultatively anaerobic bacteria which can grow with fermentative energy under anaerobic conditions, as for example *Escherichia coli* and *Enterobacter aerogenes*, can also derive energy gain from the presence of nitrate. They are able to transfer the substrate-derived electrons to nitrate to produce nitrite. This step which is catalysed by nitrate reductase A is coupled to electron-transport phosphorylation and energy gain.

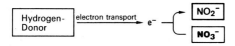

Nitrite may accumulate in the medium, but there is no evolution of N_2. Instead, the nitrate can be reduced to ammonium by the assimilatory pathway, with the ammonium being excreted. This reduction of nitrite to ammonium does not entail any energy gain. It is rather akin to a fermentation process in which nitrite functions as an exogenous nitrogen acceptor. The organisms gain an advantage from this because during the fermentation of glucose some of the reducing equivalents can be fed to nitrite reduction with a corresponding increase in acetate liberation (see beginning of Chapter 8, reaction 3).

Nitrate assimilation.   Nitrate respiration (or **dissimilatory nitrate reduction**) can now be contrasted with nitrate assimilation (or **assimilatory nitrate reduction**). Apart from ammonia, nitrate is the most ubiquitous nitrogen source for plants and bacteria. Most bacteria can produce the enzymes of nitrate assimilation. They are induced, both aerobically and anaerobically, when no other nitrogen source is present, apart from nitrate. The presence of ammonium usually represses the formation of the assimilatory nitrate reducing enzymes. Assimilatory nitrate reduction leads to the formation of ammonium and uses much reducing power:

$$8[H] + H^+ + NO_3^- \rightarrow NH_4^+ + OH^- + 2H_2O$$

Nitrogen is incorporated into amino acids and other nitrogen-containing metabolites, in the form of ammonium. This nitrate reduction proceeds via several intermediate compounds of which only nitrite is liberated, and is catalysed by two enzymes. The first step is catalysed by nitrate reductase B which is located in the cytoplasm. The resulting nitrite is then reduced by another cytoplasmic enzyme, nitrite reductase, to ammonium.

$$NO_3^- \xrightarrow{2e^-} NO_2^- \xrightarrow{2e^-} HNO \xrightarrow{2e^-} NH_2OH \xrightarrow{2e^-} NH_3$$

Nitrate-Reductase B   *Nitrite-Reductase*

This needs six electrons which are supplied via $NAD(P)H_2$ (bacteria and fungi) or ferredoxin (plants and bacteria). The enzyme is a complex, and contains apart from Fe–S centres, also iron-haem centres (sirohaem). This nitrate reductase-catalysed reaction resembles the nitrogenase and sulphite reductase-catalysed reactions, which all transfer six electrons without any intermediates being liberated.

The formation of methaemoglobin as a consequence of nitrite accumulation in drinking water and food. The consumption of nitrate-containing water (common in times of drought) and certain vegetables (e.g. over-fertilised spinach) can lead to illness, as a consequence of bacterial nitrate reduction in the intestinal tract (this can also occur in tinned foods). The uptake of nitrite into the blood causes the formation of methaemoglobin, by the binding of the nitrite to haemoglobin and the oxidation of Fe(II) to Fe(III). Methaemoglobin binds oxygen irreversibly, resulting in cyanosis, because the erythrocytes can no longer function as oxygen carriers. This illness occurs only in babies up to about 6 months old, because the nitrate-reducing bacteria can apparently pass undamaged through the stomach and proliferate in the intestinal tract. In older children and adults, the nitrate-reducing bacteria are killed by the strongly acid gastric secretion, and the nitrate ions are reabsorbed before they can be reduced in the duodenum with its favourable pH.

9.2   Hydrogen sulphide formation by sulphate reduction

The physiological group of sulphate-reducing bacteria (also called desulfuricants) is characterised by the ability to transfer substrate hydrogen to sulphate as the terminal electron acceptor with the reduction of the sulphate to sulphide. This process allows electron transport with the participation of cytochrome c, and energy gain comes from electron-transport phosphorylation under anaerobic conditions.

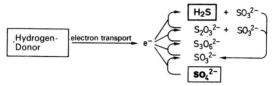

Since this kind of sulphate reduction is formally similar to respiration with oxygen, it is also called sulphate respiration or dissimilatory sulphate reduction. The main product of this reduction is hydrogen sulphide:

$$8[H] + 2H^+ + SO_4^{2-} \rightarrow H_2S + 4H_2O$$

Most of the hydrogen sulphide produced in nature is due to this reaction. The sulphate-reducing bacteria, in contrast to the nitrate-reducing ones, are obligate anaerobes and strictly dependent on anaerobic conditions.

Systematic position.   Several groups of anaerobic bacteria are able to carry out sulphate respiration. Among these are flagellated and non-flagellated eubacteria (*Desulfovibrio, Desulfobacterium, Desulfococcus, Desulfomonas, Desulfobacillus, Desulfosarcina, Thermosulfobacterium*), gram-negative gliding bacteria (*Desulfonema*), gram-positive endospore-forming eubacteria (*Desulfatomaculum*), and archaebacteria (*Archaeoglobus*). Various low molecular weight compounds can serve as hydrogen donors for different members of the group: lactate, acetate, propionate, butyrate, formate, methanol, ethanol, higher fatty acids, aromatic compounds, and molecular hydrogen. However, no species can use all these compounds, nor is any particular substrate utilised by all these organisms. This group of sulphate-respiring organisms is therefore very heterogenous with regard to substrate utilisation and metabolic pathways. The following is a brief summary of the subgroups – without going into any details.

(1) This group, discovered about a decade ago, can grow on lactate and other acids and utilise molecular hydrogen. They oxidise the H-donors incompletely and excrete acetate. the group contains species of *Desulfovibrio* and *Desulfatomaculum*.

(2) More recently species have been isolated that utilise acetate, short and long-chain fatty acids, alcohols, aromatic compounds and molecular hydrogen as H-donors. They include *Desulfatomaculum acetooxidans, Desulfobacter, Desulfonema* and others.

(3) A few species are able to grow autotrophically with molecular hydrogen and thiosulphate. This group includes strains of *Desulfovibrio, Desulfobacterium, Desulfococcus, Desulfobacter* and *Desulfatomaculum* as well as *Archaeglobus* which is a hyperthermophilic archaebacterium.

(4) A newly discovered isolate, *Desulfovibrio dismutans* carries out the surprising energy-providing dismutation between thiosulphate or sulphite to sulphate and H_2S. Various strains grow autotrophically or in the presence of acetate as chemolithoheterotrophs. Their metabolism can be regarded as 'inorganic fermentation'.

Sulphate reduction.   Nearly all bacteria, as well as fungi and green plants, can grow with sulphate as their source of sulphur. They produce the sulphide which is necessary for the synthesis of sulphur-containing amino acids by 'assimilatory sulphate reduction'. The first step is common to dissimilatory and assimilatory sulphate reduction. However, whereas in the former process activated sulphate is reduced directly, a second activation step is involved in the assimilatory process. The cell must initiate the reduction of sulphate with a fairly high energy-demanding activation of the sulphate by ATP (Fig. 9.3); an ATP sulfurylase (sulphate-adenyl transferase) exchanges the diphosphate of ATP for sulphate:

$$ATP + SO_4^{2-} \rightleftharpoons \text{adenosine-5'-phosphosulphate} + PP_i$$

The diphosphate is hydrolysed by diphosphatase and adenosine-5'-phosphosulphate (APS) is the activated product. The further steps are different. In the assimilatory sulphate reduction, APS is phosphorylated by APS kinase and another mole of ATP to phosphoadenosine-phosphosulphate (PAPS). Only this doubly activated sulphate can then be reduced to sulphide via sulphite. In the dissimilatory sulphate reduction, the APS is reduced by APS reductase with the formation of AMP and sulphite.

The **reduction of sulphite** to sulphide is carried out in different ways by different bacteria. Sulphite reductase can reduce sulphite in a six-electron step directly to sulphide without the liberation of intermediary products. This kind of reduction, as well as the assimilatory sulphite reduction, generally seems to involve iron–porphyrin compounds (desulphoviridin, desulphorubidin). In the second mechanism, sulphite is reduced in three successive steps in which free intermediates are produced (trithionate and thiosulphate) (Fig. 9.3). It is thought that the electrons for the reduction of sulphite are supplied via cytochromes (cytochrome *b* in some bacteria, cytochrome *c* in others).

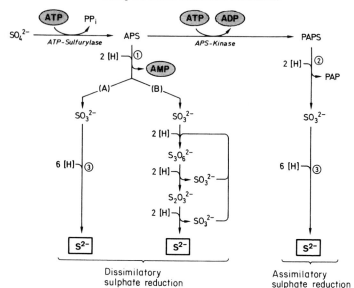

Fig. 9.3. *Diagrams of dissimilatory sulphate reduction (sulphate respiration) and assimilatory sulphate reduction.*

APS, adenosine-5'-phosphosulphate; PAPS, phosphoadenosine-5'-phosphosulphate; PAP, phospho-adenosine-5'-phosphate.

Enzymes: (1) APS reductase; (2) PAPS reductase; (3) sulphite reductase (bisulphite reductase).

Electron-transport phosphorylation. The assumption that electron-transport phosphorylation occurs in desulphuricants is based on the demonstration that cytochromes and iron–sulphur proteins are present in and on their cytoplasmic membranes; there are also considerable energy yields. Cytochrome c_3 has an extremely low redox potential (E_0', − 205 mV) compared with other cytochromes, and it is localised on the outside of the cytoplasmic membrane or in the periplasmic space.

The genera of sulphate-reducing bacteria that have been studied so far have a constitutive hydrogenase (H_2:cytochrome c_3 oxidoreductase), which can function in the uptake and activation of hydrogen as well as in its liberation. Some sulphate-reducing bacteria grow with hydrogen and sulphate as their only energy source. The ability to reduce sulphate with molecular hydrogen with the accumulation of large amounts of H_2S but without significant growth, is probably common to most of the sulphate-reducing bacteria. Electron transport with molecular hydrogen as the donor and the reduction of one mole of sulphate to sulphide is probably coupled with the regeneration of three moles of ATP, of which two must be used for the activation of the sulphate.

Autotrophic CO_2 assimilation. During the last 40 years the ability of microorganisms to grow autotrophically has been demonstrated on numerous occasions. The evidence, though never complete, can be quantitated. The pathways of this CO_2 fixation are those of the **reductive acetyl-CoA** pathway, or the **reductive tricarboxylic acid cycle** but not those of the Calvin cycle (Ch. 11.5).

Oxidation of organic substrates. The classical sulphate reducers, such as *Desulfovibrio vulgaris*, do not have a complete TCA cycle, and excrete acetate. Among the species which can utilise acetate are those which oxidise it via the oxidative TCA cycle (*Desulfobacter postgatei*), and others which oxidise it via the oxidative acetyl-CoA pathway (*Desulfobacterium, Desulfosarcina, Desulfococcus, Desulfatomaculum*). These strains thus utilise, in reverse, the same pathways for acetate oxidation, as those used in the reductive direction for CO_2 fixation. Most of the newly isolated bacteria can utilise acetate and long-chain fatty acids as well as aromatic compounds.

Assimilation of organic substrate. The metabolic energy gained by electron-transport phosphorylation allows the assimilation of organic substances (organic acids, amino acids, and complex mixtures). Some strains are able to synthesise their cellular constituents from acetate and carbon dioxide when molecular hydrogen functions as the hydrogen donor. Such assimilation of organic substances during oxidation of an inorganic hydrogen donor can be regarded as 'chemolithoheterotrophy'. CO_2 fixation via the Calvin cycle has not been demonstrated; it probably occurs via the acetyl-CoA pathway (see Section 9.5 of this chapter).

Fermentation without sulphate. Some of the desulphurising bacteria are also able to metabolise lactate or pyruvate in the absence of sulphate. Oxidation of pyruvate according to the equation:

$$4\,CH_3-CO-COOH + H_2SO_4 \rightarrow 4\,CH_3-COOH + 4\,CO_2 + H_2S$$

is replaced by a fermentative reaction with evolution of hydrogen:

$$CH_3-CO-COOH + H_2O \rightarrow CH_3-COOH + CO_2 + H_2$$

The fermentation of lactate identifies the desulphurising bacteria as potentially fermentative.

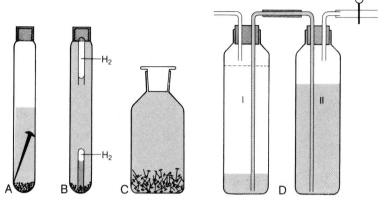

Fig. 9.4. *Enrichment cultures of sulphate-reducing bacteria.*

Growth after inoculation with decaying mud. A, Nutrient solution containing lactate and sulphate; the iron nail provides a sufficiently low redox potential by cathodic polarisation. B, Demonstration of H_2 consumption by sulphate-reducing bacteria; Durham tube filled with H_2, floating before incubation, and sunk to the bottom after incubation. C, Growth with traces of organic substances, during sulphate reduction and corrosion of iron in a stoppered flask.
D, Enrichment of sulphate-reducing bacteria in a double flask of *Söhngen*. Flask II is first filled with a nutrient solution containing lactate and sulphate; inflow of hydrogen then displaced the liquid into flask I (levels indicated by dotted lines). During incubation for 2 days at 30 °C, a large proportion of the hydrogen has been consumed.

Enrichment and isolation. For the enrichment culture of sulphate-reducing bacteria, the nutrient medium must contain a suitable hydrogen donor, assimilable substrate, mineral salts, and sulphate; anaerobic conditions and a sufficiently low redox potential (E_0', – 200 mV) are also required (Fig. 9.4).

Distribution and role of desulphurising bacteria in nature. The sulphate-reducing bacteria occur predominantly in decomposing sediments and black mud where organic materials undergo anaerobic degradation. The desulphurisers seem to be especially adapted to the products of incomplete carbohydrate metabolism, i.e. fatty acids, oxyacids, alcohols and hydrogen from fermentations. The mass of hydrogen sulphide occurring in nature can be regarded as the end product of sulphate respiration. Contaminated waters often contain 10^4 – 10^6, and black mud 10^7, sulphate-reducing organisms/ml.

Most of the utilisable sulphur deposits (in Texas, Louisiana and Mexico) are not of volcanic origin, but are accumulated during geological time. Hydrogen sulphide and sulphur can also be obtained by reduction of marine sulphate deposits with waste waters containing *Desulfovibrio*. However, *Desulfovibrio* also causes an indirect anaerobic corrosion of iron; this corrosion is of great economic importance. In a moist atmosphere the following reactions take place:

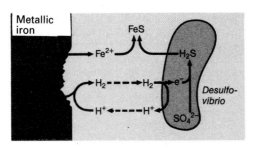

(1) Iron oxidation:

$$4\,Fe + 8\,H^+ \rightarrow 4\,Fe^{2+} + 4\,H_2$$

Normally, the iron is protected from further corrosion by the film of hydrogen. When sulphate and desulphurising bacteria are present, they cause a cathodic depolarisation, and the iron is oxidised even in the absence of oxygen:

(2) Sulphate reduction:

$$4\,H_2 + SO_4^{2-} \rightarrow H_2S + 2\,H_2O + 2\,OH^-$$

(3) Precipitation of iron:

$$4\,Fe^{2+} + H_2S + 2\,OH^- + 4\,H_2O \rightarrow FeS + 3\,Fe(OH)_2 + 6\,H^+$$

The sum of these three reactions:

$$4\,Fe + SO_4^{2-} + 2\,H_2O + 2\,H^+ \rightarrow FeS + 3\,Fe(OH)_2$$

Considerable damage to pipelines is produced in this way. The ability of the sulphate-reducing bacteria to utilise organic acids, alcohol, and hydrogen, including the hydrogen produced by the polarisation of iron, can be exploited for setting up enrichment cultures (Fig. 9.4).

Desulfovibrio has even been held responsible for the high hydrogen sulphide content at the bottom (below 200 m) of the Black Sea and for its black colour, due to iron corrosion.

Finally, the black paint on the gondolas of the Canale Grande in

Venice has been thought of as a protective measure against discoloration of white lead-based paints by H_2S.

Desulfoatomaculum ruminis participates in the formation of H_2S in the rumen of ruminants (see Ch. 14.1).

9.3   Reduction of sulphur to hydrogen sulphide

It has been known for quite a long time that on addition of 'flowers of sulphur' to a yeast suspension fermenting sugar, the sulphur 'enters the stream of biological reductions' and is converted to hydrogen sulphide. It has been discovered only recently, however, that some bacteria can grow with inorganic sulphur as the hydrogen acceptor for anaerobic electron transport. The sulphur is reduced to hydrogen sulphide in this process, which has been designated as 'sulphur respiration'.

The organism characterised in this way (until now) is *Desulfuromonas acetoxidans*. This bacterium, motile by virtue of a laterally inserted flagellum, can be enriched and isolated from seawater by anaerobic cultivation in a mineral salts solution containing acetate and elementary sulphur. *D. acetoxidans* oxidises acetate or ethanol to carbon dioxide. It is distinguished from most species of the genus *Desulfovibrio* by its ability to reduce sulphur and to oxidise organic substrates to completion, whereas the other species of this genus can reduce only sulphate or sulphite, but not sulphur, and oxidise, for example, lactate with the formation of acetate. *D. acetoxidans* contains a cytochrome c_7, which has a very low redox potential, and a 4Fe–4S protein. It also has the enzymes of the tricarboxylic acid cycle.

This organism can live in a syntrophic association with phototrophic green sulphur bacteria which, in the light, oxidise hydrogen sulphide to sulphur and fix carbon dioxide (Fig. 9.5).

Sulphur reduction in Archaebacteria.   Several of the extremely thermophilic and hyperthermophilic bacteria, most of which are also acidophilic and strict anaerobes, belong to the metabolic type capable of sulphur respiration. They were isolated only recently from hot springs and solar ponds. *Pyrodictium* (*P. occultum, P. brockii*) is a bacterium that grows at temperatures up to 110 °C and is strictly anaerobic. It grows autotrophically with H_2 as H-donor and sulphur as hydrogen acceptor, though it can also grow mixotrophically. Species of *Acedianus*, on the other hand (*A. brierleyi, A. ambivalens*), are surprisingly versatile. They can grow aerobically with oxidation of sulphur to sulphate, but can also reduce sulphur to hydrogen sulphide with molecular hydrogen as H-donor; that is, they can carry out sulphur respiration anaerobically.

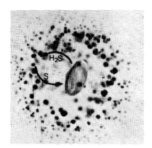 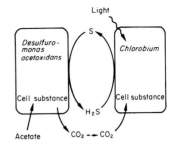

Fig. 9.5. *Mixed culture of a sulphate-reducing bacterium* (Desulfuromas acetoxidans) *and a green phototrophic bacterium* (Chlorobium) *on a nutrient agar plate.*

In the large central colony of *Desulfuromonas acetoxidans*, acetate is oxidised and sulphate is reduced. The hydrogen sulphide diffuses into the environment and serves as hydrogen donor for the cells of *Chlorobium*. The excreted sulphur diffuses, probably in the form of polysulphide, into the central colony, where it functions as hydrogen acceptor and is again reduced. The mixed growth of these two bacteria is a prime example of a syntrophic association with bidirectional transfer of substrate.

9.4   The formation of methane by reduction of carbonate

Methane is produced during the anaerobic catabolism of organic substances. The amounts of methane formed are considerable; it can be estimated that 1–1.5% of the carbon liberated as atmospheric carbon dioxide, by the mineralisation of organic substances, reaches the atmosphere first as methane, which is then converted, via CO, to CO_2 by hydroxyl radicals (OH·). The ecosystems where methane production occurs are the great tundras and swampy regions (the origin of the name 'swamp gas' for methane), rice fields, sediments of lakes, ponds and puddles; salt marshes, estuaries and sandy lagoons; sewage digesters and the rumen of the more than 10^9 ruminants on the earth. In such anaerobic locations organic substrates are first fermented to acetate, carbon dioxide, and molecular hydrogen (via several intermediary stages). It is these products of the primary and secondary breakdown that are utilised by the methane-producing bacteria (methanogens). About 70% of the total methane produced is derived from acetate, and 30% from CO_2 and H_2O.

Systematic position.   The following methane bacteria are classified morphologically: rod-shaped (*Methanobacterium*), coccoid (*Methanococcus*), sarcina-like (*Methanosarcina*), and spirillar (*Methanospirillum*).

The methanogens belong to a special group of bacteria (the archaebacteria). They differ from other bacteria not only by their type of metabolism, but also by a number of characteristic features in the composition of their cell constituents. They lack a typical peptidoglycan skeleton. *Methanococcus* has only a protein envelope, a peptide sheath is found in *Methanospirillum*, whilst the cell wall of *Methanosarcina barkeri* consists of a polysaccharide composed of uronic acids, neutral sugars, and amino sugars. The methanogenic bacteria are not subject to growth inhibition by penicillin.

The cytoplasmic membrane of the methanogens contains lipids consisting of glycerol ethers of isoprenoid hydrocarbons (see Ch. 3.13). Their ribosomes are similar in size to those of eubacteria (70S ribosomes) but the base sequence of their ribosomal RNA, especially that of 16S rRNA, is quite different. In this respect the methanogens differ more from *E. coli* than do the cyanobacteria. In addition, their method of ribosomal translation is insensitive to antibiotics that inhibit protein synthesis in eubacteria. On the basis of these and other differences within the prokaryotes, the methanogens are assigned to the archaebacteria (Ch. 3.13).

Physiology.   The methanogens are strict anaerobes; exposure to air is lethal. They contain neither catalase nor superoxide dismutase. Their extreme sensitivity to oxygen is the cause of the scarcity of existing knowledge about their biochemistry, physiology, and ecology. A special methodology, the Hungate technique, was developed to allow the inoculation and isolation of methanobacteria under conditions that exclude oxygen.

Most of the methanogens isolated and kept in pure culture up to now can use molecular hydrogen as hydrogen donor; some can also use formate, methanol, acetate, or methylamine. In some anaerobic ecosystems, acetate is known to be the main substrate for methane formation. The spectrum of substrates is very narrow.

The methanogenic bacteria are the last link in an anaerobic nutritional chain (see Chapter 8) that starts with polysaccharides (cellulose, starch), proteins, and lipids and in which a number of fermentative bacteria participate: (1) bacteria that ferment cellulose to succinate, propionate, butyrate, lactate, acetate, alcohols, CO_2 and H_2, (2) acetogenic bacteria, which ferment these primary products to acetate, formate, CO_2 and H_2. These products are the substrates for the methanogenic bacteria.

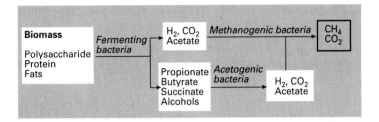

Methane-producing bacteria occur in close association with hydrogen-producing organisms (Fig. 9.6). In the microhabitats, hydrogen is rarely liberated in gaseous form. Rather, the excreted hydrogen, dissolved in the medium, is directly assimilated by the methanogenic bacteria. It is known that a high partial pressure of hydrogen is inhibitory for the metabolism and growth of the hydrogen-producing organisms. This means that not only do the methanogens depend on the hydrogen-producing bacteria, but also the latter depend on their hydrogen-utilising partners. This is therefore an association that amounts to a mutual symbiosis.

Methane bacteria are able to activate hydrogen and to couple its oxidation to the reduction of carbon dioxide. Since they can synthesise all their cell substance using carbon dioxide as sole carbon source, their mode of life is evidently to be regarded as chemoautotrophic. As the carbon dioxide is also used as a hydrogen acceptor in the generation of energy, with the production of methane, this methane formation can therefore be regarded, by analogy, as **carbonate respiration**.

$$4H_2 + CO_2 \rightarrow CH_4 + 2H_2O;$$
$$\Delta G_o = -131 \text{ kJ/mol} \ (-31.3 \text{ kcal/mol})$$

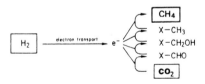

Some methanogenic bacteria can also convert carbon monoxide to methane, with the intermediary formation of carbon dioxide and hydrogen:

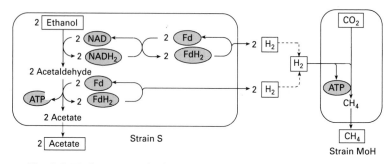

Fig. 9.6. *Hydrogen transfer between two bacterial species.*

This is shown in the example of the components of a *Methanobacterium omelianskii* culture. The culture of this bacterium was regarded as a pure culture for 30 years. and only in 1967 was it separated into a strain MoH (methanobacterium-oxidising hydrogen) and the accompanying bacterium S.

$$4\,CO + 4\,H_2O \rightarrow 4\,CO_2 + 4\,H_2$$
$$\underline{CO_2 + 4\,H_2 \rightarrow CH_4 + 2\,H_2O}$$
$$4\,CO + 2\,H_2O \rightarrow CH_4 + 3\,CO_2$$

Biochemistry of methane formation and energy gain. The biochemical conversions of H_2 and CO_2 to methane, and of acetate to methane and CO_2, involve a number of coenzymes and prosthetic groups that have been found, so far, only in methanogenic bacteria; the deazariboflavin derivative E_{420}, methanopterin, methanofuran, the nickel-tetrapyrrol factor F_{430}, and coenzyme M (mercaptoethane sulphonate). Their basic structures are shown in Fig. 9.7.

The probable pathways for the formation of methane from acetate and from hydrogen and carbon dioxide are shown below.

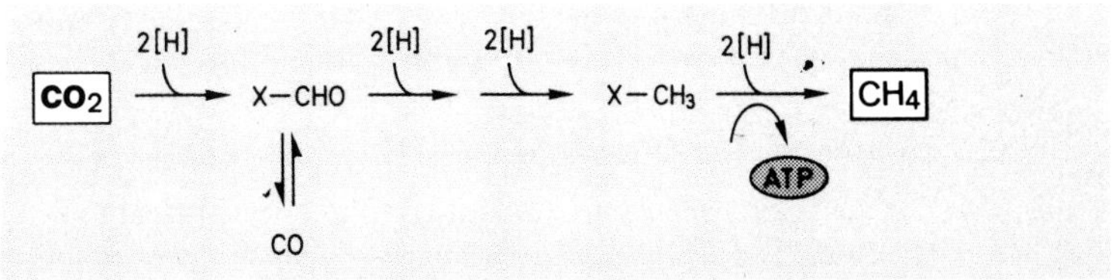

$$CO_2 \xrightarrow{2[H]} X—CHO \xrightarrow{2[H]} \xrightarrow{2[H]} X—CH_3 \xrightarrow{2[H]} CH_4$$

CO

ATP

Very little is yet known about the enzymes involved in the individual reactions, and the mechanisms of ATP regeneration are also still unsettled. Only the last step in the formation of methane has the thermo-

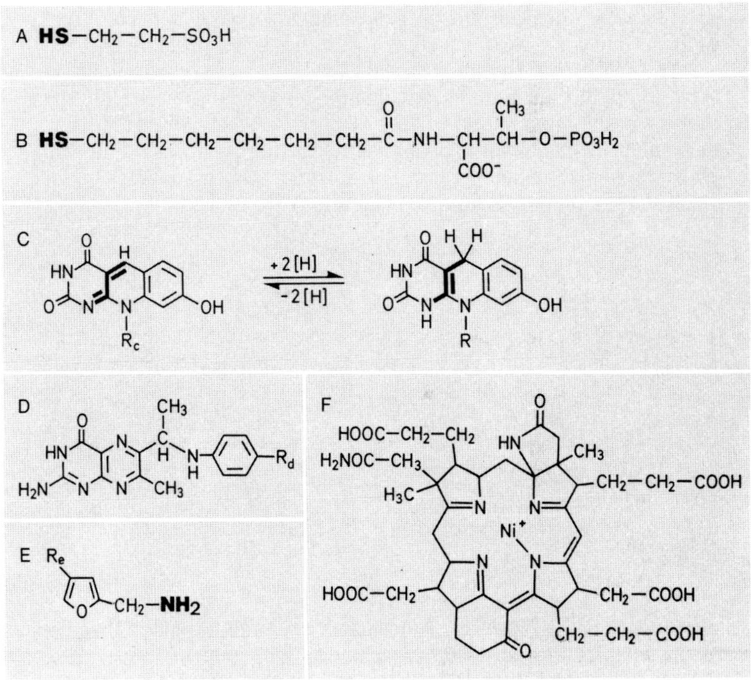

A $HS—CH_2—CH_2—SO_3H$

B $HS—CH_2—CH_2—CH_2—CH_2—CH_2—CH_2—\overset{O}{\overset{\|}{C}}—NH—CH—\overset{CH_3}{\overset{|}{CH}}—O—PO_3H_2$
$\overset{|}{COO^-}$

C

$\xrightarrow[-2[H]]{+2[H]}$

D

E R_e
$CH_2—NH_2$

F

Fig. 9.7. *Coenzymes and prosthetic groups of methanogenic bacteria.*

(a) Coenzyme M; (b) HS-HTP;
(c) F_{420} (deazariboflavine derivative);
(d) methanopterin; (e) methanofuran;
(f) factor F_{430} (after dissociation of methyl-coenzyme M methyl-

reductase). The reactive groups of the compounds (d) and (f) are not indicated. R_{a-e}, various side chains consisting of several components.

dynamic potential for the regeneration of ATP. Experiments with *Methanosarcina barkeri*, which can produce methane from methanol and hydrogen,

$$CH_3OH + H_2 \rightarrow CH_4 + H_2O$$

have yielded some clear-cut results. Addition of both substrates to bacterial suspension leads to proton extrusion, methane formation, and regeneration of ATP. The enzyme methyl transferase converts methanol directly to methyl-coenzyme M, which is reduced with the liberation of methane:

$$CH_3–S–CoM + H_2 \rightarrow CH_4 + HS–CoM$$

The reducing enzyme methyl-coenzyme M methyl reductase is a multienzyme complex which contains, besides other proteins, F_{420}, F_{430}, and hydrogenase. Most probably the reaction is accompanied by the extrusion of protons from the cell, and the resulting proton potential can then drive the regeneration of ATP. Generalising from these results, it seems that the methanogenic bacteria regenerate ATP not by substrate phosphorylation, but by electron-transport phosphorylation under anaerobic conditions (anaerobic respiration).

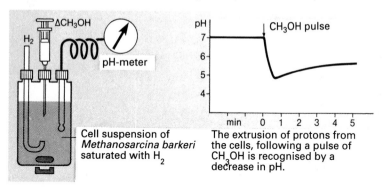

Cell suspension of *Methanosarcina barkeri* saturated with H_2

The extrusion of protons from the cells, following a pulse of CH_3OH is recognised by a decrease in pH.

Biochemistry of carbon dioxide assimilation. The autotrophic CO_2 fixation of the methanogenic bacteria (in common with that of the sulphate-reducing (Section 9.2) and the acetogenic (Section 9.5), anaerobic, hydrogen-utilising bacteria) does not involve the reactions of the ribulose-bisphosphate cycle. Rather, the synthesis of cell material from carbon dioxide proceeds via acetyl-CoA and pyruvate. The reactions involved in this have been demonstrated in experiments with radioactive compounds and by enzyme studies on *Methanobacterium thermo-*

acetotrophicum; the mechanisms are still under intensive study: carbon dioxide is reduced to the level of methanol (in bound form). A second molecule of CO_2 is reduced to carbon monoxide by a carbon monoxide dehydrogenase. The reducing equivalents are provided via activation of H_2 by hydrogenases and transferred by enzymes that react with factor F_{420} or NADP. The carboxylation of methyl-X leads to acetyl-X, and the reductive carboxylation of acetyl-CoA by pyruvate synthase leads to pyruvate, from which cell materials can be synthesised via known pathways.

Applications. Digestion tanks for the degradation of organic materials in sewage treatment are a normal part of communal water purification. In the industrial countries fermentation processes (of sediments) are used to stabilise primary sediments and those sediments precipitated from aerobic processes of waste water purification. The methane produced in this process is partly used and partly flared. In agriculture, 'bio-gas' fermenters or 'rotting pits' are used to ferment animal excreta together with cellulose-containing wastes. The bio-gas process has the advantage that, on the one hand, the nitrogen contained in animal excreta (and hence its fertiliser potential) is preserved in the rotting sediment, and on the other hand, the 'bio-gas' methane that is formed can be used as an energy source for agricultural and domestic purposes.

9.5   The formation of acetate by reduction of carbonate

In several habitats where methane is produced, acetate is also formed. Bacteria probably contribute to the acidification in digestion tanks of sewage treatment plants by metabolising carbon dioxide and molecular hydrogen according to the following equation:

$$4\,H_2 + 2\,CO_2 \rightarrow CH_3\text{--}COOH + 2\,H_2O;$$
$$\Delta G_0' = -111 \text{ kJ/mol } (-26.6 \text{ kcal/mol})$$

Some organisms that can grow autotrophically with H_2 and CO_2 have been isolated from rotting sediments and freshwater and marine muds by enrichment in a medium containing only the necessary inorganic salts and vitamins and gassing with CO_2 and H_2. They are gram-positive rods such as *Clostridium aceticum, C. thermoaceticum* and *Acetobacterium woodii* (Ch. 8.6). The acetogenic bacteria should be regarded as anaerobic, hydrogen-oxidising chemolithoautotrophs that derive their metabolic energy from a kind of anaerobic respiration, a 'carbonate respiration'. They synthesise their cell material via acetyl-CoA and pyruvate. During this assimilatory acetate synthesis, carbon dioxide is reduced to methyl-FH_4 via formate with tetrahydrofolate as coenzyme. The subsequent reactions are probably similar to the pathways of acetate synthesis by *Methanobacterium thermoacetotrophicum*. The reductive carboxylation of acetyl-CoA produces pyruvate from which cell substance can be synthesised by the usual pathways.

During growth on carbon dioxide and hydrogen, the carbonate-respiring organisms excrete large quantities of acetate. It is assumed that the synthesis of acetate proceeds via the assimilatory pathway and that the energy-rich bond of acetyl-CoA is used for ATP regeneration. The various reactions and their occurrence in different organisms have not yet been fully established.

Some extremely thermophilic and strictly anaerobic eubacteria, which were recently isolated from hot springs, can grow in mineral media under an atmosphere of pure carbon monoxide. They generate molecular hydrogen and carbon dioxide as the only metabolic products and are assumed to synthesise their cellular substance via the reductive acetyl-CoA pathway.

9.6   The formation of succinate by reduction of fumarate

Succinate has been mentioned a number of times already as a fermentation product. It has not been noted, however, that the formation of succinate can be coupled with an electron-transport phosphorylation. Succinate is the product of fumarate reduction.

$$2\,[H] + \text{fumarate} \rightarrow \text{succinate}$$

The function of fumarate can extend beyond that of a mere acceptor for the reducing equivalents ($NADH_2$) produced during the initial stages of hexose catabolism. It has a relatively high redox potential (E_4' of

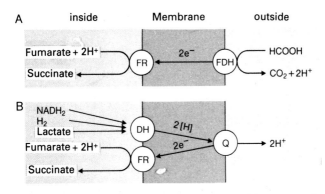

Fig. 9.8. *The electrons required for the reduction of fumarate reductase (FR) can be supplied (a) via the oxidation of formate by formate dehydrogenase (FDH) to CO_2, or (b) via the oxidation of $NADH_2$, H_2 or lactate by the corresponding dehydrogenases (DH). Both reactions lead to the formation of a proton potential across the cytoplasmic membrane and thus allow electron transport phosphorylation.*

fumarate/succinate, -30 mV). It can therefore accept electrons that are supplied by hydrogen-transferring coenzymes and that have already passed through a portion of the electron-transport chain. Fumarate reduction (by a suitable carrier) can allow electron-transport phosphorylation, and such electron-transport phosphorylation with fumarate as the final electron acceptor can therefore be classified as anaerobic respiration, called fumarate respiration (Fig. 9.8).

In fact, 'fumarate respiration' is widely distributed among chemo-organotrophic anaerobic bacteria. The addition of fumarate to nutrient media produces faster growth and higher cell yields in many bacteria. This indicates that fumarate affords effective regeneration of ATP. Such observations have been made with enterobacteria (*Escherichia, Proteus, Salmonella, Klebsiella*) and with *Bacteroides, Propionibacterium* and *Vibrio succinogenes* (see Fig. 8.8 with *R. albus*). Whilst fumarate can be supplied exogenously as a terminal electron acceptor under anaerobic conditions, it can also be formed endogenously from carbohydrates and many other substrates, via oxaloacetate and malate (Fig. 7.13).

> The localisation of fumarate reductase in the cell accords with its function in electron transport; the enzyme is membrane bound. The reduction of fumarate is a proton-consuming process. The idea that fumarate reduction is coupled to the production of a proton potential (positive on the outside) demands that the enzyme is localised on the inner membrane

surface. This is most probably the case. Measurements have shown that the reduction of one mol of fumarate regenerates about one mol of ATP.

It may also be assumed that most of the fermentations that are accompanied by formation of succinate involve the participation of fumarate reductase and, hence, an additional gain of ATP.

As mentioned above, fumarate reductase takes part in many fermentation processes; for example, the formation of succinate by *E. coli* and the formation of propionate by *Propionibacterium*. However, the importance of fumarate respiration is not limited to prokaryotes. There are several facultative worms (*Ascaris lumbricoides, Fasciola hepatica, Trichuris vulpis, Arenicola marina*) that can live under anaerobic conditions. These organisms excrete succinate and propionate. The formation of propionate is via the methylmalonyl-CoA pathway (Fig. 8.3). It seems that the formation of succinate and propionate in lower animals plays a similar role to lactate fermentation in mammalian muscle. These fermentations and 'fumarate respiration' allow a modest energy gain even in strictly aerobic organisms, thus conferring tolerance towards transient periods of anoxia.

9.7   Reduction of iron(III) to iron(II) ions

Mixed cultures of soil bacteria can reduce iron(III) to iron(II) ions. If, in addition to the iron(III) ions, nitrate or nitrite ions are also present, they are reduced to nitrite and molecular nitrogen (denitrification) before reduction of the iron(III) ions. It is assumed that nitrate reductase A transfers the electrons to iron(III). Since nitrate reduction is coupled to electron-transport phosphorylation, it seems possible that the reduction of iron(III) also allows anaerobic respiration. The redox potential E_0' of + 770 mV for Fe(III)/Fe(II) makes the reaction thermodynamically feasible. Indeed, a bacterium that carries out dissimilatory iron reduction has recently been discovered. In the absence of oxygen, this strain of *Alteromonas*, GS-15, uses acetate as carbon source and H-donor, and Fe(III) as H-acceptor. During the reduction of ferric iron by acetate a mixture of Fe^{2+} and Fe^{3+} is formed which is transformed to the oxide Fe_3O_4 (= magnetite) which is strongly ferromagnetic. The metabolic products of these iron-reducing organisms can therefore be detected with a magnet! Since iron(III) oxide is practically insoluble and must be converted to a soluble and cell-permeable form, probably by siderophores, growth under these conditions is very slow and scant.

10 Incomplete oxidations and microbial biotechnology

Most aerobic microorganisms oxidise their organic nutrients to carbon dioxide and water via their respiratory metabolism. Since the carbon in carbon dioxide is in its most oxidised form, this type of metabolism is referred to as 'complete oxidation'. In contrast to the classical fermentations which occur under anaerobic conditions (see Chapter 8), fermentations that can proceed in the presence of oxygen are known as 'oxidative fermentations' or **incomplete oxidations**. The end products of these processes include acetate, gluconate, ketoacids, oxyacids, fumarate, citrate, glutamate, lactate, etc.

In the last 50 years the number of such microbial products obtained under aerobic conditions has greatly increased, and most industrial fermentations nowadays are aerobic. This chapter, therefore, deals not only with 'aerobic fermentations' in the strict sense, but also with microorganisms and processes which are employed in industrial microbiology, nowadays referred to as **Microbial Biotechnology**. (Processes which have been described already in Chapter 8 are not repeated.) The new designation, 'microbial biotechnology' indicates a novel meaning. The microorganisms formerly used in industrial processes were either natural strains, or those selected after mutations. However, at present and increasingly in the future, microorganisms can be used which have been altered in much more profound ways as a consequence of the new developments in biochemistry and molecular genetics. The methods of **gene technology** (see Ch. 15.3.6 and 16) enable new metabolites, secondary products and foreign proteins (insulin, somatostatin, etc.) to be produced in microorganisms.

10.1 Acetic acid formation and acetic acid bacteria

The acetic acid bacteria share the ability to form acids by incomplete oxidation of sugars or alcohols and to excrete these acids, either transiently or into the medium as non-utilisable end products. Acetic acid bacteria include gram-negative rods with limited motility by virtue of peritrichous

357

(*Acetobacter*) or polar (*Gluonobacter*, formerly *Acetomonas*) flagellation. They resemble the pseudomonads but are distinguishable by their high acid tolerance, low peptolytic activity, limited motility, and lack of coloured pigments. The natural habitats of acetic acid bacteria are plants. Wherever sugar-containing sap or secretions occur, acetic acid bacteria can be found in association with yeasts.

The question of whether a given bacterium belongs to the peroxidans group, which accumulates acetate only transiently, or to the suboxidans group, which cannot metabolise acetate any further, can be determined by simple experiments. The organism can be grown on a milky (turbid) 'chalk agar' (ethanol–yeast extract plus calcium carbonate) medium. Acid secretion by growing colonies produces a clear circular zone by dissolving the calcium carbonate. Whereas this clear zone is permanent for the suboxidans group, for the peroxidans varieties the eventual further oxidation of the acetate leads to renewed turbidity by reprecipitation of the calcium carbonate. The peroxidans group includes *Acetobacter aceti* and *A. pasteurianum*. *Gluconobacter oxydans* is the prototype of the suboxidans group. Between these is a spectrum of intermediate types. *Acetobacter xylinum*, *A. aceti* and *A. acidophilum* oxidise acetate very slowly. Most acetic acid bacteria require complex nutrient media.

Acetic acid bacteria oxidise primary alcohols to the corresponding fatty acids:

$$CH_3-CH_2OH \rightarrow CH_3-COOH$$
$$CH_3-CH_2-CH_2OH \rightarrow CH_3-CH_3-COOH$$

They oxidise secondary alcohols to ketones:

$$CH_3-CHOH-CH_3 \rightarrow CH_3-CO-CH_3$$
$$CH_2OH-CHOH-CH_2OH \rightarrow CH_2OH-CO-CH_2OH$$

Sugar alcohols are oxidised to aldoses and ketoses, for example, sorbitol to sorbose. This oxidation is of great practical importance as a partial reaction in the preparative pathway from glucose to ascorbic acid. D-sorbitol is available by electrolytic reduction of glucose, and *Gluconobacter oxydans* can convert sorbitol, from solutions containing up to 30%, to sorbose, with approximately 90% yield. Glycerol, tetritols, pentitols, hexitols and heptitols can also be oxidised in an analogous manner; for example, D-mannitol to D-fructose.

D-Sorbitol   D-Sorbose   L-ascorbic acid

Aldehydes, aldoses and ketoses are oxidised to their respective acids, for example:

$$\text{glycolaldehyde} \rightarrow \text{glycollate}$$
$$\text{L-xylose} \rightarrow \text{L-xylonate}$$
$$\text{D-glucose} \rightarrow \text{D-gluconate}$$
$$\text{D-gluconate} \rightarrow \text{ketogluconates}$$

Various strains of acetic acid bacteria differ by their ability to form either 2- or 5-ketogluconate. *Gluconobacter melanogenum* produces 2,5-diketogluconate via 2-ketogluconate. This diketo acid, which is unstable at pH 4.5, is thought to be responsible for the black-brown coloration of *G. melanogenum* (hence the name) colonies on glucose agar.

Technology of vinegar production. The production of vinegar from wine is largely a problem of aeration technology (see Ch. 6.2). The technical processes all aim at bringing the bacteria and the liquids to be oxidised into intimate contact with atmospheric oxygen. Three types of procedures are distinguished by their aeration techniques: the traditional Orleans process or surface procedure, the chaining procedure, and submerged fermentations. The surface procedure is very ancient and has been standardised as the 'Orleans method'. If wine is exposed in flat dishes or fermentation vats and allowed to be 'inoculated' by *Drosophila*, a pellicle is formed on the surface, called **micoderma aceti**, which consists of cells of *Acetobacter xylinum* which are immobilised by cellulose fibrils. The acidification is very slow, but the process can be used on a domestic scale. The term 'chaining procedure' comprises those processes in which the bacteria are attached (chained) to a solid carrier material (grape stalks, husks), in casks that are frequently moved and aerated. In the 'rapid acidification' process the alcoholic liquid is repeatedly trickled through tanks that are filled with beechwood shavings. These columns of immobilised bacteria are aerated from below. This process has the advantage that the resulting vinegar is suitable for domestic consumption with hardly any further filtration because the bacteria are immobilised. Some columns have been in use for 50 years, and are still productive. However, these traditional procedures are increasingly being replaced by submerged fermentations. In these, fermenters are used which allow aeration and heat dissipation.

Biochemistry of acetic acid formation. *Acetobacter* and *Gluconobacter* produce alcohol dehydrogenase, glucose dehydrogenase, and other polyol dehydrogenases, which contain a recently discovered prosthetic group, methoxatine or pyrrolquinoline quinone (PQQ). The enzymes are localised on the outer surface of the cytoplasmic membrane and catalyse the oxidation of ethanol, glycerol, or glucose to the respective acids (acetic, glyceric, and gluconic acids). In these reactions, the electrons are fed into the electron-transport chain, and the protons are extruded into the periplasmic space. Methoxatine can also reach the nutrient medium and can be found in vinegar.

10.2   Production of other organic acids by fungi

Several organic acids are produced on an industrial scale by fungi. The advantages in using fungi for the production of citric, itaconic, gluconic, malic and other acids, have long been recognised. They lie largely in the ease of separating the organisms from the liquid. Whilst the separation of bacteria from liquid needs high speed centrifuges and a high energy input, yeasts and other fungi can be separated by low-cost filtration methods.

10.2.1   Physiology and biotechnology

Fungal metabolism is strictly aerobic. That does not mean that fungi are unable to break down carbohydrates anaerobically (yeast fermentations!); but under anaerobic conditions, they cannot grow for any length of time, and only ethanol and lactic acid are formed as end products. All other organic acids are excreted only under aerobic conditions.

In the natural habitat of fungi, that is in the soil, there is no significant excretion of intermediate product. In cases of nutrient shortage, fungi gain the maximum energy and cell material by complete oxidation and assimilation of substrates. The excretion of many metabolic products in the laboratory and in industrial practice is due to the excess of carbohydrates and a certain 'disorganisation of metabolism', which is often (deliberately) exacerbated by lack of trace elements in the nutrient media. The fungi are said to have a 'strong glycolytic system'. Intermediates accumulate at the bottle-necks in the reaction sequences of intermediary metabolism, and these are then excreted, either directly or after slight modification. J. W. Foster coined the term 'overflow metabolism'. Most of the 'oxidative fermentations' are probably due to disturbances in metabolic regulation.

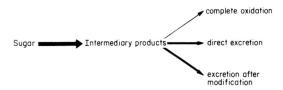

In many cases it is sufficient to exclude one trace element from the nutrient medium to induce accumulation of an intermediate product by a fungus. Zinc, iron, manganese, copper, magnesium, potassium and calcium each have notable effects (Fig. 10.1).

Lactic acid   is excreted mainly by Mucorales (*Rhizopus nodosus, R. oryzae, R. arrhizus, R. nigricans*) and other phycomycetes (*Allomyces, Saprolegnia, Blastocladiella*). It is never the only metabolic product though, as it is in the homofermentative lactic acid bacteria; apart from lactic acid, smaller amounts of fumaric, succinic, malic, formic and acetic acids, as well as ethanol, are also produced. Maximal yields of lactic acid by fungi are only reached in the presence of oxygen. Since fungi do not require complex nutrient media and can grow with urea as sole source of nitrogen, the isolation of lactic acid in practically pure form presents fewer problems than in the case of lactic acid fermentation by lactobacilli.

Fumarate production is a typical property of several genera of Mucorales (*Mucor, Cunninghamella, Circinella, Rhizopus*).

Gluconic acid is produced by many aspergilli and penicillia. Its production is due to the enzymatic oxidation of glucose by a glucose oxidase that is secreted into the medium. *Aspergillus niger* can utilise a 30–50% glucose solution, giving a high yield of gluconate provided that calcium carbonate is present to neutralise the acid.

β-D-Glucose → (Glucose-Oxidase) → Gluconolactone → (+ H_2O) → Gluconate

FAD   FADH₂

O_2 H_2O_2 → (Catalase) → H_2O + 1/2 O_2

Glucose oxidase is an enzyme which uses FAD as prosthetic group. During glucose oxidation the primary oxidation product is β-D-glucono-

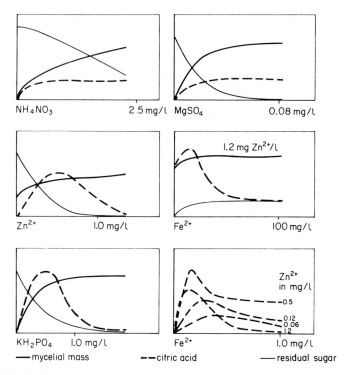

NH$_4$NO$_3$ 2.5 mg/l   MgSO$_4$ 0.08 mg/l

Zn^{2+} 1.0 mg/l   Fe^{2+} 100 mg/l

1.2 mg Zn^{2+}/l

KH$_2$PO$_4$ 1.0 mg/l   Fe^{2+} 1.0 mg/l

Zn^{2+} in mg/l
—0.5
—0.12
—0.06
—1.2

—mycelial mass   --citric acid   —residual sugar

Fig. 10.1. *Dependence of mycelial mass and amount of citric acid produced on composition of the nutrient medium, in* Aspergillus niger *grown for 9 days.*

The complete medium has the following composition (in g/l): glucose, 140; nitrogen 1.05; KH$_2$PO$_4$, 2.5; MgSO$_4$·7H$_2$O, 0.5; iron, 0.01; zinc, 0.0025; pH 3.8 (from Shu, P. & Johnson, M. J. (1948). *J. Bacteriol.* **56**, 577).

β-lactone, which either spontaneously or by a second enzyme, gluconolactonase, takes up water to yield gluconate. The reduced glucose oxidase transfers the hydrogen to atmospheric oxygen with the formation of hydrogen peroxide, which is then converted to H$_2$O and oxygen by the enzyme catalase.

Oxalic acid is excreted by many fungi. Its formation is promoted by an alkaline nutrient medium.

The formation of **citric acid** by fungi has been extensively investigated, especially with regard to the practical and economic aspects. After C. Wehmer had found citric acid in cultures of penicillia (*Citromyces pfefferianus*) in 1893, Currie (1917) laid down the basis for the industrial production of citric acid with the discovery that *Aspergillus niger* can grow abundantly in a nutrient medium with an initial pH of 2.5–3.5; while doing so, it excretes large amounts of citric acid. With increasing pH, gluconic acid and oxalic acids eventually appear. The low initial pH has the advantage that contamination of the cultures by bacteria need hardly be contemplated.

> For many years the industrial production of citric acid was carried out, without sterile precautions, in pans. Aluminium troughs ($2 \times 2.5 \times 0.15$ m) placed in fermentation chambers are filled to a height of about 8 cm with a molasses mixture, inoculated, and kept for 9–11 days at a temperature of 30 °C. The yield is high. After draining off the spent medium, fresh nutrient medium can be introduced below the mycelial mat and the process repeated. Citric acid is precipitated from the spent liquor by calcium carbonate, recrystallised, and liberated by the addition of sulphuric acid.

In the industrialised countries, citric acid production is carried out nowadays exclusively by submerged fermentation. Fermenters of 300 000–400 000 l capacity are operated aseptically. Raw sugar or hydrolysed starch are used as the substrate in places of molasses.

Citric acid production by *Aspergillus niger* depends markedly on the composition of the medium. This becomes evident when the supply of only one component is varied whilst all other conditions are held constant. Thus, when single components at known concentrations are added to nutrient medium that has been freed of trace elements by precipitation with aluminium hydroxide, the determination of mycelial mass, residual sugar, and citric acid, after inoculaion and incubation for nine days with agitation, gives a number of relationships which are shown in Fig. 10.1. The curves in the diagrammatic plots show the following: (1) Ammonium nitrate and magnesium sulphate have no specific effects on the yield of citrate; they only influence mycelial growth. (2) Typical 'optimum curves' are characteristic for the dependence of citrate production on the concentrations of zinc, iron and phosphate. When these elements allow only sub-optimal growth, the yield of citric acid is increased. At even lower concentrations, however, limitation of mycelial growth also limits the production of citric acid. (3) Particularly high yields of citrate can be obtained when the two elements iron and zinc are present in limiting amounts.

Manganese has a decidely inhibitory effect; 3 μg Mn^{2+}/l of medium are sufficient to reduce the yield. (A purified commercial glucose preparation can add 10 μg Mn^{2+}/140 g glucose to one litre of nutrient solution.) The fact that lack of iron promotes the excretion of citrate is most probably due to the function of iron as a cofactor of aconitase. Copper antagonises the effect of iron on aconitase. A new 'trick' to increase the yield of citric acid is based on this. Even with a low concentration of ferrous iron in the molasses mixture (about 10 mg/l), maximal yields can be achieved by adding excess of copper to the nutrient medium (150 mg/l).

Itaconic acid is produced by only a few strains of *Aspergillus itaconicus* and *A. terreus*. The production of itaconic acid also proceeds at pH values of about 2.0.

10.2.2 Chemistry of acid formation by fungi

There is no doubt that reactions of the tricarboxylic acid cycle play a part in the formation of the acids excreted by fungi during metabolism of glucose. It can be assumed that malate, fumarate, succinate and citrate are produced by the reactions of the tricarboxylic acid cycle and are excreted directly (Fig. 10.2).

Oxalic acid is produced from oxaloacetate by oxaloacetate hydrolase.

$$\begin{array}{c} \text{CO–COOH} \\ | \\ \text{CH}_2\text{–COOH} \end{array} + \text{H}_2\text{O} \xrightarrow{\textit{Oxaloacetate hydrolase}} \begin{array}{c} \text{HOOC–COOH} \\ + \\ \text{CH}_3\text{–COOH} \end{array}$$

The formation of **itaconic acid** starts from *cis*-aconitic acid. During the decarboxylation reaction, electrons in the carbon skeleton migrate so that the double bond moves from the 2–3 to the 3–4 position:

$$\begin{array}{c} \text{CH}_3\text{–COOH} \\ + \\ \text{CO–COOH} \\ | \\ \text{CH}_2\text{–COOH} \end{array} \longrightarrow \begin{array}{c} \text{CH}_2\text{–COOH} \\ | \\ \text{HO–C–COOH} \\ | \\ \text{CH}_2\text{–COOH} \end{array} \longrightarrow \begin{array}{c} \text{CH}_2\text{–COOH} \\ | \\ \text{C–COOH} \\ || \\ \text{CH–COOH} \end{array} \xrightarrow{\text{CO}_2} \begin{array}{c} \text{CH}_2 \\ || \\ \text{C–COOH} \\ | \\ \text{CH}_2\text{–COOH} \end{array}$$

The tricarboxylic acid cycle has a primarily catabolic function. In addition, though, it can also be viewed as a distribution cycle that supplies precursors for a great number of building blocks for the cell. However, if intermediary products are thus withdrawn at any point in the TCA cycle, other reactions will need to replenish oxaloacetate or a direct precursor. Of the two anaplerotic (replenishment) sequences (Fig. 7.7), namely, the conversion of isocitrate via glyoxylate with acetyl-CoA to malate and the carboxylation of pyruvate to oxaloacetate, the carboxylation reaction is the more important. The glyoxylate cycle serves primarily for the utilisation of acetate, long-chain fatty acids, and hydrocarbons, as well as some other substrates that are broken down via acetyl-CoA. Glucose represses the synthesis of key enzymes in the glyoxylate cycle (isocitrate lyase and malate synthase).

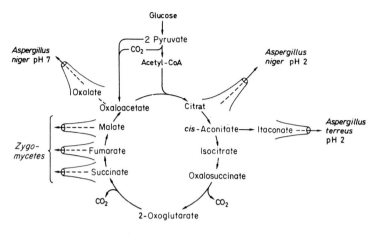

Fig. 10.2. *Production of organic acids by fungi.*

If **citric acid** were synthesised exclusively from acetyl-CoA, one mol glucose would yield only $\frac{2}{3}$ mol citrate; 100 g glucose would give only 71.1 g citrate. However, yields of 75–87 g citrate/100 g glucose can be achieved on occasions. Investigations have shown that large amounts of carbon dioxide are fixed. Added $^{14}CO_2$ is found in C-6 of citric acid. The metabolism of glucose to citric acid can therefore be represented by the following scheme:

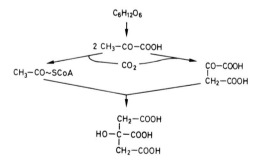

10.3   Production of amino acids

The discovery of *Corynebacterium glutamicum* by Kinoshita (1957) opened up a new era in the development of industrially useful incomplete oxidation processes. A bacterium excreting L-glutamic acid was isolated by a simple screening technique, a 'bioautography' method. In this method, a large number of soil bacteria are transferred by replica plating (see Ch. 15.1.1) to a number of different nutrient media, allowed to grow up, and then killed by UV irradiation. The plates are then overlaid with a basal medium containing a bacterial strain requiring glutamic acid. After suitable incubation this indicator strain shows which of the original colonies excreted glutamic acid.

> L-glutamate is only produced under strictly aerobic conditions. In fermenters of 50 m^3 capacity containing a nutrient solution with urea as sole source of nitrogen and 10% glucose, incubation (of the above organism) for 40 hours at 30 °C led to the accumulation of 50 g L-glutamic acid. This is a yield of 0.6 mol glutamate/mol glucose.

The degradation of glucose apparently proceeds via the fructose-bisphosphate pathway and then via citrate and 2-oxoglutarate to L-glutamate. Carboxylation of pyruvate, as in the production of citrate by *Aspergillus niger*, is the main route for the provision of oxaloacetate, rather than the glyoxylate cycle. $^{14}CO_2$ added to the nutrient medium is found almost exclusively in the α-carboxyl group of glutamic acid. Excretion apparently depends on an accumulation of 2-oxoglutarate due to a deficiency in 2-oxoglutarate dehydrogenase. In the absence of ammonium, the 2-oxoglutarate is excreted. In the industrial production of glutamate, acetate has recently been substituted for glucose as the substrate.

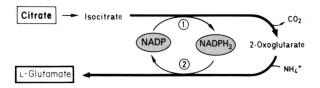

The glutamic acid-secreting strains of *Corynebacterium glutamicum* and *Brevibacterium divaricatum* require biotin. The concentration of biotin is very important for the accumulation of acid: 2.5 μg biotin/l of nutrient solution is optimal. At lower concentrations of biotin, growth is inhibited; higher biotin concentrations increased growth, but decreased the yield of glutamic acid (Fig. 10.3).

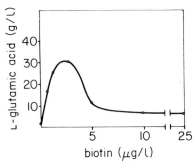

Fig. 10.3. *Formation of L-glutamic acid by* Corynebacterium glutamicum *in relation to the biotin concentration in the nutrient medium.*

(From Huang, H. T. (1964). *Progr. industr. Microbiol.* **5**, 57).

Auxotrophic mutants can be used for the production of other amino acids. Homoserine-requiring mutants may excrete 20 g L-lysine/l of medium, under suitable conditions. Other mutants of *C. glutamicum*, as well as enterobacteria and pseudomonads, produce L-homoserine, L-valine, L-isoleucine, L-tryptophan, L-tyrosine, and other amino acids.

Processes for the production of inosinic acid and guanylic acid have been developed in Japan. These 5'-nucleotides are used as spices and flavouring agents.

10.4   Interconversions of products by microorganisms

The high specificity and yields of oxidations carried out by acetic acid bacteria, and the economic benefits of these, especially in the production of sorbose, has led to intensive investigations, during the last 50 years into the catalytic properties of microorganisms. Catalytic reactions that could be useful in the conversion of natural materials to desired products, and also those reactions that involved substances extraneous to the organisms, were looked for.

Microorganisms carry out highly specific reactions on a host of substances; such reactions include oxidations, hydrogenations, hydrolyses, esterifications, methylations, decarboxylations, aminations and deaminations, dehydrations, and many other kinds of reactions. These abilities are found in actinomycetes and other bacteria, as well as in lower and higher fungi. The microbial synthesis of steroids has been one of the outstanding success stories. The chemical synthesis of cortisol and hydrocortisone comprises more than 30 steps, and the yield is poor. By using microorganisms, the process has been reduced to 13 steps. One of the most difficult reactions in the synthesis is the introduction of the hydroxy group in position 11 of the steroid skeleton. This can be carried out by the lower fungi (*Rhizopus arrhizus, Curvularia lunata,*

Cunninghamella blackesleeana) and *Streptomyces fradiae*. The conversion of Reichstein's compound S to hydrocortisone is shown below as a classic example of a specific oxygenation.

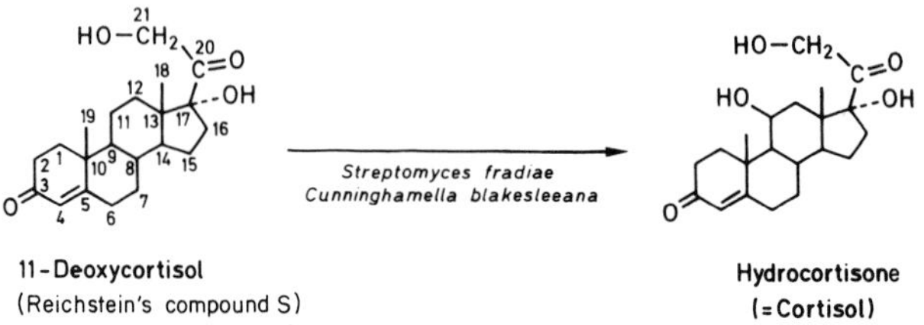

11–Deoxycortisol
(Reichstein's compound S)

Hydrocortisone
(=Cortisol)

Apart from this oxygenation, many fungi can carry out hydroxylations at almost all sites in the steroid molecule by means of stereospecific oxygenases.

Other microbial enzyme reactions concern dehydrogenation of alcoholic hydroxy groups, introduction of double bonds, reduction of keto and oxo groups, etc.

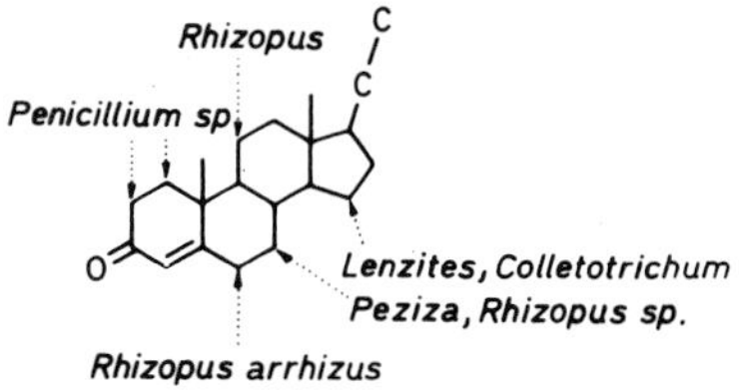

The synthesis of phenylacetyl carbinol can be cited as an example of an **addition reaction**. This compound is an important intermediate in the synthesis of ephedrine. Benzaldehyde is added to a fermenting yeast culture where it is apparently acylated, analogous to the formation of acetoin, by the transfer of 'active acetaldehyde' (Fig. 7.6, 2) to the benzaldehyde.

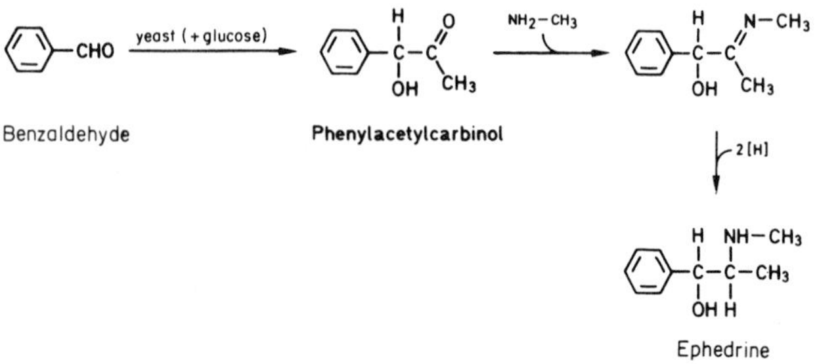

Benzaldehyde

Phenylacetylcarbinol

Ephedrine

The subsequent conversions of the phenylacetyl carbinol so formed are purely chemical.

benzaldehyde $\xrightarrow{\text{microbial}}$ phenylacetyl carbinol $\xrightarrow{\text{chemical}}$ ephedrine

The production of 6-aminopenicillanic acid can serve as an example of a specifically directed enzymatic cleavage of a substance with the aid of microorganisms. Several fungi and bacteria contain specific acylases that can hydrolyse natural penicillins to 6-aminopenicillanic acid, which is the starting material for semi-synthetic penicillins.

Benzylpenicillin (Penicillin G)

6-Aminopenicillanic acid

10.5   Production of antibiotics

Many microorganisms and plants excrete products that are not related to the basic metabolism of the producing organism; these products are called secondary metabolites. Bacteria and fungi produce a host of substances termed 'secondary metabolites'. Many of these substances play important roles as therapeutics, stimulants, feed additives, etc. and consequently, microorganisms have gained great economic importance. The discovery of penicillin and other antibiotics has opened up a wide new area for industrial microbiology. The discovery and investigation of antibiotics and the development of semi-synthetic derivatives of antibiotics have been of immense benefit in therapeutic medicine. There are practically no limits to new discoveries, modifications, and applications of secondary metabolites from microorganisms. Further opportunities for discovery and application of secondary metabolites are provided by the selection of mutants bearing alterations in metabolic regulation mechanisms (Chapter 16).

10.5.1   Organisms and discovery

Symbiotic as well as antagonistic relations between microorganisms have been known since the nineteenth century. The starting point for the elucidation of the principles concerned in antibiosis was the observation by A. Fleming (1928) that a fungal colony (*Penicillum notatum*) inhibited the growth of staphylococci. The compound excreted by this

Penicillium could diffuse in the agar and was named penicillin. Since then a great many compounds with antibiotic actions have been isolated. **Antibiotics** are defined as substances of biological origin which, at low concentrations, can inhibit the growth of microorganisms. A distinction has been made between the growth-inhibitory action (bacteriostatic effect) and a so-called 'killing' action (bactericidal effect) that results in a reduction in viable counts.

Microorganisms that produce antibiotics.   The ability to produce antibiotics has been found mainly in fungi of the group Aspergillales, in actinomycetes, and in a few other bacteria. The streptomycetes are remarkable for the chemical diversity of antibiotics that they produce. Altogether about 2000 antibiotics have been characterised so far; but only about 50 are used therapeutically. The total number of antibiotics that have been described is greater than 2000 and several groups of microorganisms, among them bacteria that are difficult to cultivate and some of the lower fungi, have not been tested yet for antibiotic production.

The significance of antibiotics for the producing organisms.   The significance of antibiotics for the producing organisms in their soil habitat is almost completely unknown. Antibiotics are generally produced by special synthetic pathways, which are included in what is known as secondary metabolism.   Secondary   metabolites   are   produced   by   synthetic mechanisms and enzymes that are not essential for the growth and maintenance of the cell. Hence, the genetic apparatus for the synthesis of antibiotics would appear to be a burden to the organism, and it is expected that such a burden would be eliminated during evolution. Proceeding from the premise, therefore, that only useful features are conserved, antibiotics must confer some advantages to their producers in their natural habitat, perhaps by favouring them in competition for limited substrates. However, such antagonistic relationships are almost impossible to demonstrate in the soil since the actual amounts of antibiotics produced are very small and, in many cases, are even growth-inhibitory for the producing organisms.

Gradually, the concept that during evolution some useless genetic material is sometimes carried along, even if it seems to represent a burden to the organism under the experimental conditions available, is coming to be accepted. Perhaps nature is somewhat more conservative than was assumed in the early period of molecular biology. Presently, antibiotics and other secondary metabolites, whose immediate usefulness to the producing organisms is not discernable, tend to be counted among the products 'made on the playground of metabolism' or the 'wood-

Fig. 10.4. *The excretion of antibiotics by bacteria or fungi is demonstrated by inhibitory zones on agar plates, evenly inoculated with indicator bacteria* Staphylococcus aureus.

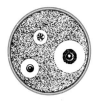

shavings (by-products) of metabolism'. However, such products show that even the secondary metabolism of bacteria, fungi, and plants can be fruitful subjects for research aimed at understanding the evolution of microorganisms.

Demonstration of antibiotic production. The first antibiotics were discovered more or less by chance because of the production of inhibition zones in the growth of target organisms. Thus, on a nutrient agar plate densely inoculated with a test organism (indicator strain), growth was suppressed in the vicinity of the fungal or streptomycete colony. The antibiotic, diffusing from the producing organism into the agar, caused the appearance of a **zone of inhibition** in the confluent growth of the bacterial test strain (Fig. 10.4). A number of representative microorganisms are used as test organisms. Qualitative demonstration of an antibiotic producer can be carried out by inoculating it in the centre of a suitable nutrient agar plate, and then applying a series of indicator strains in radiating lines from the centre (Fig. 10.5). After suitable incubation, determination of inhibition lines for the various indicator strains gives evidence of the action spectrum for the antibiotic. Antibiotics differ in characteristic ways in their effectiveness against gram-positive and gram-negative bacteria, yeasts, dermatophytes and other microorganisms.

Most antibiotics have been discovered in the course of screening programmes. The stages of such a procedure, from inoculation of the original soil sample to animal experiments, are shown in Fig. 10.6.

Quantitative determinations. Methods used for the quantitative estimation of antibiotic potency include the plate diffusion test (Fig. 10.7), the serial dilution test (less accurate), as well as others. For the plate **diffusion test**, plates are filled with an appropriate agar medium containing the test organism (as an inoculum) to a precise height (level). After the agar has set, the antibiotic solutions to be tested are applied to the agar surface, by pipetting either into a pattern of holes stamped in the agar or into glass or metal cylinders on top of the agar. A third method employs filter paper discs that have adsorbed the antibiotic solutions. In a positive reaction, zones of inhibition appear after suitable incubation; the diameter of a zone is proportional to the logarithm of the antibiotic

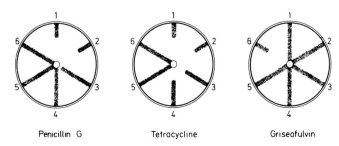

Penicillin G   Tetracycline   Griseofulvin

Fig. 10.5. *Streak test to survey the action spectra of three antibiotics.*

(1) *Staphylococcus aureus*; (2) *Streptococcus*; (3) *Escherichia coli*; (4) *Pseudomonas aeruginosa*; (5) *Candida albicans*; (6) *Trichophyton rubrum*. A filter disc containing 10 μg of the antibiotic under test is placed in the middle of a peptonecasein hydrolysate agar plate. Suspensions of the test organisms (1) to (6) were streaked out radially. Some of the organisms did not grow in the diffusion zone of the antibiotics. (From Wallhäusser, K. H. & Schmidt, H. (1967). *Sterilisation, disinfection, conservation, chemotherapy.* Stuttgart: Thieme.)

concentration, provided all relevant conditions are controlled, i.e. composition of the medium, thickness of the agar layer, concentration of the test organism in the inoculum, incubation time and temperature, etc. (Fig. 10.7).

In the **serial dilution test** the antibiotic to be tested is diluted in a 1:2 series in the inoculated nutrient solution, which is then incubated. At the end of a suitable incubation period, the minimum dilution at which no growth has occurred is recorded as the 'minimal inhibitory concentration' of the antibiotic (against the particular test organism).

Various other methods have been developed to determine synergistic or antagonistic effects of various substances and to test for effectiveness against other organisms (i.e. protozoa, algae, worms, tissue culture cells, viruses, etc.).

10.5.2   Some therapeutically important antibiotics

Only a few of the therapeutically useful antibiotics will be discussed here. The first place is still occupied by **penicillin** (a β-lactam), which is produced by *Penicillium notatum, P. chrysogenum*, and a few other fungi, especially since the introduction of the semi-synthetic penicillins. These are made by splitting the molecule with penicillin acylase and adding one of a series of other side chains to the resulting 6-aminopenicillanic

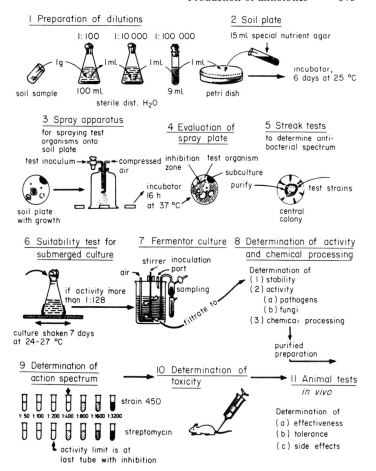

Fig. 10.6. *Work schedule of an antibiotic-screening programme.*
(From Wallhäuser, K. H. & Schmidt, H. (1967). *Sterilisation, disinfection, conservation, chemotherapy.* Stuttgart: Thieme.)

acid (Fig. 10.8). The target reaction of penicillin in bacterial metabolism has already been discussed (Ch. 2.2.4). Penicillin is practically non-toxic to humans, except for a small percentage of those treated who develop allergic reactions. Many bacteria can produce the enzyme penicillinase (β-lactamase), which cleaves the β-lactam ring of penicillin and renders

Fig. 10.7. Plate diffusion test for the quantitative determination of an antibiotic.

The filter discs applied to the agar surface contain different quantities of the antibiotic. The diameter of the inhibition zone is a measure of the antibiotic concentration. (From Zähner, H. (1965). *Biologie der Antibiotica.* Berlin: Springer.)

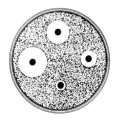

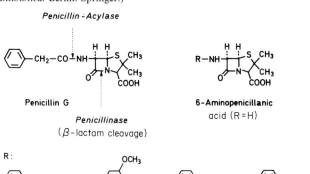

Fig. 10.8. *Target sites for the bacterial enzymes penicillinase and penicillin acylase in the molecule of penicillin G.*

The semisynthetic penicillins phenethicillin, methicillin, ampicillin and carbenicillin are prepared by reaction of 6-aminopenicillanic acid (substituent R) with the chlorides of the acidic groups indicated.

it ineffective. Many of the semisynthetic penicillins, which are produced by combination of 6-aminopenicillanic acid with various acid chlorides to give a large number of derivatives, are not attacked by penicillinase. In addition, most are sufficiently acid stable to be administered orally.

The **cephalosporins** are excreted by a species of the fungus *Cephalosporium*. Cephalosporin C contains a β-lactam ring and is similar to penicillin; it is included in the β-lactam group of antibiotics (Fig. 10.9). Several semisynthetic cephalosporins (e.g. cephalothin, cephaloridin) are produced by substitution of 7-aminocephalosporamic acid, obtained from cephalosporin, with various side chains. These semisynthetic cephalosporins resemble the semisynthetic penicillins in their action.

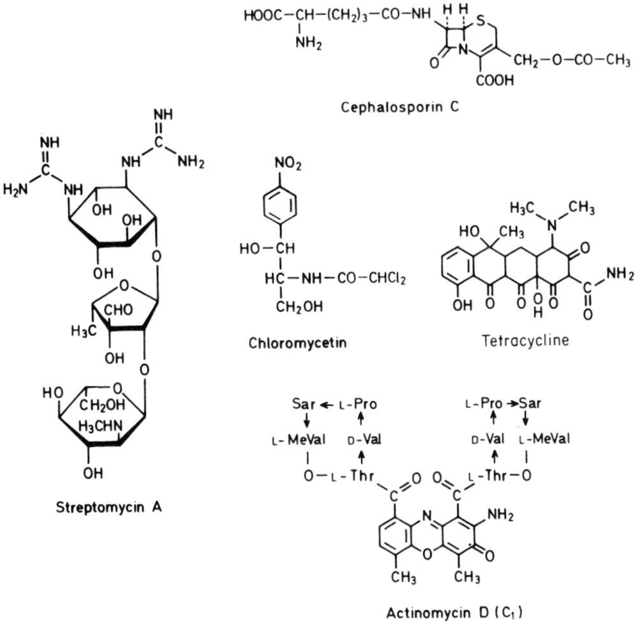

Fig. 10.9. *Structural formulae of cephalosporin C, streptomycin A, chloromycetin (chloramphenicol), tetracycline, and actinomycin D (actinomycin C_1).*
L-thr, L-threonine; D-val, D-valine;
L-pro, L-proline; Sar, sarcosine;
L-MeVal, *N*-methyl-L-valine.

Streptomycin was isolated from the culture medium of *Streptomyces griseus* and is also produced by other species of *Streptomyces*. It consists of three groups: *N*-methyl-L-2-glucosamine, a methyl pentose, and an inositol derivative with two guanidyl residues (Fig. 10.9). Streptomycin achieved its clinical success because it was effective against a series of acid-fast and gram-negative bacteria that were not sensitive to penicillin. It can give rise to quite marked allergic side reactions in humans. Streptomycin is also used in veterinary medicine and against plant infections.

Chloromycetin (chloramphicol) was first discovered in cultures of *Streptomyces venezuelae*, but it is also produced synthetically (Fig. 10.9). It is very stable and effective against many gram-negative bacteria, spiorchaetes, rickettsiae, actinomycetes and large viruses.

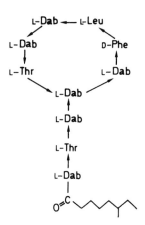

Fig. 10.10. *Polymyxin B.*

L-Dab, 2,4-diaminobutyric acid; L-
leu, L-leucine; D-Phe,
D-phenylalanine; L-Thr, L-threonine;
the aliphatic side chain is the 6-
methyloctanoic acid.

The **tetracyclines** are excreted by a number of streptomycetes, including *Streptomyces aureofaciens*. They are closely related chemically, being
derived from a naphthacene skeleton. The best known are chlortetracycline
(aureomycin), oxytetracycline (terramycine), and tetracycline. They have
a wide spread spectrum of effectiveness and are well tolerated by
humans.

The **macrolide** antibiotics (erythromycin, carbomycin A, picromycin,
etc.) are of diverse origin and have a relatively high molecular weight,
being characterised by the presence of a macrocyclic lactone ring.

Actinomycin was isolated in 1940 as the first of the antibiotics produced by streptomycetes. **Actinomycin** is actually a mixture of several
compounds, all of which contain a phenoxazone chromophore, but all
are substituted with different polypeptide chains (Fig. 10.9).

The last group to be mentioned is that of the **polypeptide antibiotics**
(gramicidin S, polymyxins, bacitracin, ristocetin, etc.). Polymyxin B consists of a ring of seven amino acids, with a side chain attached by a
peptide bond (Fig. 10.10). The polypeptide antibiotics have a high affinity for the cytoplasmic membrane and are therefore toxic for bacteria as
well as for eukaryotes; this characteristic makes their clinical usefulness
very restricted. Some of the polypeptide antibiotics are used in research
as ionophores because of their capacity for selective ion transport through

biological membranes (Ch. 7.7). **Valinomycin**, for example, promotes the transport of potassium through membranes. Valinomycin consists of a 12-membered ring containing valine and 2-hydroxyisovalerate; its configuration is such that the K^+ ion fits into the inside of the molecule. Because of its valine and isovalerate content, the valinomycin–K^+ complex is lipophilic on its exterior surface and, hence, easily transported through the membrane lipid layer. Addition of valinomycin to a cell suspension therefore leads to a loss of potassium ions.

The pharmaceutical industry engaged in the 'high technology' production of antibiotics never uses the original organisms, but mutants that produce much higher yields. Fleming's mould produced about 3 μg penicillin/ml of culture, whereas currently used strains have at least 2000 times greater yields. This increase in yield is the result of mutations and selection of more active strains, improvements in culture media, and research into the optimal conditions for antibiotic production. As the biosynthetic pathways for the production of many antibiotics have become known, further research to increase yields by isolation and selection of mutants continues.

10.5.3   Mycotoxins

The mycotoxins are secondary metabolites of fungi which are poisonous to man and animals. One of the mycotoxin producers, for example is the ergot fungus, *Claviceps purpurea* (Ch. 5.4). It produces alkaloids, derivatives of lysergic acid (ergotamine, ergotoxin) which are of considerable importance in the treatment of cardiovascular conditions, migraine and as hallucinogens (inducers of hallucinations). Whilst ergot is for the most part still produced by the artificial inoculation of rye plants with *C. purpurea*, submerged culture of other strains, including *C. paspali*, is beginning to be of economic interest. Many fungi, including some of the conspicuous basidiomycetes and the inconspicuous myxomycetes are producers of highly potent toxins, as well as of some, chemically not yet investigated, organic compounds which may reveal other interesting effects. The toxins include that of the poisonous basidiomycete *Amanita phalloides* (amanitatoxin), *A. patherina, A. muscaria* and *Inocyte patouillardi* (pilzatropin and muscarin). Research on the seconary metabolites of fungi has only just begun. Mycotoxins became objects of general public interest recently, when thousands of young turkeys died from aflatoxin poisoning.

Aflatoxin B₁

Aflatoxins   are derivatives of coumarine and are produced by several strains of *Aspergillus flavus, A. parasiticus, A. oryzae* and other fungi. They can be present in all kinds of mouldy foodstuffs, such as groundnuts, grain, oil seeds and fodder. They are also carcinogenic.

10.6   Vitamins

Vitamins are nowadays added routinely to food and fodder, and therefore produced in large quantities. Although many vitamins are chemically synthesised, production of riboflavine, vitamin B_{12}, and vitamin C (ascorbic acid) are still dependent on microorganisms.

Riboflavine is excreted by Ascomycetes (*Ashbya gossypi* and *Eremothecium ashbyii*) and is also produced by yeasts (*Candida*) and bacteria (*Clostridium*) in gram quantities per litre.

Vitamin B_{12} is synthesised only by microorganisms and is essential for animals. They therefore have to obtain it via their food or as vitamin supplements. The vitamin produced by the microorganisms (including *E. coli*) inside the intestine cannot be absorbed by the animal. The common habit of rodents, therefore, to eat their own faeces (coprophagy) can be regarded as an adaptive behaviour to obtain the vitamins contained in the intestinal contents. Bacteria in which corrinoids are metabolically important, for example, propionibacteria, clostridia, streptomycetes and methanogens are suitable for the industrial production of vitamin B_{12}.

Carotenoids.   These are added to animal foodstuffs and give the yellow coloration to egg-yolk, even in winter. They are isolated from the mycelium of Zygomycetes (*Blakesleea trispora* and *Choanephora circinans*). Their chemical synthesis now competes with the microbial biotechnology.

The insertion of a bioconversion step, namely the oxidation of D-sorbitol to L-sorbose, in the synthesis of vitamin C, has already been mentioned (see Ch. 10.1). Construction of a strain of *Erwinia* which can convert glucose directly to 2-keto-L-gulonic acid is being attempted by means of gene technology. Acidification of 2-keto-L-gulonic acid converts it directly to ascorbic acid.

Procedures and processes developed for the large-scale cultivation of bacteria, yeasts, and fungi are being increasingly applied to the culture of animal and plant cells. Thus, techniques for the growth of isolated plant cells in synthetic nutrient solutions have been worked out; these techniques allow plant cells to be cultured in fermentors of several thousand litres' capacity. Under these conditions, plant cells can produce enzymes or secondary metabolites in concentrations that are one or two orders of magnitude higher than those in intact plants. Surprisingly, even substances that are produced in only very small amounts by intact plants can be accumulated by such tissue cultures of plant cells. It is to be expected, therefore, that it will be possible in future to produce alkaloids, glycosides, steroids, organic acids, and other secondary metabolites with the help of plant cells in tissue culture, especially with the advent of the new techniques of protoplast fusion and genetic manipulation.

10.7　Exopolysaccharides

Plant mucus has long been used as a 'thickening agent' to increase the viscosity of liquids. This is now being superceded by several exopolysaccharides of bacterial origin (Ch. 2.2.5) (Table 10.1). Alginates are used as additives for ice creams, puddings, creams, etc. and as a hydrophilic cover to conserve moisture in roots. The polysaccharides derived from marine algae are increasingly being replaced by products obtained from *Azotobacter* and *Pseudomonas*. Numerous applications have been found for the slime produced by the plant-pathogenic bacterium *Xanthomonas campestris*, i.e. the xanthans. They consist of $1,4$-β-glycosidically linked chains of glucose (i.e. like cellulose) that bear trisaccharide side chains. Xanthans are used as thickening agents in the food industry and in cosmetics, as emulsifying additives in paints and printing inks, and even as additives to improve water-flooding techniques for tertiary oil recovery. Curdlan is used for the preparation of desserts and low-calorie soups because it is not broken down in the human digestive tract. The use of dextran as a blood plasma expander, and as the basis for **adsorbents** known as Sephadex, has already been discussed in Ch. 2.2.

10.8　Enzymes

Rennin, obtained from the lining of calves' stomachs, was traditionally employed for the curdling of milk used in cheese making, whilst proteases, used in tanning of leather, were isolated from dried dog faeces.

Table 10.1. *Microbially produced exopolysaccharides and their utilisation*

Product	Microbial origin	Uses
Dextran (α-1,6-glucan)	*Leuconostoc mesenteroides*, *Klebsiella*, *Acetobacter*, streptococci	Blood plasma replacement; adsorbant in the biochemical industry
Alginate (1,4-glycosidically joined mannuronic and glucuronic acids)	*Azotobacter vinelandii*, *Pseudomonas aeruginosa*	Ice cream, instant puddings and creams; dressing agent for textiles and paper; hydrophilic cover for plant roots, wounds and Christmas trees
Xanthan (cellulose with trisaccharide side-chain substituents)	*Xanthomonas campestris*	Additive for drinks and soft cheeses; whipping cream, instant puddings; French Dressing; emulsion stabiliser
Pullulan (β-1,6-glycosidically joined malto-triose groups)	*Aureobasidium*, *Pullularia* (*Dematium*) *pullulans*	Covering agent for food products
Curdlan (β-1,3-glucan)	*Alcaligenes faecalis* var. *myxogenes*	Gelling agent for puddings; not digested in the intestinal tract, hence of low calorific value

Microbial processes have facilitated the utilisation of such enzymes, and have extended the list of enzymes which can be used in biotechnology (Table 10.2). Thus the calves' renin needed for the curdling of milk can be replaced with rennin excreted by *Mucor rouxii* and other fungi. Similarly, the breakdown of starch to sugar in the course of alcohol production no longer requires addition of fermented barley but can be accomplished by treatment of starch with fungal amylases. In order to obtain fructose, which is sweeter than sucrose or glucose, the starch is converted to glucose by α-amylase and glucoamylase and fructose then

Table 10.2. *Microbially produced enzymes and their uses*

Enzyme and reactions catalysed	Microbial origin	Uses
Invertase hydrolysis of sucrose	*Aspergillus oryzae,* yeasts and other fungi	Production of invert sugar for sweets
Proteases hydrolysis of proteins	*Bacillus subtilis* and other bacteria, also fungi	Additives for detergents, and in tanning
Pectinolytic enzymes hydrolysis of pectins	fungi and *Erwinia*	Clarifying of fruit juices
Lipase hydrolysis of lipids	fungi and *Pseudomonas*	Additive for detergents, and in tanning
Glucose oxidase oxidation of glucose to gluconate	*Aspergillus niger, Gluconobacter oxydans*	Preparation of gluconic acid
Hexose isomerase isomerisation of fructose	*Streptomyces*	Preparation of fructose from glucose
Amylase hydrolysis of starch	*Bacillus subtilis, Aspergillus* species, and other fungi	Preparation of glucose syrup; removal of starch dressing agents
Cellulases hydrolysis of cellulose	*Trichoderma viride, Penicillium*	Preparation of glucose from cellulose

obtained from the glucose, in high yields, by the action of glucose isomerase. Another enzyme used for the breakdown of starch to sugars is pullulanase which can split both 1,4-α-glucosidic and 1,6-α-glucosidic bonds. Various preparations of these enzymes, including some that are relatively thermotolerant, can be isolated from bacilli, clostridia, streptomycetes and lactobacteria. Proteases and lipases are used as additives in washing powders. Another aim is to use microbial cellulase, which can convert cheap cellulose from wood or straw to sugars, so as to feed this into alcohol production. All these enzymes so far mentioned are **exoenzymes**; they are excreted by the microorganisms and isolated from the culture medium. Among enzymes isolated from cellular systems, mainly from bacteria, and made available by the biochemical industry are the endonucleases and other enzymes used in cloning techniques. Gene technology has opened up further possibilities of utilising microbial enzymes.

In addition to the traditional products of microbial processes, the first foreign proteins have been obtained during the last few years. Molecular cloning techniques (see Ch. 15.3.6) now make it possible to incorporate foreign DNA into plasmids and to transfer these to bacteria (or yeasts) by transformation techniques. Provided that there is good expression of the foreign genes, this leads to the formation of foreign proteins by the bacteria or yeasts. The industrial production of therapeutic substances and vitamins, such as interferon, insulin, somatostatin, urokinase, viral proteins and vaccines – as well as others – has already begun.

Investigations on industrially useful enzymes nowadays also includes their suitability for **immobilisation**, i.e. their capacity to bind to cellulose, agarose, alginates or glass pellets, or their inclusion in capsules. By these means, several enzymes can be significantly stabilised.

10.9   Biomass

Microorganisms are also produced in considerable quantities for use as nutrients or fodder (yeasts, bacteria, edible fungi), inocula for plants (*Rhizobium*), or as raising agents in bakeries (baker's yeast), as inocula for sour-milk products, in the production of some sausages and for many other purposes. The cultivation of feed yeasts (*Candida*) on sulphite effluents from the synthetic fibre industry goes back to the 1930s. Following the preparation of yeast protein for human consumption during times of scarcity – even in Central Europe – several processes for the mass production of **single-cell proteins** have been developed in the 1970s. Substrates and organisms which have been tested include petrol and pure hydrocarbons (*Candida lipolytica*), hydrogen and carbon dioxide (*Alcaligenes eutrophus*), methanol (*Methylomonas*), ethanol, and some valuable organic compounds which occur as waste products in chemical syntheses. The 'green revolution', however, and the optimisation of agricultural cultivation methods have inhibited the further development of relevant processes for the time being. New interest in biomass arose with the realisation that the bacterial storage product, poly-β-hydroxybutyrate (PHB) has thermoplastic properties (like polypropylene and polyethylene). It can be worked into sheets, fibres and hollow bodies like bottles and mugs, and it is biologically degradable. Some bacteria can accumulate large quantities of PHB intracellularly under suitable culture conditions, with a sugar substrate. *Alcaligenes autrophus* could easily reach a PHB content of more than 90% (w/w) of its dry weight. Following further investigations to determine conditions under which, besides PHB, poly-β-OH-valeric acid and poly-γ-OH-valeric acid can be produced, as well as – by other bacteria – poly-β-OH-octanoate and other poly-hydroxy alkanoates (PHA), the microbial production of these environmentally friendly homo- and hetero-polymers should have a bright and assured future.

A wider overview can be obtained by the study of textbooks on biotechnology and of journals orientated to applied topics or commercial reports about market and product analyses.

11 Inorganic hydrogen donors: aerobic chemolithotrophic bacteria

Several groups of soil and aquatic bacteria are able to use inorganic compounds or ions (ammonium, nitrite, sulphide, thiosulphate, sulphite and ferrous iron) as well as elemental sulphur, hydrogen, or carbon monoxide as electron or hydrogen donors, gaining energy and reducing equivalents for synthetic processes by their oxidation. Energy is usually obtained by respiration with oxygen as the final electron acceptor. Only a few 'specialists' in this group can grow with nitrate, nitrite, or nitrous oxide as hydrogen acceptors, i.e. anaerobic respiration. This mode of life with inorganic hydrogen donors is called **chemolithotrophy**.

Aerobic chemolithoautotrophic bacteria

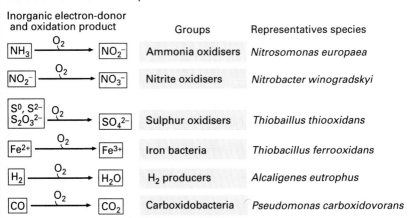

Inorganic electron-donor and oxidation product	Groups	Representatives species
$NH_3 \xrightarrow{O_2} NO_2^-$	Ammonia oxidisers	*Nitrosomonas europaea*
$NO_2^- \xrightarrow{O_2} NO_3^-$	Nitrite oxidisers	*Nitrobacter winogradskyi*
$S^0, S^{2-}, S_2O_3^{2-} \xrightarrow{O_2} SO_4^{2-}$	Sulphur oxidisers	*Thiobaillus thiooxidans*
$Fe^{2+} \xrightarrow{O_2} Fe^{3+}$	Iron bacteria	*Thiobacillus ferrooxidans*
$H_2 \xrightarrow{O_2} H_2O$	H_2 producers	*Alcaligenes eutrophus*
$CO \xrightarrow{O_2} CO_2$	Carboxidobacteria	*Pseudomonas carboxidovorans*

Most of the bacteria belonging to this metabolic type grow with **carbon dioxide** as their sole, or major, source of carbon for cell synthesis. They are therefore also **autotrophs** (chemolithoautotrophs). All the chemolithotrophic bacteria so far examined assimilate their carbon from CO_2 by fixation via the ribulose-bisphosphate cycle; the mechanism of this CO_2 fixation will therefore be discussed later in this chapter. In this respect some chemolithotrophic bacteria are obligate; others have the alternative of growing as chemo-organoheterotrophs, i.e. they are facultatively chemolithotrophic. Many of the chemolithoautotrophs are highly specialised and occupy a decided monopoly position. The oxidation of ammonium, nitrite and inorganic sulphur compounds in nature is due in the first place to the activities of the nitrifying and sulphur-oxidising bacteria.

11.1   Ammonium and nitrite oxidation: nitrification

In the course of aerobic or anaerobic degradation of nitrogen-containing substances, the nitrogen is liberated in the form of ammonium. The formation of saltpetre (potassium nitrate) during the composting of animal manure is a very old observation. The bloom of saltpetre found on the stone walls of manure pits was used for the manufacture of gunpowder in the middle ages. According to ancient instructions for 'saltpetre works', beds constructed from soil, limestone and nitrogen-containing substances were moistened with blood and urine and kept well aerated. The ammonium liberated during microbial degradation of the organic material diffused into the soil where it was oxidised by atmospheric oxygen to yield nitrate. This soil cover was the starting material for the saltpetre production. It was soaked in water, and the resulting solution was evaporated to obtain the saltpetre.

The conversion of ammonium to nitrite, i.e. nitrification, is carried out in soil by nitrifying bacteria. There is no known bacterium that converts ammonium directly to nitrate; two kinds of bacteria are always involved in this oxidation: the ammonium oxidisers form nitrite and the nitrite oxidisers produce nitrate. The best-known species are *Nitrosomonas europaea* and *Nitrobacter winogradskyi* (Table 11.1). According to more recent investigations, however, *Nitrosolobus* species, rather than *Nitrosomonas*, are the main ammonium-oxidising organisms in agricultural soils. Both genera are highly specialised for the oxidations shown in Table 11.1. The organisms that oxidise ammonium furnish the substrate for those that oxidise nitrite. Since high concentrations of ammonium in alkaline soils have a toxic effect on *Nitrobacter*, *Nitrosomonas* and *Nitrosolobus* also serve to improve the environment for the nitrite oxidisers, by both utilising the ammonium and increasing the acidity (exchanging a cation for an anion).

The **nitrifiers** are gram-negative bacteria that are collected in the family Nitrobacteriaceae. *Nitrosomonas europaea* is an oval bacterium with polar flagella. In marine habitats, *Nitrosococcus oceanus* (Fig. 2.22) seems to be the organism responsible for the oxidation of ammonium. The nitrifying bacteria can be cultured in purely mineral salts solutions but grow rather slowly, with generation times of 10–20 hours. Up to

Table 11.1. *Nitrifying bacteria*

Ammonium-oxidising (nitroso-) $NH_4^+ + 1\frac{1}{2} O_2 \rightarrow NO_2^- + 2 H^+ + H_2O$	Nitrite-oxidising (nitro-) $NO_2^- + \frac{1}{2} O_2 \rightarrow NO_3^-$
Nitrosomonas europaea	*Nitrobacter winogradskyi*
Nitrosococcus oceanus	*Nitrobacter agilis*
Nitrosospira briensis	*Nitrobacter hamburgensis*
Nitrosolobus multiformis	*Nitrococcus mobilis*

now the nitrifying bacteria were considered as strictly obligate chemolithoautotrophs that did not utilise organic substances added to their media. However, this strict abstinence is now somewhat in doubt, and more detailed investigations are being undertaken. Thus *N. winogradskyi* was shown to incorporate acetate from the medium into cell material, i.e. protein and poly-β-hydroxybutyrate.

Reaction pathway in the oxidation of ammonium.   The following intermediate steps are most probably involved in the oxidation of ammonium:

$$NH_3 \rightarrow NH_2OH \rightarrow (NOH) \rightarrow NO_2^- \rightarrow NO_3^-$$

The first step is endergonic and is catalysed by an ammonium monooxygenase; the oxygen atom of NH_2OH comes from molecular oxygen. The second step is catalysed by a hydroxylamine oxidoreductase.

In the oxidation of nitrite the electrons are transferred to a cytochrome a_1. Only the oxidation steps from hydroxylamine to nitrite and from nitrite to nitrate yield utilisable energy.

The role of nitrification in soils.   The ammonium ions liberated by the mineralisation of nitrogen-containing substances are rapidly oxidised in well-aerated soils. The conversion of a cation to an anion effects an acidification of the soil and hence leads to an increased solubility of minerals (potassium, calcium, magnesium and phosphates). The nitrifying microflora was therefore regarded as a significant factor in soil fertility. This view has undergone changes, however. Ammonium ions are much more tenaciously retained by soils than nitrate, especially by adsorption to clay minerals and more or less tight binding to, and in, humus components. Nitrate, on the other hand, is easily leached out. Thus, there have been attempts recently to suppress nitrification in areas of agricultural use, and to search for agents that specifically inhibit the growth of nitrifying bacteria. Such substances, it is thought, could serve as nitrogen-conserving agents in agricultural practice (e.g. 'N-serve' = Nitrapyrin = 2-chloro-6-trichloromethyl-pyridine).

On the other hand, growth and metabolism of the autotrophic nitrifying bacteria have a narrow pH optimum between 7 and 8. The pH range of the complete nitrification of ammonium to nitrate is therefore quite narrow, since free ammonia (in alkaline soils) and nitrous acid (in the acid range) are toxic for *Nitrobacter*. The concentrations of free NH_3 and free HNO_2 are known to be pH dependent.

The nitrifying bacteria are also indirectly involved in the destruction of limestone and cement (e.g. in motorways, buildings) because they oxidise any ammonium derived from the atmosphere or animal excreta to nitric acid.

The group of ammonium oxidisers is of great ecological importance, even beyond their known functions. Soils which have been treated with ammonium salt fertilisers release nitrogen oxides (NO, NO_2), especially under conditions of oxygen limitation (waterlogged soils). Investigations have shown that *Nitrosomonas* and *Nitrosovibrio* can carry out nitrate respiration (denitrification), and NO and NO_2 are therefore produced by reduction of nitrite which is derived from the oxidation of ammonia (Ch. 9.11).

A number of other abilities have also been demonstrated among the ammonia-oxidising organisms: they are able to oxidise methane, methanol, carbon monoxide, ethylene, propylene, cyclohexane, benzyl alcohol and phenol. In other words, they have great oxidising potential. They belong to the autochthonous soil flora and are probably involved in the slow oxidation of the intermediary products released during degradation of organic substances.

Another problem that has been investigated is the question whether methane-oxidising methylotrophic bacteria (Ch. 14.11.1), which oxidise their substrate by initial action of a monooxygenase, are able to oxidise ammonium as well as methane. This has been found to be the case, although the methylotrophic bacteria cannot use ammonia as a substrate for growth. The reaction belongs to the group of heterotrophic nitrifications.

Heterotrophic nitrification.   The question of whether autotrophic nitrifiers occupy a real monopoly position in nature or whether heterotrophic bacteria and fungi play a part in the conversion of ammonium to nitrate is still wide open. In pure cultures, only strains of *Arthrobacter* are able to form nitrite from nitrogen-containing substances. Some fungi can oxidise amino-nitrogen or ammonium to nitrate. In contrast to autotrophic nitrification, however, these heterotrophic reactions are not coupled to growth and biomass production; they are probably a kind of co-oxidation of ammonium and organic substances. In addition, the rate of heterotrophic nitrification is lower than that of autotrophic nitrification by a factor of 10^3–10^4. The heterotrophic nitrifiers therefore constitute no serious threat to the monopoly position of the autotrophic ones. The modest nitrification by heterotrophs, however, offers an explanation for the observation that even in acid soils (e.g. tea plantations, pine forests) where autotrophic nitrifiers have no chance, there is some nitrification.

Reverse electron transport and cell yields.   The oxidation of ammonium, nitrite, sulphur compounds, or iron by autotrophic bacteria is energetically very unfavourable. Their substrates have a very positive redox potential. The normal potential E_0' for NH_4^+/NH_2OH is $+ 889$ mV; for NO_3^-/NO_2^-, $+ 420$ mV; for NO_2^-/NH_2OH, $+ 66$ mV; for Fe^{3+}/Fe^{2+}, $+ 770$ mV; in comparison to $- 320$ mV for $NAD^+/NADH_2$. Therefore, the oxidation of these substrates cannot be directly coupled to the reduction of NAD^+. But reduced NAD^+ is essential for the reduction of CO_2 in the ribulose-bisphosphate cycle. There is evidence that the electrons from the oxidation of inorganic substrates enter the respiratory chain at the level of cytochrome c or a; the energy yield is correspondingly small because only one phosphorylation step (of the respiratory chain) can be utilised. Moreover, a part of this energy is then used to drive electrons entering at the cytochrome level in the reverse direction of the respiratory chain to the level of the pyridine nucleotides which are thus reduced. This reverse electron transport is an essential mechanism for these bacteria to gain reducing equivalents that are required for synthetic processes (Ch. 7.4).

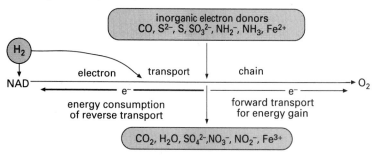

The very small amounts of energy that can be obtained by the oxidation of the inorganic substances mentioned are in agreement with the very low cell yields. The synthesis of one gram of cellular dry weight requires the consumption of far greater amounts of substrates than is known for other organisms (Table 11.2). Several of these bacteria also carry out uncoupled oxidation reactions, i.e. they oxidise substrates without simultaneous synthesis of cell material ('metabolic idling'). It is therefore

Table 11.2. *Comparison of cell yields with the primary energy source to be converted in different autotrophic and organotrophic microorganisms*

For the synthesis of 1 g cells (dry weight), microorganisms must convert:

Thiobacillus ferrooxidans	156 g Fe^{2+}	*Alcaligenes eutrophus*	0.5 g H_2
Thiobacillus neapolitanus	30 g $S_2O_3^{2-}$	*Escherichia coli*	2 g glucose
Nitrosomonas	30 g NH3	Yeast	1 g petroleum

not surprising that nitrification reactions in soil and water are carried out by relatively small populations of bacteria.

11.2   Oxidation of reduced sulphur compounds

The ability to obtain energy by oxidation of reduced sulphur compounds is the property of a group of gram-negative bacteria with polar flagella; these bacteria constitute the genus *Thiobacillus*. Quite recently, a bipolarly flagellated spirillum (*Thiomicrospira*) and a non-motile thermophilic bacterium (*Sulfolobus*) with this capacity were discovered (Table 11.3). Most of the thiobacilli can oxidise several sulphur compounds and form sulphate as the end product.

$$S^{2-} + 2O_2 \rightarrow SO_4^{2-}$$
$$S + H_2O + 1\tfrac{1}{2}O_2 \rightarrow SO_4^{2-} + 2H^+$$
$$S_2O_3^{2-} + H_2O + 2O_2 \rightarrow 2SO_4^{2-} + 2H^+$$

Most of the thiobacilli (*T. thiooxidans*, *T. thioparus*, *T. denitrificans*) are obligate chemolithoautotrophs and depend on CO_2 fixation. Others can also grow with organic compounds as energy and carbon sources (*T. novellus*, *T. intermedius*).

T. thiooxidans produces large amounts of sulphuric acid and is specifically adapted to growth at low pH; it can tolerate 1 N sulphuric acid. This acidification can be exploited in a number of ways. Addition of elementary sulphur can be used for de-alkalisation of chalky soils; the sulphuric acid produced by thiobacilli converts calcium carbonate to the more soluble calcium sulphate, which is readily leached out. In a similar way, the acidophobic organism that causes potato scab can be combated. Whereas the above-named thiobacilli live aerobically, *T. denitrificans* can utilise nitrate as hydrogen acceptor and thus carry out anaerobic

Table 11.3. *Sulphur-oxidising bacteria*

Species	pH of growth	Electron donor	Type[a]
Thiobacillus thiooxidans	2–5	S^{2-}, $S_2O_3^{2-}$, S	o
Thiobacillus ferrooxidans	2–6	Fe_2+, $S_2O_3^{2-}$, S	f
Thiobacillus thioparus	6–8	CNS–, $S_2O_3^{2-}$, S	o
Thiobacillus denitrificans	6–8	CNS–, $S_2O_3^{2-}$, S	o
Thiobacillus intermedius	2–6	$S_2O_3^{2-}$, S, glutamate	f
Thiobacillus novellus	6–8	$S_2O_3^{2-}$, S, glutamate	f
Thiomicrospira pelophila	6–8	S^{2-}, $S_2O_3^{2-}$, S	o
Sulfolobus acidocaldarius	2–3	S, glutamate, peptone	f

[a] o, Obligately autotrophic; f, facultatively autotrophic.

respiration. This organism denitrifies nitrate but cannot carry out as-similatory reduction to ammonium; hence it is dependent on ammonium salts as nitrogen source.

Sulfolobus acidocaldarius and *Caldariella acidophila* belong to the Archaebacteria and occupy extreme ecosystems. They inhabit acid hot springs where mainly volcanic hydrogen sulphide is oxidised. *S. acidocaldarius* is a thermophilic, facultatively chemolithotrophic bacterium that oxidises elemental sulphur to sulphuric acid and grows optimally at pH 2–3 and temperatures of 70–75 °C, though it can tolerate even 90 °C.

Reaction pathways in the oxidation of sulphur compounds.   It has been difficult to establish the steps in the reaction pathway of sulphur oxidation because hydrogen sulphide, as well as sulphur in aqueous solutions, is oxidised non-biologically, albeit slowly. The scheme shown in Fig. 11.1 includes the most important enzyme-catalysed reactions. The yellow sulphur (flowers of sulphur) exists as an eight-membered ring (S_8) which is moderately soluble in water (0.176 mg sulphur/l).

It is assumed that the electrons obtained in the oxidation of sulphite to sulphate enter the respiratory chain at the level of cytochrome *c*. At least some thiobacilli (*T. thioparus*, *T. denitrificans*) can utilise the energy available from the oxidation of sulphite to sulphate by a substrate-level phosphorylation (Fig. 11.1: 5,6).

(1) $SO_3^{2-} + AMP \xrightarrow{\text{APS reductase}} APS + 2e^-$

(2) $APS + P \xrightarrow{\text{ADP sulfurylase}} ADP + SO_4^{2-}$

(3) $2\,ADP \xrightarrow{\text{adenylate kinase}} ATP + AMP$

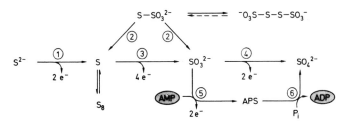

Fig. 11.1. *The most important reactions in the oxidation of sulphur compounds by sulphur-oxidising bacteria.*

Enzymes: (1) sulphide oxidase; (2) thiosulphate-cleaving enzymes (rhodanese); (3) sulphur-oxidising enzyme (sulphur oxidase); (4) sulphite oxidase; (5) APS reductase; (6) ADP sulphurylase (sulphate adenylyl transferase).

Reactions (1) and (2) are in the opposite direction to those involved in the dissimilatory sulphate reduction (Fig. 9.3).

Filamentous and other sulphur bacteria. In the sediments of ponds and puddles or slowly moving waters where hydrogen sulphide is formed, the colourless filamentous sulphur bacteria *Beggiatoa, Thiothrix* and *Thioplaca* (Fig. 2.44), as well as the large unicellular forms *Achromatium oxaliferum* and *Thiovolum* (Fig. 2.44), are found. S. N. Winogradsky used *Beggiatoa* to carry out his investigations that led to the concept of chemoautotrophy. Up to now, however, none of these 'classic sulphur bacteria' has been obtained in pure culture, nor can their biochemical and physiological properties be investigated. The failure to grow these bacteria in pure culture in the laboratory is apparently due to their very special growth requirements. On the one hand they require hydrogen sulphide, and on the other hand, they require oxygen, which they can tolerate only at very low concentrations. It would take great patience and very special experimental tricks to satisfy these requirements.

Hydrogen sulphide as the basis for an ecosystem without light. The life of all higher heterotrophic organisms is based on the biomass provided by photosynthesis. An exception to this rule was discovered a few years ago. In the ocean depths where no light can penetrate, water at 350 °C arises from the sea floor in places where the continents separate. The water of these hot springs contains many minerals in solution and also H$_2$S. In places where this water makes contact with the cold seawater containing oxygen, bacteria that can oxidise sulphur or hydrogen sulphide are able to grow. They serve as food for crabs and worms. A worm of the group Pogonophora, *Riftia pachyptila*, is highly adapted to this ecosystem; this worm has neither a mouth nor an anus, but possesses an organ called a trophosome in which H_2S-oxidising bacteria grow as endosymbionts. This organ is provided with H_2S and O_2 by the worm's blood. thus, in the neighbourhood of the hot springs of the ocean floor there exists an ecosystem that is not based on biomass production by photosynthesis, but by chemolithoautotrophy.

11.3   Oxidation of iron(II)

The iron bacterium *Thiobacillus ferrooxidans* oxidises ferrous to ferric iron:

$$4Fe^{2+} + 4H^+ + O_2 \rightarrow 4Fe^{3+} + 2H_2O$$

This bacterium is very similar to *T. thiooxidans*, tolerating pH values of 2.5, but being able to obtain energy not only by the oxidation of reduced sulphur compounds but also by oxidation of ferrous ions. The habitat of these iron bacteria is in acid waters of iron ore mines which contain metal sulphides as well as iron pyrites (FeS_2). The acidophilic iron bacteria have been shown unequivocally to be capable of chemoautotrophic growth.

Most recently, thermophilic strains of iron- and sulphur-oxidising thiobacilli have been discovered, and even strains of the thermophile *Sulfolobus acidocaldarius* can oxidise ferrous iron. An antimony-oxidising bacterium, *Stibiobacter senarmontii*, which can oxidise Sb^{3+} to Sb^{5+}, has been isolated from antimony-containing soils.

Leaching of ores.   The ability of some acidophilic iron- and sulphur-oxidising bacteria to convert sulphide ores to water-soluble heavy-metal sulphates is utilised for the leaching of low-grade ores, and to obtain copper, nickel, zinc, molybdenum and uranium. Leaching processes are in large-scale use for reclaiming ores from slag-heaps and might also be useful in deep-mining operations. In its simplest form, water is allowed to percolate through columns of broken up ore-containing rocks, for example iron pyrites (FeS_2) and associated metal sulphides such as Cu_2S, CuS, ZnS, NiS, MoS_2, Sb_2S_3, CoS and PbS, and the sulphate-containing solutions are collected. The various metals are then obtained by concentration and precipitation. Bringing the heavy metals into solution is the result of several associated processes: bacterial oxidations of reduced sulphur compounds (1) or elementary sulphur (2) to sulphuric acid and of Fe^{2+} to Fe^{3+} (3), and also by chemical oxidation of insoluble heavy-metal salts to soluble metal sulphates and sulphur (4).

(1) $FeS_2 + 3\frac{1}{2} O_2 + H_2O \rightarrow FeSO_4 + H_2SO_4$

(2) $S + 1\frac{1}{2} O_2 + H_2O \rightarrow H_2SO_4$

(3) $2FeSO_4 + \frac{1}{2} O_2 + H_2SO_4 \rightarrow Fe_2(SO_4)_3 + H_2O$

(4) $MoS + 2Fe^{3+} \rightarrow Mo^{2+} + 2Fe^{2+} + S$

The bacteria are responsible for the supply of sulphuric acid and for the regeneration of Fe^{3+}; both these components are consumed in the solubilisation of the ores. These conversions are carried out by *Thiobacillus thiooxidans* and *T. ferrooxidans*. The strains involved are remarkably tolerant to the prevailing concentrations of Cu^{2+}, Co^{2+}, Zn^{2+}, Ni^{2+} and other heavy-metal ions. Strains of *Sulfolobus* that oxidise iron and sulphur also take part in the leaching of metal ores.

Other iron bacteria.   *Gallionella ferruginea* (Fig. 3.19) and *Leptothrix ochracea* belong to the best-known and most easily recognised iron bacteria. They are found in drainpipes and mountain streams associated with flakes and thick coverings of iron oxides. Until a few years ago it was not known whether they could use the energy available from the oxidation of Fe^{2+} to Fe^{3+} and thus grow autotrophically. Quite recently ribulose-bisphosphate carboxylase was demonstrated in *Gallionella* which is therefore now included in the group of lithoautotrophic bacteria.

Apart from iron, this group of bacteria can also oxidise manganese. The sheathed bacterium *Leptothrix discophorus* can oxidise Mn^{2+} to Mn^{4+} but it is uncertain whether it can utilise the energy released in this reaction for metabolism.

> **Obligate autotrophy.**   Obligate autotrophy is the expression of an extreme specialisation and adaptation to the respiration of inorganic substrates. Several hypotheses have been advanced and examined to explain this phenomenon.
>
> (1) One can start with the assumption that the tricarboxylic acid cycle is not essential for the oxidation of inorganic substrates (in analogy to fermentative metabolism). After all, reducing equivalents are obtained by the oxidation of the inorganic substrate and can enter the respiratory chain. Only the synthetic functions of the tricarboxylic acid cycle (supply of 2-oxoglutarate and succinate) need to be safeguarded, but this does not require the enzyme 2-oxoglutarate dehydrogenase. Investigations have shown that this enzyme is indeed lacking in a number of obligate autotrophs. Even in a number of facultatively autotrophic bacteria this enzyme is not demonstrable when the cells have been grown on an inorganic substrate. A mutant of such a facultative organism that has lost the ability to produce 2-oxoglutarate dehydrogenase, therefore should behave more or less like an obligate autotroph.
>
> (2) Since the nitrifying as well as the sulphur- and iron-oxidising bacteria have a 'branched' respiratory chain, it seems possible that in some

obligate autotrophs the first section of the respiratory chain contains an irreversible step which prevents the oxidation of $NADH_2$; this is more easily envisaged because this section is only used for reverse electron transport. A possible inhibition of reversibility by enzyme regulation would lead also to conservation of the reducing power ($NADH_2$) that must be generated with such great expenditure of energy.

Up to now there is no unitary explanation for the phenomenon of obligate autotrophy. Its origin may differ in different physiological groups of organisms.

11.4 Oxidation of molecular hydrogen

Hydrogen is produced during the anaerobic degradation of organic substances in sediments and anaerobic microhabitats in soil. Many bacteria have the capacity to utilise this hydrogen. A large part of it is metabolised by bacteria that are associated with the hydrogen-producing fermentative organisms and oxidise H_2 with reduction of sulphate to sulphide or carbon dioxide to methane (see Ch. 9.4). Hydrogen is also produced in well-aerated ecosystems, for instance, in soils growing leguminous plants (e.g. soybeans, beans, clover). It arises in the nitrogenase reaction (Ch. 13.3) and diffuses into the environment from the bacteroids of the root nodules, many of which do not produce hydrogenase. Some members of all bacterial groups that can generate ATP via electron-transport phosphorylation under anaerobic conditions (anaerobic respiration) are able to use molecular hydrogen as hydrogen donor (Chapter 9).

Anaerobic chemolithoautotrophic bacteria

Electron donors and reduction products	Group designation	Representative species
$H_2 \xrightarrow{CO_2} CH_4$	Methanogens (carbonate respiring)	*Methanobacterium thermoautotrophicum*
$H_2 \xrightarrow{CO_2} CH_3\text{–}COOH$	Acetogens (carbonate respiring)	*Acetobacterium woodii*
$H_2 \xrightarrow{SO_4^{2-}} H_2S$	Sulphidogens (sulphate respiring)	*Desuslfovibrio desulfuricans*
$H_2 \xrightarrow{S^0} H_2S$	Sulphidogens (sulphur respiring)	*Desulfomonas acetoxidans*
$H_2 \xrightarrow{NO_3^-} N_2$	Denitrifiers (nitrate respiring)	*Paracoccus denitrificans*
$CO \xrightarrow{NO_3^-} N_2$	Denitrifiers (nitrate respiring)	*Pseudomonas carboxydovorans*
$CO \xrightarrow{SO_4^{2-}} H_2S$	Sulphidogens (sulphate respiring)	*Desulfobacterium autotrophicum*

Aerobic hydrogen-oxidising bacteria.   Those bacteria that oxidise hydrogen aerobically with oxygen as the terminal electron acceptor are collected under the designation of aerobic hydrogen-oxidising bacteria. All of these are able to fix carbon dioxide and are thus autotrophs. On the other hand, all of these are also able to utilise organic substrates. Thus the hydrogen-oxidising bacteria are facultative chemolithoautotrophs.

A few aerobic hydrogen-oxidising bacteria can also oxidise carbon monoxide and can grow with this as the only electron donor and carbon source.

Isolation and growth.   The aerobic hydrogen-oxidising bacteria grow in a simple nutrient solution containing only inorganic salts, under a gas mixture of 70% H_2 + 20% O_2 + 10% CO_2 (v/v). The gases are metabolised approximately according to the following stoichiometry:

$$6H_2 + 2O_2 + CO_2 \rightarrow \langle CH_2O \rangle + 5H_2O$$

$\langle CH_2O \rangle$ is the approximate composition of cell material in terms of C, H and O.

Under the above conditions, these bacteria are easily brought into enrichment culture and isolated from a soil inoculum. They include the most rapidly growing autotrophs with a doubling time of about 3 hours and some thermophiles with a doubling time of only 1 hour. Some strains can grow heterotrophically at even faster rates. Under favourable conditions, cell yields of 20 g dry weight per litre of nutrient medium can be achieved.

Systematics.   The aerobic hydrogen-oxidising bacteria are taxonomically extremely heterogeneous. Most species can be classified with the gram-negative genera *Pseudomonas*, *Alcaligenes*, *Aquaspirillum*, *Paracoccus* and *Xanthobacter*, whilst some belong to the gram-positive genera *Nocardia*, *Mycobacterium* and *Bacillus* (Table 11.4). More recently, the ability to grow as autotrophs aerobically with hydrogen has been discovered also in other genera (*Rhizobium*, *Derxia*). The possession of enzymes that can activate hydrogen and the ability to fix CO_2 is therefore distributed among several taxonomic groups of bacteria.

Utilisation of hydrogen and energy metabolism.   Hydrogen enters metabolism by means of hydrogenases. Two types of hydrogenases are found in aerobic hydrogen-oxidising bacteria: a soluble, NAD^+-reducing hydrogenase (H_2:NAD^+ oxidoreductase) localised in the cytoplasm, and a membrane-bound hydrogenase. Only a few bacteria (*Alcaligenes eutrophus*, *A. hydrogenophilus*) possess both kinds of enzymes. *Nocardia*

Table 11.4. *Some species of aerobic hydrogen-oxidising bacteria*

| Species | Hydrogenase | | Nitrogen fixation | Gram stain |
	Soluble	Membrane-bound		
Alcaligenes eutrophus	+	+	−	−
Pseudomonas facilis	−	+	−	−
Pseudomonas saccharophila	−	+	−	−
Pseudomonas carboxydovorans	−	+	−	−
Pseudomonas pseudoflava	−	+	−	−
Pseudomonas carboxidoflava	−	+	−	−
Aquaspirillum autotrophicum	−	+	−	−
Paracoccus denitrificans	−	+	−	−
Xanthobacter autotrophicus	−	+	+	−
Nocardia opaca	+	−	−	+
Mycobacterium gordonae	−	+	−	+
Bacillus sp.	−	+	−	+

contains only the soluble enzyme whilst the majority of the other bacteria in this group have only the membrane-bound enzyme. Both kinds of hydrogenase can catalyse the entry of hydrogen into the respiratory chain. The process of ATP generation is very efficient; the composition of the respiratory chain in *Alcaligenes eutrophus* and *Paracoccus denitrificans* is almost the same as that in mitochondria.

Heterotrophic and mixotrophic modes of nutrition.   Many hydrogen bacteria catabolise hexoses and gluconate via the Entner–Doudoroff pathway and oxidise the substrate to CO_2 and water. These bacteria can usually also utilise a large number of other organic compounds including branched-chain fatty acids, aromatic and heterocyclic ring systems, and even testosterone. Poly-β-hydroxybutyrate and glycogen are found as storage materials. Some hydrogen bacteria can exhibit mixotrophic nutrition when the inorganic substrates (carbon dioxide and hydrogen) are present at the same time as organic substrate. This means that the organic nutrients are assimilated for the formation of cell material, whilst the energy required for synthetic processes is derived from the oxidation of hydrogen. Under these conditions, none of the organic nutrients need to be oxidised to completion. This capacity for a mixotrophic nutrition is found in many facultatively autotrophic organisms, where the energy required for synthetic reactions may be supplied by oxidation of various reduced inorganic compounds (hydrogen sulphide or sulphur in sulphur bacteria) or by photosynthesis (in green algae and plants).

Regulation of substrate utilisation.   In some hydrogen-oxidising bacteria the utilisation of substrates is very strictly regulated. For example, autotrophically grown cells of *Alcaligenes eutrophus* do not contain the enzymes for fructose utilisation. If such cells are inoculated into a medium containing fructose and incubated aerobically, they will form the enzymes of the Entner–Doudoroff pathway and will grow. However, if incubation is in the presence of a gas mixture of 80% H_2 and 20% CO_2, the cells do not grow nor do they produce the enzymes. Thus, hydrogen apparently represses the formation of enzymes required for the utilisation of fructose. If experiments are carried out with cells that contain the enzymes of fructose catabolism as well as hydrogenase and the cells are incubated in a gas mixture of hydrogen and oxygen, fructose catabolism occurs at a very low rate; hydrogen also inhibits fructose catabolism. The control point is the enzyme glucose-6-phosphate dehydrogenase. The drastic reduction in the rate of fructose catabolism *in vivo* (by $H_2 + O_2$) could be traced back to inhibition of the above enzyme by NADH. In these experiments glucose-6-phosphate dehydrogenase was shown to be the regulatory enzyme of the Entner–Doudoroff pathway, analogous to the function iof phosphofructokinase in the fructose-bisphosphate pathway (see Ch. 16.2.2).

Carbon monoxide-utilising bacteria (carboxidobacteria).   Carbon monoxide occurs in nature under aerobic and anaerobic conditions. Neither the biochemical mechanisms nor the microorganisms involved in this production are known in any detail. It is known, on the other hand, that several bacterial species can oxidise carbon monoxide to carbon dioxide. The ability to grow with carbon monoxide as the sole electron donor and the only source of carbon, however, is restricted to aerobic bacteria. *Pseudomonas carboxydovorans* metabolises carbon monoxide during growth according to the following equation:

$$7\,CO + 2\tfrac{1}{2}\,O_2 + H_2O \rightarrow \langle CH_2O \rangle + 6\,CO_2$$

The assimilation of carbon occurs by carbon dioxide fixation via the ribulose-bisphosphate cycle. Oxidation of CO is catalysed by an enzyme containing molybdenum; therefore growth on CO requires molybdenum as a trace element, whereas growth on organic substrates does not. The carbon monoxide-utilising bacteria, also called carboxidobacteria, possess a membrane-bound hydrogenase and can also grow as hydrogen bacteria.

11.5   Carbon dioxide fixation

Most organisms that can grow with carbon dioxide as the only carbon source fix this via the **ribulose-bisphosphate cycle** (Calvin–Bassham cycle). These organisms include the aerobic chemolithoautotrophic bacteria, almost all phototrophic bacteria, the cyanobacteria, and green plants. It is certain that the cycle is not involved in the CO_2 fixation by methanogenic and acetogenic bacteria, which also belong, by definition, to the chemolithoautotrophs. Two enzymes are characteristic for the ribulose-bisphosphate cycle and are not involved in any other metabolic pathways: phosphoribulokinase and ribulose-bisphosphate carboxylase. The latter enzyme is quantitatively the most predominant protein on this planet.

The cycle represents a reductive sequence in which carbon dioxide is reduced to the level of carbohydrates. Three stages can be distinguished: (1) the carboxylation reaction, (2) the reduction and, (3) the regeneration of the CO_2-acceptor molecule.

The carboxylation reaction.   Ribulose-1,5-bisphosphate is converted with fixation of carbon dioxide by ribulose-bisphosphate carboxylase to two molecules of 3-phosphoglycerate.

Ribulose-bisphosphate carboxylase

This enzyme can catalyse a second reaction. In the absence of carbon dioxide and the presence of oxygen, it converts ribulose-bisphosphate by oxygenation to phosphoglycollate and 3-phosphoglycerate (its oxygenase activity). This reaction participates in the formation of glycollate by autotrophic bacteria and green plants and, hence, in 'light respiration'.

Ribulose-bisphosphate Carboxylase / Oxygenase

The reduction reaction.   The carboxylation reaction is immediately followed by the reduction of the carboxy group in 3-phosphoglycerate to the aldehyde group. This conversion involves reactions known from the fructose-bisphosphate pathway (Ch. 7.2.1), namely, the phosphorylation from ATP by 3-phosphoglycerate kinase and the reduction from NAD(P)H by glyceraldehyde-3-phosphate dehydrogenase. This last reaction is specific for NADH in bacteria and for NADPH in plants.

The reduction of 3-phosphoglycerate is the CO_2-fixation step that requires energy and reducing power. The subsequent steps are not important energetically, and they proceed at a more or less constant energy level.

Regeneration of the CO_2-acceptor molecule.   Glyceraldehyde-3-phosphate is in equilibrium with dihydroxyacetone-phosphate by triose-phosphate isomerase, and both triose-phosphates are in turn kept in equilibrium with fructose-1,6-bisphosphate by fructose-bisphosphate aldolase.

Fructose-bisphosphate is dephosphorylated to fructose-6-phosphate by fructose-bisphosphatase. The conversion of one molecule of fructose-6-phosphate and three molecules of triose-phosphate to three molecules of ribulose-5-phosphate is carried out by some of the enzymes known from the oxidative pentose-phosphate cycle as well as some other enzymes. The reaction sequence is initiated by transketolase (Fig. 11.2, right-hand side), which catalyses the transfer of a glycolyl group from a ketomonophosphate to an aldose-phosphate. The glycolaldehyde, functioning as the coenzyme, is transiently bound as 'active aldehyde' to thiamine diphosphate (TPP).

The tetrose-phosphate (erythrose-4-phosphate) produced by the transketolase reaction is then converted in an aldolase reaction with dehydroxyacetone phosphate, to yield sedoheptulose-1,7-bisphosphate. This is dephosphorylated in the 1-position by a fructose-bisphosphatase to produce sedoheptulose-7-phosphate (Shu-7-P). This step of a phosphate ester hydrolysis is irreversible and bestows irreversibility on the whole reaction sequence. It therefore affords the possibility of regulating the metabolite flux at this point. It has been ascertained that, in plants, photosynthetic regeneration of ribulose-5-phosphate occurs via sedoheptulose-1,7-bisphosphate (Fig. 11.2, right-hand side) but that the synthesis of pentose-phosphates in the dark proceeds via a transaldolase reaction direct to sedoheptulose-7-phosphate (Fig. 11.2, left-hand side). From sedoheptulose-7-phosphate, transketolase then transfers a glycolyl group to glyceraldehyde-3-phosphate, thus producing two molecules of pentose-phosphates. The pentose-phosphates, ribose-5-phosphate and xylulose 5-phosphate, are in enzymatic equilibrium with ribulose-5-phosphate (see Fig. 7.4 where these reactions have been presented within the

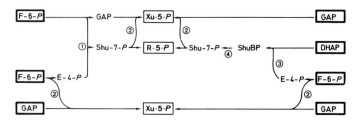

Fig. 11.2. *Diagrammatic scheme showing two possibilities for the regeneration of pentose phosphate from triose-phosphates and fructose-6-phosphate.*

The left side summarises the reaction steps involve din the synthesis of nucleic acid pentoses (ribose, deoxyribose) in which transaldolase plays a part. The right side summarises the reaction steps involved in the regeneration of the CO_2 acceptor in CO_2 fixation (ribulose-1,5-bisphosphate); in these steps, sedoheptulose-1,7-bisphosphate and aldolase participate, but not transaldolase. F-6-P, fructose-6- phosphate; GAP, glyceraldehyde-3-phosphate; DHAP, dihydroxyacetone phosphate; E-4-P, erythrose-4-phosphate; Shu-7-P, sedoheptulose-7-phosphate; ShuBP, sedoheptulose-1,7-bisphosphate; Xu-5-P, xylulose-5-phosphate; R-5-P, ribose-5-phosphate; (1) transaldolase; (2) transketolase; (3) fructose-bisphosphate aldolase; (4) fructose-bisphosphatase.

oxidative pentose-phosphate pathway). The phosphorylation of ribulose-5-phosphate with ATP to ribulose-1,5-bisphosphate by phosphoribulo-kinase is the last reaction in the ribulose-bisphosphate cycle.

Balance sheet of the ribulose-bisphosphate cycle.   To synthesise one mol hexose from 6 mol carbon dioxide requires six turns of the cycle. The balance sheet of the cycle for the fixation of CO_2 can therefore be stated by the following equation:

$$6\,CO_2 + 18\,ATP + 12\,NAD(P)H_2 \rightarrow F\text{-}6\text{-}P + 18\,ADP$$
$$+\,12\,NAD(P) + 17\,P_i$$

This presentation as a closed cycle should not be allowed to obscure the fact that several intermediary products are important precursors for the synthesis of cell material; 3-phosphoglycerate leads to pyruvate and acetyl-CoA; erythrose-4-phosphate leads to the synthesis of aromatic amino acids; ribose-5-phosphate is the precursor for the synthesis of nucleotides; and hexose-phosphate is the precursor of various polymers.

Regulation of the activity of some of the participating enzymes ensures that, on the one hand, not too much energy (ATP) is withdrawn

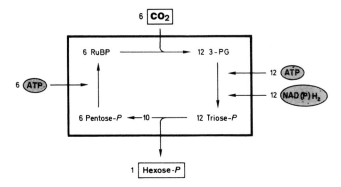

from cell metabolism by the relatively large energy demands of CO_2 fixation, and, on the other hand, that the withdrawal of intermediary products for synthesis of cell material does not bring the cycle to a standstill (see Ch. 16.2.2).

Other pathways of autotrophic carbon dioxide fixation.   Although carbon dioxide fixation via the ribulose-bisphosphate cycle is the most important pathway for the synthesis of organic substances from CO_2 in the biosphere today, it is not the only one (Table 11.5). Anaerobic autotrophic bacteria have two further mechanisms of CO_2 assimilation. The methanogenic, acetogenic, and sulphate-reducing (sulphidogenic) bacteria that can utilise hydrogen or carbon monoxide as hydrogen donor reduce CO_2 via the anaerobic acetyl-CoA pathway, i.e. to acetyl-CoA and pyruvate (Ch. 9.4). The pyruvate then feeds into the central synthetic pathways by well-known reactions.

The green sulphur bacteria (*Chlorobium thiosulfatophilum*) fix CO_2 exclusively via the reactions of the reductive tricarboxylic acid cycle; in this cycle, CO_2 is fixed by reductive carboxylation of succinyl-CoA.

> A comparison of the three types of autotrophic CO_2 fixation shows that the anaerobic processes work more economically than the aerobic process. The synthesis of one mol triose-phosphate from 3 mol CO_2 via the anaerobic acetyl-CoA pathway probably requires only 3 mol ATP; via the reductive tricarboxylic acid cycle this requires approximately 5 mol ATP; and via the ribulose-bisphosphate cycle, this requires 9 mol ATP.

General reactions of carbon dioxide fixation.   It has been mentioned on several occasions already that heterotrophic organisms also require carbon dioxide and incorporate it into their cellular metabolism. The role of the carboxylation of pyruvate and phosphoenolpyruvate in the

Table 11.5. *The three pathways of autotrophic CO_2 fixation*

Reductive acetyl-CoA pathway	Reductive TCA cycle	Calvin cycle
Homoacetogenic fermentors *Clostridium thermoaceticum* *Acetobacter woodii* *Sporomusa* sp.	**Green sulphur bacteria** *Chlorobium limicola*	**Anoxygenic phototrophic bacteria** *Chromatium vinosum* *Rhodospirillum rubrum*
Most sulphate reducing bacteria *Desulfobacterium autotrophicum* *Desulfovibrio baarsii*	**Thermophilic hydrogen bacteria** *Hydrogenobacter thermophilus* **Few sulphate-reducing bacteria** *Desulfobacter hydrogenophilus*	**Chemolithoautotrophic bacteria: Nitrifiers, sulphur oxidisers, hydrogen and carboxydo bacteria, iron oxidisers**
Methanogens *Methanobacterium thermoautotrophicum* *Methanosarcina barkeri*		**Oxygenic phototrophic bacteria, algae and higher plants**

replenishment of the tricarboxylic acid cycle (anaplerotic sequences) has been discussed in detail (see Ch. 7.5). The following diagram shows the intermediary metabolites that can have carbon dioxide incorporated.

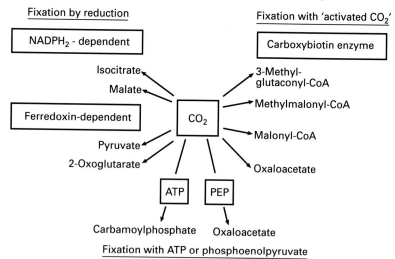

The various CO_2-fixing reactions shown play different parts and are not of equal importance in different organisms. Some serve only for the activation of metabolites or for the replenishment of central metabolic pathways. The ferrodoxin-dependent reductive carboxylation reactions are found only in some anaerobic and phototrophic bacteria.

12 Phototrophic bacteria and photosynthesis

Two groups of bacteria have the ability to use light as an energy source for growth. The two groups are fundamentally different.

The **purple bacteria** and the **green bacteria** can be regarded as relics from the earliest period in the evolution of photosynthesis. They are not able to utilise water as the hydrogen donor, as are green plants; they are obliged to use more reduced hydrogen donors (H_2S, H_2 or organic compounds). In consequence, these bacteria also do not evolve any oxygen during **photosynthesis**. They carry out anoxygenic photosynthesis. They are typical aquatic bacteria, widely distributed in freshwater and seawater. They are unicellular with red, orange, or green pigmentation, depending on their content of bacteriochlorophyll and carotenoids.

The **cyanobacteria** do utilise water as hydrogen donor and evolve oxygen in the light; that is, they carry out **oxygenic photosynthesis.** Their pigment system includes chlorophyll a, carotenoids, and phycobilins. Since their photosynthetic process is basically the same as that of green plants, they were formerly discussed together with the photosynthetic eukaryotes and were referred to as 'blue-green algae'. However, their cell structure is typical of prokaryotes. The cyanobacteria have been described in detail in Ch. 3.21 and will not be discussed here.

12.1 Purple sulphur bacteria, non-sulphur purple bacteria and green sulphur bacteria

The photosynthetic bacteria that carry out anoxygenic photosynthesis have been divided into three large groups; the purple sulphur bacteria, the purple non-sulphur bacteria and the green bacteria. The representatives of these three orders are distinguished by their cytological and physiological properties as well as by their pigmentation (Table 12.1; Figs 12.1, 12.6, 12.10).

All members of the purple bacteria have in common the localisation of the whole photosynthetic apparatus (the light-harvesting or antenna system and the reaction centre) on the intracytoplasmic membranes (the thylakoids). With a few exceptions, they all contain bacteriochlorophyll a (Bchl a) and they can all fix carbon dioxide via the ribulose-bisphosphate

Table 12.1. *The four families of anaerobic phototrophic bacteria*

Order	Group	Type species	Growth (aerobic dark)	Growth (anaerobic light)	H₂S oxidation	S deposition	Pigments	Photosynthetic apparatus	Growth factors
Anaerobic phototrophic bacteria — Purple bacteria	Chromatiaceae (sulphur purple bacteria)	*Chromatium vinosum*	–	+	+	intracellular	Bchl *a* (Bchl *b*)	thylakoids	none or B$_{12}$
	Rhodospirillaceae (non-sulphur purple bacteria)	*Rhodospirillum rubrum*	(+)	+	–(+)	extracellular	Bchl *a* (Bchl *b*)	thylakoids	pABS, thiamine, biotin, nicotinic acid
Green sulphur bacteria	Chlorobiaceae (green sulphur bacteria)	*Chlorobium limicola*	–	+	+	extracellular	Bchl *a* Bchl *c* Bchl *d* Bchl *e*	Cm chlorosomes	none or B$_{12}$
	Chloroflexaceae (*Chloroflexus* group)	*Chloroflexus aurantiacus*	+	+	(+)		Bchl *a* Bchl *c*	Cm chlorosomes	

Bchl, bacteriochlorophyll; pABS, 4-aminobenzoic acid; Cm, cytoplasmic membrane.

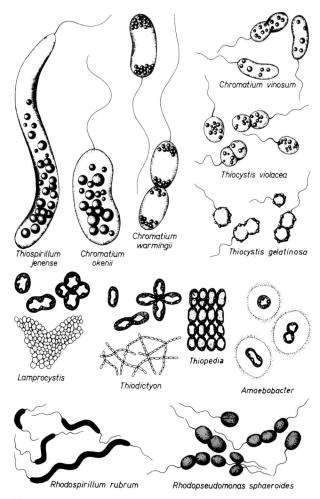

Fig. 12.1. *Some sulphur purple bacteria (Chromatiaceae) and non-sulphur purple bacteria (Rhodospirillaceae).*

cycle and utilise organic compounds as hydrogen donors and/or carbon source. Within the purple bacteria, two families are distinguished by their ability or inability to utilise sulphur as the hydrogen donor; they are the purple sulphur bacteria or Chromatiaceae (formerly

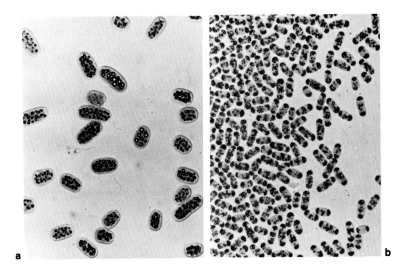

Fig. 12.2. Chromatium okenii *(a)* and Chromatium warmingii *(b)*.
Bright-field illumination,   (Photos: N. Pfennig.)
magnification × 800.

Thiorhodaceae) and the non-sulphur purple bacteria or Rhodospirillaceae
(formerly Athiorhodaceae).

Chromatiaceae.   The majority of the purple sulphur bacteria are easily
recognised by their intracellular presence of highly refractile sulphur
globules. (Figs 2.43, 12.2, 12.3). *Chromatium okenii* (5 μm diameter and
20 μm length) and *Thiospirillum jenense* (3.5 μm diameter and 50 μm
length) belong to the giants among bacteria (Figs 12.1, 12.2, 12.3). They
have always attracted the attention of microscopists and have been used
for investigations on flagellar movements and phototactic responses.
Chromatium warmingii can be distinguished from *C. okenii* by its slightly
smaller dimensions and by the polar location of its sulphur globules
(Fig. 12.2). The large chromatia are kidney-shaped, whereas the smaller
ones are like short rods. *Chromatium vinosum* belongs to the latter and was
the object of important investigations on bacterial photosynthesis. The
genus *Thiocystis* (*T. violaceas, T. gelatinosa*) is characterised by spherical
motile cells, whereas the cells of *Thiocapsa roseopersicina* and *T. pfennigü*
are also spherical but non-motile. Several species of Chromatiaceae contains gas vacuoles; *Lamprocystis roseopersicina*, with motile spherical

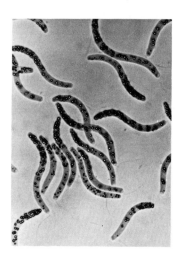

Fig. 12.3. Thiospirillum jenense *with monopolar polytrichous flagellation and sulphur inclusions.*

Bright-field illumination, magnifica-   (Photo: N. Pfennig.)
tion about × 700.

cells, as well as the non-motile genera *Amoebobacter* (spherical), *Thiopedia* (elliptical) and *Thiodictyon* (rod-shaped), belong to these.

The typical feature of the Chromatiaceae is the intermediary deposition of intracellular sulphur during the oxidation of hydrogen sulphide. Members of the genus *Ectothiorhodospira* (*E. mobilis*, *E. halophila*) accumulate the sulphur on the outside of the cell, where it is further oxidised extracellularly. All the Chromatiaceae possess vesicular thylakoids (chromatophores) which almost fill the cell. Only two exceptions are known so far: *Ectothiorhodospira* species and *Thiocapsa pfennigii*, which have tubular thylakoids.

Rhodospirillaceae.   The known non-sulphur purple bacteria are presently assigned to five genera. Those with spiral shape belong to the genus *Rhodospirillum*. In this genus *R. rubrum*, *R. fulvum* (Fig. 12.4), *R. molischianum* and *R. photometricum* are distinguished by their colour and size. The rod-shaped species belong to the genera *Rhodopseudomonas* (*R. palustris*, *R. viridis*, *R. acidophila* and *R. sulfoviridi*) and *Rhodobacter* (*R. capsulatus*, *R. sphaeroides* and *R. sulfidophilus*). Bent rods are designated *Rhodocyclus* (*R. purpureus*, *R. gelatinosus* and *R. tenuis*). The al-

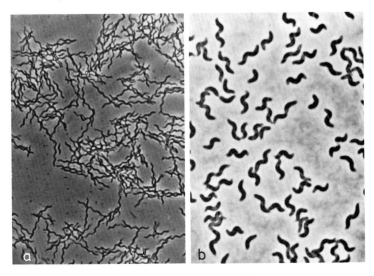

Fig. 12.4. Rhodospirillum rubrum *(a)* *and* Rhodospirillum fulvum *(b)*. Bright-field illumination, magnification approximately × 1200 and × 1800, respectively.

most spherical motile organisms form a genus *Rhodopila* with only one species *R. globiformis*. The non-sulphur purple bacteria are found to contain all the known thylakoid structures. The two species *Rhodomicrobium vannielii* and *Rhodocyclus purpureus* occupy a special position. *Rhodomicrobium vannielii* (Fig. 12.5) multiplies by budding, the buds remaining attached to the mother cell by hypha-like stalks, or being liberated as peritrichously flagellated swarmers. *Rhodocyclus purpureus* is the only non-motile form in this family. Its cells are semicircular. The photosynthetic membrane is probably identical with the cytoplasmic membrane, which shows only a few small invaginations.

The growth of most non-sulphur purple bacteria is inhibited by hydrogen sulphide, although some species can tolerate or even use it as hydrogen donor for the fixation of CO_2. *Rhodopseudomonas sulfidophila* and *R. palustris* can oxidise hydrogen sulphide to sulphate without the intermediary formation of sulphur.

Green sulphur bacteria.   The members of the green sulphur bacteria are characterised by the possession of pigmented organelles immediately adjacent to the cytoplasmic membranes, the so-called **chlorosomes**

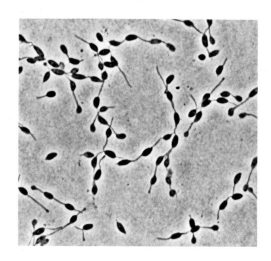

Fig. 12.5. Rhodomicrobium vannielii, *a budding hyphae-forming non-sulphur purple bacterium.*

Bright-field illumination, magnification   (Photo: N. Pfennig.)
approximately × 1200

(formerly *Chlorobium* vesicles). These contain the bacteriochlorophyll characteristic for this group, bacteriochlorophyll *c*, *d* or *e* (Bchl *c*, *d*, *e*), i.e. the antenna pigment. In addition, these bacteria also contain small amounts of Bchl *a*, which is directly connected to the photosynthetic reaction centre and localised in the cytoplasmic membrane.

The green sulphur bacteria are also distinguished from the purple bacteria by the absence of the enzyme Ribulose-bisphosphate carboxylase. They are therefore unable to fix carbon dioxide via the ribulose-bisphosphate cycle. The two families of the green sulphur bacteria Chlorobiaceae and Chlorofexaceae, are phylogentically unrelated according to 16S RNA data.

They also differ in their cell wall composition; gram-negative in the Chlorobiaceae and gram-positive in the Chloroflexaceae.

Chlorobiaceae   The green sulphur bacteria (Figs 12.6-12.9) comprise green- (*Chlorobium vibrioforme, C. limicola*) as well as brown-pigmented strains (*Chlorobium phaeobacteriodes*), star-shaped aggregations (*Prosthecochloris*), and net-forming organisms (*Pelodictyon clathratiforme*). *Chlorochromatium aggregatum* is a symbiotic association of two bacterial species; a colourless, chemo-organotrophic rod, motile by a long

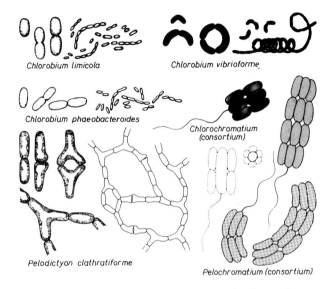

Fig. 12.6. *Phototrophic green sulphur bacteria (Chlorobiaceae).*

polar flagellum has green, phototrophic bacteria attached as ectosymbionts to its outer surface. *Pelochromatium roseum* is similarly constituted; the ectosymbiotic bacteria have a brown pigmentation. The marine bacterium *Chloroherpeton thalassium* is distinguished from the *Chlorobium* strains by its filamentous cell shape and creeping motility.

Chloroflexaceae. The phototrophic green bacterium *Chloroflexus* belongs to the filamentous gliding bacteria according to its shape and type of motility. However, it contains bacteriochlorophylls *c* and *a*, and possesses chlorosomes corresponding to those of the green sulphur bacteria. *Chloroflexus* differs from *Chlorobium* species, on the other hand, by its capacity for aerobic, heterotrophic growth in complex media in the dark as well as in the light. In contrast to the Chlorobiaceae, photoautotrophic growth with CO_2 and H_2S is hardly demonstrable. The Chloroflexaceae are therefore more nearly photoheterotrophs. *Chloroflexus aurantiacus* is a bacterium of world-wide distribution and constitutes the main component of the green and orange mats found at the bottom of channels and in effluents of hot springs.

Heliobacteria. The Heliobacteria are a quite new and different group of anoxygenic phototrophs. So far only three representatives have been

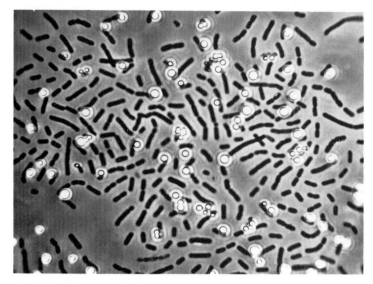

Fig. 12.7. Chlorobium limicola, *young culture with extracellularly deposited sulphur.*

Bright-field illumination, magnification approximately × 1000.   (Photo: N. Pfennig.)

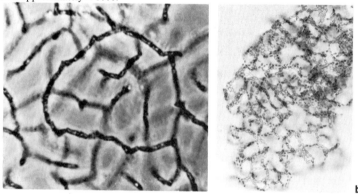

Fig. 12.8. Pelodictyon clathratiforme *(a), a green sulphur bacterium forming networks; (b) the purple sulphur bacterium* Thiodictyon elegans, *which forms loose networks.*

Bright-field illumination, magnification: (a) × 1500; (b) × 400.   (Photos: N. Pfennig.)

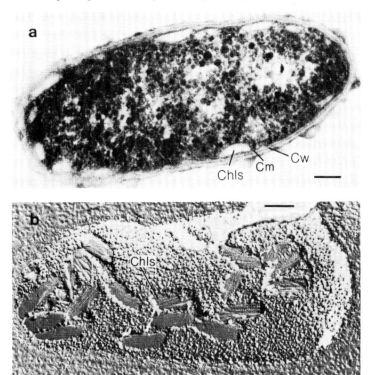

Fig. 12.9. *Electron micrographs of* Chlorobium limicola.

(a) Ultrathin section; (b) freeze-etched preparation showing chlorosomes. Chls, chlorosomes; Cm, cytoplasmic membrane; Cw, cell wall. Bars, 100 nm. (Photos: Staehelin, L. A., Golecki, J. R. & Drews, G. (1980). *Biochim. Biophys. Acta.* **589**, 30.)

discovered. *Heliobacterium* is a gliding bacterium, *Heliospirillum* a large, very motile spirillum, and *Heliobacillus* a motile rod. They contain bacteriochlorophyll *g*; this differs only slightly from bacteriochlorophyll (Fig. 12.11). The most fundamental difference from the purple bacteria already described – which are all gram-negative – lies in their gram-positive character, and in their position on the phylogenetic tree. This shows them as a separate group of gram-positive Eubacteria, close to the genus *Clostridium*.

12.1.1   Pigments of the photosynthetic apparatus

Heavy suspensions of photosynthetic bacteria appear green, blue-green, purple, violet, red, brown or salmon-coloured to the eye, according to their content of photosynthetic pigments. These differences in coloration are due to the nature and the quantitative composition of the pigments. The pigment components can be recognised readily by the absorption spectra of intact cells (Fig. 12.10). Absorption maxima in the blue (< 450 nm) and the red, as well as infra-red, spectra (650–1000 nm) are due to chlorophylls. Absorption in the range 400–550 nm is mainly due to carotenoids, and that of cyanobacteria in the range 550–650 nm is due to the phycobiliproteins.

The various chlorophyll types differ from each other chiefly by the presence or absence of a double bond between carbon atoms 3 and 4 and by the substituents on the porphyrin skeleton (Fig. 12.11). These differences are responsible for the absorption maxima in the near infra-red. They can be recognised clearly in spectra of intact cells and isolated photosynthetic membranes where the pigments are present in specific pigment-protein complexes (Fig. 12.10). Thus, the main absorption maximum of chlorophyll a in green algae and cyanobacteria lies between 680 and 685 nm; that of bacteriochlorophylls c , d, and e in green sulphur bacteria and *Chloroflexus* is between 715 and 755 nm, and that of bacteriochlorophyll a of most purple bacteria is between 850 and 890 nm. Bacteriochlorophyll b, which has so far been found only in *Rhodopseudomonas viridis*, *Ectothiorhodospira halochloris* and *Thiocapsa pfennigii*, absorbs between 1020 and 1035 nm.

The Bchl a of the purple bacteria occurs in four spectral forms: B800, B820, B850 and B870-890. These differences in absorption spectra are caused by the kind of binding and the position of the bacteriochlorophyll molecule in the pigment-protein complexes of the photosynthetic apparatus. The number of peaks and the heights of the peaks relative to each other differ from species to species, and with many organisms these peaks can also be influenced by culture conditions.

Apart from their characteristics chlorophyll components, Bchl c, d or e, the Chlorobiaceae also contain, in each case, a small amount of Bchl a, with only one peak at 810 nm. In the cells of *Chloroflexus*, however, the Bchl a spectrum has two distinct maxima at 808 and 868 nm.

The coloured **carotenoids** are so-called accessory pigments of photosynthetic organisms. They absorb light in the spectral region of 400–550 nm. In purple bacteria, they are mainly aliphatic C_{40} compounds (tetraterpenoids) with tertiary hydroxy or methoxy groups (lycopene, rhodopin, spirilloxanthin, spheroidene). The presence of an oxo or alde-hyde group can give them a deep red coloration (spheroidenone, okenone,

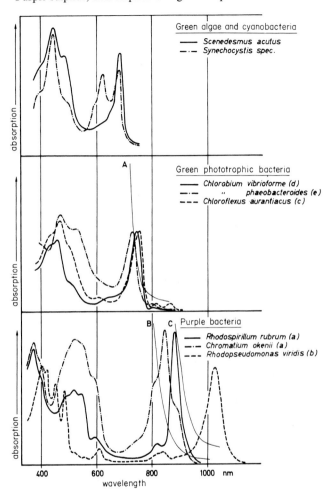

Fig. 12.10. *Absorption spectra of intact cells of phototrophic bacteria, cyanobacteria and green algae.*

The species of characteristic bacteriochlorophylls are given in brackets. Also shown are the absorption properties of the infra-red filters used for the enrichment cultures of chlorobacteria and purple bacteria (A), purple bacteria (B), and purple bacteria containing bacteriochlorophyll *b* (C). (After Pfennig, N. (1967). *Ann. Rev. Microbiol.* **21**, 285.)

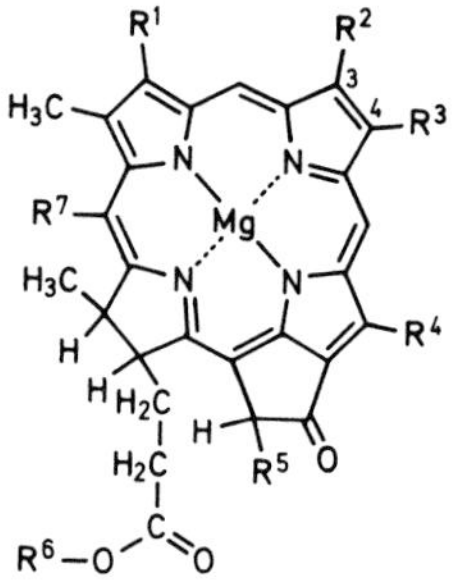

Fig. 12.11. *Relation between chlorophyll* a *and the bacteriochlorophylls* a, b, c, d, e *and* g.

Pigment	R^1	R^2	R^3	R^4	R^5	R^6	R^7
Chloro-phyll a	$-CH=CH_2$	$-CH_3$	$-CH_2-CH_3$	$-CH_3$	$O=C\diagdown^{OCH_3}$	Phytol	$-H$
Bacterio-chlorophyll a	$O=C\diagup^{CH_3}$	$-CH_3^*$	$-CH_2-CH_3^*$	$-CH_3$	$O=C\diagdown^{OCH_3}$	Phytol or Geranyl-geraniol	$-H$
Bacterio-chlorophyll b	$O=C\diagup^{CH_3}$	$-CH_3^*$	$=C\diagdown^{CH_3^*}_{H}$	$-CH_3$	$O=C\diagdown^{OCH_3}$	Phytol	$-H$
Bacterio-chlorophyll c	$-CH-CH_3$ $\mid$ OH	$-CH_3$	$-C_2H_5$ $-C_3H_7$ $-i\text{-}C_4H_9$	$-C_2H_5$ $-CH_3$	$O=C\diagdown^{OCH_3}$	Farnesol	$-CH_3$
Bacterio-chlorophyll d	$-CH-CH_3$ $\mid$ OH	$-CH_3$	$-C_2H_5$ $-C_3H_7$ $-i\text{-}C_4H_9$	$-C_2H_5$ $-CH_3$	$-H$	Farnesol	$-H$
Bacterio-chlorophyll e	$-CH-CH_3$ $\mid$ OH	$-CHO$	$-C_2H_5$ $-C_3H_7$ $-i\text{-}C_4H_9$	$-C_2H_5$	$-H$	Farnesol	$-CH_3$
Bacterio-chlorophyll g	$-CH=CH_2$	$-CH_3$	$=C\diagdown^{CH_3}_{H}$	$-CH_3$	$-H$	Phytol	$-H$

rhodopinal). Carotenoids with aromatic rings (arylcarotenoids) derived from γ- or β-carotene are also found. These are restricted to a few families (okenone occurs in a few species of Chromatiaceae, chlorobactene is the typical carotenoid of the green Chlorobiaceae, and isorenieratene is that of the brown Chlorobiaceae).

The carotenoids fulfil two functions. On the one hand, they are photosynthetically active and belong to the antenna pigments which channel energy to the chlorophylls. On the other hand, they have a protective function: they shield the chlorophylls from photo-oxidative damage. Carotenoid-free blue-green mutants of purple bacteria can grow only in dim light and are killed by high light intensities.

The differences in the absorption spectra of green algae, cyanobacteria, purple bacteria and green bacteria lead to the conclusion that the individual groups of phototrophic organisms utilise different spectral components of light for photosynthesis. These differences correlate with the light conditions in the natural habitats of the phototrophic organisms. The differences can also be exploited for the selective cultivation of individual phototrophic organisms (see Fig. 12.13).

Localisation of the pigments.   The photosynthetic pigments in purple bacteria are bound to intracytoplasmic membranes (thylakoids). These originate as vesicular or tubular invaginations of the cytoplasmic membrane into the cell interior and remain connected. The membranes of different species occur in different forms and can be present as tubules, vesicles, and as concentrically or cylindrically arranged lamellar stacks, occupying most of the cell interior (see Fig. 2.24). The vesicular membrane fragments that can be isolated from broken cells by differential centrifugation are called 'chromatophores'. In the cells of the green sulphur bacteria the photosynthetic pigments are bound to two separate cell structures: the antenna pigments are localised in the chlorosomes, whereas the pigments of the reaction centre are in the cytoplasmic membrane (Fig 12.9).

Regulation of pigment and thylakoid synthesis.   The synthesis of photopigments is dependent on several growth conditions: in the first place, on the extent and degree of illumination, and, in the facultative aerobes, on the presence of oxygen. In an intermediate range of illumination, the pigment content of the cells increases with decreasing light intensity during cell growth. The presence of oxygen also exerts an influence on the formation of pigment; high light intensities and oxygen repress the formation of the pigment-bearing membrane structures, and thereby repress the synthesis of bacteriochlorophylls and carotenoids. The variations in the number of tubules and vesicles that can be demonstrated microscopically parallel the variations in concentrations of photosynthetic pigments. Oxygen has an additional inhibitory effect on some enzyme reactions in the synthesis of bacteriochlorophyll. The highest concentrations of photosynthetic pigments and of pigment-containing vesicles and tubules are found in cells that have been grown anaerobically at low light intensities.

12.1.2   Metabolism

The metabolism of phototrophic bacteria presents a large number of questions. Many of the non-sulphur purple bacteria and the Chloroflexaceae are able to grow anaerobically in the light, as well as aerobically in the dark. Other groups are strict anaerobes and obligate phototrophs. Many utilise hydrogen; some use hydrogen sulphide or sulphur as hydrogen donor. Both carbon dioxide fixation and assimilation of organic substrates occur; a modest amount of energy can even be obtained by fermentation, anaerobically in the dark, though this does not support any cellular growth. Altogether, the phototrophic bacteria belong to the physiologically most versatile organisms. It is therefore possible only to give an overview of their physiological capabilities.

Carbon dioxide fixation.   Nearly all of the photosynthetic bacteria so far examined can fix carbon dioxide via the ribulose-bisphosphate pathway. However, they use $NADH_2$ rather than $NADPH_2$ as is the case in green plants, for the reduction of 3-phosphoglycerate. In addition, ferredoxin- or NADP-dependent reductive carboxylations are also used for the assimilation of carbon. The fixation of CO_2 can either support completely autotrophic growth or serve to equalise the redox balance in the presence of very reduced organic compounds. *Chlorobium* fixes CO_2 via the reductive tricarboxylic acid cycle.

Hydrogen donors.   The anaerobic phototrophs are dependent on an external hydrogen donor. They can use gaseous hydrogen itself, or hydrogen sulphide, elemental sulphur, thiosulphate, organic acids, alcohols, sugars, and even some aromatic compounds. Hydrogen is used by a great many, but by no means all, phototrophic bacteria. Small chromatia, *Rhodobacter* species (e.g. *R. capsulatus*), rhodospirilla and chlorobia can grow in the light with only H_2 and CO_2. The quantum yield in this case is almost the same as in oxygenic photosynthesis. In the case of *Rhodopseudomonas acidophila* and also in the cyanobacterium *Anabaena cylindrica*, this has been determined as 8 mol (Einstein) quanta/mol of carbon dioxide fixed. The purple and the green sulphur bacteria, as well as a few of the non-sulphur purple bacteria, oxidise hydrogen sulphide to sulphate. Most of the sulphur purple bacteria can accumulate elemental sulphur transiently inside the cell during this process. This capacity for rapid hydrogen sulphide oxidation in the light, with the intracellular accumulation of sulphur, may account for the quantitative preponderance of the large chromatia in ponds and puddles; the intracellular sulphur can serve as stored reducing equivalents, which allow the fixation of carbon dioxide in the light, even in the absence of external hydrogen donors. In the utilisation of thiosulphate, sulphane- and sulphone-sulphur can be distinguished; only the sulphane-sulphur is stored whereas the sulphone-sulphur appears immediately as sulphate in the medium. Some chlorobia oxidise hydrogen sulphide only to sulphur, which is excreted. These bacteria flourish especially in association with *Desulfuromonas acetoxidans*; the latter organisms, which respire anaerobically, reduce sulphur to hydrogen sulphide with the oxidation of ethanol to acetate. *Chlorobium* and *Desulfuromonas* together are a model example of the functional association, syntrophy, between two microorganisms (see Ch. 9.3).

Dark metabolism. Many of the non-sulphur purple bacteria and *Chloroflexus* can grow aerobically in the dark at the expense of organic substrates. This shows that they must possess the components of respiratory metabolism, including the tricarboxylic acid cycle. The latter is also involved in anaerobic metabolism in the light. The utilisation of a large number of organic acids and sugars by some Chromatiaceae and Rhodospirillaceae leads to the conclusion that the basic metabolism of the phototrophic bacteria, though varying in detail is principally that of the known pathways (fructose-bisphosphate, Entner–Doudoroff, tricarboxylic acid cycle, etc.).

A modest energy gain is also possible in the dark under anaerobic conditions. This is not really surprising since phototrophic bacteria need to survive during the night! Fermentation reactions may take place at the expense of reserve materials being used as the hydrogen donor and with sulphur as the hydrogen acceptor; carbon dioxide, acetate, proprionate and hydrogen sulphide have been demonstrated as end products of this anaerobic metabolism. However, no growth of these organisms occurs in the dark under anaerobic conditions.

Photoproduction of hydrogen. In the presence of suitable organic or inorganic hydrogen donors, some representatives of the Rhodospirillinaeae and the Chlorobiaceae can produce molecular hydrogen in the light. This formation of H_2 is dependent on the carbon to nitrogen ratio of the medium and is inhibited by free ammonium ions. It is also reversibly inhibited by N_2. The photoproduction of hydrogen has been attributed to a secondary function of nitrogenase, i.e. the ability to reduce protons as well as N_2 and thus to liberate H_2. The presence of excess energy and reducing power, therefore, leads to the evolution of hydrogen.

Nitrogen fixation. The vast majority of the phototrophic bacteria so far examined are able to fix nitrogen. Their growth rates, however, are usually lower in this case than in the presence of ammonium ions.

Storage materials. The following typical storage products occur in phototrophic bacteria: poly-β-hydroxybutyrate, polysaccharides and polyphosphate. Under some growth conditions, chromatia contain inclusions of sulphur present in the orthorhombic form inside vacuoles.

12.1.3   Distribution of the phototrophic bacteria

Distribution. Phototrophic bacteria have their habitats in the anaerobic zones of many aquatic locations; in shallow ponds, slowly flowing waters, lakes, and estuaries. The purple sulphur bacteria often occur as salmon-coloured to dark burgundy coverings on mud and decomposing plant materials. Sometimes they spread in 10-cm-high layers over the black mud. Such water 'blooms' in ponds (Fig. 12.12) are due mainly to the giant Chromatiaceae (*Chromatium okenii, C. warmingii, C, weissei, Thiospirillum jenense*), but are also due to some small chromatia and Chlorobiaceae. The purple bacteria also grow prolifically in shallow ponds when the surface is covered by a thick layer of duckweed (*Lemna*) or by the leaves of water-lilies. This biological filter apparently absorbs the spectral components that can be utilised by green algae and cyanobacteria, but it transmits the spectral components that are absorbed by the bacteriochlorophylls and the dark red carotenoids. Hence, the anoxygenic photobacteria can grow underneath the *Lemna* cover, but cyanobacteria and green algae cannot (Fig. 12.12). Some species, therefore, occur as almost pure cultures in their natural habitat. Rhodospirillaceae are almost always present, but they rarely accumulate.

A seasonal mass proliferation of purple sulphur bacteria also occurs in the anaerobic zones of lakes below the chemocline (see Fig. 17.2). Hydrogen sulphide, carbon dioxide and organic compounds are available in this layer. Although the infra-red spectral components of sunlight do not reach to a depth of 10–30 m, the maximum of the spectral energy distribution in the blue to blue-green range (450–500 nm) occurs here; this is the range in which carotenoids absorb. This explains the relatively high carotenoid content of the purple bacteria and actually determines their colour. The carotenoids (like the phycoerythrins in red algae and some cyanobacteria) enable the purple bacteria to carry out photometabolism at these greater depths of water. For the same reason, the carotenoid-rich brown-coloured species of the green sulphur bacteria (*Chlorobium phaeobacteriodes, C. phaeovibrioides, Pelochromatium*) also predominate at these depths.

Enrichment culture. Enrichment culture of anaerobic phototrophic bacteria is based on the above observation, i.e. that purple sulphur bacteria proliferate in shallow ponds and under coverings of *Lemna*. Selective

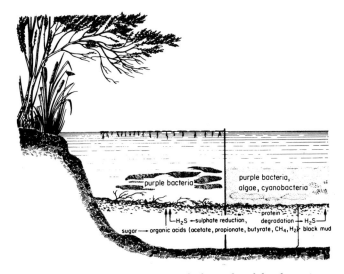

Fig. 12.12. *Edge of shallow water in which purple sulphur bacteria can grow profusely.*

culture conditions for the green sulphur bacteria, as well as for the purple bacteria containing Bchl *a* and Bchl *b*, can be established by the use of filters that absorb light in the short-wave range but transmit only in the infra-red region that is appropriate for the various groups.

In addition it is the available hydrogen donor and the concentration of hydrogen sulphide that determine whether Rhodospirillaceae, Chromatiaceae or Chlorobiaceae will predominate in such an enrichment culture (Winogradsky column, Fig. 12.13). On inoculation of such a column (containing protein, soil and sand, and filled with water) with a sample from the natural habitat, non-sulphur purple bacteria multiply in the light. Addition of calcium sulphate can provide for a continuous supply of hydrogen sulphide by the reduction of sulphate; this inhibits the growth of the non-sulphur purple bacteria, and sulphur bacteria come to predominate. In a synthetic medium containing vitamin B_{12}, many different species of green and purple bacteria can be enriched by careful manipulation of hydrogen sulphide and nutrient salt concentrations, pH, temperature, and light intensities. The nature of the hydrogen donor and presence of some vitamins (biotin, 4-aminobenzoic acid, thiamine, nicotinic acid) also play decisive roles in the selective enrichment of individual non-sulphur purple bacteria.

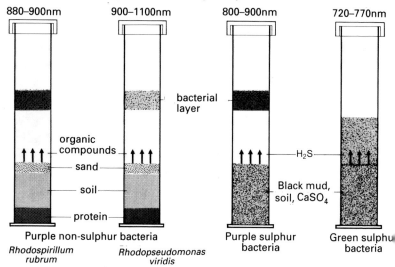

Fig. 12.13. *Enrichment cultures (Winogradsky columns) for phototrophic bacteria.*

The spectral transmission regions of the light filters behind which the cited bacterial species and groups develop preferentially are shown at the top. Some days after start of the culture and inoculation with pond water and mud, red and green bacterial layers respectively, form in the water columns.

12.2   The elementary processes of photosynthesis

Photosynthesis is defined as the **conversion of light energy** to biochemically utilisable energy (**ATP**) and **reducing power** (NAD(P)H) in the cells of phototrophic organisms for the synthesis of cell material. The photosynthetic phosphorylation and the photosynthetic pyridine nucleotide reduction are the elementary processes of photosynthesis.

This knowledge is the result of experiments and their interpretation based on comparisons of bacterial photosynthesis with the photosynthesis of green plants. Winogradsky (1888) recognised from his experiments with sulphur bacteria that the assimilation of CO_2 is not obligatorily coupled to light as energy source. Engelmann (1883–8) described purple bacteria as being phototrophic on the basis of stimulus-response experiments. Buder (1919) then showed that the purple bacteria represented a new metabolic type: sulphur and non-sulphur purple bacteria assimilate carbon dioxide and organic substances, respectively, in the light. This type of photosynthesis, however, is basically quite different from that of the higher plants: (a) by the inability to use water as the hydrogen donor for photosynthesis and hence the absence of any oxygen evolution; (b) by the utilisation of hydrogen sulphide or organic substances as hydrogen donors (an ability not shared by green plants).The quantitative investigations on purple sulphur bacteria (by van Niel in 1931) then led to the formulation of the following equation:

$$CO_2 + 2H_2S \xrightarrow{h\nu} \langle CH_2O \rangle + H_2O + 2S$$

$$2CO_2 + H_2S + 2H_2O \xrightarrow{h\nu} 2\langle CH_2O \rangle + H_2SO_4$$

On comparing the first of these equations with the equation for green plant photosynthesis, a striking analogy was found:

Chromatium:

$$CO_2 + 2H_2S \xrightarrow{h\nu} \langle CH_2O \rangle + H_2O + 2S$$

Green plants:

$$CO_2 + 2H_2O \xrightarrow{h\nu} \langle CH_2O \rangle + H_2O + 2O$$

This suggested that in bacterial photosynthesis, hydrogen sulphide plays the role that water plays in green plant photosynthesis. The general equation of photosynthesis, based on this analogy,

$$CO_2 + H_2A \xrightarrow{h\nu} \langle CH_2O \rangle + H_2O + 2A$$

then led to the hypothesis that all photosynthesis is based on the same elementary process, and that the various types differ only by the nature of their hydrogen donor (i.e. water, hydrogen sulphide or organic material). The common elementary process was seen as a photolytic cleavage (photolysis) of water ($H_2O + h\nu \rightarrow [H] + [OH]$) into a reducing and an oxidising component. In this scheme, bacteria are dependent on an external hydrogen donor, H_2A, with which the oxidising component can be reduced to water, whereas the green plants have gained the ability to liberate oxygen from the oxidising component ($4[OH] \rightarrow 2H_2O + O_2$). Although this concept of the photolysis of water as the primary elementary process in photosynthesis had to be abandoned, the principle of a light-driven transport of reducing equivalents, is still maintained in the modern representation of the electron flux theory of photosynthesis.

The **products of photosynthesis** are ATP and reducing equivalents. These products can be demonstrated in intact cells and in the chloroplasts isolated from these (in green plants), as well as in suspensions of photosynthetic membrane vesicles from purple bacteria. CO_2 fixation is not obligatorily coupled to the light reaction and can take place as a 'dark reaction' independent of the pigment-carrying structures, provided that

ATP and $NAD(P)H_2$ are available. The two processes are also spatially separate: photosynthesis is localised in the membranes, whereas CO_2 fixation occurs in the cytoplasm and the chloroplast stroma, respectively. As has already been discussed, the oxygenic photosynthesis of green plants and cyanobacteria differs from the anoxygenic photosynthesis of the anaerobic phototrophic bacteria by the nature of the utilisable hydrogen donors. Two successive photoreactions are required for the utilisation of water as the hydrogen donor, whereas a single photoreaction is sufficient for the utilisation of hydrogen donors with more negative redox potentials than water. Since the elementary processes of oxygenic photosynthesis are known in more detail than those of anoxygenic photosynthesis, the former will be discussed first.

The photoreactions.   The photoreactions are the primary elementary processes in photosynthesis. These photochemical redox reactions take place in the **photochemical reaction centres**, which consist of several components, the primary electron donor (P) (a special chlorophyll–protein complex) and the primary electron acceptor (X) being the most important. Both are redox systems. The donor system (P/P^+) always has a positive potential, and the acceptor system (X/X^-) a negative potential. The energy input leads to the transfer of an electron.

$$\text{donor (reduced)} + \text{acceptor (oxidised)} \xrightarrow{\ hv\ } \text{donor (oxidised)} \\ + \text{acceptor (reduced)}$$

Alternatively, this can be written

$$P + X \xrightarrow{\ hv\ } P^+ + X^-$$

The first photoreaction can therefore be formulated as follows:

$$\text{Chl } a + X \xrightarrow{\ hv\ } \text{Chl } a^+ + X^-$$

The photoreaction of the purple bacteria can be described analogously as

$$\text{Bchl } a + X \xrightarrow{\ hv\ } \text{Bchl } a^+ + X^-$$

The photochemical redox reaction in which 'P' is oxidised and 'X' reduced is illustrated in the accompanying diagram. This photoreaction causes an electron gap at the donor; this gap must be re-filled. According to the origin of the replenishing electrons, an **open chain** and a **cyclic electron flow** can be distinguished. In the open chain electron flow electrons

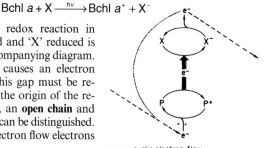

·········· cyclic electron flow
– – – – – open chain electron flow

are supplied by external donor; in the case of the first photoreaction, the electron-transport chain connects the two photosystems, whereas in the case of the second photoreaction, the electron donor is H_2O. In cyclic electron flow, the electrons are passed back from the reduced acceptor (X) to the oxidised donor.

Whereas the open chain electron flow causes a reduction of NADP as well as proton translocation at the membrane, the cyclic electron flow results only in proton translocation.

12.2.1   Anoxygenic photosynthesis

The photosynthetic electron transport of the anaerobic phototrophic bacteria differs in several respects from that discussed above. Only a single light reaction participates in anoxygenic photosynthesis and drives a cyclic electron transport. The electrons that are withdrawn from the cycle for the reduction of NAD cannot be replaced by the cleavage of water. This photosynthesis, therefore, depends on the presence of reduced substances in the medium, and no oxygen is evolved. Although the light reaction proper is analogous to the light reaction I of green plants, it probably leads only to the creation of a proton potential, and hence the trapping of energy (ATP), but not to the reduction of NAD. There is no 'open chain' electron transport (from a donor to pyridine nucleotide); $NADH_2$ is apparently formed in a dark reaction in the course of an energy-driven reverse electron transport. In addition, the differences between the various groups of phototrophic bacteria with regard to their pigment composition and photosynthetic mechanisms are far greater than those between different groups of green plants. In the overall presentation below, the green bacteria have not been included.

Photoreaction of the purple bacteria.   As has already been mentioned, the pigments and electron-transport components of the purple bacteria are also localised in membranes. The pigment complex of the photochemical reaction centre can be separated from antenna pigments. The energy absorbed by the antenna pigments (bacteriochlorophylls and carotenoids) is channelled to the reaction centre. Isolated reaction centres consist of a protein complex containing Bchl a, bacteriophaeophytin, carotenoid, ubiquinone, and iron-sulphur proteins. The reaction centre pigment is designated P 870 according to the wavelength of the maximal absorption decrease on illumination. P 870 is oxidised to P 870$^+$ on illumination. The redox potential of this electron donor is in the region +450 to +490 mV. A complex of ubiquinone and Fe–S protein probably functions as the primary electron acceptor. This complex seems to

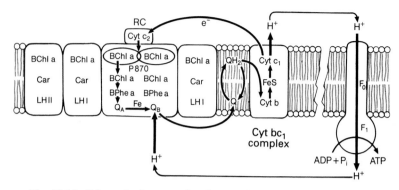

Fig. 12.14. *Schematic diagram of a photosynthetic membrane from a purple bacterium with cyclical electron transport.*

LHI = Antennapigment complex I (B 870); LHII = Antennapigment complex II (B 800–850); BChl a = Bacteriochlorophyll *a*; BPhe a = Bacteriophaeophytin a; Q_A = Quinone A; Q_B; Quinone B; Q = Quinone 'pool'; P 870 = Pigment 870 (Bchl *a*, special pair); RC = Reaction centre;

Car = Carotenoid; Cyt b = cytochrome *b*; Cyt c_1 = cytochrome c_1; FeS = Iron-sulphur centre (Rieske-protein); Cyt c_2 = cytochrome c_2; F_0 = F_0-component of ATP synthase; F_1 = F1 component of ATP synthase; Cyt. bc_1 = cytochrome b_1 complex.

have a potential of only –100 mV, and it is therefore improbable that the electrons emitted by the light reaction can reduce NAD. Rather, the electrons are transferred back to P 870$^+$ via ubiquinone, cytochromes *b* and c_2, and possibly Fe–S proteins (Fig. 12.14). It is thought, therefore, that the electrons required for the reduction of NAD are withdrawn from the cyclic electron flow and are transferred via an energy-dependent reverse electron-transport flow to NAD. This is an important difference from the otherwise analogous first photoreaction in oxygenic photosynthesis. To fill the electron gap in the cycle, the purple bacteria must rely on external electron donors: hydrogen sulphide, sulphur, or thiosulphate, in the case of the purple sulphur bacteria, and organic compounds (malate, succinate) or hydrogen in both groups of purple bacteria.

It has been shown experimentally that the photosynthetic electron transport in purple bacteria also leads to the creation of a proton gradient. Intact cells respond to illumination by extrusion of protons (acidification of the medium). In suspensions of photosynthetic membrane vesicles (chromoatophores), illumination causes transport of protons into

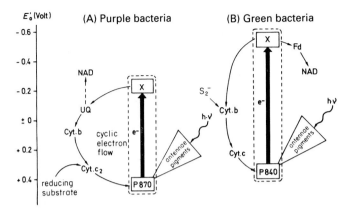

Fig. 12.15. *Scheme for the photosynthetic electron transport in Rhodospirillaceae and Chlorobiaceae in a redox potential diagram.*

Cyt, cytochrome; Fd, ferredoxin; UQ, ubiquinone; P 870 or P 840, BChl a (electron donor of the reaction centre); X, electron acceptor of the reaction centre. The photochemical reaction centre is ringed by a broken line. See text for further explanations.

the vesicles. The polarity of the vesicles and thylakoid membranes is therefore the same as that of sub-mitochondrial vesicles. This polarity is explained by the fact that these membranes originated from invagination of cytoplasmic or inner chloroplast membranes to the inside. Although the individual membrane components have not yet been localised, it can be assumed that hydrogen- and electron- transporting components in the membranes of the anaerobic phototrophic bacteria are also arranged so as to effect proton translocation. In the vesicles, the electrons are transferred to the outside and the protons to the inside. This proton potential is the force driving photosynthetic phosphorylation.

Photoreaction of Chlorobiaceae.   The photoreaction of the green bacteria has not yet been fully elucidated. There are indications that the primary electron acceptor of the light reaction has a potential of about -500 mV (compared with -100 mV in the purple bacteria). With such a strongly negative potential, electrons from the primary acceptor can be used directly for the reduction of ferredoxin and pyridine nucleotides (Fig. 12.15). Thus the Chlorobiaceae are probably not dependent on an energy-driven reverse electron transport, and this independence would constitute a very important difference from the photosynthetic mechanism of the purple bacteria. The yield of the photoreaction in the

Chlorobiaceae would then be completely equivalent to that of the first photoreaction in cyanobacteria. From an evolutionary point of view, this would place photosynthesis of Chlorobiaceae as the connecting link between photosynthesis in purple bacteria and that in cyanobacteria and green plants.

12.2.2   Oxygenic photosynthesis

The elementary processes of photosynthesis take place in the thylakoids. These are flattened, completely closed membrane vesicles and are contained in the cells of cyanobacteria and in the chloroplasts of green algae and higher plants.

The thylakoid membrane and antenna pigments.   The thylakoid membranes of chloroplasts contain chlorophyll (Chl) a and b, carotenoids, electron carriers, and enzymes. The vast majority of the chlorophyll molecules (99.5%), as well as accessory pigments (carotenoids, phycobiliproteins), serve for light absorption and energy transfer. They constitute the antenna pigment system. Only a very small fraction of chlorophyll a serves as the photochemical reaction centre, which is where the photochemical redox reaction proper takes place. The antenna pigments harvest the light (energy) and channel it to the reaction centre chlorophyll (carotenoid $\rightarrow$ carotenoid*; chlorophyll + carotenoid* $\rightarrow$ chlorophyll* + carotenoid). The carotenoids also have a protective function. In glaring sunlight they act as a buffer: they convert the excess light energy to heat, which is dissipated, thus protecting the chlorophylls from destructive photo-oxidation. The antenna pigment system and the photochemically active reaction centre constitute the photosynthetic unit.

Two photoreactions at two pigments systems.   In oxygenic photosynthesis, two pigment systems are placed in series (Fig. 12.16). The pigment system responsive to the longer wavelengths ($\lambda < 730$ nm) is known as photosystem I, and the pigment system responsive to the shorter wavelenths ($\lambda < 700$ nm) is known as photosystem II. The photochemical reaction centre of system I contains Chl a_1 (P 700) which functions as the primary electron donor for the first photoreactions. The Chl a_1 is activated by the light energy absorbed by the antenna pigments of system I. This activation causes the oxidation of Chl a_1 to Chl a_1^+, that is, the emission of an electron, whereby Chl a_1 to Chl a_1^+. In other words, the emission of an electron in the reaction centre produces an electron deficit. This electron gap is then immediately filled by another electron which is passed on via an electron-transport chain. The acceptor of the

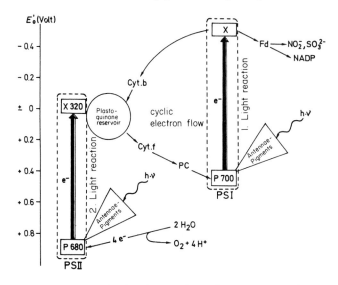

Fig. 12.16. *Z-scheme for the photosynthetic electron transport in a redox potential diagram.*

P 700, Chl a_I (electron donor of pigment system I (PSI)); P 680, Chl a_{II} (electron donor of pigment system II (PSII)); X320, electron acceptor of PSII; X, electron acceptor of PSI, an iron–sulphur protein; Fd, ferredoxin;

PC, plastocyanine; Cyt, cytochrome. The photochemical reaction centres are ringed by broken line. See text for explanations.

electron emitted by Chl a_I is probably an iron–sulphur protein ('X'). This has an even more negative redox potential than –420 mV, possibly –530 mV. The acceptor transfers the electron to ferredoxin, and from ferredoxin (reduced) the reducing power can be transferred to NADP or other acceptors. Alternatively, the electron can pass from 'X' via plastoquinone, cytochrome, and plastocyanine in a cyclic electron flow back to the reaction centre chlorophyll a_I^+ and, thus, replenish the electron gap.

The reaction centre of photosystem II contains Chl a_{II} (P 860), which is the primary electron donor of the second photoreaction. Chl a_{II} is excited by the energy absorbed by the antenna pigments of photosystem II. The activation of Chl a_{II} causes the emission of an electron; this is accepted by a specific plastoquinone molecule (X 320), which is thereby reduced to a semiquinone. The transferred electron is only weakly reducing (E_0', ~0 mV). The electron donor for photosystem II is water. The electron gap localised at Chl a_{II} is filled by one of the electrons released from H_2O in the formation of O_2 ($2\,H_2O \rightarrow O_2 + 4\,H^+ + 4e^-$). The splitting of water is carried out with the participation of manganese.

The two pigment systems are connected by an electron-transport chain and cooperate in series. The essential connecting link in this chain is plastoquinone. It is present in large excess and functions as an electron reservoir, rather like ubiquinone in the respiratory electron-transport chain. This reservoir accepts electrons from X320, and is in turn oxidised by photosystem I. After being transferred via the redox carriers cytochrome f (a membrane-bound c-type cytochrome) and plastocyanine (a soluble copper-containing protein), the electrons of the plastoquinone reservoir serve to replenish the electron gap of Chl a_i^+. This plastoquinone reservoir has the important function of collecting and distributing the electrons from several sources; at least ten electron transport chains are joined via this common electron reservoir.

The main electron-transport pathways of the primary photosynthetic processes are presented in an energy diagram (Fig. 12.16). This well-known Z-scheme of electron flow is the result of investigations using light-flash spectrophotometry with artificial electron donors and acceptors, as well as specific inhibitors. It takes account of the redox potentials of individual pigments and electron-transfer agents, as well as of the time sequence of their oxidation and reduction. However, it does not give any information about the localisation of these components in the membrane.

Localisation of pigments and electron carriers in the membrane.   Clues about the precise localisation of individual pigments and electron-transport components have been obtained by means of functional tests of thylakoids in the presence of antibodies or of lipophilic or hydrophilic artificial redox system. The antibodies against individual purified components of the photosynthetic electron-transport system cannot traverse the membrane and therefore can react only with components on the outer surface of the thylakoid membrane. The antibodies against ferredoxin and ferredoxin-NADP reductase, for example, inhibit the function of photosystem I, indicating that these components must be situated on the outer surface of the thylakoid. The site of the electron donor, on the other hand, is on the inner surface. Although there are still contradictory observations and doubts regarding the localisation and orientation of photosystem II, Fig. 12.17 ventures a schematic representation. This Z-scheme of the photosynthetic electron-transport system must be distinguished from that of the redox potential diagram (Fig. 12.16). Figure 12.17 shows that the electrons obtained from the cleavage of water are transferred from inside the thylakoid membrane to the stroma.

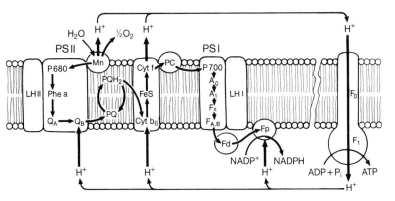

Fig. 12.17. *Schematic diagram of a photosynthetic membrane from a green plant with both Photosystems, PS I and PS II.*

The components are arranged in the thylakoid membrane in such a way as to produce vectorial electron flux (e^-) through the membrane. A_0 = Primary acceptor (chlorophyll) of PS I; A_1 = Secondary acceptor (phylloquinone) of PS I; Cyt b_6 = cytochrome b_6; Cyt f = cytochrome f; F_1 = F1 component of ATP synthase; $F_{A,B}$ = Iron–sulphur centre A and B; F_d = Ferredoxin; FeS = Iron–sulphur centre; F_0 = F_0 component of ATP synthase; Fp = Flavoprotein (ferredoxin-NADP oxidoreductase); F_x = Iron–sulphur centre X; LHI = Antennapigment complex I; LHII = Antennapigment complex II; Mn = Manganese-containing hydrolysis complex; P680 = pigment 680 (chlorophyll *a*, special pair); P700 = pigment 700 (chlorophyll *a*, special pair); PC = Plastocyanine; Phe a = Phaeophytin *a* (Primary acceptor of PSII); PQ = Plastoquinone; Q_A = Secondary acceptor (quinone A) of PS II; Q_B = Quinone B.

Vectorial electron transport and formation of a proton gradient.   The suggested localisation of the photosynthetic electron-transport components is in agreement with physiological observations and measurements. Illumination of a suspension of broken chloroplasts or thylakoids leads to an increase in the pH of the external medium, followed by a decrease in pH when the illumination is terminated. Thus, illumination causes transport of protons into the thylakoids (Fig. 12.18). In other words, light energy can be utilised to establish a proton gradient across the thylakoid membranes. It had already been shown some time ago that thylakoid suspensions can synthesise ATP in the dark if the pH of the medium is increased from 4 to 8. Such experiments were among the first to support the chemiosmotic theory of energy conversion. More detailed investigations showed that the transport of one electron by the two light

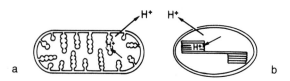

Fig. 12.18. *Proton transport in illuminated cells and organelles.*

(a) *Rhodopseudomonas sphaeroides*;
(b) chloroplasts. See text for details.

reactions resulted in the transport of two protons to the inside of the thylakoid. It is therefore assumed that the two photoreactions together with an electron-transport chain cause a vectorial electron flow from water on the inside of the thylakoid membrane to NADP on the outside. The photoreactions thus lead to reduction of NADP and charging of the membrane. In other words, the light reactions function as a light-driven proton pump (positive charge inside the thylakoid) and lead to the formation of a proton gradient. The proton potential causes the generation of ATP; it couples photosynthetic electron transport to phosphorylation in the same manner in which respiratory electron transport is tied to phosphorylation.

12.2.3   Summary

Photosynthesis converts light energy into chemical energy. The primary action of light is the transfer of electrons, in the photochemical reaction centres, from a donor to an acceptor against a thermodynamic gradient. At least some of these electrons return to the reaction centre via an electron-transport chain. By virtue of an appropriate arrangement of the electron-transport chain components in the membrane, this leads to translocation of protons and the establishment of a proton gradient across the membrane. The photosynthetic apparatus can therefore be regarded primarily as a 'light-driven proton pump'. The proton potential is a prerequisite for the conversion of energy by phosphorylation. This regeneration of ATP occurs by a mechanism similar to that in the membranes of respiring bacteria and mitochondria. As far as the conversion of radiant energy to biochemically utilisable energy (ATP) is concerned, there is in principle little difference between the photosynthesis of phototrophic bacteria and that of green plants: in the purple bacteria, photosynthesis is apparently only just sufficient to support this generation of utilisable energy. Photosynthesis in the cyanobacteria and green plants can be regarded in evolutionary terms as more developed

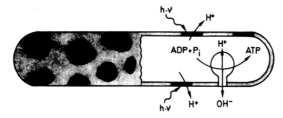

Fig. 12.19. Halobacterium halobium.

The red cytoplasmic membrane and the patches of purple membrane are shown on the left, and the function of the purple membrane as a light-driven proton pump is shown on the right.

processes; the sequential arrangement of two light reactions has made it possible to activate electrons in the first reaction to a level sufficient for the reduction of ferredoxin and NADP. A second light reaction then allows the utilisation of water as an electron source. This combination therefore provides for the reduction of NADP and the evolution of oxygen in addition to generating utilisable energy.

The process of photosynthesis is the most frequently occurring chemical reaction on earth. Not only does it provide for the continuous *de novo* synthesis of organic materials, it is also the source of fossil energy in the form of coal, petroleum, and natural gas.

The effort and expense invested in the attempts to unravel the mysteries of photosynthesis is therefore fully justified. Apart from the facts that have been demonstrated experimentally, the model of photosynthesis described above still incorporates many hypotheses; further investigation is required for their proof.

12.3   Utilisation of light energy by halobacteria

The species of the genus *Halobacterium* (*H. halobium*, *H. cutirubrum*) are a physiologically highly specialised group. They have their habitat in very concentrated or saturated salt solutions, such as the great salt lakes of Utah, or the salterns in which seawater is evaporated to obtain salts. These bacteria are well adapted to their extreme habitats by having intracellular salt concentrations similar to those in the medium. They grow optimally in the presence of 3.5–5.0 M NaCl. Enzymes isolated from these cells also require salt concentrations of 2 M for their activity and stability. The halobacteria belong to the archaebacteria.

The rod-shaped motile cells of *H. halobium* are pigmented red, orange or yellow by virtue of their carotenoid content. Their cytoplasmic membrane shows dark red patches about 0.5 μm in diameter, the total area of which occupies about half of the cell surface (Fig. 12.19). These pigmented areas constitute the so-called purple membrane; their colour is due to the presence of **bacteriorhodopsin** which resembles the rhodopsin in the visual cells of animals. This pigment effects a proton gradient between the inner and outer surface of the membrane during illumination. The purple membrane thus acts as a 'light-driven proton pump' and leads to the establishment of an electrochemical membrane potential. Its equilibration can be accompanied by the generation of ATP. The purple membrane thus facilitates a special kind of photo-phosphorylation. The energy obtained by this in the light complements that obtained from aerobic substrate oxidation.

13 Fixation of molecular nitrogen

Prokaryotes are the only organisms that are able to tap the nitrogen reservoir of the atmosphere and fix molecular nitrogen. Either as free-living organisms or in symbiosis with higher plants, they can carry out reactions that result in the incorporation of N_2 into organic compounds and hence, directly or via plant substance, into the protein reservoir of the soil. The symbiotic nitrogen fixation of leguminous plants can produce a nitrogen yield of 100–300 kg N/hectare (ha)/annum. The free-living organisms are estimated to contribute about 1–3 kg N/ha/annum (see 'The nitrogen cycle', Chapter I). In addition, significant amounts of bound nitrogen may reach the soil via precipitation from the atmosphere; according to the degree of atmospheric pollution, this can amount to 3–30 kg N/ha/annum. It has been estimated from overall measurements and calculations that the total global nitrogen fixation during 1974 produced 175×10^6 tonnes (t), of which 90×10^6 t were fixed in cultivated soil. The Haber–Bosch process fixed 40×10^6 t, but the main part of the fixed nitrogen was contributed by rhizobial symbiosis.

Biological nitrogen fixation is a reductive process. The nitrogenase system transfers a total 6[H] to N_2 and releases 2[H] as molecular hydrogen (H_2). Ammonia is the first identifiable product of this enzyme reaction:

$$N \equiv N + 8\,[H] \longrightarrow HN = NH \longrightarrow H_2N-NH_2 \longrightarrow 2\,NH_3 + H_2$$

| Nitrogen | Diimide | Hydrazine | Ammonia |

Diimide and hydrazine are suggested only as illustration of possible enzyme-bound intermediates.

All the nitrogenase enzyme systems isolated so far from many N_2-fixing bacteria show extensive similarities. Their most remarkable property is their exquisite sensitivity to oxygen *in vivo* as well as *in vitro*. This has to be remembered in all investigations and formulation of hypotheses.

13.1   Nitrogen fixation by symbiotic bacteria

Because of its high yield, the symbiotic fixation of nitrogen was noticed long ago and exploited in agriculture by crop rotations, in which leguminous crops were ploughed into the soil to add organic nitrogen.

> The first evidence that clover and bean crops yielded a gain in nitrogen was provided by Boussingault, Hellriegel and Wilfarth (1886–8) who pointed out the connection between the leguminous root nodules and nitrogen fixation. Bean plants can grow without a supply of fixed nitrogen only when their roots bear nodules; the nodules are the result of infection of the root hairs by soil bacteria (Fig. 13.1).

13.1.1   Root nodules of leguminous plants

The bacteria responsible for the formation of root nodules in leguminous plants belong to the genus *Rhizobium*. They occur as free-living, strictly aerobic, gram-negative rods in soil and grow on organic nutrients. There are some strains (*Bradyrhizobium*) which are able to grow autotrophically with H_2. Three groups can be distinguished according to their host specificity and their growth (Table 13.1) which have been given a number of generic names. Group (1) *Rhizobium* includes the fastest growing nodule bacteria of the indigenous cultivated plants. Group (2) *Bradyrhizobium japonicum* is the group of slow-growing symbionts of soybeans. Group (3) *Azorhizobium caulinodans* is a bacterium that forms stem nodules.

Table 13.1. *Subgroups of leguminous nodule-forming bacteria*

Genus and species	Plant host
Rhizobium leguminosarum	Peas
Rhizobium meliloti	Lucerne
Rhizobium trifolii	Clover
Rhizobium phaseoli	Beans
Rhizobium lupini	Lupins
Bradyrhizobium japonicum	Soybeans
Azorhizobium caulinodans	Sesbania

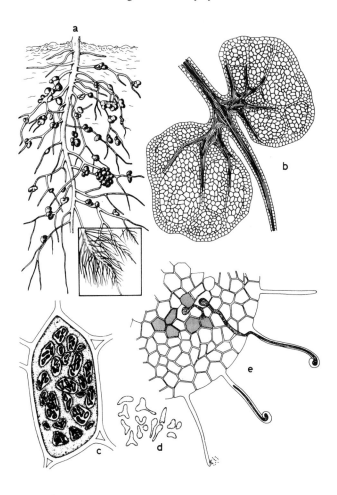

Fig. 13.1. *Symbiotic nitrogen fixation in the root nodules of leguminous plants.*

(a) Root of pea with nodules.
(b) Section through fully developed nodules. (c) Section through a cell filled with rhizobia. (d) The bacteria inside the cells have various shapes (bacteroids). (e) Penetration of the bacteria at the tips of the root hairs and growth of the infection thread through the root cortex.

Nearly all leguminous plants can form nodules with rhizobia, and a given *Rhizobium* species can usually form a symbiotic relationship with a number of leguminous plants.

Stages in root nodule formation.   The bacteria enter young root hairs from the soil. Initial contact between the partners is followed by **recognition**. Leguminous plants contain **lectins**. These are glycoproteins that bind specific polysaccharides. Lectins are ubiquitously distributed in nature and probably have general recognition functions. The interactions between the lectins on the outer wall of the young root hairs and the polysaccharides on the outer cell wall of rhizobia have been investigated in the case of *R. trifolium*, infecting white clover. Binding occurs only between compatible partners; not any *Rhizobium* can bind to any leguminous plant or vice versa. When binding has occurred, the tip of the root hair bends and the bacteria penetrate and grow in the form of an 'infection tube' – which is surrounded by the root cells with a cellulose membrane – towards the base (i.e. upwards), and infects further cells of the root epidermis. Normal diploid cells are destroyed but in tetraploid cells, of which there are always some present, the rhizobia multiply. Growth hormones are produced and the root epidermal cells undergo multiplication. The **root nodule** is the result of this tissue proliferation induced by the rhizobia via growth promoters, probably **cytokines**. The rapidly dividing bacteria grow into deformed cells, the **bacteroids**, which can have more than ten times the volume of a rhizobium. The bacteroids, singly or in groups, surrounded by peribacteroid membranes, inhabit the cytoplasm of the plant cells. The tissue containing the bacteroids is red because it contains **leghaemoglobin**. The nodules turn green during ageing due to the breakdown of the leghaemoglobin to green bile pigments (biliverdins). When the nodule dies, stationary-phase rhizobia, which are still present in considerable numbers, are released and can multiply by using the degradation products of the nodule as substrates.

The function of the bacteroids and leghaemoglobin.   The bacteroids fix nitrogen. During the nitrogen-fixing phase they are supplied with C_4-dicarboxylic acids (malate, succinate, fumarate, etc.) by the plant cell. In contrast to the free-living rhizobia, the bacteroids are unable to utilise sugars. They secrete ammonium ions which are apparently incorporated into organic compounds by glutamine synthase present in the surrounding plant cell (Ch. 7.6). The relationship between the plant and *Rhizobium* is thus a true mutual symbiosis. This mutual dependence of the two partners is even more explicit in the role played by leghaemoglobin in the fixation of nitrogen. The formation of leghaemoglobin is a specific effect of the symbiosis. The prosthetic group, protohaem, is synthesised by the bacteroids, whilst the synthesis of the protein part involves the plant cells.

Leghaemoglobin resembles myoglobin. It is present in the nodules predominantly in the iron (II) oxyform and has a very high affinity for oxygen. The pigment is localised in the cytoplasm of the plant cell, and not in the peribacteroid space. It is assumed that the leghaemoglobin facilitates the **transport of oxygen** through the plant cells to the bacteroids, i.e. that it increases the rate of oxygen transport. Its properties ensure that the bacteroids have sufficient oxygen for their energy requirements without producing excessive partial pressures of O_2 which would inhibit nitrogen fixation. The presence of the leghaemoglobin seems to provide full protection against oxygen damage for the N_2-fixing enzymes (Ch. 13.3). Rhizobia are the only nitrogen fixing bacteria of which not all strains possess the enzyme hydrogenase, which also has a protective function against oxygen.

It is thought improbable that free-living rhizobia in soil can fix nitrogen. Demonstration of nitrogenase during growth on nutrient agar plates has been possible in only a few strains of *Rhizobium*. Formation of nitrogenase depends on the partial pressure of oxygen inside the colonies.

Stem nodules. In some leguminous plants nodules occur on the stem. They contain strains of rhizobia which belong to the genus designated *Azorhizobium caulinodans*. These leguminous plants, for example *Sesbania rostrata*, grow in damp habitats in tropical Africa and India. The nodules appear on submerged stems and on those above soil level. Knowledge regarding this stem symbiosis is only very recent. It is expected that these nitrogen-fixing systems will show less oxygen sensitivity than the other N_2-fixing systems.

13.1.2   Root nodules in non-leguminous plants

A number of dicotyledonous higher plants, that are not members of the Leguminosae also contain root nodules with the ability to fix nitrogen. This nitrogen fixation is also due to a symbiotic partnership with prokaryotes. In most cases these endosymbionts are actinomycetes and members of the genus *Frankia*. The host plants of such actinomyctes include trees, shrubs, and herbaceous plants. They are widely distributed and often occur as pioneer plants in nitrogen-poor habitats. The nitrogen yield of at least a few of these plants amounts to 150–300 kg N/ha/annum and is thus of considerable economic importance. The following plants belong to the most effective nitrogen fixers: *Casuarina equisetifolia,*

Alnus, Hippophae and *Ceanothus*. *Myrica*, *Dryas*, *Elaeagnus* and *Shepherdia* are somewhat less effective as nitrogen fixers.

The root nodules of woody plants can attain the size of tennis balls. They consist of densely packed, coral-like, branching roots that have ceased to grow. In *Casuarina* the nodules consist of a loose bundle of thickened rootlets whose growth is negatively geotropic. Only the outer parenchyma cells are infected by the symbionts. Infection of the roots occurs from the soil, via the root hairs, as in the Leguminosae. They also share the presence of leghaemoglobin with the nodules of the Leguminosae. Most recently, a strain of *Rhizobium* was identified as the endosymbiont in a non-leguminous plant, *Parasponia parviflora*. This strain was transferred to bean plants, and the resulting nodules were active in N_2 fixation.

13.1.3   Symbiosis with nitrogen-fixing cyanobacteria

Cyanobacteria can also occur as nitrogen-fixing partners in symbiosis with higher plants. In the water fern *Azolla*, which grows on the surface of static tropical waters, cyanobacteria are contained in the tissue spaces of leaves. This symbiotic partner is *Anabaena azollae*. Whilst free-living *Anabaena* contain only a few (5%) heterocysts, 15–20% of the symbiotic *Anabaena* trichomes have heterocysts. This is indicative of effective nitrogen fixation. Measurements of nitrogenase activity support this assumption. *Azolla* grows in flooded rice fields, and with suitable cultivation methods it can supply the total nitrogen demand of the rice field. The nitrogen yield of the symbiosis of *Azolla* with *Anabaena* is approximately 300 kg N/ha/annum. A similar symbiosis occurs between liverworts (*Blasia pusilla*, *Anthoceros punctatus*, *Peltigera*) and *Nostoc*. In the tropical shrub *Gunnera macrophylla*, *Nostoc punctiforme* is contained in the lower stem in special glands at the leaf nodes. This *Nostoc* also produces heterocysts and nitrogenase.

13.2   Nitrogen fixation by free-living bacteria and cyanobacteria

The ability to fix nitrogen is fairly widely distributed among soil and water bacteria. Nearly all physiological groups have some representatives which can fix N_2 with greater or lesser efficiency.

Among the large groups of the phototrophic Prokaryotes, the purple sulphur bacteria, the non-sulphur purple bacteria and the cyanobacteria, the majority are able to fix nitrogen (Table 13.2). This ability is of ecological importance. Among the autotrophic bacteria able to fix nitrogen are *Xanthobacter autotrophicus*, *Alcaligenes latus* and *Derxia gummosa*.

Table 13.2. *Some free-living nitrogen fixing bacteria. Physiological groups, genera and species*

Strictly aerobic respiration	Anaerobically respiring	Phototrophs
Azotobacter chroococcum	**Desulphurisers**	**Anoxygenic**
Azotobacter vinelandii	*Desulfovibrio*	*Chromatium*
Azomonas agilis	*Desulfotomaculum*	*Rhodospirillum*
Alcaligenes latus	**Methanogens**	*Rhodopseudomonas*
Xanthobacter autotrophicus	*Methanobacterium*	*Rhodobacter*
Beijerinckia indica	*Methanosarcina*	*Heliobacter*
Derxia gummona	**Obligate fermenters**	*Chlorobium*
Azospirillum lipoferum	*Clostridium*	**Oxygenic**
Several methylotrophs		most of the
Facultative anaerobes		Cyanobacteria
Klebsiella pneumoniae		
Bacillus polymyxa		

Among the facultative anaerobes are found *Klebsiella pneumoniae* and *Bacillus polymyxa*, and among the obligate anaerobes clostridia, methanogens and sulfidogenic bacteria have been found able to fix nitrogen. The unequivocal demonstration of N_2 fixation by archaebacterial methanogens was a surprise. Introduction of isotopic techniques (demonstration of ^{15}N) and gas chromatography, which allows the ready demonstration of ethylene produced from acetylene by nitrogen fixers, has facilitated the examination of a large number of bacteria. However, in the last analysis, final proof of nitrogen fixation still rests on growth experiments. It would seem quite possible that a majority of bacteria possess the genetic information for nitrogen fixation, but that the genes are not expressed under the conditions prevailing in the habitat to which the organisms have become adapted.

Whilst most of the aerobic nitrogen fixers can carry out the fixation only under reduced partial pressures of oxygen, the Azotobacter group is fully adapted to atmospheric oxygen. *Azotobacter chroococcum, A. vinelandii, Beijerinckia indica, Derxia gummosa* and *Azomonas agilis* belong to bacteria which can be easily isolated by inoculation of soil or water into nutrient media lacking bound nitrogen, and aerobic incubation. *A. chroococcum* is found in much larger numbers in soils which are nitrogen deficient, than in well-fertilised, nitrogen-rich soils.

The rhizospheres of some plants contain accumulations of nitrogen-fixing bacteria, such as *Azotobacter paspali* on the root surfaces of the sand grass *Paspalum notatum*, and *Azospirillum lipoferum* in the rhizosphere of *Digitaria decumbens*. Since both partners benefit from the associations, these can be considered as symbioses.

Nitrogen fixation by free-living cyanobacteria is of considerable importance, at least in rice fields (30–50 kg n/ha/annum). The ability to fix nitrogen has been demonstrated in at least 40 species of cyanobacteria in pure cultures. Cyanobacteria are counted as pioneering species in the colonisation of poor soils (for example, volcanic soils) and are found in extreme habitats, such as in Antarctica, at temperatures near freezing, as well as in hot springs. They grow alone, or in symbiotic association with fungi, as blue-algal lichen. In inland waters and in some parts of the oceans the annual mass proliferation of cyanobacteria gives rise to the so-called 'algal blooms'. It has not yet been possible to estimate the proportion of biomass production and nitrogen gain of the oceans that is due to the cyanobacteria.

Trace elements in nitrogen fixation.   Molybdenum and nickel are required for nitrogen fixation. Two of the bacterial processes require **molybdenum**: **nitrogen fixation** and **nitrate reduction**. The key enzymes in both these systems are **molybdoproteins**. **Nickel** is a component of the enzyme hydrogenase. The fact that all nitrogen fixers (with the exception of a few rhizobia) contain hydrogenase makes nickel an essential element for these organisms.

The role of molybdenum as an essential component in nitrogen fixation was discovered some 50 years ago by H. Bortels. In a few cases it may be replaced by vanadium. Genetic studies have now shown that *Azotobacter vinelandii* and *Xanthobacter autotrophicum* have two groups of genes, of which one codes for molybdenum-containing nitrogenase and the other for a vanadium-containing nitrogenase. The subsequent discovery that these two trace elements are actually not essential was a surprise. Apparently *A. vinelandii* can still carry out nitrogen fixation when both genes have been deleted. In that case a simple iron–sulphur *Nitrogenase* is produced.

13.3   Biochemistry of nitrogen fixation

Nitrogen fixation is mediated by an enzyme system, the **nitrogenase system**, which has two components: nitrogenase and nitrogenase reductase (Fig. 13.2). Both these associated components are located in the cytoplasm and are extremely sensitive to oxygen. This property is the reason why facultative anaerobes can fix nitrogen only under anoxic conditions, cyanobacteria only in heterocysts, and why rhizobia can fix nitrogen

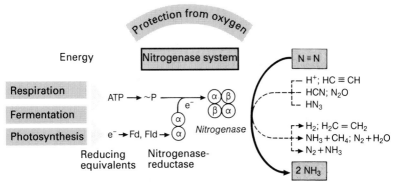

Fig. 13.2. *General scheme for nitrogen fixation.*
Fd, ferredoxin; Fld, flavodoxin.

only in the presence of leghaemoglobin. Both components are iron–sulphur proteins. Nitrogenase is the larger component and consists of four subunits, α_2 and β_2), each of which contains one atom of molybdenum. The proteins have a negative redox potential. Electrons are supplied via ferredoxin and flavodoxin, first to the nitrogenase reductase, and then, with the consumption of 16 mol ATP per mol N_2, to nitrogenase. It is the molybdenum protein which catalyses the actual reduction of nitrogen. At the same time $2H^+$ are reduced to H_2. The enzyme system is able to reduce not only molecular nitrogen, but also acetylene, azide, NO_2, cyanide, nitrile, isonitrile and protons. The methodologically simplest technique for demonstrating nitrogenase is based on its ability to reduce acetylene to ethylene, which can be easily quantitated by gas chromatography. Up to now, all nitrogen-fixing bacteria and symbiotic systems have been found to be able to reduce acetylene. The alternative nitrogenase system, which contains vanadium as its heavy metal component, can reduce acetylene a step further, to ethane. This allows differentiation of the two enzymes, even *in vivo*.

The energy – in form of ATP – required for nitrogen fixation can be derived from fermentation, respiration or photosynthesis (Fig. 13.2). The amounts of reducing power and ATP required are sufficiently large to be reflected in the growth yield. Thus, if cultures of nitrogen-fixing bacteria are grown with a limiting amount of sugar (or carbon substrate) a supply of ammonia will allow a higher cell yield than growth dependent entirely on nitrogen fixation.

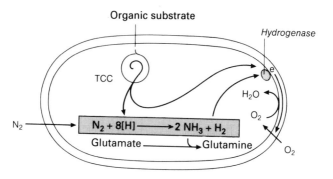

Fig. 13.3. *Nitrogen fixation in an aerobic respiring cell.*

The catabolism of the substrate, the reactions catalysed by the nitrogenase system (in box), as well as the transfer of NH_3 into organic compounds and the role of H_2, are indicated. H_2 increases the consumption of oxygen diffusing into the cell and thus contributes to the protection of nitrogenase.

Role of hydrogenase.   The discovery that the nitrogenase systems of practically all bacteria produced some H_2 in addition to NH_3 was at first rather unexpected, especially as it seemed to waste valuable reducing power. However, the fact that all these bacteria also possessed a membrane-bound hydrogenase, indicated that hydrogen might have a **protective function**, i.e. that it might be a **protective gas** for the oxygen-sensitive nitrogenase. It seems that hydrogen serves to reduce any oxygen diffusing into the cell, thus 'detoxifying' it in the form of water (Fig. 13.3).

Without the enzyme hydrogenase, hydrogen cannot be activated. The demonstration of molecular hydrogen in the atmosphere immediately above fields of clover would lend support to this suggestion. It is due to the fact that many rhizobia, including *Rhizobium trifolii* do not contain hydrogenase and therefore cannot activate H_2, which is consequently released into the plant cell, and hence into the atmosphere. The lack of hydrogenase in many rhizobia can be explained by their possession of leghaemoglobin, which functions as a protective device against oxygen damage. There would therefore be no selection pressure for the maintenance of a second protective mechanism. Yield estimates on soybeans that had been inoculated with (1) a hydrogenase-forming strain of *Bradyrhizobium japonicum* and (2) a mutant of the same strain lacking hydrogenase, indicated that the intracellular utilisation of the hydrogen produced by the nitrogenase system led to an energy gain and higher yield. This increased energetic efficiency, though, is probably not the main reason for the simultaneous presence of nitrogenase and hydrogenase in all nitrogen-fixing bacteria (with the exception of the rhizobia). The most important effect is the protective action.

Regulation of nitrogen fixation.   In many bacteria, nitrogenase is only produced under conditions where it is essential for growth, i.e. in the absence of a utilisable source of fixed nitrogen. Ammonium ions repress the synthesis of nitrogenase. In some organisms, the activity of the enzyme when present is also inhibited by ammonium ions. The enzyme glutamine synthetase apparently plays an important role in the regulation of nitrogenase synthesis (Ch. 7.6). Glutamine synthetase and glutamate synthase are the two enzymes that enable the bacteria to incorporate ammonium ions into organic compounds when the ions are present at low concentrations. This system has a low affinity for ammonium ions and keeps their cellular concentration low. Increase in ammonium ion concentrations in the environment and, hence, intracellularly as well, leads to repression of glutamine synthetase formation and, in consequence, also to repression of nitrogenase synthesis.

Genetic transfer of the *nif* gene.   It has been possible to transfer the ability to fix nitrogen from one bacterium to another by direct cell contact. This transfer of the *nif* gene from *Klebsiella pneumoniae* to *Escherichia coli* by conjugation, and the localisation of the *nif* gene on a plasmid, raised the hope of transferring it also to other bacteria and eventually even to eukaryotes. However, since nitrogen fixation also requires, apart from the nitrogenase complex, another specific iron–sulphur protein and the protection of the nitrogenase system from oxygen, such experimental investigations face considerable difficulties.

14 Degradation of natural substances

Although green plants have been synthesising organic materials from carbon dioxide for millions of years, such substances have not accumulated to any marked extent. Only a small fraction has been conserved as highly reduced carbon compounds (coal, petroleum, natural gas) under complete exclusion of air. All the biosynthetically formed compounds are degradable under aerobic conditions (and some under anaerobic conditions). This means that for every compound, however complicated, there exist one or more microorganisms that have the ability to degrade it either completely or partially; the fragments that are produced can then be utilised by other organisms. In their totality, therefore, the microorganisms appear to be **biochemically omnipotent**, and this has been referred to as the principle of 'microbial infallibility'. More recently this principle has come to require limitations. Several of the synthetic and designed low molecular weight compounds and highly polymerised materials are resistant to bacterial attack as far can be determined after several years of observation and research.

Knowledge of the microorganisms that attack, degrade, and metabolise individual natural substances is based largely on experiments with enrichment cultures. Simple solutions of basic nutrients with the material to be investigated as the only energy (and/or carbon) source allow the growth of only those organisms with relatively undemanding nutrient requirements; in liquid enrichment cultures the organisms that can grow fastest under the conditions applied come to predominate. It is therefore somewhat doubtful whether these organisms can be regarded as typical representatives of the organisms that carry out the degradative process being investigated under natural conditions. Many organisms with different growth requirements and physiological properties may have remained unrecognised. Not only bacteria, but also eukaryotic microorganisms and small animals (worms, molluscs, insects) take part in the decomposition of organic substances in soil (Fig. 14.1). One of the aims of microbial ecology is the elucidation of the aerobic food chain.

Decomposition under anaerobic and aerobic conditions.   A large proportion of the biomass produced by photosynthesis is mineralised under **anaerobic conditions**. Anoxic ecosystems comprise, apart from the al-

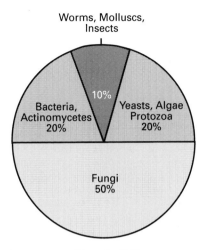

Fig. 14.1. *Approximate composition of soil biomass.*

ready mentioned sediments of still waters, rice fields, marshes and tundra, also waterlogged soils, waste deposits, silos and the intestinal tracts of animals. The microorganisms involved in these anaerobic decomposition processes have been extensively investigated and can be presented as an anaerobic food chain (Ch. 9.3). The interactions between the organisms involved have been described as symbioses, syntrophy, interspecies hydrogen transfer and co-metabolism and a fairly complete picture has been obtained. This achievement is due to the fact that bacteria are the almost exclusive participants in this anaerobic metabolic process.

On the other hand, the predominant part of the biomass is decomposed **aerobically**. These aerobic processes are carried out by prokaryotes and eukaryotes with the latter being predominant, with respect both to the number of organisms involved and to the amount of biomass turned over. The flow of this aerobic degradation is therefore far more branched than the anaerobic food chain. Because of this it should be thought of not as a food chain, but rather as a **food network**. A number of small animals, mainly invertebrates such as worms, molluscs, insects and their larvae, occupy a considerable space in this net. On the other hand, it should not be forgotten that microorganisms always play a part in the digestion of food and nutrients in the intestinal tracts of animals, not least in the breakdown of fibrous substances, such as lignocellulose and cellulose, which constitute more than half of the photosynthetic biomass. Unfortunately, the processes and organisms that occur in animal intestines have not been much investigated up to now, whether descriptively or biochemically, or in terms of population dynamics. The intestine of termites is a welcome exception. Increased attention focused on the aerobic breakdown of the primary biomass would seem, therefore, to be of some urgency.

14.1   Cellulose

Cellulose is the basic component of plant material, and is produced in greater quantities than any other substance. Thus, about half of photosynthetically produced biomass consists of cellulose. Plant residues in soil consist of 45% (average) to 90% (cotton) cellulose which is therefore of central importance – next to carbon dioxide – in the carbon cycle.

> Cellulose consists of chains of β-D-glucopyranose units in 1,4-glycosidic linkage. It has polymerisation numbers (glucose units per molecule of cellulose) of up to 14 000 in plants and 3500 in *Acetobacter xylinum*. In the green alga *Valonia* the polymerisation number was found to be 25 000. In relation to the structural conformation of cellulose, however, the dissacharide cellobiose, rather than the monosaccharide glucose, has to be regarded as the elementary unit. Cellulose is partially crystalline; that is, crystalline regions alternate with amorphous areas. The crystalline regions of cellulose show definite polymorphism; thus cellulose I (i.e. natural cellulose) and cellulose II (mercerised cotton) are distinguished by different arrangements of their glucose chains in the crystal lattice. The high mechanical strength and the insolubility of cellulose are due, at the molecular level, to the presence of inter- and intra-molecular hydrogen bridges. They serve to **link single chains**. The single chains themselves are stabilised by the **intramolecular** H-bridges (2 per glucose unit). The result is a 2-dimensional network of H-bridges. The strong cohesion between individual levels of the network is due to Van der Waals' forces (cellulose I) and in the case of cellulose II again to H-bridge bonding. This then produces a 3-dimensional network.

The **enzymatic cleavage** of cellulose is catalysed by cellulase. According to investigations on fungi, the cellulase system consists of at least three enzymes. (1) Endo-β-1,4-glucanases attack the β-1,4 bonds in the centre of the macromolecule and produce long-chain fragments with free ends. (2) The exo-β-1,4-glucanases remove the dissacharide cellobiose from the ends of the cellulose chains. (3) The β-glucosidases hydrolyse cellobiose with formation of glucose.

The regulation of cellulose synthesis.   This can be brought about either by catabolite repression or through substrate induction by cellobiose,

Table 14.1. *Cellulose-digesting microorganisms*

Eukaryotes		Prokaryotes	
Aspergillus fumigatus	a	*Cytophaga*	a
Aspergillus nidulans	a	*Sporocytophaga*	a
Botrytis cinerea	a	*Archangium, Sorangium*	a
Chaetomium globosum	a	*Polyangium*	a
Fusarium	a	*Pseudomonas fluorescens*	
Myrothecium verrucaria	a	var. *cellulosa*	a
Trichoderma viride	a	*Cellulomonas flmi*	a
Trichoderma reesei	a	Streptomycetes, several	a
Rhizoctonia solani	a	*Clostridium thermocellum*	b
Neocallimastix frontalis	b	*Clostridium cellobioparum*	b
Diplodinium	b	*Ruminococcus albus,*	
Entodinium	b	*R. flavefaciens*	b
		Bacteroides succinogenes	b
		Butyrivibrio fibrisolvens	b
		Eubacterium cellulosolvens	b
		Cellvibrio flavescens	a

a, Aerobic growth; b, anaerobic growth.

whilst small amounts of cellulose are produced constitutively. The concentrations of cellobiose that have inducing or repressing effects vary in different organisms. In general, low concentrations of cellobiose act as inducer, and relatively high concentrations have repressor action. In addition, cellobiose can also act as a competitive inhibitor at the enzymic level. Cellulose itself, as it is water-insoluble, has no direct effect on the synthesis, and can influence it only indirectly via the cellobiose produced by its hydrolysis. This can account for the apparent inducing action of crystalline cellulose.

Degradation under aerobic conditions.   Cellulose is degraded and utilised in well-aerated soils by aerobic microorganisms (fungi, myxobacteria and other eubacteria) and under anaerobic conditions by bacteria, a few anaerobic fungi and protozoa (Table 14.1).

The fungi play a significant part in the degradation of cellulose under aerobic conditions. They are more successful than bacteria in acid soils and in the degradation of cellulose embedded in lignin (i.e. in wood). Species of the genera *Fusarium* and *Chaetomium* are prominent. Others known to be cellulolytic are *Aspergillus fumigatus* and *A. nidulans, Botrytis cinerea, Rhizoctonia solani, Trichoderma viride, Chaetomium globosum* and *Myrothecium verrucaria*. The last three species named are used as test organisms for the demonstration of cellulolytic activity, respectively, for testing impregnation media used on cloths and coverings to prevent damage by cellulolytic microorganisms. The fungi excrete cellulases which can be isolated from the mycelium and the culture medium.

Cytophaga and *Sporocytophaga* are the most easily isolated of the aerobic cellulolytic bacteria; this is done by enrichment culture in liquid medium. Very little is known about the utilisation and initial attack of cellulose by myxobacteria. No extracellular cellulase or initial cleavage products of cellulose have ever been demonstrated. The bacterial cells are attached to the cellulose fibre, with their longitudinal axis parallel to that of the fibre; they apparently hydrolyse cellulose only when they are in close contact with it, and they immediately absorb the hydrolysis products. In addition to *Cytophaga* species, myxobacteria producing fruiting bodies, of the genera *Polyangium, Sorangium* and *Archangium*, are also able to grow on cellulose.

The ability to grow on cellulose as substrate is also quite common among many aerobic bacteria which could almost be considered 'omnivores'. Some of these attack cellulose only in the absence of other carbon sources. Some *Pseudomonas*-like bacteria were formerly collected in a *Cellvibrio* group. *Pseudomonas fluorescens* var. *cellulosa* has been described only recently. *Cellulomonas* should be mentioned among the coryneform bacteria.

Only a few cellulolytic species have been described among the actinomycetes: *Micromonospora chalcea, Streptomyces cellulosae, S. sporangium.*

Degradation under anaerobic conditions.   Under anaerobic conditions cellulose is degraded by mesophilic and thermophilic eubacteria and a few fungi and protozoa. The thermophile *Clostridum thermocellum* grows in a simple synthetic medium with cellulose or celliobiose as substrate and ammonium salts as the only nitrogen source; glucose and many other sugars cannot be metabolised. The degradation of cellulose is preceded by the secretion of a yellowish, carotinoid-like substance, as has been observed in other cellulolytic bacteria. This increases the affinity of the cellulolytic enzyme for cellulose. The yellow coloration of the cellulase is a good indicator for the initiation of cellulose hydrolysis. In the case of *C. thermocellum* the multienzyme complexes described above are organised in so-called cellulosomes which can have molecular weights of several million.

The products of this cellulose fermentations are ethanol, acetate, lactate, formate, molecular hydrogen, and carbon dioxide. Extracellularly, the cellulose is probably converted to glucose. Similar fermentation products occur in the fermentation of cellulose by the mesophile *Clostridium*

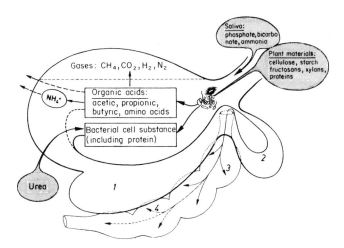

Fig. 14.2. *Microbial conversions in the rumen.*
(1) Rumen; (2) omentum; (3)   for explanations.
omasum; (4) abomasum. See text

cellobioparum. The long rods known as *Bacillus cellulosae-dissolvens* appear closely apposed to cellulose fibres, similar to those of *Cytophaga* species, and do not excrete any cellulase into the medium.

Microbial conversion of cellulose in the rumen.   Cellulose is degraded in the rumen by anaerobic bacteria, fungi and protozoa. The main carbohydrate sources for ruminants are hay, straw, and grass. About 50% of dry grass consists of fructosans and xylans and the rest of the carbohydrates is present as cellulose. This cellulose component of their food would be useless to ruminants if they had not achieved, in the course of evolution, a symbiotic relationship with microorganisms, some of which are able to degrade cellulose (Fig. 14.2).

> The first two sections of the ruminant stomach, i.e. the rumen and the reticulum, represent a large fermentation chamber with a volume of 100–250 litres. This provides ideal conditions for the growth of several types of microorganisms. The contribution of the animal to this symbiosis consists of a constant temperature between 37 and 39 °C; a continuous supply of a well-buffered (by bicarbonate and phosphate, pH 5.8–7.3) solution of minerals (about 100–200 1 saliva/day); a periodic supply of nutrient substrates in the form of small pieces of cellulose-containing foods; and mechanical mixing by movement of the rumen. The rumen thus resembles a semi-continuous microbial culture.

Protozoa and bacteria predominate among the rumen microorganisms. One millilitre of rumen contents has about 10^5 protozoa, mainly ciliates of the genera *Diplodinium* and *Entodinium*. These species are specialised and rarely found outside the rumen. They account for about 6–10% of the weight of rumen contents and some part of their weight is due to stored polysaccharides. Their role in the rumen does not appear to be essential. The functionally most important inhabitants of the rumen are bacteria. They are present at concentrations of 10^{11} cells/ml of rumen fluid and account for 5–10% of the dry mass of rumen contents. The rumen-specific bacteria are all strict anaerobes.

The bacteria catalyse the breakdown of the polymeric carbohydrates of fodder to simple compounds such as fatty acids and alcohols. Cellulose, starch, fructosan and xylan are preferentially catabolised to fatty acids. According to carbon balance determinations, 90% by weight of the cellulose taken up is metabolised with the production of large quantities of acids. Their percentage composition (w/w) is approximately as follows: acetate (the main product), 50–70; propionate, 17–21; butyrate, 14–20; valerate and formate are produced only in small quantities. In addition, up to 900 l of gas are produced per day, with the approximate composition by volume being 65% CO_2, 27% methane 7% nitrogen, 0.18% hydrogen, and traces of hydrogen sulphide. Since cellulolytic bacteria and fungi isolated from rumen in the last few years produce the same acids in similar proportions under laboratory conditions, it can be assumed that the acids in the rumen are produced during the degradation of cellulose. Organisms that can degrade cellulose in the rumen are: *Ruminococcus albus* and *R. flavefaciens* which are gram-negative cocci; *Fibrobacter succinogenes*, a gram-negative, non-motile rod which forms predominantly acetate and succinate; *Butyrivibrio fibrisolvens*; *Clostridium cellobioparum*. The absence of lactate from the rumen is due to the presence of *Veillonella alcalescens (Micrococcus lactilyticus)*, which ferments lactate to acetate, propionate, and carbon dioxide. The methane produced is formed from fatty acids and from molecular hydrogen and carbon dioxide (Ch. 9.4). The formation of hydrogen sulphide in the rumen is due to the reduction of sulphate by *Desulfotomaculum ruminantium*. *Selenomonas ruminantium* (Fig. 2.37b) ferments glucose to lactate, acetate and propionate.

Amongst the fungi present in the rumen, *Neocallimastix frontalis* (Chytridiomycetes) is the most extensively investigated. It hydrolyses cellulose to glucose and ferments glucose to acetate, formate, ethanol, lactate, CO_2 and H_2.

The food of ruminants in their natural habitat, i.e. in the savannahs and steppes, is very poor in nitrogen and protein. To provide for the protein synthesis of the rumen symbionts, ruminants seem to have developed an appropriate cycle, the rumino-hepatic circulation. The urea produced by the liver for the detoxification of ammonium is only partially excreted in the urine; part of the urea finds its way into the ruminant stomach via secretions from the salivary glands and by transfer across the rumen wall and thus becomes accessible for protein synthesis by the rumen flora (Fig. 14.2). The symbiosis with the microflora inhabiting the rumen renders the ruminants independent of protein supply. It has been shown repeatedly that cattle can be maintained on protein-free diets.

The bacteria support the nutrition of ruminants in two ways: the acids produced in the catabolism of polysaccharides are reabsorbed in the rumen; the cell substance of the bacteria, migrating along with the rumen contents, through the digestive tract is digested in the intestine and is also reabsorbed.

Lysis of the bacteria involves the enzyme *Lysozyme* which is secreted by the rumen epithelium. Since the bacteria growing in the rumen can utilise inorganic nitrogen, they afford a significant gain of protein for the animal.

Hardening of fats. Plant fatty acids differ from those in animal fats by their low degree of saturation: they contain oleic acid, olelinic and linoleic acid, linolenic acid and arachidonic acid. Plant fats are thus of a softer consistency (lower melting point). In animals which do not possess a rumen (pigs, geese, rodents) the fatty acids derived from plants are taken up by the intestines and used unaltered in the deposition of storage fat. These storage fats are therefore of a soft consistency. In ruminants, however, the plant fatty acids in the rumen are extensively hydrated (saturated) by the bacterial rumen flora and the saturated fats are then absorbed from the intestine and built into the storage fats. Beef fat (butter, suet) is therefore of a firm consistency. Since these alterations are brought about by bacteria, and considering that 60–90% of beef protein is also of bacterial origin, consumption of a steak is, in the final analysis, at the expense of bacteria, and consumption of a pork chop at the expense of fodder plants.

14.2   Xylan

Xylan is the next most abundant and widely distributed carbohydrate after cellulose. Straw and bark consist of up to 30% xylan; conifer woods is 7–12% xylan and deciduous wood is 20–25% xylan.

Xylan is one of the carbohydrates that are also designated 'hemicelluloses'. They are not structurally related to cellulose, nor do they contain the same building blocks, but they are, at least partially, soluble in water or alkali. The hemicelluloses consist of either pentoses (xylose, arabinose) or of hexoses (glucose, mannose, galactose), as well as uronic acids. They function as storage and supporting substances in plants. The designation 'hemicelluloses' has been discontinued since a large number of similar polysaccharides were discovered in fungi and bacteria.

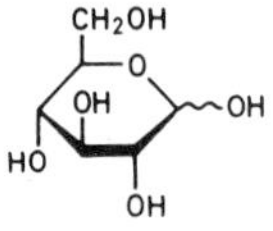

D - Glucose

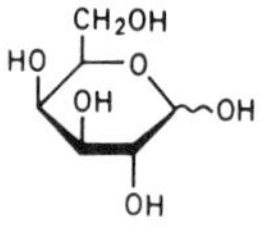

D - Galactose

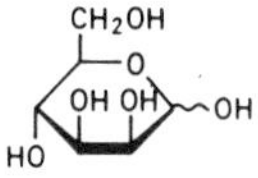

D - Mannose

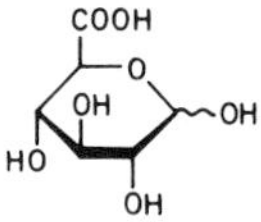

D - Glucuronic acid

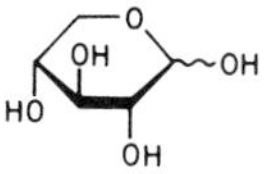

D - Xylose

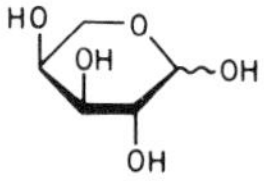

L - Arabinose

The xylan chain consists of 1,4-glycosidically linked β-D-xylose. It can be derived from a cellulose chain by substituting hydrogen atoms for the CH_2–OH groups, but its polymer size (number of units per polymer) is considerably lower (30–100). Some xylans also contain arabinose, glucose, galactose and glucuronate. They thus have a complex structure, in contrast to cellulose, and are highly branched.

Xylan is more rapidly degraded by a large number of microorganisms than cellulose. Many cellulose-degrading organisms also produce xylanase. Even *Sporocytophaga myxococcoides*, which attacks cellulose only when it is in contact with cellulose fibres and *Neocallimastix*, excretes xylanase. Which organisms first attack xylans in soil depends on environmental factors. In acid soils fungi predominate, whereas in alkaline or neutral soils bacilli, *Sporocytophaga*, and other bacteria are dominant. The ability to utilise xylans is very common among fungi. Xylan is even an excellent substrate for the cultivation of mushrooms.

In the bacteria, xylanase is formed constitutively in some organisms (clostridia) and in others it is inducible by xylan. The action of cell-free xylanase produces, apart from xylose, xylobiose and larger fragments. The enzyme can apparently attack the molecule in many places simultaneously; it is probably an enzyme system, containing several enzymes.

14.3   Starch and other glucans

Starch is the predominant storage material in plants. It is usually present as granules, which may be spherical, lens-shaped or egg-shaped, and which have a distinctly layered structure. Plant starch is composed of two glucans, amylose and amylopectin. Amylose is soluble, without swelling, in hot water and is responsible for the typical blue coloration with iodine. It consists of helically wound, unbranched chains of D-glucose, in 1,4-α-glycosidic linkage. There are about 200–500 units per chain. Amylopectin swells in water and on heating forms a starch paste. It reacts with iodine to give a violet-to-brown coloration. It is also a poly-1,4-α-D-glucose, but, like glycogen, it is branched in 1,6-positions at approximately every 25th glucose molecule. In addition, it contains phosphate residues, and magnesium and calcium ions. Starches from different sources differ considerably in their branching, the number of units per chain, and other properties. Starch can be converted to glucose by acid hydrolysis or enzymatically. There are three types of enzymatic degradation of glucans: (1) phosphorolysis, (2) hydrolysis, and (3) transglycosylation.

> *Phosphorolysis.* The conversion of starch, glycogen, and similar polysaccharides to glucose-l-phosphate is catalysed by α-1,4-glucan phosphorylases (phosphorylases). Although the reaction is reversible, it occurs intracellularly only in catabolism of polysaccharides, and it plays no part in synthesis. The phosphorolysis starts at the free, non-reducing terminus of the amylose chains and liberates one glucose-l-phosphate. In amylopectin the phosphorolysis stops at the 1,6-branching points and resumes after amylo-1,6-glucosidase has cleaved these. The phosphorylases play an important role in the mobilisation and utilisation of intracellularly stored polysaccharides (glucans).

Amylose (n + 2)   Glucose-1-P

> **Hydrolysis.** Polysaccharides are attacked extracellularly by the hydrolytic action of amylases. α-Amylase occurs in plants, animals, and microorganisms. It rapidly liquefies starch, simultaneously attacking many 1,4-glycosidic bonds, including those in the centre of the chain (it is therefore also known as endoamylase). It produces maltose, glucose and oligomers with three to seven glucose residues. Because of its rapid breakdown of the macromolecular structure, the viscosity of the solution and its ability

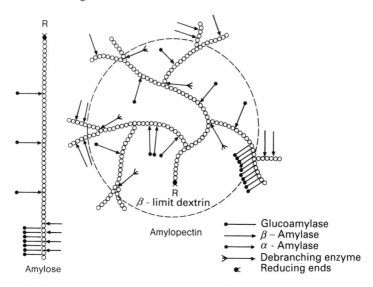

Fig. 14.3. *Target sites of the enzymes degrading amylose and amylopectin.*

to react with iodine also decline rapidly, whilst fermentable sugars (glucose, maltose, maltobiose) appear gradually. When a debranching enzyme like pullulanase or isoamylase is present in addition to the α-amylase, dextrins can also be cleaved (Fig. 14.3).

β-Amylases occur mainly in plants (barley, wheat, among others) as well as in bacteria. In contrast to α-amylase, they start at the free, non-reducing ends of the macromolecule. Their action on starch, therefore, leads to rapid accumulation of sugars whilst reactivity with iodine continues. The hydrolysis stops at the branching points. The residue is known as 'limit dextrins'. When the presence of debranching enzyme ensures the cleavage of the branch points, hydrolysis proceeds as far as the complete conversion to maltose. This can then be hydrolysed extracellularly by maltase. If appropriate permeases are present, maltose and other oligomers can be transported into the cells and cleaved phosphorolytically.

Transglycosylation. Schardinger discovered crystalline compounds in starch-containing media after growth of *Bacillus macerans*. These compounds consisted of closed circular chains of glucose in α-1,4-glycosidic linkage. These α-, β- or γ-cyclodextrins contain six, seven or eight molecules of glucose in the ring and are produced from starch by the action of transglycosylases.

Fungi and bacteria produce γ-amylases. The ability to degrade starch by amylolytic exoenzymes is very common in microorganisms: there is no specific starch-degrading microflora. Many soil fungi are active producers of amylases. Technical preparations of amylases are produced commercially by use of *Aspergillus oryzae*, *A. niger* and *A. wentii*. Taka-amylase or Taka-diastase, for example, are commercial crude preparations from cultures of *A. oryzae*; they hydrolyse starch to glucose. Among bacteria, the bacilli (*Bacillus macerans*, *B. polymyxa*, *B. subtilis*), pseudomonads, and several streptomycetes are active producers of α-amylases. The enzymes excreted by *B. stearothermophilus* and *B. licheniformis* can be heated to 100 °C for a short period without loss of activity. Some thermophilic clostridia such as *Clostridium thermosulfurogenes* and *C. thermohydrosulfuricum* also excrete thermostable α-amylases and pullulanases. Since alcohol-producing yeasts do not excrete amylases, the hydrolysis of starch to sugar (in beer making) is dependent on the amylases contained in the malt, or those obtained from *Aspergillus oryzae*.

In anaerobic, waterlogged soils recently fertilised with carbohydrates, starch is mainly degraded by saccharolytic clostridia. Since these also fix molecular nitrogen, such anaerobic decomposition of polysaccharide-rich plant remains in soil can give a high nitrogen yield.

Other glucans.   Bacteria and fungi contain a large number of glucans, some with structural functions and others with storage functions. Many of the slimes excreted by microorganisms are among these. The best known is dextran which is produced in large quantities by the exoenzyme dextran sucrase, excreted, for example, by *Leuconostoc mesenteroides* or *L. dextranicum* growing in sucrose-containing medium (see Ch. 2.2.5).

> The supporting skeleton of yeast cell walls contains β-1,6-glucan. The exact structure of this insoluble supporting structure, cross-linked with small blocks of β-1,3-units, is not yet known. Yeast cell walls, like many other glucans, are degraded by the gastric juice (hepatopancreatic secretion) of snails. The secretion contains a mixture of 30 or more enzymes, among them cellulase, mannase, gluconase, chitinase and lipases. It is a useful agent for preparing protoplasts of yeasts and of other fungal and algal cells.
>
> The smut fungus *Aurebasidium (Pullularia) pullulans*, whose growth resembles that of yeast, excretes **pullulans** during growth on glucose- and sucrose-containing media. This glucan consists of maltotriose units in 1,6-α-glycosidic linkage (poly-α-1,6-maltotriose). Pullulan is broken down by pullulanase.

14.4   Fructans

Some plant families store fructans (also called polyfructosans) in place of, or in addition to, starch (glucan). Whereas inulin, the fructan of the

Compositae (dahlia tubers), is quantitatively of little importance, the phlein-type fructans (*Phleum pratense*, timothy grass) deserve some detailed consideration. They are found in pasture grasses where they represent up to 12–15% of the dry weight. Hydrolysing enzymes have been isolated from *Aspergillus niger* and from bacteria, and they seem to be widely distributed.

Fructans, which are also found as exopolysaccharides (Chapter 10.7 and Table 10.1), are produced by a number of bacteria on sucrose-containing media. The process of laevan formation is analogous to that of dextran synthesis and is catalysed by an extracellular laevan sucrase.

$$n \text{ sucrose} \rightarrow \text{laevan} + n \text{ glucose}$$

This enzymatic synthesis of laevan can be seen as the appearance of small laevan drops in the vicinity of colonies growing on sucrose-containing media. It can be easily observed in strains of *Bacillus subtilis*, *B. cereus* and *Azotobacter chroococcum*. *Streptococcus salivarius*, *S. mutans*, many strains of fluorescent and phytopathogenic pseudomonads, bacilli, and *Enterobacter* are also able to produce laevans. Some strains make use of the laevan they have synthesised by hydrolysing it when the sucrose has become exhausted.

14.5   Mannan

Mannan is found in some conifer timber, constituting up to 11% of the dry weight. It also occurs in yeast cells as a soluble polysaccharide that can be extracted with aqueous alcohol or by autoclaving a yeast suspension. The yeast *Hansenula holstii* excretes a soluble mannan, 20% esterified with phosphate, during growth on glucose.

14.6   Pectin

Pectins are found as intercellular substances in the tissues of young plants and are especially abundant in berries and fruit. Their importance rests not so much on their quantitative role but rather on the functional part they play in plant stability and solidity. They are components of the middle lamella found between the cell wall and adjacent cells.

> Pectins are polygalacturonides. They consist of unbranched chains of α-1,4-glycosidically linked D-galacturonic acids. The carboxy groups are either partly or completely esterified with methanol. In the insoluble pectins, the chains are largely cross-linked. Microbial degradation of pectins involves pectinolytic enzymes (esterases and depolymerases). Pectin esterases

split methyl-ester bonds and liberate methanol. The residual polygalacturonic acids are hydrolysed by polygalacturonases with the liberation of monomers and oligomers of D-galacturonic acid. The polygalacturonic acids, in the form of their calcium salts, are used as setting agents for solidifying fruit gels, jams, and marmalade.

Many bacteria and fungi have the capacity to metabolise pectins. The pathogenicity to plants of some microorganisms (*Botrytis cinerea. Fusarium oxysporum, F. lycopersici*) is due to their ability to excrete pectin-dissolving enzymes. *Erwinia carotovora* causes dissolution of tissues in lettuce, carrots, celery, and other plants. The number of pectin decomposers in soil is very large (10^5 cells/g soil). Spore formers like *Bacillus macerans* and *B. polymyxa* belong to the most active decomposers of pectins. Many pseudomonads (*Pseudomonas fluorescens*), rumen bacteria, actinomycetes, thermophilic clostridia and lactic acid bacteria break down pectins. Among the fungi, *Aspergillus niger, Penicillium italicum, Aureobasidium pullulans, Fusarium* and *Rhizoctonia solani* should be mentioned.

The pectin-decomposing organisms are of technical importance in the retting of flax and hemp. This process aims at freeing the bundles of cellulose fibres from their association with the plant tissue. The aerobic process involves fungi, whereas the anaerobic process of water-retting involves mainly bacteria. Among the latter, the butyric acid-forming, pectinase producers *Clostridium pectinovorum* and *C. felsineum* appear to be the most important. Pectinolytic enzymes for technical purposes, such as clarification of fruit juices and wine, are mainly obtained from fungi that have been grown on pectin-containing media.

14.7   Agar

Agar is a mixture of agarose and agaropectin. The main polysaccharide consists of D-galactose and 3,6-anhydrogalactose in linear chains with alternating β-1,4 and β-1,3 linkage. Agaropectin has a more complicated structure and contains D-galactose, 3,6-anhydrogalactose, the corresponding uronic acids, and sulphate. Most of the red algae contain agar, which is obtained commercially from *Gelidium* species.

Agar is not attacked by the vast majority of microorganisms. Only a few bacterial species that can hydrolyse agar have been isolated from seawater and seaweed. The decomposition of agar (by microorganisms) can be recognised by the sinking of colonies into the agar medium (Fig. 14.4). Agar-decomposing bacteria are found mainly in marine environments. In the tidal zones, up to 10^7 agar deomposors/g silt can be demonstrated; this is about 2–4% of the aerobic bacteria found in this habitat. Agar

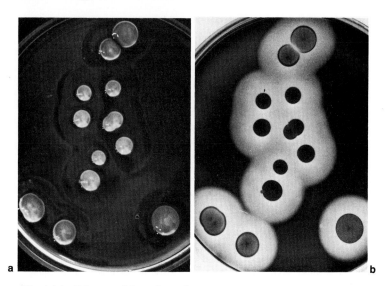

Fig. 14.4. *Colonies of* Cytophaga fermentans *var.* agarovorans *on agar plates.*

(a) Degradation of the agar can be recognised by the sinking of the colonies into the agar. (b) Diffusion zones, due to the exoenzymes hydrolysing agar, are made visible by flooding the plate with potassium iodide solution. (From Veldkamp, H. (1961). *J. gen. Microbiol.* **26**, 331.)

decomposers are found in the genera *Cytophaga, Flavobacterium, Bacillus, Pseudomonas* and *Alcaligenes*.

14.8   Chitin

Chitin can be regarded as the second most common polysaccharide on earth, after cellulose. Formally, chitin can be derived from cellulose by substitution of the hydroxy group on carbon atom 2 of glucose with an acetylated amino group (see Chapter 2.2.4). Chitin's pronounced stability is based on the hydrogen bonding of the *N*-acetyl side chains. Chitin occurs as a support medium in the animal as well as in the plant kingdom and forms the exoskeleton of many non-vertebrates. Chitin is also continuously produced in soil as the main cell wall component of many Basidiomycetes and Ascomycetes.

It is hardly surprising, in view of the above, that a large number of soil and aquatic bacteria can utilise chitin. Among 50 chitin-decomposing bacteria isolated from agricultural soil, the following genera are represented: *Flavobacterium*, *Bacillus*, *Cytophaga*, *Pseudomonas*, *Streptomyces*, *Nocardia* and *Micromonospora*. Among the fungi that can decompose chitin, *Aspergillus*, *Mucor* and *Mortierella* species are included. Up to 10^6 organisms/g agricultural soil are able to utilise chitin. Such large proportions of chitin-utilising microorganisms in soil indicate that chitin may be a constantly available substrate. The addition of finely divided chitin to soil produces a rapid response of accelerated growth in actinomycetes. Therefore, media with chitin as the sole source of carbon and nitrogen are especially suitable as selective media for streptomycetes. Anaerobically, chitin is broken down by some highly specialised chitinolytic, obligately anaerobic bacteria. Further knowledge about chitin breakdown in the gastric tract of copepods, shrimps and crab-eating marine animals, as well as in sediments, would be of great interest.

Extracellular enzymes of microbial origin also contribute to the attack on chitin. Those excreted by *Streptomyces griseus* could be separated into chitinase and chitobiase. Degradation apparently occurs by simultaneous attack of chitinase at many points along the polymer, yielding little *N*-acetyl-glucosamine and predominantly chitobiose and chitotriose as the products. The latter are then converted to monomers by chitobiase.

Chitin can also be broken down to **chitosan** by *Absidia coerula*. Chitosan is a polyglucosamine and is produced by deacetylation of chitin. It is already an important product of biotechnology and is used as an adhesive for wound dressings, as a chelator and as additive for soil and animal feeds.

14.9   Lignin

Lignin is quantitatively the most important component of plants, after cellulose and hemicellulose. The lignin content of woody tissue varies between 18 and 30% of the dry weight. The lignin is embedded in the plant tissue and is situated within the secondary lamellae of the cell walls. Lignin is the most slowly biodegradable component of plants. It is therefore the major source of the slowly decomposing organic substances in soil, especially of the humic acids.

Lignin is not uniform chemically, but is, instead, a **very complex compound** (Fig. 14.5). The complexity is not due to a large number of different monomeric building blocks: the basic units are all derivatives of phenyl propane, predominantly coniferyl alcohol. Instead, the complexity results from the large number of different bonds by which the monomeric

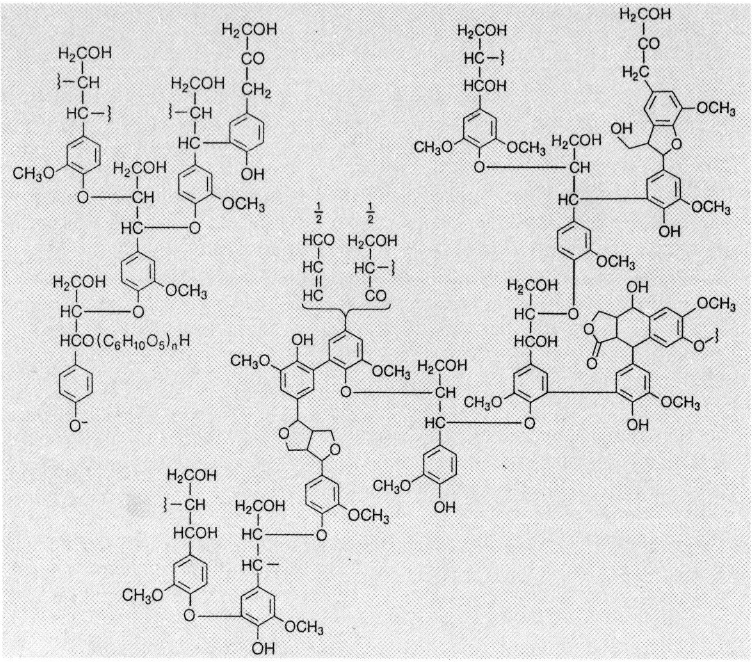

Fig. 14.5. *Section of conifer wood lignin.*

The schematic drawings have to be
interpreted in 3-dimensional
perspective.

building blocks are linked. This irregular structure of lignin is in accord-
ance with the idea that the enzymatic process of lignin synthesis is restricted to the formation of coniferyl alcohol radicals. These radicals then
undergo spontaneous linkages whose nature and possibilities are dependent on the mesomeric conditions of the radicals.

A number of dimers and oligomers of coniferyl alcohol have been isolated as intermediate products in lignin synthesis (Fig. 14.6). Whereas
the lignin of spruce (pine) is predominantly composed of coniferyl alcohol, the lignin of deciduous wood contains coniferyl and sinapyl alcohol,
whilst that of the Gramineae contains coumaryl alcohol. The differences
in lignin composition are expressed mainly in the content of methoxy
groups: lignin of deciduous wood contains 20.5–21%, that of spruce
contains 15–16%, and that of Gramineae contains 14–15%.

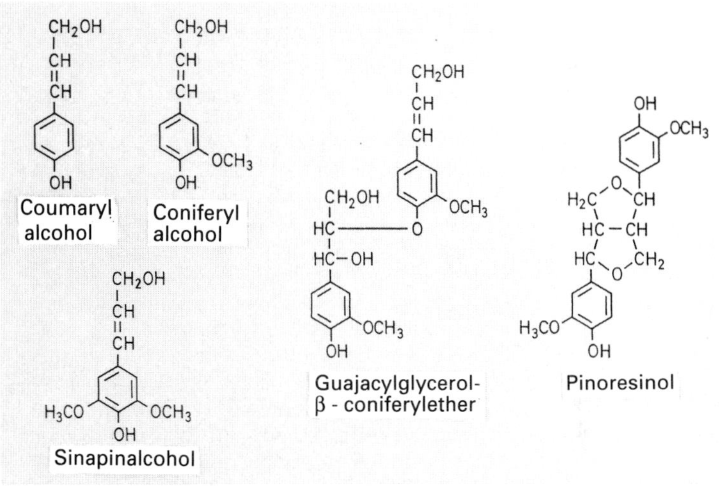

Fig. 14.6. *Precursors for the biosynthesis of lignin and dimers of coniferylalcohols which are intermediates in the synthesis and degradation of lignin.*

The phenyl-propane building blocks in lignin are multiply cross-linked by ether and carbon–carbon bonds (Fig. 14.6). These bonds are extremely resistant to enzymatic attack. In plants, lignin is an inert end product of metabolism; lignin is not re-utilised in metabolism and fulfils only structural functions. It is subject only to microbial attack. Compared to cellulose or hemicellulose, the decomposition of lignin is extraordinarily slow and is carried out by wood-destroying fungi, as well as by bacteria and fungi in soil.

Lignin degradation.   Some fungi can degrade lignin even in the living plant. Two groups are distinguished among the wood-destroying Basidiomycetes. Those that cause **brown rot** convert the wood into a reddish-brown mass; they preferentially degrade the cellulose and hemicellulose components of the wood and leave the phenyl-propane polymers as residues. Those fungi that cause '**white rot**' of wood leave a white mass. They attack mainly lignin and, at first, leave most of the cellulose intact. The fungi that primarily attack lignin include *Polystictus versicolor, Stereum hirsutum* and *Phanerochaete chrysosporium*. Other fungi attack lignin and cellulose simultaneously (*Pleurotus ostreatus, Ganoderma applanatum, Polyporus adustus, Armillaria mellea*). The decomposition of wood by pure cultures of fungi is so slow that such experiments take months or even years. By using various methods, lignin decomposition can also be demonstrated in members of the following genera: *Pholiota, Clitocybe, Lenzites Panus, Poria, Trametes* and others.

One of the most active white-rot fungi and presently the model organism for investigations on fungal lignin breakdown is *Phanerochaete chrysosporium*. Degradation of lignin occurs only in the presence of oxygen and glucose. There is no anaerobic breakdown. The breakdown is catalysed by an enzyme system that used to be called ligninase. This contains peroxidases, including two haem protein peroxidases, a 'lignin peroxidase and a manganese-dependent peroxidase, which are well understood. Peroxidases require H_2O_2 for their function and catalyse the oxidative cleavage of β-O-4 ether bonds and C–C bonds in lignin and model compounds. The necessary hydrogen peroxide is probably supplied by the oxidation of glucose (described for cellulose) by glucose oxidase. The formation of peroxidases is promoted by nitrogen limitation. This regulation of peroxidase formation supports the interpretation that the breakdown of lignin by fungi does not serve the purpose of obtaining metabolic energy, but may be aimed primarily at the release of nitrogenous components of wood which would otherwise be inaccessible.

Data on isolated peroxidases are available and are of general interest because the breakdown is initiated by the transfer of one electron. This electron produces relatively stable aromatic cation-radicals in the lignin skeleton. These can then function as further one-electron oxidants and can act at a distance from the enzyme. In this way numerous radicals can be produced in a snowball reaction. These radicals then effect the cleavage of the C–C-ether bonds and therefore the collapse of the lignin skeleton (structure) into low molecular weight phenolic compounds, which are then further oxidised by phenol oxidases. Intermediary formation of radicals is well known in the function of oxygenases. It is doubtful, though, whether the mechanism of lignin degradation will ever be fully elucidated, especially in view of the large number of phenolic compounds that can arise in the breakdown of lignin complexes. The intermediary formation of radicals, already known to play a part in the electron transfer catalysed by oxygenases, therefore merits further study. There is no doubt that lignin can be degraded not only by fungi but also by bacteria. However, the decomposition is so slow that it seems negligible compared to other metabolic activities. There is, therefore, a continuing search for microorganisms able to decompose lignin or to alter it in such a way that it can then be oxidised by other microorganisms.

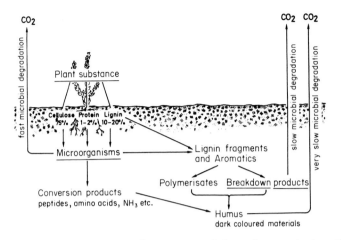

Fig. 14.7. *Decomposition and conversions of plant substances in the soil and the formation of humus.*

(Modified from Flaig, W. (1968).
Landw. Forsch. **21**, 103.)

14.10   Formation of humus

Decomposition of most dead plant and animal matter occurs in the soil (Fig. 14.7). The more easily degradable substances are rapidly and more or less completely oxidised. The compounds that are less amenable to microbial degradation remain for a time as organic components of the soil. The organic soil components consist partly of incompletely decomposed plant residues and partly of humus. Humus is the name applied to amorphous organic substances in the soil; it is usually dark in colour and derived from organisms. It contains those materials that are not easily attacked by microorganisms, primarily lignin, but also fats, waxes, carbohydrates, and protein components. These are converted into chemically ill-defined polymeric substances. The formation of humus involves not only bacteria and fungi, but also protozoa and lower and higher worms.

The conversion of plant materials to humus is accompanied by an accumulation of nitrogen. Whereas the C/N ratio in plant residues is about 40:1, that in humus is about 10:1. A large part of the nitrogen is incorporated in organic compounds, and, in this form, it is not available to plants. Lignin is a particularly effective nitrogen-consuming compound and a source of lignoproteins and of heterocylically bound nitrogen. The soil humus is in a 'steady state': on the one hand, it is continuously replenished by incorporation of organic residues, and on the other hand, part of it is oxidised to completion. The humus content of a soil is highest under conditions that are favourable for its formation and unfavourable for its decomposition. The low humus content of tropical soils, for example, is due to the rapid degradation of all organic substances by the many small living organisms favoured by a tropical climate. The black soil of steppe and prairie has been formed in regions subjected to long cold winters and dry summers. The amount of humus accumulating depends not only on factors of soil and climate, however, but also on the nature of plant substances. Thus, the straw of cereal grasses and prairie plants supplies an easily digestible humus, whereas the wood of forests, especially litter of pine forests, yields humus that is difficult to degrade.

> A large number of carboxy groups are formed or exposed in organic substances during the formation of humus. Hence the presence or absence of cations is of great importance for the quality of the humus and the speed with which it can be decomposed by microorganisms. In mineral-poor and alkali-poor soils (podsol, heath, coniferous forests), brown humic acid (acid humus) accumulates. When basic minerals are present in adequate amounts, base-saturated humus colloids constitute the so-called 'adsorption complexes' of soil. The organic part of such adsorption complexes can be regarded as a natural high molecular weight ion exchanger that can provide an ionic equilibrium suitable for soil organisms, plants, and microbes. Formation of a mild humus leads to an active soil; fungal hyphae and mucus keep the soil particles together and produce a desirable crumb structure.

Whereas a purely mineral soil is poor in microorganisms, humus-rich soils contain a microflora of great species diversity. This soil microflora, existing without addition of nutrients, is called autochthonous, in contrast to zymogenous microorganisms that become dominant on addition of organic nutrients. The stabilising effect of the humus fraction on soil dynamics is also due to the maintenance of a complex microflora.

14.11   Hydrocarbons

Even such chemically stable materials as paraffins, mineral oil, and rubber undergo microbial degradation. Only the absence of oxygen, as in oil deposits, or the special conditions of coal seams ensure the absence of significant degradation.

The following questions are of great practical importance. Can crude oil that has reached soil or water be biologically oxidised? Is there a specific hydrocarbon-utilising microflora? Can the presence of a number of hydrocarbon-oxidising microorganisms be indicative of oil or natural gas deposits?

> Hydrocarbon-utilising bacteria are widely distributed; they can be isolated from all arable, pasture, and forest soils. Nor is the ability to utilise mineral oils as an energy source restricted to a few specialists among microorganisms; it is found in numerous species of fungi and bacteria. These findings are also in accord with new analytical data about the composition of bacteria, plants, and animals. Hydrocarbons are present in many organisms and are constantly synthesised by bacteria and plants; they belong, for example, to the wax-like substances that cover the leaves of plants. Hydrocarbons, therefore, should not be regarded solely as fossil relics of primary production by plants in prehistoric times, but also as secondary metabolites that are still being synthesised in considerable quantities by green plants.

The breakdown of hydrocarbons usually requires the presence of oxygen. This is true for the aliphatic hydrocarbons – from gaseous methane, ethane, and propane, up to the solid paraffins – and for the aromatic hydrocarbons, from benzol and naphthol to anthracene and the polycyclic compounds. All these substances are fed into the central metabolic pathways only after preliminary oxidative reactions. These reactions are characterised by the incorporation of molecular oxygen into the organic molecule. The initial step is designated an **oxygenation**, and the enzymes involved as **oxygenases**. When only one oxygen atom is introduced the enzyme is known as a mono-oxygenase and when both atoms of oxygen are incorporated it is called dioxygenase. These enzymes are quite different from the oxidases which transfer hydrogen atoms from a hydrogen donor to oxygen, thus reducing the latter to water, but never incorporate it into organic molecules or cellular substance.

14.11.1 Methane

Methane occupies an exceptional place among the hydrocarbons. It can be utilised and oxidised by bacteria that are unable to degrade long-chain hydrocarbons. The methane-utilising bacteria should therefore be regarded not so much as hydrocarbon-utilising bacteria, but rather as an extremely specialised group of one-carbon compound utilisers. They are thus members of the methylotrophic group of organisms, that is, the bacteria (and some yeasts) that can utilise methanol, methylated amines, dimethyl ether, formaldehde, and formate. Enrichment cultures that

contain methane as the sole carbon and energy source support the growth
of bacteria belonging to several genera: *Methylomonas, Methylococcus,
Methylosinus*. Some can grow only with methane, methanol or dimethyl
ether as substrate and are unable to use sugars, organic acids or other
alcohols.

Energy gain.   Reducing equivalents for the provision of energy can be
obtained by oxidation of methane, via methanol, formaldehyde, and
formate to carbon dioxide. The oxidation of methane to methanol involves the incorporation of molecular oxygen into the molecule and is
catalysed by a methane oxygenase.

$$CH_4 \xrightarrow[\text{H}_2\text{O} + \text{X}]{\text{O}_2 + \text{XH}_2} CH_3OH \xrightarrow[2\,[\text{H}]]{} HCHO \xrightarrow[2\,[\text{H}]]{\text{H}_2\text{O}} HCOOH \xrightarrow[2\,[\text{H}]]{} CO_2$$

The synthesis of cell material.   The synthesis of cell material usually
starts from formaldehyde, the intermediary product of methane oxidation. It can occur in several ways of which the ribuolose-monophosphate
cycle of formaldehyde fixation and the serine pathway are the best known.
In the ribulose-monophosphate cycle, the formaldehyde produced as an
intermediate in methane oxidation undergoes an aldol condensation with
ribulose-5-phosphate to arabino-3-hexulose-6-phosphate, which is then
converted to fructose-6-phosphate by an isomerase reaction (Fig. 14.8).
The latter is then re-converted to pentose-phosphate as in the ribulose-5-

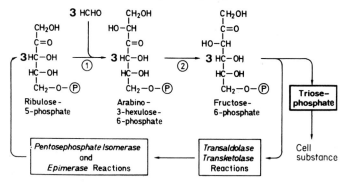

Fig. 14.8. *Ribulose-monophosphate cycle of formaldehyde fixation.*
Key enzymes: (1) hexulose-
phosphate synthase; (2) hexulose-
phosphate isomerase. (After Strom,
Ferrenci & Quayle (1974). *Biochem.
J.* **144**, 465.)

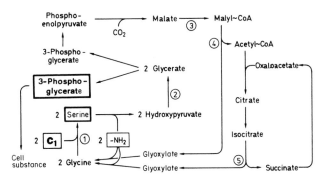

Fig. 14.9. *The assimilation of* C_1 *compounds via the serine pathway.*

The C_1 compound is incorporated into serine with the participation of tetrahydrofolate. The further reaction sequence serves for the synthesis of central intermediary products (phosphoenolpyruvate and pyruvate) and finally cell material, as well as for the regeneration of glycine. Key enzymes involved:

(1) serine hydroxymethyl transferase; (2) hydroxypyruvate reductase; (3) malate thiokinase; (4) malyl-CoA lyase; (5) isocitrate lyase. (After Bellion & Hersh (1972). *Arch. Biochem. Biophys.* **153**, 368; Harder, Attwood & Quayle (1973). *J. gen. Microbiol.* **78**, 155.)

bisphosphate cycle of carbon dioxide fixation. The cycle proceeds as shown on the left-hand side of Fig. 11.2 (see Ch. 11.5), i.e. without involvement of the sedoheptulose-1,7-bisphosphatase reaction.

The serine pathway (Fig. 14.9) was elucidated by studies of *Pseudomonas* MA and *Hyphomicrobium* X. Quite probably, modifications of this scheme occur in other microorganisms. Glycine functions as the acceptor for formaldehyde. In organisms that assimilate one-carbon compounds via this pathway, the enzymes hydroxypyruvate reductase, malate thiokinase, malyl-CoA lyase and isocitrate lyase should be demonstrable.

Utilisation of methanol.   Apart from the methane-utilising bacteria, many other bacterial strains as well as some yeasts can utilise methanol. For example, *Methylobacterium extorquens*, *Methylomonas clara*, *Xanthobacter autotrophicus*, *Paracoccus denitrificans*, *Hyphomicrobium* and *Rhodococcus erythropolis*, and among the yeasts *Hansenula polymorpha* and *Candida boidinii*. As with the methanotrophs, the methanol-utilising bacteria include many species with diverse nutritional and metabolic capacities, as well as some that are obligate methanol users. Some bacteria grow so well on methanol that they can be exploited for large-scale technical production of biomass, namely for the production of single-cell protein.

The utilisation of methanol in bacteria is initiated by a methanol dehydrogenase. This enzyme contains pyrroloquinoline-quinone (PQQ) (methoxatin) as prothetic group. PQQ has now been recognised as a component of many membrane-bound alcohol dehydrogenases and amino acid oxidases. It is also found in eukaryotes, including humans.

> Yeasts can utilise only methanol and not methane. In these yeasts (*Candida boidinii, Hansenula polymorpha*), the incorporation of methanol into the cell substance also involves formaldehyde, but a different pentose-phosphate, i.e. xylulose-5-phosphate. In this xylulose-monophosphate cycle of formaldehyde fixation, formaldehyde and xylulose-5-phosphate are converted to glyceraldehyde phosphate and dihydroxyacetone by a special transketolase. The dihydroxyacetone is phosphorylated by thiokinase and both products then enter the synthetic pathways.

14.11.2   Ethane, propane and butane

Enrichment cultures containing only pure methane plus carbon dioxide and oxygen yielded *Methylomonas methanica* as the predominant organism, but cultures with natural gas, which contains ethane as well as methane, yielded only oxidising organisms. The ability to oxidise ethane is found in a much larger number of species than the ability to utilise methane. Most of the ethane oxidisers belong to the genera *Mycobacterium*, *Flavobacterium* and *Nocardia*. Some ethane-utilising bacteria can also oxidise gaseous hydrogen. Enrichment cultures with propane allow even larger numbers of bacterial species to be cultivated. Some butane-oxidising bacteria have also been isolated.

14.11.3   Long-chain alkanes

Long-chain hydrocarbons (alkanes) can be utilised by a large number of bacteria. The actual chain length is of decisive importance. The number of species that can utilise them and the vigour with which these species attack increases for paraffins of increasing chain length. Mycobacteria, nocardiae, and corynebacteria take part in the degradation. The interest in hydrocarbon-oxidising bacteria was aroused by two observations. Around 1950, two yeasts were isolated at the Institute for Fermentation Technology, Berlin, from enrichment cultures using the products of fractional distillation of hydrocarbons as the energy source. These yeasts were *Candida lipolytica* and *C. tropicalis*. *C. lipolytica* can utilise chains of 15 carbon atoms and all higher homologues. In the meantime it was also shown that most *Candida* species can oxidise hydrocarbons. Sur-

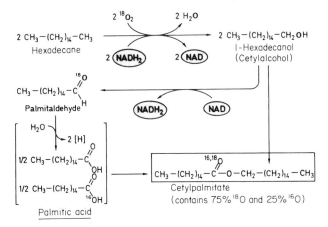

Fig. 14.10. *The formation of cetylpalmitate from hexadecane by* Acinetobacter calcoaceticus.

During growth in normal water ($H_2{}^{16}O$) but in an atmosphere containing ${}^{18}O_2$, cetylpalmitate is produced with 75% of its oxygen as ${}^{18}O$. This observation is consistent with an initial alkane oxidation by an alkane oxidase at the terminal carbon.

veys of yeast collections have indicated that the ability to utilise hydrocarbons is widely distributed among yeasts. This utilisation proceeds with an unusually high yield coefficient. Carbohydrate substrates give Y-values of 0.5, but hydrocarbons show Y-values of 0.7–1.0.

Mechanism. Many pseudomonads oxidise hydrocarbons so completely that no intermediate products are accumulated. Only *Acinetobacter calcoaceticus* excretes oxidation products, and *Nocardia* accumulates such products intracellularly. The nature of the products accumulated depends on the actual substrates. When *A. calcoaceticus* is grown on hexadecane, cetyl palmitate can be isolated from the culture medium. Cetyl plamitate is the ester of palmitic acid and cetyl alcohol (hexadecanol). Both of these are oxidation products of hexadecane. The experiment sketched in Fig. 14.10 provides evidence for the suggestion that breakdown of paraffins is initiated by oxidation of the terminal carbon.

Oxygen takes part in the initial attack on the hydrocarbon chain; no oxidation of paraffins occurs in the absence of molecular oxygen. The oxidation is catalysed by a mono-oxygenase (alkane oxygenase).

$$paraffin + O_2 + NADH_2 \rightarrow paraffin\ alcohol + NAD + H_2O$$

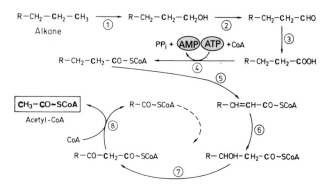

Fig. 14.11. *Degradation of alkanes (paraffins) via terminal oxidation by mono-oxygenase and β-oxidation to acetyl-CoA.*

Enzymes involved:
(1) mono-oxygenase (alkane-1-hydroxylase); (2) alcohol dehydrogenase; (3) aldehyde dehydrogenase; (4) acyl-CoA synthetase; (5) acyl-CoA dehydrogenase; (6) 3-hydroxyacyl-CoA hydroxylase; (7) 3-hydroxyacyl-CoA dehydrogenase; (8) β-ketothiolase.

The further oxidation of the paraffins then proceeds by β-oxidation, i.e. the reactions known from the oxidation of long-chain fatty acids (Fig. 14.11). If heptane-oxidising pseudomonads are exposed to lowered partial pressures of oxygen, C_3, C_5 and C_7 fatty acids accumulate in the nutrient medium. When cells grown on hexane are incubated with heptane, propionate is accumulated. This accumulation of propionate is due to the fact that hexane-grown cells apparently lack the enzymes for the utilisation of propionate via methylmalonyl-CoA.

14.11.4 Aromatic hydrocarbons

Plants produce many organic compounds that contain aromatic rings. The quantitatively predominant compound is lignin, which accounts for about 20% (by weight) of wood. Many bacteria and fungi are able to cleave the aromatic ring.

Some pseudomonads grow more rapidly on benzoate than on sugars. The presence of oxygen, however, is a precondition for the rapid degradation of aromatic compounds. The pathways involved in these degradations are described below. According to recent investigations degradation of aromatic compounds can also occur under anaerobic conditions, but this pathway will not be described at present.

Preparations for ring cleavage. Most of the aromatic compounds in nature are initially degraded by bacteria to one of two compounds: catechol or protocatechuate. Many singly substituted or 1,2-di-substituted aromatic rings, for example, mandelate, phenylalanine, toluol, benzoate, salicylate, phenol and benzene, are degraded to catechol.

Aromatic rings di-substituted in positions 1,3 and 1,4 and multiply substituted rings, for example, 4-hydroxybenzoate, quinate, vanillate, and shikimate, are degraded to protocatechuate. In all cases hydroxy groups are incorporated into the ring. The oxygen comes from molecular oxygen. In non-phenolic aromatics, the 1,3-dihydroxybenzene structure necessary for ring cleavage is achieved by double hydroxylation.

Benzene   *Dioxygenase*   *cis*-1,2-Dihydro-   *Dehydrogenase*   Catechol
1,2-dihydroxy-
benzene

The unsubstituted ring of benzene, for example, is hydroxylated by a dioxygenase (double hydroxylase) to *cis*-1,2-dihydro-1,2-dihydroxy-benzene, which is then dehydrated to protocatechuate.

In contrast, phenolic aromatics are further hydroxylated by mono-oxygenases. One of the oxygen atoms of molecular oxygen is incorporated and the other is reduced to water. Reduced pyridine nucleotides can function as hydrogen donors.

Phenol   *Mono-oxygenase*   Catechol

The substituents on the aromatic ring are often, but not always, removed before ring cleavage. Chloro substitutents and nitro and sulphonate groups can be replaced by hydroxy groups. Aliphatic side chains can be modified and shortened in many ways or can remain intact.

Ring cleavage. The cleavage of the aromatic ring is carried out by dioxygenases. In the course of this, molecular oxygen is incorporated. The cleavage occurs either between two neighbouring hydroxy groups, or between the hydroxylated and the neighbouring non-hydroxylated carbon atoms. The most extensively investigated enzymes have been isolated from *Pseudomonas* species. The most important types of ring openings are presented in Fig. 14.12.

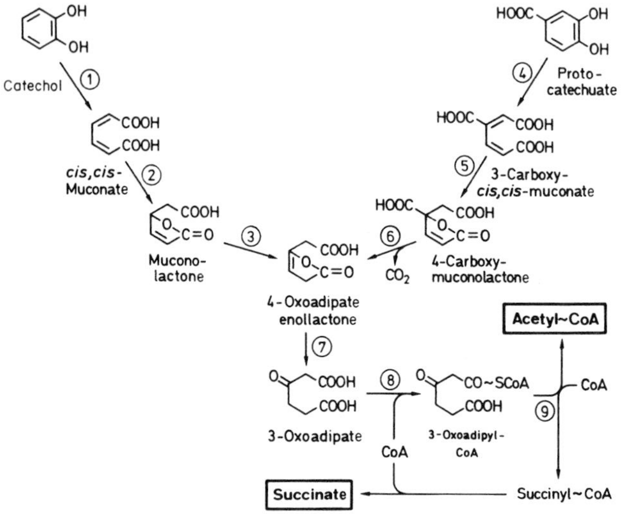

Fig. 14.12. *Ortho cleavage of the aromatic ring and the 3-oxoadipate pathway.*

Enzymes involved: (1) pyrocatechase (catechol-1,2-dioxygenase); (2) muconate cycloisomerase; (3) muconolactone isomerase; (4) protocatecuate-3,4-dioxygenase; (5) 3-carboxymuconate cycloisomerase; (6) 4-carboxymuconolactone decarboxylase; (7) 4-oxoadipatenollactone hydrolase; (8) 3-oxoadipate-succinyl-CoA transferase; (9) 3-oxoadipyl-CoA thiolase.

Ortho or intradiol cleavage is the cleavage between two neighbouring hydroxylated carbon atoms and it leads to dicarboxylic acids. Presumably, there is a primary addition of the O_2 molecule to the carbon atoms next to the hydroxy group with the formation of a cyclic peroxide. Intramolecular rearrangement then dissolves the C–C bond with the formation of *cis,cis*-muconic acid.

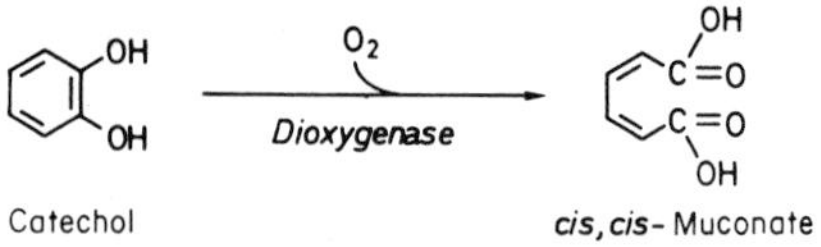

Catechol is cleaved by ortho-pyrocatechase (catechol-1,2-dioxygenase) and protocatechuate is cleaved by protocatechuate-,3,4-dioxygenase. The

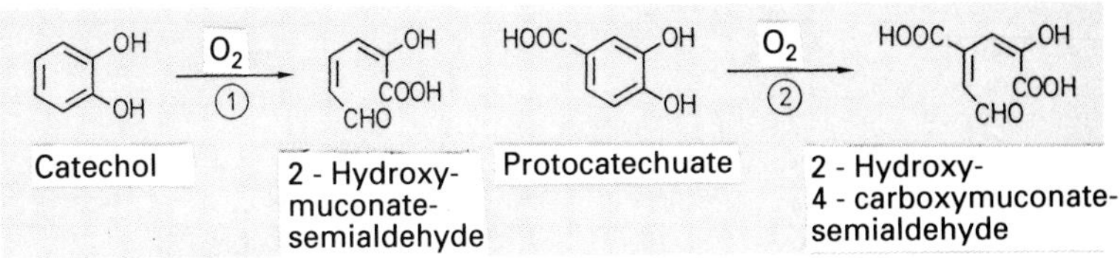

Catechol   2 - Hydroxy-muconate-semialdehyde   Protocatechuate   2 - Hydroxy-4 - carboxymuconate-semialdehyde

Fig. 14.13. *Meta cleavage of the aromatic ring.*

Enzymes involved: (1) metapyrocatechase (catechol-2,3- dioxygenase); (2) protocatechuate-4,5-dioxygenase.

products of these two enzyme reactions, *cis,cis*-muconate and 3-carboxy-*cis,cis*-muconate, are further metabolised via the common intermediate, 3-oxoadipate. The latter is activated by a CoA-transferase and split into succinyl-CoA and acetyl-CoA, which are metabolised via the pathways of intermediary metabolism (Fig. 14.12).

Meta or extradiol cleavage is the cleavage of the ring between the hydroxylated and non-hydroxylated carbon atoms and it is also catalysed by dioxygenases. The cleavage products are 2-hydroxy-muconate-semialdehydes, which then enter the pathways of intermediary metabolism via pyruvate, acetaldehyde, oxaloacetate, acetoacetate, fumarate, or succinate, according to the substituents on the aliphatic acids produced (Fig. 14.13).

Experimental investigations have shown that the catabolic pathways for aromatic compounds vary considerably in the methods of ring cleavage, as above, and also in the preparatory reactions leading to cleavage of the aromatic ring. In some bacteria even the growth phase and growth conditions determine whether the enzymes for the ortho or meta cleavage are produced. In some pseudomonads, the aromatic compounds catabolised via catechol undergo ring cleavage by the ortho method, whereas those catabolised via protocatechuate undergo meta cleavage and metabolism.

Convergent pathways. The catabolism of various aromatic compounds involves a relatively large number of reactions. The pathways eventually converge in the formation of catechol or protocatechuate (Figs 14.14, 14.15). These catabolic pathways were very useful in the elucidation of regulatory mechanisms for convergent catabolic pathways (see Ch. 16.1.1).

Naphthalene, anthracene, and polyaromatic compounds. Some bacteria can degrade poylcyclic hydrocarbons, of which only naphthalene, anthracene, and phenanthrene will be mentioned here. When these bacteria are grown in media containing one of these substrates, salicyclate is often

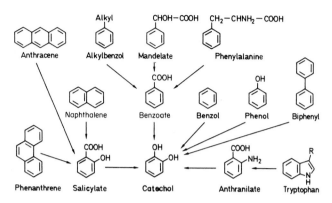

Fig. 14.14. *Degradative pathways of aromatic compounds leading to catechol.*

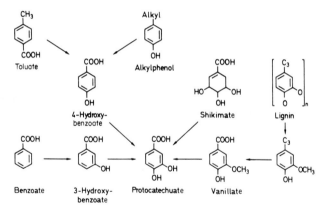

Fig. 14.15. *Degradative pathways of aromatic compounds leading to protocatechuate.*

found in the culture medium. This suggests that the reactions described for the catabolism of monocyclic compounds are involved (Fig. 14.15).

It can finally be said that the naturally occurring hydrocarbons can be altered and either partially or completely oxidised by microorganisms. Even asphalt can be degraded, though extremely slowly, under suitable environmental conditions, and graphite, too, can be oxidised in microbially active soils.

Oil spillage and contamination.   Regarding contamination of soil with petroleum, it should be borne in mind that hydrocarbons are rapidly and completely degraded in well-aerated active soils. Only when the contamination is severe or under anaerobiosis, or if the oil has penetrated to great depths, is there any danger of its conservation and contamination of drinking water. Petroleum spillage at sea presents an immediate danger to marine fauna and flora, but it is also subject to degradation by bacteria. However, residues of long-chain alkanes, polyaromatic hydrocarbons, and asphalt-like mixtures may occur which can resist biological attack for considerable periods.

Anaerobic breakdown of aromatic hydrocarbons.   Because of the involvement of molecular oxygen in the initial steps of aromatic ring cleavage, it was thought that benzol, benzoic acid, 4-hydroxybenzoic acid and many other derivatives had to be resistant to anaerobic breakdown. This premature conclusion, however, has to be revised. Phenol, as well as benzoic acid and even benzyl alcohol can be attacked under anaerobic conditions. That is, provided that H-acceptors, which allow anaerobic respiration, such as nitrate, sulphate, CO_2 or light are available. This statement is based on studies with mixed populations and defined mixed cultures, and of a few, recently isolated, bacteria. On the other hand, conclusive enzymatic studies on the detailed degradative steps and the enzymes involved are available only piecemeal or not at all. The isolation of *Rhodopseudomonas palustris* from enrichment cultures growing with benzoate in the light was demonstrated already by Van Niel in his remarkable work of 1932. Since then it has become clear that coenzyme A is involved in the initial step of benzoate activation via the formation of benzoyl-CoA. This is the intermediate which is then hydrated to a cyclohexane derivative and subsequently broken down to acetyl-CoA. The anaerobic breakdown of substituted benzyl alcohol is a reductive pathway. Much still remains to be investigated before the many possibilities of anaerobic breakdown of aromatic hydrocarbons can be fully elucidated.

Xenobiotics.   These are chemically synthesised compounds, most of which do not occur in nature. It can be considered doubtful whether organisms exist which can break down such substances. The xenobiotics include fungicides, pesticides, herbicides, insecticides, nematocides, etc. Most are substituted hydrocarbons, phenylcarbonates and similar compounds. Some of these substances, of which great quantities are applied to crops and soils are very recalcitrant and are degraded only very slowly or not at all. Others are known to disappear from the soil, but their breakdown products are not known. Some of the compounds, however, are rapidly degraded. Research in this area is full of surprises.

Above some impermeable clay soils situated under industrial build-ings, solvents like chloroform, di-, tri- and poly-perchlorethylene have accumulated in amounts that can be pumped away. But the soil has to be cleaned up and rehabilitated by chemical, physical or biotechnological means. Relevant problems of this kind are the subject of studies in microbial biodegradation.

Man-made fibres like polyethylene and polypropylene, though harm-less, are practically non-degradable. Whilst the plasticisers and softeners contained in these textiles are gradually oxidised, the polymer skeleton remains intact. It is to be hoped that these polymers may come to be replaced by biopolymers like poly(hydroxy)fatty acids or starch deriva-tives which are biodegradable.

Co-metabolism. Some substances can be degraded by microorganisms only in association with other, utilisable substrates. Metabolism that cannot by itself support cell growth but supports growth in the presence of another substance that is utilisable (a co-substrate) is called co-me-tabolism or co-oxidation. Such co-metabolism can be exploited, for ex-ample, by purification of industrial effluents that contain degradation-resistant synthetics together with domestic sewage water in a common waste water treatment plant. In some cases the mechanisms is not yet obvious. A natural variant of such metabolism can be seen in the lignin decomposition by *Phanerochaete chrysosporium*. This contains cellulose combined with lignin (lignocellulose). The formation of glucose from this yields hydrogen peroxide, hydroxyl and superoxide radicals which are needed to initiate the breakdown of the lignin skeleton. By incubat-ing xenobiotics with substrates which induce the formation of mono-oxygenase, the mono-oxygenase could be harnessed for the production of radicals.

14.12   Proteins

Organisms consist to a large extent of proteins. For most living beings a dead organism is the best substrate (food). The proteins of dead organ-isms are attacked and broken down by a large number of fungi and bacteria. Like other high molecular weight substances, proteins are first broken down outside the cell by extracellular enzymes into convenient cleavage products. The **proteases**, excreted by bacteria and fungi, hydro-lyse proteins to oligopeptides and amino acids. The proteolytic activity of microorganisms is often assayed in solid media containing gelatine, where proteolytic activity can be recognised by a clear zone around the colony in which gelatine can no longer be precipitated by acid (HCl).

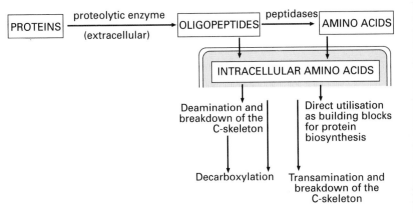

Fig. 14.16. *Schematic illustration of protein catabolism outside and inside the bacterial cell, and the possible conversions of the resulting amino acids.*

Oligopeptides and amino acids are taken into the cell by specific transport systems and the peptides broken down to amino acids by intracellular **proteinases**. The amino acids are then incorporated into cellular proteins or they are deaminated via specific pathways and then enter intermediary metabolism and its terminal oxidising system to serve as energy source (Fig. 14.16).

Proteases are enzymes which split peptide bonds. There are intracellular, as well as extracellular proteases. The former function in cellular metabolism whereas the latter function in extracellular protein breakdown.

Exo- and **endopeptidases** are distinguished by their specificities. Those enzymes with specificities determined by the carboxy- or amino-terminal of the polypeptide chains are known as exopeptidases. The endopeptidases, also called proteinases, hydrolyse the peptide bonds within the polypeptide chains. At least four groups of these can be distinguished, serine, cysteine, aspartate and zinc proteinases. These intracellular enzymes are highly specific and play important roles in the regulation of cell metabolism by, for example, hydrolysing signal peptides and activating or inactivating various enzymes.

Some of the extracellular proteases, which are excreted into the medium, act as toxins and virulence factors (subtilisin, lysotaphine, streptokinase, elastase, haemolysin and others). Large quantities of proteases are produced industrially and are used as additives to detergents, in the processing of leather and for other purposes. Thermostable proteases are produced by thermophilic bacteria (Table 10.2).

Although a large number of bacteria and fungi can produce extracellular proteases, this is by no means a universal ability of microorganisms.

> Partially digested proteins were formerly called **peptones**. This badly defined term is now only applied to the peptone used for bacteriological media. It is obtained by treating proteins with pepsin, which hydrolyses only some of the peptide bonds. Peptone consists of about 30% (by weight) amino acids, with the remainder comprising a mixture of di- and tripeptides and water-soluble, but no longer heat- or acid-precipitable, polypeptides. The much-used, undefined, complex 'nutrient broth' employed in bacteriological laboratories consists of a mixture of peptone, meat extract and yeast extract in the proportion of 7:7:2. It contains, apart from amino acids and oligopeptides, a series of sugars, organic acids and trace elements.

Protein degradation in soil is accompanied by the formation of ammonia. It is therefore referred to as mineralisation of nitrogen or ammonification. Many fungi and bacteria take part in the decomposition of proteins, including *Bacillus cereus* var. *mycoides*, pseudomonads, *Proteus vulgaris*, and others.

The first catabolic reaction attacking an amino acid can be either a decarboxylation or a deamination. Decarboxylases are produced mainly in acid conditions. The decarboxylation products of amino acids are carbon dioxide and primary amines (biogenic amines). The best known of these bases (formerly called ptomaines) are cadaverine, putrescine, and agmatine; they are produced from lysine, ornithine, and arginine, respectively. These primary amines occur during normal intestinal digestion and other anaerobic degradations of proteinaceous materials.

$$H_2N-(CH_2)_4-CHNH_2-COOH \longrightarrow H_2N-(CH_2)_4-CH_2NH_2 + CO_2$$

Lysine   Cadaverine

$$H_2N-(CH_2)_3-CHNH_2-COOH \longrightarrow H_2N-(CH_2)_3-CH_2NH_2 + CO_2$$

Ornithine   Putrescine

$$\underset{H_2N}{\overset{HN}{>}}C-NH-(CH_2)_3-CHNH_2-COOH \longrightarrow \underset{H_2N}{\overset{HN}{>}}C-NH-(CH_2)_3-CH_2NH_2 + CO_2$$

Arginine   Agmatine

Deamination means the liberation of ammonia from an amino acid. Oxidative, desaturative, and hydrolytic deaminations are distinguished according to the fate of the carbon skeleton.

Oxidative deamination is the most common type of amino acid

catabolism. Glutamic acid is oxidatively deaminated by glutamate dehydrogenase to 2-oxoglutarate. The reaction is reversible and is the most important in the metabolism of amino acids. The equilibrium is towards glutamic acid.

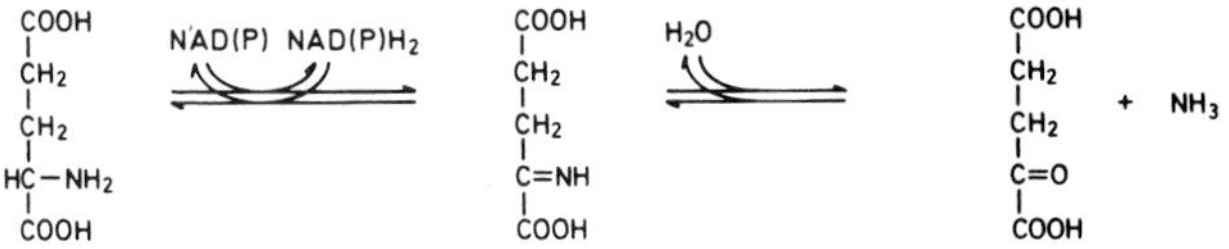

The desaturative deamination of aspartic acid yields fumarate.

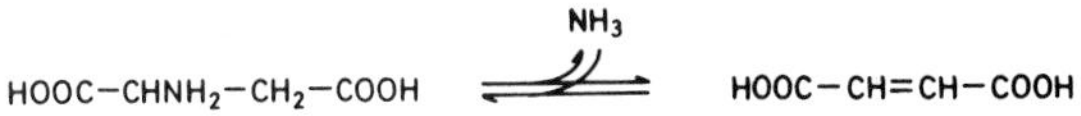

This reaction is catalysed by aspartase and is also reversible.

The hydrolysis of urea is regarded as a **hydrolytic deamination**. A large number of bacteria can utilise urea as a nitrogen source, the urea being hydrolysed by the enzyme urease.

$$H_2N–CO–NH_2 + H_2O \rightarrow 2NH_3 + CO_2$$

In most bacteria the formation of urease is repressed by ammonium ions. By this means, the amount of ammonium produced and excreted into the medium is kept at the level necessary for protein synthesis. In a few bacteria known as 'urea splitting organisms' (*Bacillus pasteurii, Sporosarcina urea, Proteus vulgaris*), the urease is constitutive; its formation does not depend on the presence of urea, nor is it repressed by ammonium. These bacteria, therefore, hydrolyse all the urea present (in stables, for instance) to ammonium, producing a pH of 9–10, to which they are adapted.

In **transamination** the amino group of an amino acid is transferred to a 2-oxoacid by transaminases.

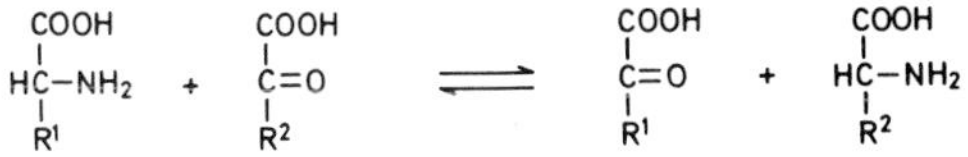

Transamination thus serves for the synthesis of some amino acids that cannot be directly aminated by ammonium and, at the same time, serves for the catabolism of other amino acids. Pyridoxal phosphate is involved in the above reactions of decarboxylation and transamination (Fig. 14.17). This coenzyme of amino acid metabolism is related to pyridoxal, known as vitamin B_6. The reactive group of pyridoxal phosphate is the aldehyde

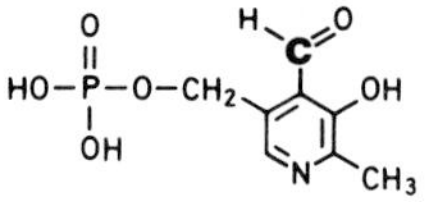

$$HO-\overset{\overset{\displaystyle O}{\|}}{\underset{\underset{\displaystyle OH}{|}}{P}}-O-CH_2$$

Pyridoxal phosphate

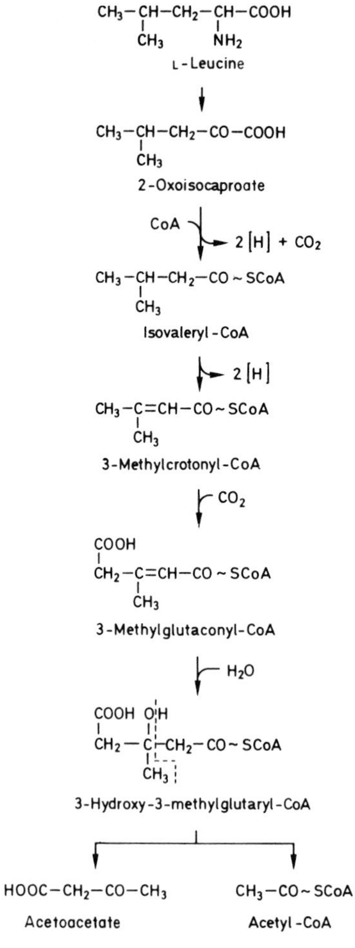

$$CH_3-\overset{\overset{\displaystyle }{}}{\underset{\underset{\displaystyle CH_3}{|}}{CH}}-CH_2-\overset{\overset{\displaystyle }{}}{\underset{\underset{\displaystyle NH_2}{|}}{CH}}-COOH$$

L-Leucine

$$CH_3-\underset{\underset{\displaystyle CH_3}{|}}{CH}-CH_2-CO-COOH$$

2-Oxoisocaproate

CoA ⟶ 2 [H] + CO_2

$$CH_3-\underset{\underset{\displaystyle CH_3}{|}}{CH}-CH_2-CO \sim SCoA$$

Isovaleryl-CoA

2 [H]

$$CH_3-\underset{\underset{\displaystyle CH_3}{|}}{C}=CH-CO \sim SCoA$$

3-Methylcrotonyl-CoA

CO_2

$$\underset{\underset{\displaystyle CH_3}{|}}{\overset{\overset{\displaystyle COOH}{|}}{CH_2-C}}=CH-CO \sim SCoA$$

3-Methylglutaconyl-CoA

H_2O

$$\overset{\overset{\displaystyle COOH}{|}}{CH_2}-\overset{\overset{\displaystyle OH}{|}}{\underset{\underset{\displaystyle CH_3}{|}}{C}}-CH_2-CO \sim SCoA$$

3-Hydroxy-3-methylglutaryl-CoA

Fig. 14.17. *Catabolic pathway of leucine.*

Initially L-leucine is converted to a 2-oxoacid by transamination. The oxoacid is oxidatively decarboxylated with formation of a CoA derivate. Dehydrogenation then leads to formation of 3-methyl-crotonyl-CoA. 3-hydroxy-3-methylglutaryl-CoA is formed from this by a biotin-dependent carboxylation and a hydroxylation. The cleavage products acetoacetate and acetyl-CoA are metabolised by the well-known pathways. The example of leucine catabolism demonstrates that carboxylation reactions can occur in catabolic pathways. Reduction of the carbon dioxide content of the environment below a certain threshold value can lead to cessation of growth in many microorganisms.

$$HOOC-CH_2-CO-CH_3$$
Acetoacetate

$$CH_3-CO \sim SCoA$$
Acetyl-CoA

group; it participates with the amino group of an amino acid in the formation of a Schiff base. In transamination, the amino group remains on the pyridoxal phosphate whilst the carbon skeleton is liberated as a 2-oxoacid; the pyridoxal phosphate is then regenerated in the reaction with the (receptor) oxoacid. In the decarboxylation, the Schiff base liberates carbon dioxide.

The further fate of the carbon skeleton varies in the different amino acids. Only a few of the deamination products are intermediates of the central metabolic pathways (pyruvate, 2-oxoglutarate, oxaloacetate). Other carbon skeletons enter intermediate metabolism via specific catabolic reactions. It would go beyond the framework of this presentation to detail all these catabolic pathways. A representative example, the catabolism of leucine, is shown in Fig. 14.17. Attention should be drawn to the occurrence of 3-hydroxy-3-methylglutaryl-CoA, which is an important intermediate in the synthesis of steroids and carotenoids.

15 Constancy, change, recombination and transfer of genetic information

Each living organism resembles its ancestors in most of its characters. The maintenance of specific properties, that is, the constancy of characters over the generations, is called **heredity**. **Genetics** is concerned with the transfer of these characters and with the laws of heredity. Each genetic character can be assigned to a **gene** which carries the information. Classical genetics already regarded the genes as situated in the cell nucleus of eukaryotic organisms, and it was concluded that the genes must be arranged linearly. For a long time it was thought that genetic information was associated with the protein components of the nucleoplasm. Eventually, the successful transfer of genetic information (transformation) by DNA demonstrated that this must be the material equivalent of hereditary characters. It was further demonstrated, first with insects and later with microorganisms, that the expression of genetic characters is due to the action of enzymes. In microorganisms, enzymes could be described as biochemically identifiable characters. The **'one gene, one enzyme' hypothesis** states that one gene contains the information necessary for one specific enzyme; today this is stated more accurately; that each structural gene codes for a specific polypeptide chain. Changes in, or of, a gene by mutation lead to a loss of the enzyme or to production of an altered enzyme, and hence to a recognisable change in the hereditary character. Thus, the gene is recognised by its mutation. The term mutation was coined by De Vries who studied variation and heredity in plants and found sudden, discontinuous changes in hereditary characters. Beijerinck then applied the term also to bacteria. Genetics is based on studies of differences in hereditary characters resulting from alternative (allelic) forms of a gene. Genetic investigations are therefore studies of mutants. The naturally occurring strain is called the wild type and the product of the mutation, the mutant. Microorganisms offer great advantages as research material for genetics. A very large number of individuals can be dealt with in a limited space (and time). Bacteria were included in genetic research, though, only after certain dogmatic assumptions had been overcome.

15.1   The origins of mutation

15.1.1   The undirected nature of mutation

The view that microorganisms can mutate and change their hereditary characters was not accepted for a long time. Before the development of pure culture techniques, many groups of microbiologists (Nägeli, Zopf) thought that bacteria were morphologically and physiologically variable. One of the ideas was that the large numbers of bacterial types found in nature represented different stages in the life cycle of a small number of species (**pleomorphism**). Cohn and Koch, however, on the basis of their improved methodology and experience with pure cultures, defended the opposite view of **monomorphism**. This states that morphological and physiological characters of bacteria are constant and can serve for identification and classification. Eventually, the difference between genotype and phenotype had to be recognised in bacteria (as in other organisms). **Genotype** refers to the genetic constitution of a cell, whereas phenotype describes its actual, observed properties. The **phenotypic** expression of a given genotypic constitution is governed by environmental factors and conditions.

The most remarkable variants among bacteria are those that arise in the presence of toxic compounds. Such toxin-resistant cells were at first assumed to be the products of adaptation. It seemed difficult to distinguish between **phenotypic adaptation** to changes in the environment and **genotypic changes**, although the criteria are simple: in phenotypic adaptation all the cells in a culture adapt, whereas genotypic changes occur in only a few cells of a culture; these are then selected by an environment to which they are better adapted. Thus, genotypically toxin-resistant cells outgrow the parent culture in the presence of the toxin.

Another question about genotypic changes concerned their origin. Were they in fact caused by the selective agent in the environment and thus were 'aimed' in a certain direction, or did mutations occur at random without any directive influence by the environment?

In the case of higher organisms, the views of Darwin – that new types and species arise by random mutations and subsequent selection of the fittest – had been generally accepted, and Lamarck's theories about the heredity of adaptively acquired characters forced to be abandoned.

A number of notable experiments eventually proved that bacterial mutations also occur at random and are non-directed. In this chapter we present one of the classic experiments; it is easy to follow and demonstrates the use of the much-practised technique of replica plating.

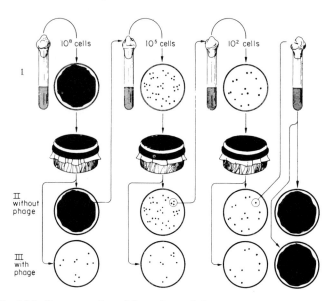

Fig. 15.1. *Demonstration of the undirected character of mutation in bacteria by the replica plating method.*

See text for explanation.

Indirect selection of mutants by replica plating.   Lederberg's experiments in 1952 provided unassailable proof for selection of mutants. He also demonstrated for the first time the technique of sterile replica plating, which has since become widely established. A sterile velvet pad, of a slightly smaller diameter than the petri dish, is pressed onto the surface of an agar plate on which colonies have been grown. The velvet pile is thus charged with inocula from all the colonies on the plate; by immediately pressing the velvet pad onto the surface of an uninoculated agar plate, this plate is inoculated with the exact colonial pattern of the original plate.

Organisms from a plate covered with a confluent growth of **phage-sensitive bacteria** (Fig. 15.1, plate I) were transferred by means of a velvet pad to another ordinary agar plate (II) and to a plate already seeded with the phage (III). After incubation of all the plates, some phage-resistant colonies appeared on plate III. An area of the normal plate (II) which corresponded to the area where a resistant colony had appeared on the phage plate (III) was then harvested, allowed to multiply in a liquid medium without phage, and again plated onto a fresh agar plate without phage. After incubation, the resulting colonies were again replica-plated onto normal (II) and phage-seeded agar plates (III). The procedure was repeated several times, and eventually a fully phage-resistant culture was obtained whose ancestors had never been in contact with any phage. This experiment provided convincing proof that resistant mutants can arise spontaneously in the absence of any contact with the selective agent.

15.1.2   Mutations and their frequency

Spontaneous mutations.   Bacterial populations are subject to mutations occurring at certain rates without any outside intervention. These are called spontaneous mutations, and the mutated cells are called spontaneous mutants.

Mutant frequency and mutation rate.   The numerical proportion of mutants in a cell population is called the **mutant frequency**. This differs greatly for individual characters, from 10^{-4} to 10^{-11}. The actual numbers of mutants in a population depends on environmental conditions, age of the population, and other factors. The probability of a given mutation occurring per cell and per generation is called the **mutation rate**. Mutation rates are usually determined on cells in exponential growth under optimal conditions. The spontaneous mutation rate for a gene is of the order of 10^{-5} and for a given nucleotide pair is of the order of 10^{-8}.

Silent mutations.   At the molecular level every heritable, stable change in DNA is a mutation, although it must be clear already from the degeneracy of the genetic code that not every such mutation is phenotypically expressed. In many triplet codons, for example, a change in the third base is without phenotypic consequences (silent mutations). Even a replacement of the first or second base of a triplet does not need to have phenotypically recognisable consequences. Although the primary structure (amino acid sequence) of a protein determines its higher order (secondary, tertiary) structure, alterations of individual amino acids can have very different effects on protein structure. For example, a transition from AUC to GUC would lead to the substitution of an isoleucine by a valine, that is, of one non-polar, hydrophobic amino acid by another with similar properties. However, if CUU is changed to CCU, the non-polar amino acid leucine is exchanged for the polar amino acid proline. This substitution produces a kink in the polypeptide chain; such a kink could profoundly influence the higher order conformation. It is clear, therefore, that in a set of mutants bearing changes in the structural gene of the same enzyme, a whole range of altered enzyme activities can be found; from a barely measurable decline in activity to a complete loss of activity.

Back mutation or reversion.   Against this background (of spontaneous mutations) it has become obvious that many – though not all – mutants can back mutate and regain the wild-type character. Two types of such back-mutants can be distinguished: (1) **revertants**, in which a second mutation at the same gene establishes exactly the same genotype, i.e. the wild type that existed before the first mutation; (2) **functional revertants**, that still have the original mutation, but have regained the original phenotype via a second mutation, outside the original gene locus (either intra- or extragenic). This group includes **suppressor mutants**, in which a new mutation suppresses the original defect in an indirect way. The suppression can be brought about by alteration of a transfer-RNA anticodon (see Chapter 2) which now recognises the mutated codon and inserts the original amino acid into the polypeptide chain. Suppressor mutants often grow more slowly than the genuine wild-type strain because they still tend to incorporate a wrong amino acid now and again, owing to the fact that most amino acids have several cognate tRNAs.

15.1.3   Types of mutation

Three types of mutation can be distinguished on the basis of the molecular alteration, namely, **point mutations, deletions and insertions**, and **frameshift mutations**.

Point mutations.   These are characterised by an exchange of individual bases. When a purine (for example adenine) is replaced by another purine (i.e. guanine), or a pyrimidine (for example thymine) by another pyrimidine (i.e. cytosine), the exchange is called a **transition**. Exchange of a purine for a pyrimidine base is called **transversion**. In general, the product of a point mutation is most frequently the substitution of the normal 'sense' codon by a **'mis-sense'** codon (see Chapter 2) and therefore the production of a polypeptide chain containing a different amino acid. However, in some cases the replacement of a base can give rise to the substitution of a **nonsense** or '**terminator**' codon for the normal, sense codon, which leads to premature termination of translation and an incomplete protein. Point mutations are characterised by high reversion frequencies.

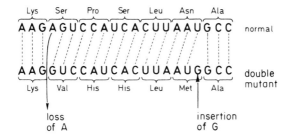

Fig. 15.2. *Shift in the triplet arrangement of the nucleotide sequence by a frame-shift mutation.*

The bacteriophage T4 has the ability to produce lysozyme. The enzyme is coded by a phage gene. The upper row shows a part of the normal base sequence of the wild type with the corresponding amino acids indicated. The lower row shows the base sequence of a double mutant phage obtained from the wild type by two treatments with proflavin. The loss of a nucleotide means that the first base (A) in the second triplet has been lost. From this point onwards the triplets are misread; the reading frame has been shifted. After the insertion of G at the end of the fifth wrong triplet, the reading of the succeeding base sequences is again meaningful. The base sequence of the double mutant differs from that of the wild type only by the second to fifth triplet. If the amino acids coded by these triplets are not crucial for the functioning of the enzyme, the second mutation can restore the properties (phenotype) of the wild type (genetic suppression).

Deletions and insertions.   A deletion mutation means the loss of one or more bases from the DNA. The deletion can cover wide areas of DNA comprising several genes. For this reason deletions cannot usually be reversed by a second mutation. The same is true for insertion mutations: that is, the insertion of one or more bases into one (or more) genes, which are thereby inactivated.

Frame-shift mutations.   Each individual gene is strictly defined by a reading frame. During the translation of a messenger-RNA, the ribosome binds to a base sequence of about 9 base pairs (Shine–Delgarno Box) which are immediately adjacent to the **initiation codon AUG**, and complementary to the 3'-OH end of the 16S rRNA. Translation then begins at the start codon, and proceeds in a continuous 'frame' of 3 bases encoding one amino acid. Frame-shift mutations are brought about by the loss or insertion of a single base, i.e. they represent a special case of deletion or insertion mutations (Fig. 15.2). A frame-shift mutation thus distorts the reading frame of a gene and, depending on the location of the mutation, causes the cell to produce non-functional or low-activity proteins.

Polarity. If a point mutation, a deletion or an insertion leads to the formation of a 'stop codon', and hence to premature termination of the translation, the ribosome dissociates from the mRNA. According to the length of the non-translated mRNA, the subsequent genes are also affected, and form a gradient of non- and weakly-translated messages. This effect is termed 'polarity'. If a translation is interrupted at the start of a gene (i.e. the 5' end), the effect on subsequent genes is stronger, i.e. the polar effect is greater than when the interruption occurs near the end of the gene (i.e. the 3' end).

15.1.4   Mutagenic agents and their effects

The frequency of mutational events can be increased by treating cells with mutagenic (mutation inducing) agents. This is called induced mutation, and the resulting mutant cells are called induced mutants. Chemical, physical, and biological agents can be used as mutagens. The mechanism(s) by which they produce their effects will be discussed in some selected examples in the following paragraphs (Table 15.1).

Base analogues.   Base analogues are antimetabolites. Some of these are so similar to normal purines and pyrimidines that they can be taken up by the cell and incorporated into DNA, where they can function almost like normal bases. However, they usually exhibit a greater tendency to pair with the wrong partner during DNA replication. Two such base-analogue compounds used for inducing mutations are bromouracil (BU) and 2-aminopurine. Bromouracil is a structural analogue of thymine and is incorporated in its place, i.e. as a partner to adenine. BU tautomerises to the enol form more frequently than thymine. During replication of a BU-containing chain, the enol form of BU pairs like cytosine and therefore causes incorporation of guanine in place of adenine, so that the base pair AT in these cases is replaced by CG. 2-aminopurine is incorporated in place of adenine and its effect is similar. This kind of change, the replacement of a purine by another purine derivative (A $\rightarrow$ G) or of one pyrimidine by another (C $\rightarrow$ T) is called transition.

Chemical modification of bases.   Several mutation-inducing agents act by chemically altering some of the bases in DNA and thus producing

Table 15.1. *Mutagenic agents and their mode of action*

Mutagen	Structure	Mode of action
5-Bromouracil (BU)		Replaces thymine by pairing with guanine
2-Aminopurine (AP)		Replaces adenine by pairing with cytosine
Nitrous acid	HNO_2	Deamination, strand crossing over
Hydroxylamine	NH_2OH	Hydroxylation of cytosine
Ethylmethane-sulphonate	$CH_2SO_3CH_2CH_3$	Alkylation of purines, transitions
N-methyl-N'-nitro-N-nitroso-guanine (NMG)		Synthesis of methyl-guanine during replication, transitions and multiple mutations
Acridine orange		Frameshift mutations by intercalation
Ultraviolet rays (UV)	254 nm wavelength	Pyrimidine dimers, repair errors
X-rays	5 nm wavelength	Breakage of single- and double-stranded DNA

replication errors. A very clearly recognisable change of this kind is produced by nitrite. This deaminates adenine, guanine, or cytosine without causing breakage or other alterations in the DNA chain. Substitution of the amine group by a hydroxy group converts adenine to hypoxanthine, which pairs with cytosine instead of thymine, and thus produces a transition AT → GC. On deamination of cytosine to uracil, this pairs with adenine instead of guanine and thus produces a transition GC → AT. On the other hand, guanine conversion to xanthine does not result in a mutation because the xanthine continues to pair with cytosine.

Hydroxylamine reacts predominantly with cytosine and alters it so that it pairs with adenine, thus also causing a transition CG → AT.

Alkylating agents.   Ethyl- and methyl-methanesulphonate, dimethyl and diethyl sulphate, nitrogen mustard, as well as *N*-methyl-*N'*-nitro-*N*-nitroso-guanidine belong to the most effective mutagenic agents. Ethyl methane-sulphonate predominantly ethylates the N-7 atom of guanine. The N-7 alkylguanine is cleaved from the chain, creating a gap. At the next rep-lication a wrong base is frequently inserted at this place.

Intercalating dyes.   Proflavine and other **acridine dyes** act in a different manner. The acridine molecule apparently inserts itself between neigh-bouring bases (**intercalation**), increasing their distance from each other. This steric alteration can give rise to two kinds of error during DNA replication. It can cause the loss of a nucleotide or the insertion of an additional base pair. This kind of mutation has very far-reaching conse-quences; it leads to a frame-shift mutation, as described above (Fig. 15.2).

Ultraviolet light and ionising radiations.   UV light, X-rays and other ionising radiations have mutagenic effects on microorganisms, in addi-tion to their lethal action. Their specific actions are not yet well under-stood. The far-reaching agreement between the absorption spectrum of nucleic acids and the action spectrum of the lethal effect and mutant frequencies suggest that UV radiation predominantly attacks nucleic acid. Radiation in the near ultraviolet, around 260 nm, is the most effec-tive (Fig. 15.3). Toxic side effects are slight. UV damage occurs mainly to the pyrimidine bases. For example, two neighbouring thymine bases in DNA become covalently bound. These thymine dimers then cause errors in replication (Fig. 15.4).

Transposons.   The method of inducing mutagenesis by transposons is becoming a standard technique in bacterial genetics. Transposons (Tn elements) are short sections of double-stranded DNA, consisting of more than 2000 base pairs. They usually code for resistance to one or some-times several antibiotics. Transposons are able to move or **jump** within the genome, even between a bacterial chromosome and a plasmid, and they are able to become integrated in a number of different sites on the genome (see Section 15.2.1 on genetic recombination). Insertion of a

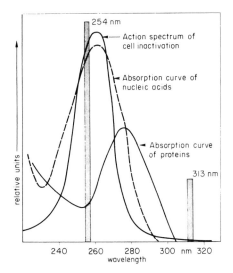

Fig. 15.3. *Basis for the use of the low-pressure mercury lamp for mutagenesis and 'killing' of microorganisms.*

The absorption curve of nucleic acid and the action spectrum of cell inactivation show a maximum at 260 nm. The low-pressure Hg lamp has a strong emission band in this wavelength region (254 nm). It has a germicidal effect.

transposon within a structural gene thus interrupts the normal nucleotide sequence of the gene so that it can no longer deliver the information for the synthesis of the normal, functionally potent polypeptide. Transposons thus serve primarily for production of insertion mutants.

Transposons cannot replicate autonomously and need a carrier or vector for transmission between different bacterial cells. Plasmids and bacteriophages are suitable vectors. In this connection it is noteworthy that the coliphage Mu (mutator phage) has the ability, similar to a transposon, to integrate at a number of different sites on the bacterial chromosome, thus causing mutations. Phage Mu has become known as 'giant transposon' and can be used as a mutagenic agent for *E. coli* strains.

Directed mutagenesis.   The *in vivo* mutagenising procedures described above result in random mutations. It has now become possible, thanks to DNA recombination techniques and DNA sequencing, as well as

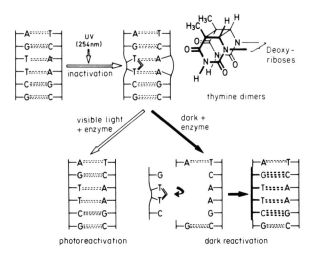

Fig. 15.4. *The changes in DNA produced by UV irradiation and the processes of photo- and dark reactivation.*

See text for explanation (Section 15.1.6).

nucleotide synthesising methods, (Section 15.5) to carry out *in vitro* **directed mutations**. These can be targeted at the molecular level and produce insertions, deletions or substitutions of specific bases at defined loci of a DNA segment (see Section 15.2). Such a mutated gene can be reincorporated into the host cell via use of a vector (plasmid or phage) and the consequences of the mutation then analysed. The tools and methodologies for carrying out such *in vitro* mutagenesis will be discussed in the section on molecular cloning techniques (Section 15.5).

15.1.5   Expression and selection of specific mutant phenotypes

Expression of mutations.   The phenotypic expression of a mutation needs a number of sequential processes which can require several cell divisions, depending on the type of mutation and the cell. Thus, if there is a 'gain' mutation, such as the reversion from an amino acid requirement (auxotrophy) to the restoration of the ability to synthesise the amino acid (prototrophy), the genotypic change can be immediately recognised phenotypically under suitable conditions. A loss mutation, however, such as an amino acid auxotrophy, where the ability to synthesise a given

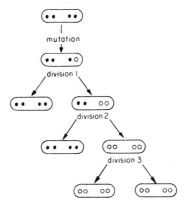

Fig. 15.5. *Chromosomal segregation during multiplication of bacteria with more than one chromosome.*

A genetically pure clone is only produced after the third division. The phenotypic expression of the mutation may take further genera- tions (i.e. to dilute out the gene product originating from the parent cell).

amino acid is lost, may be recognised only after allowing several genera- tions of growth. This delayed phenotypic expression of a loss mutation is due to the persistence and continued function of pre-existing enzyme(s), even though synthesis of new enzyme is no longer possible. The pre- existing enzyme must be 'diluted out' by several cell divisions before the mutated character can be recognised. Gain and loss mutations can also be distinguished in cells with several chromosome copies. *Escherichia coli*, growing in a nutrient-rich medium at a fast rate usually contains four chromosomes (Ch. 2.2.1).

In a gain mutation the information in the mutated chromosome is dominant and immediately causes the synthesis of the new enzyme, and hence the expression of the new phenotype. A loss mutation in a cell with several chromosomes, however, behaves as a recessive. In the course of several successive cell divisions, the chromosomes are distributed among the different individuals (chromosome segregation: Fig. 15.5). Only a cell in which all the chromosomes carry the mutated gene can express the defect. The progeny of such a cell represents a genetic clone.

Selection of mutants.   Mutants that are resistant to antibiotics, toxins or bacteriophages (Table 15.2) can be easily identified. The selective agent

Table 15.2. *Some mutants and methods for their isolation*

Type of mutant	Selection and enrichment method
Resistance mutant Resistant to inhibitors, antibiotics, toxins or bacteriophages	Plating out a *c.* 10^8 cells on nutrient media containing the inhibitor. Resistance mutants, which do not take up or detoxify the inhibitor, survive and form colonies
Auxotrophic mutants Defective in the synthesis of vitamins, amino acids, nucleic acids or other cell building blocks	Use of penicillin selection method to eliminate wild-type cells. Plating out survivors on nutrient media containing traces of the metabolite the auxotrophs cannot synthesise. The mutants grow as micro-colonies; they cannot grow without the metabolite (Fig. 15.8)
Mutants unable to utilise substrate Defective in catabolic enzyme system. Lack of carbon and/or energy	Enrichment by penicillin selection. Direct selection technique: use of nutrient media containing indicators (e.g. eosin–methylene blue, neutral red, crystal violet, X-gal) on which acid secreting mutants change colour. Indirect selection technique: recognition of micro-colonies (Fig. 15.8)
Temperature-dependent mutants The temperature reaction of the formation or the structure of a protein is changed in such a way that it either tolerates a higher temperature (temperature-resistant) or exhibits greater heat-sensitivity (temperature-sensitive).	Enrichment by cultivation at temperatures at which the mutant grows better than the wild type. Possibly use of penicillin enrichment
Regulatory mutants Altered rate of synthesis of one or more metabolic enzymes	Mutants whose synthesis of a metabolic enzyme is no longer subject to induction/repression (Ch. 16.1.1 and 16.1.2) but synthesise the enzymes constitutively, can be enriched by: – cultivation in continuous culture with the substrate as growth-limiting factor; – alternating growth on two substrates; – growth in presence of antimetabolites which inhibit growth of wild-type

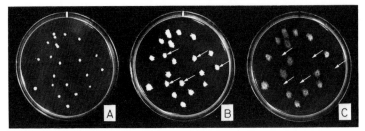

Fig. 15.6. *Recognition and isolation of mutants with biochemical defects.*

The three petri dishes show the results of an experiment to identify mutants of *Alcaligenes eutrophus* that have lost the ability to grow on fructose (Fruc⁻). The medium in plate A and B contains lactate, on which the cells of the mutant and the wild type grow equally well. Plate C contains only fructose, and the mutants cannot grow on this. A mixed suspension of mutant and wild-type cells was streaked out on A (the master plate) after enrichment of the mutants by a modified penicillin technique. After individual cells had grown into colonies, these were transferred by replica plating to plates B and C. The Fruc⁻ cells are recognised by the fact that they grow only on B and not on C. The defect-mutant colonies are marked by arrows. In this mutant the inability to utilise fructose is due to a defect of the 2-keto-3-deoxy-6-phosphogluconate aldolase. Similar methods can be used for the recognition and isolation of mutants that are auxotrophic for amino acids. (Photo: I. Sammler.)

allows only the resistant mutants to survive and eliminates the wild-type cells. Only few mutants are easily recognised by changes in pigmentation, colony form or other phenotypic characters on common solid media. Other altered characters may be made recognisable by addition of indicators or dyes. Identification of mutants that differ from their parent cells by increased or decreased nutrient requirements calls for comparisons of growth on different media. For example, loss of the ability to synthesise the amino acid leucine means that the mutant can grow only on media containing leucine. Such a mutant is called an **auxotrophic** leucine-requiring (*leu*⁻) mutant (also known as loss, defect, or deficiency mutant). The wild type as regards leucine requirement is called a **prototroph** (*leu*⁺). When *leu*⁻ mutants are present in a suspension together with *leu*⁺ prototrophs, they can be distinguished by comparison of their growth on two different nutrient media. A common technique for the recognition of such defective mutants is illustrated in Fig. 15.6.

Enrichment of mutants.   As was mentioned earlier in this chapter, the mutation rate for many characters is quite low. For the majority of metabolic and physiological characters so far examined it is between

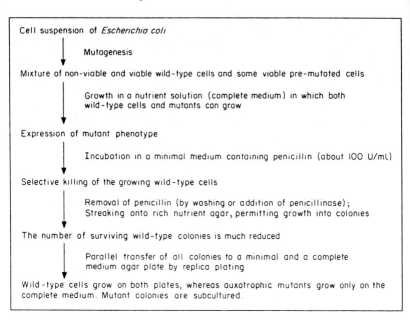

Cell suspension of *Escherichia coli*

↓ Mutagenesis

Mixture of non-viable and viable wild-type cells and some viable pre-mutated cells

↓ Growth in a nutrient solution (complete medium) in which both wild-type cells and mutants can grow

Expression of mutant phenotype

↓ Incubation in a minimal medium containing penicillin (about 100 U/mL)

Selective killing of the growing wild-type cells

↓ Removal of penicillin (by washing or addition of penicillinase); Streaking onto rich nutrient agar, permitting growth into colonies

The number of surviving wild-type colonies is much reduced

↓ Parallel transfer of all colonies to a minimal and a complete medium agar plate by replica plating

Wild-type cells grow on both plates, whereas auxotrophic mutants grow only on the complete medium. Mutant colonies are subcultured.

Fig. 15.7. *Penicillin method for the enrichment and isolation of auxotrophic mutants of* Escherichia coli *or other penicillin-sensitive bacteria.*

10^{-5} and 10^{-10}. A mutant frequency of 10^{-8} would require the screening of 100 million cells and their progeny, respectively, to discover a new mutant. Although induction of mutations with mutagens can increase mutation rates and mutant frequencies considerably, the time and effort involved in screening remains high. For this reason a technique known as **mutant enrichment**, for use before the actual mutant selection, has been developed. Enrichment of **auxotrophic mutants** is based on the principle of exposing the cell suspension to conditions under which the desired mutants do not grow, and the growing prototrophic cells can be killed off or eliminated. This selective elimination makes use of agents that act on growing cells but do not affect non-growing, resting cells. After removal of the eliminating agent and addition of the required nutrient, the auxotrophic mutants can then proliferate.

Penicillin, or the derivative ampicillin, is used for the enrichment of auxotrophic mutants in *E. coli*. When added to the prototrophic medium (i.e. medium lacking the nutrient required by the auxotroph), it 'kills' the growing wild-type cells, whilst the non-growing mutants survive (Fig. 15.7).

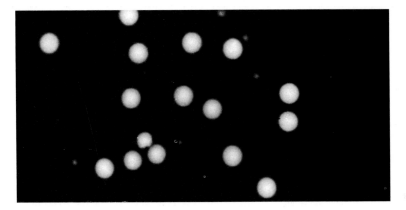

Fig. 15.8. *Wild-type colonies (of normal size) and pin-point colonies of an auxotrophic defect mutant of* Escherichia coli.

The nutrient agar contains excess glucose (0.4%) and very low concentration of nutrient broth (0.005%); this limits the growth of the mutant which is dependent on a substance contained in the nutrient broth.

After induction of mutations and several hours of subsequent growth, the bacterial suspension is incubated for several hours in a nitrogen-free, glucose-nutrient solution to deplete the cells of their soluble nitrogen compounds. Penicillin and ammonium sulphate are then added and the incubation continued for up to 24 hours. The prototrophic parental cells can grow under these conditions and are 'killed' by the penicillin, whereas the auxotrophic mutants cannot grow and are therefore not affected by the penicillin. The suspension is then freed of penicillin by washing or addition of penicillinase and plated out onto agar medium supplemented with the required nutrient (amino acid). The colonies growing on this medium consist of a high percentage of auxotrophic mutants, as well as prototrophs that have survived the penicillin treatment. For bacteria that are resistant to penicillin, other antibiotics (novobiocin, cycloserine, colistin, kanamycin) may be used. Other procedures for eliminating growing cells may utilise 'lethal synthesis'.

By means of this and similar manoeuvres, a number of mutant types with different defects can be enriched and isolated (Fig. 15.8). Such defects include defects in transport and catabolism of substrates, defects in intermediary metabolism, temperature-sensitive (conditional lethal) mutants, etc. Techniques for the isolation of other cells with altered metabolic regulation will be described further on. An overview of the procedures for isolation and recognition of a number of mutant types, including some regulation-deficient mutants, is presented in Table 15.2.

15.1.6   DNA repair

DNA is permanently exposed to cellular enzyme activities which can lead to alterations (alkylation, depurination, bond breakage) as well as energy-rich and energy-poor radiations (light, radioactive isotopes in rocks, buildings, food). Life has developed over billions of years in the presence of such radiations. It would be surprising, therefore, if no mechanisms for DNA repair had developed in cells. Such DNA repair mechanisms are mostly inducible. Organisms which have been exposed to sublethal doses of DNA-damaging agents are commonly more resistant than organisms without such exposure. Of the many known mechanisms of DNA repair only three will be described here.

Photo- and dark-reactivation.   The discovery that DNA damage is partially repairable was made during UV light treatment of bacteria. If treatment of bacterial suspensions with high doses of UV irradiation is followed by incubation in the dark, only a very small percentage of the cells can form colonies. However, if the cells are exposed to light of longer wavelenghts (< 320–384 nm) the percentage of survivors increases by orders of magnitude. This **photo-reactivation** involves an enzyme called photolyase. This gains energy from the longer wavelength light which it uses to split thymine dimers into monomers (Fig. 15.4). In this way the original state is regained, and this system of DNA repair works error-free.

Another, similarly reliable mechanisms of irradiation repair does not involve light. Dark reactivation involves the excision of defective sections of the DNA strands (excision repair) and their replacement by newly synthesised nucleotides. The process is catalysed by a correction endonuclease which represents an enzyme complex of the gene products *uvr* A, B and C. The extent to which such repair of radiation damage is effective varies in different bacterial strains. Radiation resistance of some bacteria, for example *Deinococcus radiodurans*, is due to a highly effective repair mechanism.

SOS repair.   When DNA is substantially damaged by high doses of mutagenic agents or radiation, or replication is inhibited by certain antibiotics like novobiocin or mitomycin C, an alarm reaction is elicited in the cell, called the SOS response. Extensive modifications take place; among others, the release of temperate phages (Ch. 4.2.2), delay of cell division, decreased respiration, higher protein turnover and, finally, the induced synthesis of repair enzymes. This process is regulated by two proteins, LexA and RecA. RecA normally plays a role in genetic recombination, which will be discussed below (Section 15.2). LexA is a DNA-binding protein (a repressor protein) which binds at the operator region and inhibits transcription into mRNA. LexA acts as repressor of a number of cellular functions under SOS conditions, signalled by an increase in single-stranded DNA. LexA loses its repressor function through proteolytic cleavage which abolishes its ability to bind DNA. This proteolysis is stimulated by the RecA protein, which apparently has no proteolytic activity itself. According to recent studies the SOS-induced repair system differs from the constitutive repair systems discussed earlier in its high error rate, hence error-prone repair. In this way many mutations, i.e. UV-induced mutations, occur as a consequence of incorrect repair. This is an important point in the context of cancer chemotherapy, since the agents used inhibit DNA replication and therefore cell division. But they can also cause considerable damage because of their mutagenic effects.

15.1.7   Tests for mutagenicity

Almost all DNA-attacking and carcinogenic substances are also mutagens. About 500–1000 novel compounds are artificially produced per annum. To identify those among them which could be carcinogens is a difficult problem because of the large numbers involved and the labour-intensive and time-consuming animal tests needed to gain a degree of certainty. Ames *et al.* have developed a bacteriological method which allows identification of substances causing DNA damage, and can therefore be assumed with reasonable probability to have oncogenic (carcinogenic) properties. The principle of this test is illustrated in Fig. 15.9.

The original **Ames test** has been modified and expanded to increase its reliability and sensitivity. Test organisms have been developed which carry multiple mutations that make them hypersensitive towards mutagens. This is because they lack the DNA repair mechanisms which would normally correct some of the damage. Release of a prophage in a lysogenised bacterium (see Ch. 4.2.2) by the substance under test is also used as an indicator of its mutagenicity. This testing procedure, which has drastically lowered the number of animal experiments, is now applied on a world-wide scale. The reliability is very high; of 100 substances with proven mutagenicity, 84 registered positive in a test system with *Salmonella typhimurium* and 91 with *Escherichia coli.*

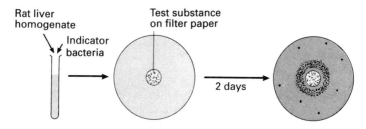

Fig. 15.9. *Ames test for the mutagenicity of a substance.*

The test bacterium is a histidine-requiring mutant of *Salmonella typhimurium* with a very low reversion frequency. The cells are mixed with rat liver extract and plated out on a mineral agar which cannot support their growth. The function of the liver extract is – as in the living organism – to supply enzymes for metabolic conversions of the test substance that could produce mutagenicity. A filter paper is saturated with the substance under test and placed on the nutrient medium. If the test substance has mutagenic effects, some mutations would restore ability of the test bacterium to synthesise histidine, and thus enable such mutants to grow, especially in the diffusion zone of the mutagen.

15.2   Transfer of characters and genetic recombination

In eukaryotic organisms, single, complete sets of genes are brought together during fertilisation and combined in the zygote. In the diploid zygote, after some mitotic divisions, a recombination between the two sets of genes and a reduction (by meiosis) to the single set of genes takes place. The gametes so formed are haploid. These sexual new combinations of genetic material are different from the parasexual processes, including the recombination of characters in prokaryotes. Bacteria are almost always haploid; they possess only one single set of genes. They can also form zygotes, but these are never the result of fusion of whole cells. Usually, only a part of the genetic material of a donor cell is transferred to a recipient (acceptor) cell, so that a partial zygote (merozygote) is produced. The chromosome of the recipient and the partial chromosome of the donor pair and exchange segments. The subsequent chromosomal and cell division results in a cell that contains only the recombined chromosome (Fig. 15.10).

Three types of transfer of genetic characters are known in bacteria: **conjugation**, **transduction** and **transformation**. In the course of all three

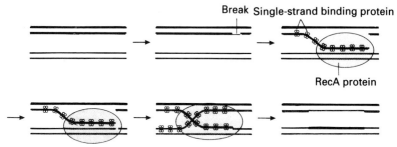

Fig. 15.10. *Model representing the mechanism of general or homologous genetic recombination.*

The exchange between a DNA segment derived from the donor with a segment of the recipient's chromosomal DNA starts with the pairing of homologous DNA and a single-strand break. This is followed by the exchange of single-strand segments between donor and recipient DNA. This process involves the RecA protein and a 'single-strand binding' protein (SSB). Only the daughter cells reveal whether recombination has taken place.

processes, DNA is transferred from a donor bacterium to a recipient bacterium. The processes differ only in the manner in which the DNA is transported. The transfer process is immediately followed by **DNA recombination** in the recipient cell. In this, the donor DNA is integrated into the DNA of the recipient bacterium. A cell in which such recombination has occurred is called a **recombinant**.

15.2.1   Genetic recombination

According to the present state of research there are two different mechanisms by which foreign DNA that has gained entry into a bacterial cell can be recombined *in vivo* into the bacterial chromosome or a plasmid: (1) general or homologous recombination, and (2) site- or sequence-specific recombination (including lambda phage).

General or homologous recombination.   General recombination is the term applied to the process by which foreign DNA that has entered the cell becomes integrated with the cellular host DNA, via pairing of homologous sequences, breaking and cross-over exchange (Fig. 15.10). The prerequisite for this is a large area of homologous base sequences between the two DNA partners. However, minor variations in the DNA molecules to be combined, such as can arise through mutations, can be tolerated. This homologous recombination can take place between wild-type and mutant DNA. The catalytic processes of general recombination involve at least six enzymes which also function in DNA repair (Section 15.1.6), and/or DNA replication (Ch. 2.2.1). The most prominent enzyme is the RecA protein. A simplified diagram of the molecular mechanism of recombination is shown in Fig. 15.10.

Site- or sequence-specific recombination.   Site- or sequence-specific recombination, in contrast to general recombination, requires only small segments of homologous DNA for recognition. This recombination is not catalysed by RecA protein, but by enzymes which are specific for the recombinant DNA molecules. When both DNA partners carry a recognition sequence, the recombination is '**double site specific**'. Examples of this are the integration of bacteriophage lambda (Fig. 15.11) and of the fertility plasmid F (Fig. 15.18) into the host genome of *E. coli*. When only one of the DNA molecules carries a recognition sequence, the process is called '**single site-specific**' recombination. Examples of this are the **transposable genetic elements** (insertion sequences, transposons, bacteriophage Mu) to be discussed later.

(a) Double specific recombination. Genetic experiments show that in the transition of lambda to the prophage state it becomes integrated at a certain site on the host chromosome, namely between the *gal* and *bio* operons (Fig. 15.11). The insertion is initiated by the strands being in close contact. It was thought earlier that this contact was due to a high degree of homology between the base sequences of the contact segments *att*P and *att*B. However, this base sequence homology is slight, extending to only 15 bp, which serve as recognition sequence for the phage-specific integrase. In this region the integrase acts similarly to a restriction endonuclease in cutting the phage and host double-stranded DNA. This produces two staggered ends which are reunited, after crossing over, by a DNA ligase. The integration of the phage is reversible, but the

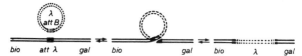

Fig. 15.11. *Site-specific recombination shown in the example of the integration of λ phage into the chromosome of the host cell.*

The circular phage chromosome attaches, via a protein, with its attachment region *att* B to the *att* λ region of the host chromosome, between the *bio* and *gal* operons.

The phage chromosome is then integrated by means of breakage and cross-wise rejoining of the double strands (see also Fig. 4.14).

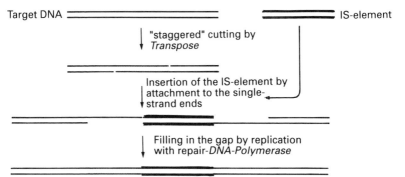

Fig. 15.12. *Model representing the insertion of an IS element into double-stranded (target) DNA.*
See text for explanation. The target DNA segment undergoing replication is shaded grey.

excision is carried out by a further phage enzyme excisionase. Both these processes, phage integration and excision, also involve the participation of a host-specific protein called 'integration host factor' (IHF). This IHF protein which consists of two gene products, *him*A and *hip*, is gaining increasing importance for interactions between DNA and proteins.

(b) Single site-specific recombination. **Insertion sequences**, called IS-elements, belong to those genetic elements which are able to carry out the process known as **transposition**. They can integrate at a large number of sites in the bacterial genome without having extensive sequence homology. This ability gives them a great genetic mobility. IS-elements were first discovered as inducing mutations in spontaneous mutants of *E. coli*, when they interrupted the continuity of individual genes by insertions (Section 15.1.3). IS-elements occur in the bacterial chromosome, in plasmids and in phages. They have also been found in many eukaryotes and in viruses. They consist of 800–1400 nucleotide pairs, and apart from their function in transposition, do not seem to have any other phenotypic characteristics. The ends of the IS-elements carry either direct or indirect 'repeats', that is, complementary, or inverse complementary, repetitive nucleotide pairs, which seem to be important for the process of transposition. This is catalysed by an IS-element-coded transposase, which recognises a certain region in the double-stranded DNA (target DNA) and the ends of the IS-element. It produces a staggered cut (Fig. 15.12). The IS-element finds and inserts into the cut

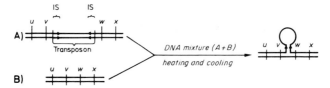

Fig. 15.13. *Electron microscience heteroduplex analysis for the recognition of transposons.*

To make the transposon visible, the DNA of the wild-type bacterium B and the transposon-carrying bacterium A are heated so that the strands separate (melting). During the subsequent slow cooling of the mixture of single strands, pairing takes place between complementary bases of the single strands of A and B; a DNA heteroduplex is formed. If the transposon is flanked by inverted repeats (IS sequences), these regions also pair and form a 'stem' on which the central part of the transposon forms a 'bubble' (lollipop structure).

target DNA. The latter duplicates nucleotide pairs at the site of insertion. It can be assumed that IS-elements play an important role in the reorientation and recombination of genetic characters.

Transposons.   Transposons (abbreviation Tn), already discussed in Section 15.1.4, also belong to the genetic elements that are able to cause mutations by transposition. They are sometimes termed 'jumping genes'. In contrast to IS-elements, they usually code for easily recognised phenotypic characters: for example resistance to antibiotics such as penicillin, tetracycline, and kannamycin, or to heavy metals, such as mercury. The resistance determinants of a transposon are flanked by two IS-elements, their position being demonstrable by electron micrographical heteroduplex analysis (Fig. 15.13). The 'jumping' or transposition of a transposon is usually the result of its **replication** and thus not connected with the loss of a transposon at its original integration site. According to one model the transposon is duplicated via contact with a target DNA, so that there is a transient, co-integrated form of the original transposon carrier and the new target DNA. The co-integrate is then 'resolved' by the enzyme resolvase so that finally there are two molecules of DNA, each of which carries a copy of the transposon.

Bacteriophage Mu.   The bacteriophage Mu shares with the IS-elements and transposons its unusual ability to integrate by transposition. It is called Mu as abbreviation for 'mutator' because the phage causes mutations in the host genome. It acts as a giant transposon. Animal retroviruses

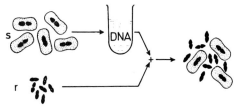

Fig. 15.14. *Transformation in* Streptococcus pneumoniae.

Transfer of the ability to form capsules by transformation of a non-capsulated strain (r, rough form) of *S. pneumoniae* with intact DNA extracted from a capsulated strain (s, smooth form). (From Nultsch, W. (1968). *Allgemeine Botanik*, 3rd edn. Stuttgart: Theime.)

seem to have similar properties (Ch. 4.3). The transposition is an obligatory step in the lytic multiplication of bacteriophage Mu whose DNA cannot be replicated outside the bacterial genome. Another interesting property which can also be demonstrated in bacteriophage Mu is that of **gene inversion**. This process, based on site-specific recombination, also called 'flip-flop' mechanism, causes the reorientation of a discrete segment of DNA within the phage genome. A segment of the bacteriophage Mu, the G-segment, has the ability to invert. It contains the code for the tail-fibre proteins. When the segment is in the G$^+$ orientation, the tail proteins S and U are produced, and the phage can infect the host, *E. coli* K 12. When the segment is inverted, in the G$^-$ orientation, another promotor becomes active and, starting from the opposite DNA strand, the genes S' and U' are transcribed. These gene products form a tail protein which alters the phage's host range. It can then adsorb onto cells of *E. coli* C and other enterobacteria. In *Salmonella*, gene inversion is responsible for a change in flagellum synthesis.

15.2.2   Transformation

Gene transfer by soluble DNA, which has been extracted, or otherwise liberated from a donor bacterium, to a recipient bacterium is called transformation. This is the longest-known and historically most important kind of gene transfer in bacteria.

Discovery of DNA as carrier of hereditary characters.   In 1928 Griffith discovered the transformation of a non-capsulated R strain of *Streptococcus pneumoniae* into a capsulated S strain (Fig. 15.14). He injected mice with a small number of avirulent R cells, together with heat-killed S cells. The R cells were derived from another S strain (SII) whose capsular material could be distinguished serologically from that of the heat-killed S strain (SIII). Virulent cocci with capsules of the SIII type could subsequently be isolated from the mice. It appeared, there-fore, that the heat-killed SIII cells had transferred their genetic character for capsule formation to the R cells which, in turn, were able to pass it on to their progeny. Eventually, Avery, Macleod and McCarty in 1944 established that the 'transforming principle' in such experiments con-sisted of DNA. This transformation provided the decisive proof at the time for the localisation of genetic information in DNA and not in protein.

Mechanisms of transformation.   Several experimental methods are now available for inserting isolated DNA into bacteria: (1) exploiting the natural competence to take up DNA of certain bacterial species; (2) induction of competence by pre-treatment of cells; (3) production of protoplasts; (4) electroporation.

(1) The normal ability to take up DNA, which is termed **competence**, has been described for a number of bacterial genera, i.e. *Acinetobacter*, *Azotobacter*, *Bacillus*, *Haemophilus*, *Mycobacterium*, *Neisseria*, *Pseudomonas*, *Streptocuccus* and *Synechococcus*. Such characters as toxin resistance and prototrophy for amino acids could be transferred in this way. Competence depends on the physiological state of the cells and the growth phase. The time and duration of competence are species-specific parameters. Competent cells have an altered cell surface; their cell wall is porous, they have increased activity of extracellular enzymes and they produce a 'competence factor' which is excreted into the medium. This mediates the alteration in properties which are characteristic for expres-sion of competence. Transformation requires only very small concentra-tions of DNA: 0.1 μg/ml cell suspension is sufficient to transform the competent recipient cells – maximally 5% of the cell population. The DNA that is to be transformed has to be double-stranded, must be of a minimum size, and is divided into approximately 15 kb size fragments by extracellular endonuclease. During the uptake of the transforming DNA, one of the two strands is digested, so that only one DNA strand reaches the interior of the cell. There, provided there is sufficient homol-ogy with the recipient DNA, it is inserted into the (recipient) genome by the mechanism of general recombination (see Section 15.2.1).

(2) The induction of competence by specific treatment of cells under laboratory conditions has been successfully achieved even in bacteria which are normally not amenable to transformation. The mostly empiri-cal methods include quite specific changes in culture conditions. Thus *E. coli* can be successfully transformed with an efficiency of 0.05

transformants per viable cell, by treatment with calcium chloride and storage in the cold. This method is of great importance for the universal application of this bacterium in the molecular cloning technique (Section 15.5).

(3) The use of protoplasts for transformation has been successfully carried out, predominantly in the case of gram-positive genera such as *Bacillus* and *Streptomyces*. In these organisms, the cell wall-less protoplasts can be induced to take up plasmid DNA by treatment with polyethyleneglycol (Section 15.3). In the case of chromosomal DNA transfer, the process is initiated by direct fusion of the protoplasts. This brings together part of the genome from both parent cells, which are then able to regenerate 'mutant' (recombinant) cells under certain experimental conditions. The recombinants obtained from such fusion exhibit properties of both parents, by virtue of homologous recombination.

(4) Experimental difficulties and unsatisfactory yields in applying transformation techniques to other test organisms have led to the development of a new method known as **electroporation**. This method of rendering biological membranes permeable and causing their fusion by application of electric fields was first carried out with eukaryotic cells, for example in the hybridisation of plant cells. In the meantime it has been possible, with the use of commercially available instruments for electroporation, to transform numerous gram-positive as well as gram-negative bacteria with plasmid DNA.

15.2.3   Transduction

Transduction is the transfer of DNA from a donor cell to a recipient cell by bacteriophages. In most cases only a small segment of the host (i.e. the donor) DNA is transferred. Two kinds of transduction can be distinguished: a non-specific (generalised) transduction which can transfer any part of the host DNA, and a specific transduction which is restricted to the transfer of specific DNA segments. In non-specific transduction the host DNA segment is integrated into the virus particle, either in addition to, or in place of (some of) the phage genome. In specific transduction some of the phage genes are replaced by the host genes. In both cases, the transducing phages are usually defective in some respect; for example, they often lose the ability to lyse host cells.

The transfer of genetic characters by transduction has been demonstrated in a large number of bacteria, including species of *Salmonella*, *Escherichia*, *Shigella*, *Bacillus*, *Pseudomonas*, *Staphylococcus*, *Vibrio* and

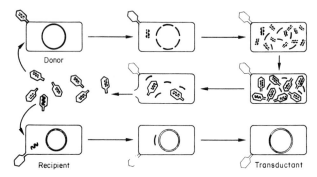

Fig. 15.15. *Non-specific transduction, a mechanism for the transfer of host DNA into a recipient bacterium.*
See text for details.

Rhizobium. However, not all phages transduce, nor can DNA be transferred by transduction in all bacteria.

Non-specific transduction.   The transfer of bacterial genes by phage was discovered by Lederberg and Zinder in 1951. In the decisive experiment (Fig. 15.15) a donor strain B^+ was infected with the temperate phage P22. After lysis of the host cells the liberated phages were separated and incubated with a suspension of the recipient strain B^-, which was distinguished from B^+ by at least one genetic character. By plating out on selective media the authors found recombinants that carried the genetic marker of the donor strain B^+. The processes that occur during this non-specific DNA transfer are rather complex.

During the lytic multiplication of the phage inside the donor strain, broken fragments of the host DNA occasionally become included in the capsids in place of phage DNA. A phage lysate thus contains a mixture of normal and defective phages. Infection of a recipient cell by a normal phage usually leads to lysis. A few cells of the recipient, however, become infected with a defective transducing phage, whose DNA can recombine with the chromosome of the recipient. Homologous DNA segments are exchanged, and this can give rise to genetic complementation of a defective gene in the recipient by an intact one of the donor. Since only small fragments of DNA are transduced, the probability of recombination for any given character is very low. It lies in the region of 10^{-6} to 10^{-8}. This also explains why the *Salmonella* phage P22, as well as the non-specifically transducing coliphage P1, can transduce only single or very closely neighbouring genes at each transduction (i.e. by one phage particle); the amount of DNA equal to the phage DNA represents only 1–2% of the bacterial DNA. The *Bacillus subtilis* phage PBS1 is an exception: it can transduce up to 8% of the host genome.

Specific transduction.   The best-known example of specific transduction is phage λ which has already been discussed in Ch. 4.2.2. Lambda normally transduces only specific genes of the *gal* (galactose utilisation) and *bio* (biotin synthesis) operons. As already described, it integrates into the host genome during its transition to the prophage state, site-specifically between the *gal* and *bio* operons. During the separation of the phage DNA from the host DNA, induced, for example, by UV irradiation, the phage DNA may not be precisely excised. It may leave a fragment in the host chromosome and acquire a neighbouring piece of the host DNA, which is then liberated together with the phage DNA.

When a transducing phage infects a recipient cell with a defect in the appropriate gene, such as gal^-, the intact transduced gene can exchange with the defective host gene. All resulting recombinants, or transductants, are then gal^+.

Gene transfer mediated by phage $\phi80$ is similar. Its DNA integrates in the neighbourhood of genes coding for tryptophan biosynthesis. Phage $\phi80$ is therefore especially suitable for transfer of *trp* genes.

Integration of the phage into the host chromosome is essential for successful gene transfer by specific transduction (in contrast to nonspecific transduction).

15.2.4   Conjugation

The transfer of genetic material from cell to cell by direct contact is called conjugation. It was suggested quite early on, on the basis of morphological indications, that bacteria might pair. Unequivocal proof of the transfer of DNA between bacteria by direct contact was obtained in experiments with multiple mutants. In 1946 Lederberg and Tatum carried out the decisive experiments with two mutants of *E. coli* K12, each of which was auxotrophic for two different amino acids (Fig. 15.16). One of the double mutants was auxotrophic for amino acids A and B, but it could synthesise amino acids C and D ($A^-B^-C^+D^+$). The other mutant was complementary (differed reciprocally) ($A^+B^+C^-D^-$). These mutants cannot grow or form colonies on a minimal medium (i.e. one lacking the amino acids) but a mixed inoculum of both mutants on the same minimal medium produced colonies. The cells of these colonies had the hereditary ability to synthesise all four amino acids and were of the genetic type $A^+B^+C^+D^+$ (i.e. prototrophs). They arose at a frequency

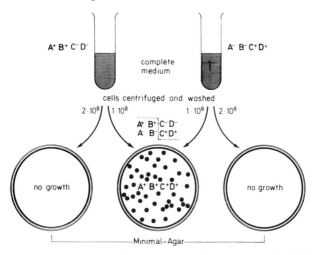

Fig. 15.16. *Recombination by conjugation of two reciprocally defective mutants of* Escherichia coli, *strain D12.*
(After Braun, W. (1965). *Bacterial Genetics.* Philadelphia: Saunders.)

of 1 in 10^6 and were called recombinants because they combined the genetic information of two reciprocally defective parent types. The use of multiple mutants as the parental organisms precludes the possibility that the colonies were revertants. The probability of simultaneous back mutations in two genes is of the order of 10^{-14} to 10^{-16} per generation.

Directed transfer from donor to recipient cells.   Double cross-over experiments between partners of which one in each case was streptomycin resistant demonstrated that the genetic material is transferred only in one direction. After mating, each mixed suspension was plated on streptomycin agar. Recombinants appeared only when one of the strains, namely the recipient, was streptomycin resistant and could therefore survive. Streptomycin sensitivity of the other donor parent (which would thus be killed) was immaterial for the appearance of recombinants, provided the genetic information had been transmitted. It was concluded from these experiments that the transfer of genetic material is unidirectional, from a **donor** to a **recipient** strain, and that the process of recombination and segregation takes place in the recipient cell.

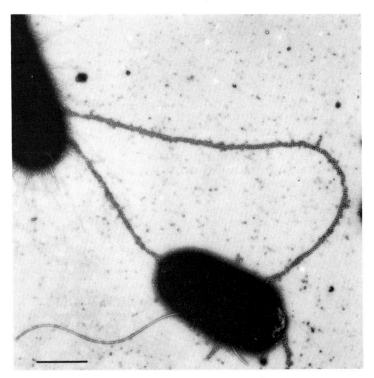

Fig. 15.17. *Two cells of* Escherichia coli *connected by F pili.*
The two F pili of the Hfr cell have been tagged with the donor-specific RNA phage MS-2. The numerous type I pili of the recipient cell (top) are short and do not adsorb the phage. Electron micrograph of cells negatively stained with phosphotungstic acid. Bar, 1 μm. (From Curtiss, R., Caro, L. G., Allison, D. P. & Stallions, D. R. (1969). *J. Bacteriol.* **100**, 1091.)

F factor and Hfr state.   It became evident during investigations on the pairing process that the donor state in bacteria is dependent on the presence of a transferable DNA element in the cell, the **sex factor** F (F for fertility). The F factor is a closed circular double-stranded DNA molecule of 100 kb size. As an extra-chromosomal, autonomously replicating DNA element, it is classified as a **plasmid**. It contains the genes responsible for the process of conjugation. To these belong the genes that determine special structures on the cell surface, such as the F pili

(Fig. 15.17). These are essential for conjugation. The hair-like pili, two or three per cell surface, serve to facilitate the contact between donor and recipient cells. During this, so-called 'cross-over aggregates' are formed, as the donor cell can be in contact with several recipient cells. The DNA of the F factor reaches the recipient via a partial fusion of the pairing partners.

Only a few bacteria in a F^+ population are able to transfer chromosomal DNA. These are cells in which the F factor has been integrated into the bacterial chromosome (Fig. 15.18). When clones of such donor cells are used in conjugation experiments, the yield of recombinants is about 1000-fold higher than with ordinary F^+ strains. Such cells are called **Hfr** (high frequency of recombinants). The integration of F factors takes place via IS-elements (see Section 15.2.1), which occur in F factors as well as in the *E. coli* chromosome. The F factor-specified IS-elements, IS2 and IS3, can integrate at all sites in the *E. coli* chromosome which carry a copy of the appropriate IS-element. The reaction is based on homologous recombination and is reversible. Since the IS-elements are capable of transposition, a co-integrate between F factor and chromosome can also occur in a RecA-independent reaction.

The transfer of chromosomal genes.   When a population of Hfr cells is mixed with an excess of F^- cells, practically all the Hfr cells find F^- partners and conjugate. In the now famous experiment on interrupted pairing, samples were removed from such a mixture at various time intervals and subjected to violent agitation in a mixer to separate conjugating pairs. The samples were then plated on suitable agar plates to isolate recombinants, and the recombinants were examined to determine which gene had been transferred from the donor to the recipient. This analysis showed a definite time of transfer from donor to recipient for each gene (Fig. 15.18). The time course of gene transfer was in agreement with the chromosomal gene sequence that had been established by genetic analysis. Hfr strains that have been isolated independently have two identifying properties. Each Hfr strain transfers the chromosome with its own specific origin and with a separate, specific orientation of the gene into the recipient cell. This shows that a given strain of Hfr cells consists of a homogeneous population in which each cell transfers its chromosome from the same 'origin' and in the same direction. During the transfer of the DNA, bacterial DNA is replicated from the insertion point of the F factor, and the 5' end of the newly synthesised strand leads the entry into the recipient cell (Fig. 15.18). The transfer process is immediately followed by the recombination of the donor and recipient DNA inside the recipient cell (homologous recombination).

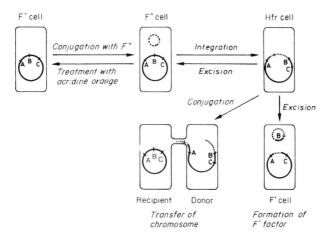

Fig. 15.18. *The relationship between the sexual types of* Escherichia coli.

The F⁻ cells can only serve as recipients. By conjugation with an F⁺ or Hfr strain they can receive the F factor and thus become F⁺. In the F⁺ cell the F factor is present as a covalently closed circular DNA molecule. It can be removed by treatment with acridine orange. Its integration into the bacterial chromosome, on the other hand, makes the cell Hfr. The insertion can occur at different sites on the chromosome and in different orientations. It determines the beginning and the direction (indicated by arrows) of chromosome transfer. Incorrect excision of the F factor from the chromosomal DNA gives rise to an F-factor containing a short piece of chromosomal DNA, this is called F' factor.

The genetic map.   The method of interrupted mating just described, by which the time course of gene transfer from donor to recipient can be determined, can be used to construct a map representing the arrangement of genes on the bacterial chromosome (Fig. 15.19). The further a gene is from the origin, the later is its time of transfer, and the less frequently does it reach the recipient cell in an uninterrupted mating. The transfer of the whole *E. coli* chromosome takes about 100 minutes. The rate of transfer remains quite constant during the whole process. Hence the times of entry of genes into the recipient cell depend on the distances between the genes on the bacterial chromosome. However, differences of less than a minute cannot be determined by this technique. Such fine-structure analysis is possible by means of coupling analysis in phage transduction experiments. The genetic map illustrated in Fig. 15.19 is considerably simplified. In the meantime positions of 1403 gene loci

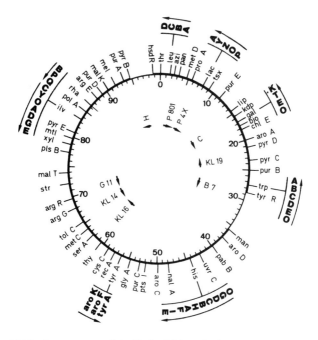

Fig. 15.19. *Genetic map of the* Escherichia coli *chromosome.*

The figures indicate the relative distances between the genes in terms of time intervals (minutes) at which the individual genes reach the recipient cell during conjugation (in nutrient broth at 37 °C). The arrows inside the circle indicate the sequence in which the genes reach the recipient bacterium during conjugation with different Hfr strains. The direction of chromosomal movement is the opposite of that indicated by the arrows. The arrows on the outside show the direction in which individual genes of an operon are read during transcription (e.g. in the *lac* operon: P, O, Z, Y, A). Genes: *azi*, azide resistance; *bio*, biotin requirement; *gal*, galactose utilisation; *his*,

histidine requirement showing the genes for the enzymes involved in histidine synthesis; *ilv*, isoleucine, valine requirement; *lac*, lactose operon with the genes P (promotor), O (operator), Z (β-galactosidase), Y (galactoside permease), A (thiogalactoside transacetylase); *ProA*, proline requirement (blocked before glutamate semialdehyde); *rec* A, ability for repair of radiation damage and genetic recombination; *thr*, threonine requirement; *trp*, tryptophan requirement. (Redrawn after Bachmann, B. J., Low, K. B & Trotter, A. L. (1976). *Bacteriol. Rev.* **40**, 116. The new (8th) version of the genetic map is given in Bachman, M. J. (1990). *Microbiol. Rev.* **54**, 130–97.)

have been established. Gene maps have also been constructed for the chromosomes of *Salmonella typhimurium*, *Streptomyces coelicolor*, *Bacillus subtilis*, *Pseudomonas aeruginosa* and some other bacteria.

Gene transfer by F' factors.   The integration of the F factor into the bacterial chromosome is reversible. The F factors can be excised from the chromosome, so that the Hfr cell reverts to a F^+ cell (Fig. 15.18). This excision occurs at about the same frequency as integration. Correct excision depends on a break occurring at the same site on the chromosome as the integration site. In rare cases, however, the break occurs at a neighbouring site, so that on excision a neighbouring segment of host DNA remains attached to the F factor. Such an F factor, containing a small piece of chromosomal DNA, is called an F' factor. The origin of an F' factor is analogous to the formation of a specific transducing phage (see Section 15.2.3).

The cell containing an F' factor is called a primary F' cell. The DNA integrated into the F' factor can now be transferred from the F' donor cell to an F^- recipient cell with the same frequency (100%) as the F factor from F^+ strains to F^- strains. The same piece of chromosomal DNA would be transferred from Hfr cells to F^- cells only with a frequency of 1%. Transfer of the F' factor from a primary F' cell in which it originated to a normal F^- cell results in a secondary F' cell. In this cell the segment of the bacterial chromosome is present twice (i.e. in the diploid state).

Occurrence of conjugation in other groups of bacteria.   Gene transfer by conjugation was discovered in *E. coli* and is very common in enterobacteria. Conjugation processes have been extensively investigated in naturally occurring *Streptomyces coelicolor*, *Nocardia* species, *Rhizobium* and other bacterial species and genera. It is probable that exchange of genes by conjugation and mobilisation of genes by plasmids is widely distributed in the prokaryotic kingdom.

15.3   Plasmids

Many bacteria can harbour extrachromosomal DNA elements – **plasmids**. These small (relative to the bacterial chromosome), circular, covalently closed, double-stranded DNA units are not essential for the growth of the cells under normal conditions: Cells which have been 'cured' of plasmids, by UV irradiation or treatment with mitomycin V or acridine dyes, grow well on normal nutrient media. Plasmids are recognised by the special characters they confer on the host cell. Some plasmids enable the host to conjugate. The prototype of such a conjugative plasmid has already been described, namely the F factor of *E. coli*. In these cases further distribution of the plasmid is also facilitated because of the direct contact between cells. Other plasmids can transiently integrate into the bacterial chromosome rather like a prophage, and thus lose their autonomous state for a period.

Plasmids can mobilise the host chromosome and can therefore contribute to exchange and recombination of genetic material under natural conditions. In genetic engineering and gene technology (Section 15.5), where plasmids are used as vectors of foreign DNA, the methods applied are analogous to natural processes.

Plasmids can also be found in eukaryotes, but have been far less intensively studied up to now.

15.3.1   Evidence for plasmids and their properties

In order to exist autonomously as an extrachromosomal DNA molecule, the plasmid requires a replication origin (Fig. 15.20) analogous to that of the bacterial chromosome. The number of copies of a given plasmid in a cell is a plasmid-specific property. As a rule of thumb, the larger the plasmid, the lower the **copy number**. The replication itself is catalysed by cell-specific proteins; plasmid-coded functions control the time of initiation and the distribution of plasmid copies to the daughter cells. Small plasmids with a high copy number undergo multiple rounds of replication during one cell cycle.

Amplification.   The best-studied plasmid, ColE1 (Fig. 15.20) (see Section 15.3.2), is a small plasmid with a size of 6646 bp. Normally, replication of chromosomal DNA in the host cell ceases about one hour after

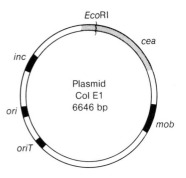

Fig. 15.20. *Genetic map of* Escherichia coli *plasmid ColE1.*

ori, replication origin; *oriT*, origin of transfer; *inc*, incompatibility; *mob*, mobility function; *cea*, structural gene for colicin E1; *EcoR1*, Cutting site for endonuclease *EcoR1*.

addition of chloramphenicol, but replication of the plasmid (ColE1) continues for another 12–15 hours. This leads to an increase in copy number from 15 to about 1200 per chromosome, and the process has been termed **amplification** of the plasmid DNA. It has also been observed in a number of other plasmids. Whereas replication of chromosomal DNA requires continuous new synthesis of proteins, the replication of plasmids which are capable of amplification only requires proteins which remain stable and hence functional in the cell for considerable periods.

Incompatibility.   Many bacteria can harbour several different plasmids. The coexistence of different plasmids in the same cell means that these plasmids must be compatible. Two related plasmids, however, cannot coexist in one cell: they are **incompatible**. It is possible to classify plasmids into incompatibility groups, abbreviated as **Inc**. Plasmids belonging to the same Inc group cannot coexist. So far, about 30 incompatibility groups have been identified for *E. coli* and about 10 for *Staphylococcus*. Compatibility is controlled by plasmid-bound determinants, localised in the so-called Inc region. (Fig. 15.20). The expression of incompatibility/compatibility is associated with the control of plasmid replication. Apparently, the incompatible plasmids exert mutual inhibition of each other's replication, in a complex manner that is not yet understood.

Physical properties.   With few exceptions, the size of a plasmid is usually less than one tenth of the *E. coli* chromosome (450 kb), although naturally occurring plasmids in the size range of 2–1200 kb have also been described. Plasmid DNA can be isolated as a covalently closed circular (ccc), double-stranded molecule. This circular double helix is also internally coiled, giving a very compact configuration, which is termed 'supercoiled'. A break in one of the two strands loosens the compact secondary structure and gives rise to an open circular form (oc) which has different physical properties. A double break transforms the plasmid DNA to a linear form which can no longer be distinguished from other linear DNA molecules that appear as chromosome fragments on lysis of the cell.

The isolation of plasmid DNA makes use of the special physical properties of the ccc molecule. Plasmid DNA sediments faster in the ultracentrifuge than linear DNA and has a lower affinity for intercalating dyes such as ethidium bromide, which reduce the density. Because of its higher density, plasmid DNA bands at a different position from chromosomal DNA in a caesium chloride gradient, and can therefore be easily isolated. Plasmid molecules of different size can be separated electrophoretically in an agarose gel. The migration of nucleic acids through the pores in a gel depends on the molecular weight and the structure of the molecule. Small plasmids migrate faster than linear DNA because of their compact conformation. Large plasmids, on the other hand, migrate more slowly. Comparison of the migration rates with those of suitable standards, whose molecular weight is known, allows estimation of plasmid size. The banding of DNA in the gel can be visualised by UV light after staining with ethidium bromide.

A more laborious technique for the demonstration of plasmids is provided by electron-microscopic analysis. This, however, also affords the possibility of measuring the contour length of individual molecules and hence a precise measure of plasmid size.

Conjugative plasmids.   In the preceding section on conjugation we have already dealt with the fertility (F) factor of *E. coli*. It can serve as an example of an autotransferable or conjugative plasmid. All the plasmids so far known as conjugative possess transfer functions based on the so-called *tra* genes. These code for the formation of sex pili which serve to make contact between the conjugating cells. *tra* genes thus mediate the transferrability of conjugative plasmids via cell contact. They also code for proteins which are required for the stabilisation of the pairing partners and for conjugative DNA transfer, together with its regulation. They are furthermore required for the exclusion of other plasmids. The *tra* region of the F factor comprises about 30 kb, and 31 genes have been located in this region.

Conjugative DNA transfer proceeds in distinct phases.

(1) A single-strand break occurs within the transfer-replication origin (*oriT*). *oriT* is a DNA sequence of 373 bp which is recognised by specific DNA-binding proteins and differs from the vegetative replication origin *ori* (Fig. 15.20).

(2) The DNA then unwinds in the 5' to 3' direction, starting from *oriT*. This process is catalysed by two transfer-specific proteins and consumes ATP.

(3) The free 5' end migrates through a pore, which connects the donor and recipient cell, into the recipient.

(4) In a concurrent process, the complementary double strand in the donor is continuously synthesised from the 3' end by what is known as a 'rolling circle' mechanism. The synthesis of the double strand in the recipient proceeds discontinuously on RNA primer fragments (Fig. 15.21).

Conjugative plasmids have been found in many gram-negative bacteria apart from E. coli. In gram-positives they have been shown to occur in the genera *Bacillus, Clostridium, Nocardia, Staphylococcus, Streptococcus*

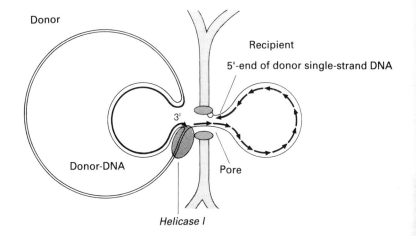

Fig. 15.21. *Model of DNA transfer from donor to recipient during conjugation.*

Following a single-strand break in the *oriT* locus, the single strand, headed by the 5' end, is transported through a connecting pore into the recipient cell. In the donor cell, the double strand is unwound by helicase I and restored by 'continuous' synthesis starting from the 3' end. In the recipient cell, the complementary strand is made by discontinuous synthesis. (According to W. Schumann, 1990.)

and *Streptomyces.* One group of conjugative plasmids of *Streptococcus faecalis*, which is transferred with high efficiency, codes for the formation of a specific pairing signal, a **sex pheromone**. It elicits the synthesis of an 'aggregation substance' in the plasmid donor. This product, which is known as **adhesin**, connects donor and recipient cells and results in the clumping of the two cell types.

Plasmids with wide host ranges.   The majority of plasmids are restricted to a very narrow host range which allows replication only in closely related species. However, some plasmids are known to have a wide host range. Among the gram-negative bacteria the conjugative resistance plasmid **RP4** which belongs to the *Inc*PI group, and the non-conjugative resistance plasmid **RSF1010** belonging to the *Inc*Q group deserve special mention. The former imparts resistance to the antibiotics ampicillin, kanamycin and tetracycline as well as to the heavy metal tellurium. The latter confers resistance to streptomycin and sulphonamides on its host. There are only a few gram-negative bacteria in which these plasmids cannot be stably established or multiply. Knowledge of plasmids with extended host range in gram-positive bacteria is still sparse. However, conjugative plasmids have been isolated from *Streptococcus faecalis* which can replicate in other species and in recipients belonging to the genera *Staphylococcus*, *Bacillus* and *Lactobacillus*. The 2.9 kb plasmid pC194 from *Staphylococcus aureus* has an exceptionally wide host range which includes other gram-positive bacteria like *Bacillus subtilis*, as well as gram-negative bacteria, i.e. *E. coli* and even eukaryotes like *Saccharomyces cerevisiae*.

The properties which confer a wide host range on plasmids are not yet completely defined. It is noticeable, however, that such plasmids code for several replication functions which might render them independent of host activities. Plasmids with restricted host ranges either do not require any plasmid-coded proteins for their replication – for example ColE1 (Fig. 15.20) – or a single plasmid-coded protein is required for the initiation of replication. Conjugative plasmids can also have a helper function in facilitating the transfer of a non-conjugative plasmid from a donor to a recipient cell. This process is termed '**plasmid mobilisation**'. It may be based on two molecular mechanisms: (1) the non-conjugative plasmid which can be mobilised is co-transferred with the conjugative plasmid without the two molecules making any connection; (2) a physical interaction between the two plasmids, i.e. recombination between the two molecules, is required. The co-integrate thus formed reaches the recipient cell in which it can be separated again into the two original plasmids. The plasmid ColE1, which can undergo mobilisation, codes in the so-called *mob*-region for three mobilisation proteins which are required for the transfer of ColE1.

Linear plasmids.   Linear plasmids, whose DNA is not covalently closed to a circular form, are the exception in prokaryotes. Up to now they have only been found in streptomycetes, streptococci and strains of *Nocardia opaca*. It is not known how their DNA is protected from attack by exonucleases.

15.3.2   Biological importance of plasmids

Plasmids are very widely distributed among bacterial species and genera. Quite often they are recognised only by their physical presence, that is without conferring recognisable phenotypic characters on their host. Such plasmids are known as 'cryptic plasmids'. A selection of plasmids which do code for phenotypically recognisable characters as well as replication, are the following:

Resistance plasmids.   Bacteria resistant to several antibiotics were first reported in the 1950s from Japan. They were strains of the dysentery-causing organism *Shigella* which had been isolated from antibiotic-treated patients. It was noted that the bacteria showed resistance to several different antibiotics, and that this property could be transferred to other bacteria, including *E. coli*, by simple cell-to-cell contact. As is now known, the resistant (R) plasmids contain genes which render the host bacterium resistant to sulphonamides, streptomycin, chloramphenicol, kanamycin and tetracycline. Some R-plasmids confer resistance to up to eight different antibiotics. Others confer resistance to toxic heavy metals, such as mercury, nickel, cobalt, cadmium, copper, zinc, chromium, arsenic, antimony, tellurium and silver. Resistance plasmids are usually mobilisable or conjugative. Some R-plasmids have an extensive host range and can be transferred between several bacterial genera, which explains their wide distribution. The transfer of R-plasmids is sometimes accompanied by the transfer of chromosomal genes which are apparently mobilised by the R-plasmid.

Plasmid-coded and chromosome-coded antibiotic resistance in bacteria seem to function by different mechanisms. An example is resistance to streptomycin. Chromosomally determined resistance is based on a change in the 30S subunit of the ribosomes, whereas the plasmid-determined resistance involves an enzymatic attack on the antibiotic molecule which is adenylated. In most cases plasmid-determined antibiotic resistance is due to enzymatic modifications of the antibiotics: chloramphenicol is acetylated, kanamycin and neomycin are phosphorylated or acetylated, and penicillin is hydrolysed by penicillinases. The widespread use of antibiotic therapy, especially in hospitals, has led to the spread of R-plasmids among pathogenic bacteria and hence to the selection and accumulation of antibiotic-resistant bacteria. The accumulation of multiple antibiotic resistance in a single plasmid is not difficult to understand in view of the high recombination potential and selection pressure. What is not understood is what part resistance plasmids may have played in therapeutic practice during the periods before antibiotics were used. They have been found in bacteria that were preserved before 1940, that is before the introduction of antibiotic therapy.

Bacteria which are resistant to heavy metals can be isolated from soil and waters which normally contain such metals or which are polluted with metals. Metal-resistant bacteria are rarely isolated from non-polluted soils. The genetic information for heavy metal resistance can be chromosomal or plasmid-coded. The resistance may be based on efflux, that is on ATPase or antiport-based export of the toxic ions from the cell interior. The habitat-dependent spread of heavy-metal-resistant bacteria indicates that selection pressure can play an important part in the maintenance of genetic information within an ecosystem.

Bacteriocin-coding plasmids.   Many bacteria produce proteins which are able to inhibit the growth of related organisms or can even 'kill' them. These **bacteriocins**, which are species-specific in their effects, are coded by bacteriocin plasmids. Bacteriocins have been isolated from *E. coli* (colicins) *Pseudomonas aeruginosa* (pyocines) *Bacillus megaterium* (megacines) and several other bacteria.

Pathogenicity- or virulence factor.   The human and animal organism offers almost ideal conditions for the growth of many microorganisms by virtue of its secretions, which can serve as nutrient media, and its relatively constant internal environment. Bacteria in tens and thousands of millions belong to the normal flora of skin and the intestinal tract. Many species have a useful or even essential role for the healthy life of the host. However, other organisms damage the host organism, i.e. they are **pathogenic**. During the course of evolution man and animals have developed a number of barriers which give protection against the entry and growth of pathogenic bacteria. These comprise the skin, the immune system and blood components. The pathogenic organisms on their part have evolved increased aggressive capacity by developing virulence and pathogenicity factors. Many of these factors are plasmid-coded, and the extra-chromosomal location contributes to their rapid spread. Colonising factors promote uninhibited colonisation of mucous surfaces, and plasmid-coded 'invasins' allow active penetration of intestinal epithelial cells by a human-specific strain of *Shigella flexneri*. Enterotoxins which exert their toxic effects inside the intestinal tract and cause diarrhoea are also often plasmid-coded. Haemolysins cause the lysis of erythrocytes. In many pathogenic strains of *E. coli* these genetic determinants are located on plasmids. Invasion of cells and tissues by many enterobacteria is dependent on the presence of ionised iron. It is therefore not entirely surprising that iron-complexing **siderophores**, such as **aerobactin**, are plasmid-coded.

An example of plasmid function in the production of plant diseases is the tumour-inducing plasmid of *Agrobacterium tumefaciens*, which has already been mentioned (Ch. 4.3). The insecticidal effect (the BT-toxin) of the protein-containing inclusion body in *Bacillus thuringiensis* (Ch. 2.2.7) is also coded by genes localised on a large (100 kb) plasmid.

Table 15.3. *Some degradative plasmids*

Substance	Designation of plasmid	Host
Toluol	TOL	*Pseudomonas putida*
Napthalene	NAH	*Pseudomonas putida*
2,4-Diclorophenoxyacetic acid	2,4-D	*Acinetobacter, Alcaligenes, Arthrobacter, Corynebacterium, Pseudomonas, Flavobacterium*
n-Alkane	OCT	*Pseudomonas putida*
Salicylate	SAL	*Pseudomonas putida, P. aeruginosa*
Terpene	CAM	*Pseudomonas putida*
Nicotine	NIC	*Arthrobacter oxydans, Pseudomonas convecta*

Degradative plasmids.   Plasmids may carry genes for special chemical reactions. In some cases these code for enzymes which can catalyse the degradation of chemically synthesised substances which do not naturally occur in the biosphere (xenobiotics). These include many aromatic and heterocyclic compounds with halogen substituents, including herbicides, fungicides and insecticides, and can be degraded only by specialised bacteria which harbour degradative plasmids. A selection of such plasmids is presented in Table 15.3.

Plasmids with other properties.   The list of properties that can be coded on plasmids has grown very long, almost too long to survey. It includes genes for complex metabolic reactions; for example, nitrogen fixation, nodule formation, production of indole acetate and diacetyl; transport of sugars and metal (nickel) ions; synthesis of hydrogenase and enzymes of denitrification. These 'metabolic' plasmids are often very large, with a size range of 300–1200 kb, and are called 'megaplasmids'.

Restriction and modification systems (see Section 15.4) which protect the bacteria from entry of foreign DNA are also sometimes plasmid-coded. It is quite typical for these bacterial properties that their genes can be chromosomally located in some strains, whilst they are carried on plasmids in others. This is true for different strains of one species but also for different strains of phylogenetically related bacteria. This alternating location (on chromosomes and plasmids) might indicate that genes, and even whole gene complexes, can be exchanged between chromosomes and plasmids, and that plasmids may have played a very important role in the evolution of the prokaryotic genome.

15.4   Restriction and modification of DNA

The observation that phages which had been grown in one strain of *E. coli* could then not grow in other strains gave the first clue to the system of restriction and modification of DNA. It was found that this restriction is due to bacterial enzymes which could recognise and split specific loci in foreign DNA, whilst the cellular (host) DNA is protected by an enzymatic modification which makes it unrecognisable to the **restriction enzyme**.

The restriction and modification system is widely distributed in microorganisms. It serves specifically to mark and protect cellular DNA and to destroy and degrade any invading foreign DNA. The system consists of two enzymic activities, an endonuclease and a methyltransferase, which can occur on a single protein or may be located on two separate proteins. Both act at a specific DNA locus, the recognition sequence, though a given nucleotide sequence is substrate for only one of the two enzymes. Cellular DNA is chemically modified by the methyltransferase, which methylates adenine in the N-6 position and cytosine either in the preferred N-5 position or in the N-4 position. This modification occurs during replication, so that the product is double-stranded DNA which is methylated on one strand. In the case of foreign DNA, the restriction endonuclease hydrolyses phosphodiester bonds. This enzyme is only activated when non-modified DNA, which alone can function as its substrate, is present in the cell.

Restriction endonucleases.   Restriction endonucleases can be coded by bacteriophages and plasmids as well as by the bacterial genome. Several classes of restriction enzymes are distinguished, all of which cut double-stranded DNA. Enzymes of class 1 recognise specific nucleotide sequences but cleave DNA non-specifically, outside the recognition zone. The restriction endonuclease of bacteriophage P1 belongs to this class. Enzymes of class 2 are characterised by having cleavage sites that are specific and located inside the DNA segment that is recognised. This leads to the formation of defined DNA fragments. The restriction endonucleases of class 2 are used in the molecular cloning technique that is described in

Table 15.4. *Some restriction endonucleases*

Host organism	Enzyme designation	Recognition sequence
Escherichia coli RY13	*Eco*RI	5' – G $\downarrow$ A – A $\overset{*}{-}$ T – T – C – 3' 3' – C – T – T $\overset{*}{-}$ A – A $-$ G – 5' $\uparrow$
Haemophylus haemolyticus	*Hha*I	5' – G – C $\overset{*}{-}$ G $\downarrow$ C – 3' 3' – C $-$ G $\overset{*}{-}$ C – G – 5' $\uparrow$
Brevibacterium albidum	*Bal*I	5' – T – G – G $\downarrow$ $\overset{*}{C}$ – C – A – 3' 3' – A – C – C $\overset{*}{-}$ G – G – T – 5' $\uparrow$
Haemophylus aegypticus	*Hae*III	5' – G – G $\downarrow$ $\overset{*}{C}$ – C – 3' 3' – C – $\overset{*}{C}$ $-$ G – G – 5' $\uparrow$

The arrows show the location of the cuts by the restriction endonucleases. The dotted line shows the rotation axis of the recognition sequence and the stars indicate the methylated bases.

the following section. Table 15.4 shows some representative members of the class 2 group of restriction endonucleases. Some of these recognise a group of four bases, whilst others recognise six bases. In the case of a four-base recognition sequence, a given DNA molecule is cut more frequently than in the case of a six-base sequence, yielding more and smaller fragments. The recognition sequence has a double rotation symmetry, whose axis is shown as a stippled line in Table 15.4. This structure is known as a **palindrome**. The cleavage sites are indicated by arrows and lie either within or outside the axis of symmetry. In a staggered cut, as for example with *Eco*RI, single-strand ends with four bases are formed. A cut within the axis of symmetry, as in the case of *Hae*III produces fragments with so-called 'blunt' ends. Up to now restriction enzymes have been isolated from hundreds of microorganisms and many are commercially available. Their nomenclature is based on the host organism from which they were isolated (this is why their names are printed in italics).

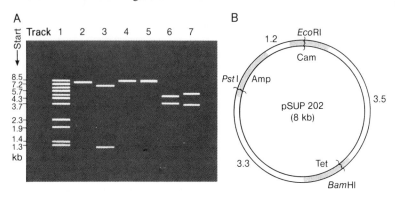

Fig. 15.22. *Assembly of a restriction map for the cloning vector pSUP202.*

(A) Gel electrophoresis of the fragments produced by cutting of SUP202-DNA with the restriction enzymes (2) *Pst*I, (4) *Eco*RI and (5) *Bam*HI, as well as double digestion with *Pst*I/*Eco*RI (3), *Bam*HI/*Eco*RI (6) and *Bam*HI/*Pst*I (7). Track 1 contains lambda DNA as size marker. Fluorescence of the fragments results from staining with ethidium bromide. (B) A circular map of the plasmid obtained by arranging overlapping fragments of the band profile in (A). The figures give the distances in kilobases (kb) between the restriction cuts situated in the antibiotic resistance gene for ampicillin (amp), chloramphenicol (cam) and tetracycline (tet).

Restriction maps.   The various DNA fragments of different sizes which are obtained by the use of restriction endonucleases can be separated by electrophoresis in agarose gels (as described in Section 15.3). This is shown in Fig. 15.22. The migration rates of the fragments are determined by their length: the smaller fragments migrate faster through the gel than larger fragments. The actual sizes of DNA fragments can then be determined by comparison with the bands obtained from DNA standards of known size. The sequence of the restriction cleavage site can be established by multiple digestion of DNA after alignment of the overlapping ends of fragments.

The construction of restriction maps, however, needs endonucleases which cut DNA relatively infrequently and therefore provide large fragments. On the other hand, restriction enzymes which can cleave large DNA molecules into small fragments are gaining increasing importance for the determination of nucleotide sequences (see Section 15.5).

15.5   Molecular cloning techniques

Molecular cloning techniques were developed in the early 1970s. They are based on the knowledge gained from many years of basic research on DNA, RNA and enzymes involved, as well as gene transfer by plasmids and viruses. This short introduction to DNA recombination technology complements the material discussed in Sections 15.1–15.4.

Cleavage of DNA and restriction analysis.   Using restriction endonucleases (Section 15.4), DNA molecules can be split into specific and, because of their small size, easily handled fragments. Endonucleases are the elementary tools of cloning techniques. A typical pattern of fragments obtained after digestion of plasmid DNA by endonucleases is shown in Fig. 15.22. Fragments of up to 1000 bp can be separated by electrophoresis in acrylamide gels. Separation of larger fragments, up to 25 kb, needs a matrix with larger pores, e.g. agarose gels. The migration rate of fragments within a certain size range is inversely proportional to the logarithm of the number of base pairs. Summation of the fragment measurements should correspond to the size of the original molecule. Employing several different endonucleases, with alignment of overlapping fragments, allows the location of individual cleavage sites to be determined, and hence the production of a restriction map for a given segment of DNA. Maps for whole chromosomes can be produced in a relatively short time by the use of pulse-field electrophoresis.

The technique of **Southern Blotting** can be used to find a DNA sequence that is complementary to a given isolated DNA fragment. After electrophoretic separation and denaturing of the DNA, single-stranded DNA fragments are transferred to a nitrocellulose membrane by '**blotting**'. They are then hybridised with the ^{32}P, or dye-labelled, DNA 'probe'. This produces DNA–DNA double strands only between homologous segments, which can be visualised in an autoradiogram or by virtue of the dye label as a specific marker.

Determination of nucleotide sequences.   The availability of restriction fragments has accelerated the development of relatively simple methods for DNA sequencing. Knowledge of a DNA sequence then allows the derivation – according to certain rules – of the coded amino acid sequence.

There are two methods for sequencing of DNA.

(i) **Chemical cleavage (Maxam–Gilbert method)**. In this, chemical reagents are used to modify the four bases of a ^{32}P-labelled DNA strand. Using specific reagents which attack guanine, guanine+adenine, thymine+cytosine, or cytosine (in parallel incubations), the bases are split from their sugar residues. The resulting gap then becomes a specific cleavage site within the DNA strand. Breakage at these sites produces fragments of different sizes which are electrophoretically separated on acrylamide gels. Comparison of the band patterns which appear in autoradiograms after treatment of samples with the different reagents can then be used to read off the positions of individual bases within the DNA molecule.

(ii) **The dideoxy method of Sanger**. This is based on the enzymic replication of a DNA strand and chain termination. Starting with a radioactively labelled short DNA fragment as **primer** (usually a commercially available oligonucleotide), the complementary strands are synthesised from the four deoxyribonucleotides by DNA polymerase in four parallel incubations. To each of these one of the four 2',3'-dideoxynucleotide base analogues is added. Their incorporation blocks further growth of the chain as no phosphodiester bonds can be formed. This produces, as in the first method, fragments of different lengths which can be separated by gel electrophoresis. Comparison of the band patterns of the four tracks in the autoradiogram then allows determination of the base sequence (Fig. 15.23).

Construction of a recombinant DNA molecule.   Molecular cloning techniques use plasmids or viruses as **vectors** to introduce foreign DNA, which may even be of eukaryotic origin, into bacterial cells. Whereas prokaryotic DNA can be directly employed for cloning, eukaryotic DNA has to be used as **cDNA**. cDNA contains only the coding sequences and is prepared by reverse transcription from mRNA using reverse transcriptase. The method of entry of foreign DNA into bacteria is usually by transformation. Animal and plant cells can also take up DNA molecules. The construction of a recombinant DNA molecule is presented in Fig. 15.24. Both the vector and the foreign DNA are first cleaved with a specific endonuclease, for example *Eco*RI. Both DNA molecules yield linear fragments with single-strand ends, whose base sequences are complementary to AATT, respectively TTAA (**sticky ends**). On mixing the thus prepared plasmid and foreign DNA fragments, hydrogen bridges are formed between the complementary single strands. The breaks can then be covalently closed by polynucleotide ligase. This step terminates the construction of a recombinant DNA molecule. The product is termed a **hybrid** DNA or **DNA chimera**.

Vectors.   A cloning vector has to fulfil two requirements. It should have only one cleavage locus for the endonuclease to be used, and provide the

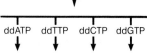

DNA-template strand

Marked starter molecule

are incubated with the four dNTPs,
DNA-Polymerase I and the four
dideoxynuleotidetriphophates.

ddATP   ddTTP   ddCTP   ddGTP

The synthesised strands are then
separated by electrophoresis on
polyacrylamide gels, and the
bands xisualised on X-ray films

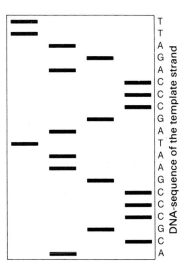

Fig. 15.23. *DNA sequencing by
the dideoxymethod according
to Sanger.*

See text for explanation.

potential for selecting the recombinant containing the foreign DNA. A
high degree of efficiency in the uptake of foreign DNA is a very desirable property of vectors employed in the setting up of gene libraries.
Mutants of phage lambda have been found very suitable for this purpose. A group of vectors derived from this phage, called **cosmids** can
take up DNA fragments of size 35–40 kb (Fig. 15.25). Cosmids are

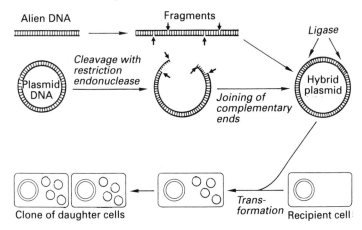

Fig. 15.24. *Simplified presentation of the method for producing hybrid DNA (or DNA chimaera) by insertion of a piece of eukaryotic DNA into a bacterial plasmid.*

Alien DNA and plasmid DNA are treated *in vitro* with the same restriction endonuclease. This produces fragments with 'sticky ends' (protruding single strands with complementary bases). Upon mixing of the two DNA preparations and treating with ligase, plasmids with inserted eukaryotic DNA are obtained. These DNA chimaeras can be introduced into transformable bacteria. They can be multiplied by mass culture of the bacterium, and the alien DNA can be isolated from the cloned culture.

vectors produced by gene technology which contain a replication function (for example from plasmid pBR322), antibiotic-resistance gene (such as tetracycline resistance), and the cohesive ends of phage λ (the so-called '*cos*' site). The latter serve as recognition sites for the cell extract present in 'λ-packaging kit'. For cloning, the foreign DNA and the cosmids are cleaved and ligated. When incubated *in vitro* with the λ-packaging extract, only those hybrid cosmids are cleaved at their *cos* sites which contain a fragment of alien DNA of 35–45 kb size. These fragments are then packed into empty phage heads. Smaller fragments are not packed, so that the cloning of long DNA fragments is favoured (Fig. 15.25).

Another elegant cloning system is provided by the phage M13. This filamentous virus has a length of 900 nm and a width of 9 nm. It invades *E. coli* via the sex pilus and does not kill the host when it replicates. M13 belongs to the single-stranded DNA viruses (Ch. 4.1). After infection,

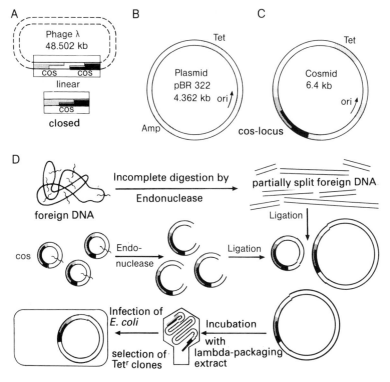

Fig. 15.25. *Cosmids as cloning vectors.*

(A) The cos loci (cohesive sites) are the single-stranded complementary ends of the lambda chromosome. (B) The cloning plasmid is PBR 322 which carries resistance genes for ampicillin (amp) and tetracycline (tet). (C) The cosmid derived from PBR 322 contains the integrated cos loci. (D) For the cloning, foreign DNA and cosmids are cut and ligated. On incubation with 'lambda packaging extract', only those hybrid cosmids which contain a foreign DNA fragment of 35–45 kb are cut at their cos loci. They are packaged into phage heads and the phage used to infect *Escherichia coli* from which tet[r] clones can then be selected. (For further explanation see text).

the plus strand is replicated, and a replicative intermediate (RF) is formed, consisting of a plus and a minus strand. Only the plus-strand is packed into phage particles. The double-stranded RF form behaves as a plasmid; it can be split by endonucleases and recombined with a foreign DNA.

After ligation of the foreign DNA fragments in both orientations, followed by phage replication, single-stranded DNA species can be isolated which contain one or the other of the recombinant DNA segments in the plus strand. This vector M13 has been proved especially useful in sequencing work. Since it yields single-stranded DNA, the DNA denaturation step can be omitted; and since the cloning site is always the same, DNA replication (by the Sanger method) can be initiated with a universal primer.

Selection of hybrid DNA-carrying clones.   Cells which carry a recombinant DNA molecule can be selected, either by virtue of a phenotypic character of the vector, or by a property of the cloned gene.

The first-named selection method is based on insertion of a foreign DNA sequence into an antibiotic-resistance gene of the vector which is thereby inactivated. Thus in the plasmid pBR322 (Fig. 15.25) the resistance towards either tetracycline or ampicillin is abolished. Bacteria which have been transformed with a recombinant DNA molecule in this way, therefore, have lost resistance to one of the two antibiotics, in contrast to cells which contain only the vector DNA.

If a particular gene in a gene library has to be identified, further methods to recognise recombinant clones can be used. If a homologous gene fragment (that is, a gene probe) is available, it can be used to screen the gene library by the 'Southern blotting' procedure already described. If the function of the gene to be cloned is known, and mutants with a defect in this gene are available, they can be genetically complemented by transfer of the cloned DNA. For example, a mutant defective in the leucine biosynthesis gene can gain the ability to grow on mineral medium without leucine by insertion of the appropriate wild-type gene. It can then be selected without difficulty.

However, cloned DNA cannot always be translated into a functioning gene product; especially when the cloning host – usually *E. coli* – is unrelated to the donor organism.

If the gene product formed in the cloning host has no catalytic activity, protein-specific antibodies can be used for its identification. This procedure can be applied even to single colonies.

Expression of cloned DNA.   In order to get eukaryotic cDNA to be expressed in bacteria, the DNA sequence must be inserted in a region of the vector which is strongly expressed in the cloning host. If, for example, insulin cDNA is to be recombined with the gene for β-lactamase or β-galactosidase, a mixed polypeptide, called a 'fusion protein' is constructed. Its expression is controlled by the appropriate bacterial promoter. The strength of the promoter and the translation efficiency govern the rate of formation of the recombinant gene product. A high yield is usually desirable. However, it is not uncommon for overexpression of a protein to lead to toxic side effects for the producing organism, or to increased breakdown of the desired product. Because of this, uncontrolled (constitutive) gene expression is undesirable. Special expression vectors have been constructed for cloning, which have very strong promoters that can be regulated, as for example the pL promoter of phage λ. This promoter provides a genetically altered regulation system which can be controlled by temperature changes. In this, the repressor which normally blocks the pL promoter, is inactivated at higher temperatures. The cells can therefore be grown at lower temperatures in non-toxic conditions, and synthesise the foreign protein only after the temperature is raised.

Insertion of DNA into animal cells is especially facilitated by retroviral vectors. A metallothioneine gene promoter derived from mouse cells allows induced expression of the protein after addition of cadmium. The cysteine-rich metallothioneine normally binds heavy metals and serves as a protective protein.

The insertion of genes into plant cells is promoted by altered Ti-plasmids (Ch. 4.3) which have been successfully employed, at least in dicotyledons. Transformation of plant protoplasts with plasmid DNA by electroporation (Section 15.2.4) appears to be a promising technique for dicotyledons and monocotyledons.

Applications.   The possibilities opened up by research on recombinant DNA are being investigated for exploitation by biotechnologically orientated industry. The aim is to prepare biological products more efficiently, in larger amounts and of greater purity. Another area of application, which is being successfully exploited since the late 1970s, is the genetically engineered manufacture of therapeutically useful proteins. These include proteohormones like human insulin which can be produced in large-scale fermentations from bacteria or yeasts, growth hormones like follicle-stimulating hormone, the pain antagonistic endorphins and anti-cancer agents like tumour necrosis factor, interleukins and interferons.

Traditional procedures for the production of vaccines are expensive and not without risks. Gene technology offers simpler and less risky methods. Thus, production of a highly effective vaccine against hepatitis B was achieved by cloning of the virus envelope protein in bacteria. Vaccines against herpes, rabies and foot-and-mouth disease have been produced in a similar manner. At the present time intensive work is going on for the development of vaccines against malaria and other parasitic diseases, against cancer and against HIV.

Thrombolytics like urokinase and tissue-specific plasminogen activators are being used in cardiovascular illnesses. Their production leads a promising application area for gene technology.

Cells which produce human monoclonal antibodies can now be obtained by means of the so-called 'hybridoma techniques'. This opens up the prospect of developing successful measures against infectious diseases for which there are no chemo- or antibiotic therapies, and against tumour cells, as well as elimination of T-lymphocytes which are mainly responsible for transplant rejection. There is some vigorous debate about the use of gene technology in the human field, for genome analysis, gene therapies in somatic cells and manipulation of germ cells.

In agriculture, the conventional methods of plant breeding (used up to now) were limited by the gene potential of cross-breeding species. DNA recombinant techniques have extended and enriched genetic variability. It has become possible to cross species barriers without decades of breeding experiments, and to introduce new genetic material into crop plants. The main focus of these efforts is to equip such plants with resistance to poisons, herbicides, metals, etc. and to increase their tolerance to environmental stresses such as dehydration, low temperature and high salt concentrations; to achieve more efficient utilisation of light and molecular nitrogen; and to test their suitability for the production of secondary metabolites and useful raw materials. Analogous efforts are being made to use gene technology for increased performance in domestic animals.

The specific use of microorganisms in the treatment of sewage and effluents goes back to the last century. This **environmental** field of applications, which include air purification, domestic and industrial waste disposal and the exploration of new energy sources and raw materials offers a wide scope for the activities of the gene technologist. Microorganisms could be constructed to have specific and highly efficient metabolic capacities which would enlarge and enrich the microbial potential so far available.

Safety aspects.   Naturally occurring gene transfer and DNA recombination can yield new combinations of genetic characters even between eukaryotes and prokaryotes, as was shown in the example of plant tumour-induced Ti-plasmids (see Ch. 4.3). The novel aspect of gene technology is its ability to target *in vitro*, and on a considerable scale, the combination of genes from unrelated organisms. Because the characters of the products can generally not be predicted in detail, gene technology entails a certain potential risk. This was pointed out at the time when the new possibilities first became known by the scientists themselves (Asilomar Conference) and counteracted by the establishment of guidelines. This voluntary system of self-regulation entails classification of experiments into safety categories and the definition of appropriate technical conditions. The latter include special equipment for laboratories that envisage working in genetic engineering and gene technology – which have to be registered in some countries – and the use of special 'safety strains' which are not viable in the natural habitat. In addition, all organisms which contain recombinant DNA have to be killed before disposal, so that their spread is prevented. Release of microorganisms which have been modified by genetic engineering into natural habitats needs special permission.

The handling of pathogenic microorganisms has been subject to safety regulations for many years. The experience of nearly 20 years' work in the field of genetic engineering and gene technology has allowed the conclusion that carriers of recombinant DNA do not carry a higher risk potential than that indicated by the characters of the donor DNA, the recipient organism, and the cloning vector. The voluntary control measures that have been in use for work with *in vitro* recombinant DNA have now been complemented by legal enforcement.

16 Regulation of metabolism

The regulation of metabolism and growth by environmental factors has been frequently mentioned in earlier chapters dealing with the metabolic activities of microorganisms. The inhibition, observed by Pasteur, of fermentation in yeast by atmospheric oxygen is an example of metabolic regulation that has been frequently observed and extensively investigated. It has also been known for a long time that some catabolic enzymes are produced only in the presence of the substrate. In the denitrifying bacteria, nitrate respiration functions only in the absence of oxygen; oxygen inhibits the formation and function of the nitrate-reducing system. pH changes in cultures of enterobacteria and clostridia determine the course of fermentation and the production of characteristic fermentation products. Oxygen and light influence the synthesis of pigments in phototrophic bacteria. These and many other environmentally determined changes can be attributed to basic regulatory mechanisms.

The multiplicity of metabolic processes required for cellular syntheses and multiplication demands their optimal co-ordination. Each metabolic pathway comprises a number of enzymatic reactions. The total of metabolic processes results in the provision of utilisable energy, the synthesis of building blocks and macromolecules, and the reduplication of the cell. Success in the competition between organisms has necessitated the evolutions of mechanisms for adaptation to changing environmental conditions, on the one hand, and for optimal tuning of the flow of metabolites through the pathways, on the other. The objects of these optimising processes are the enzymes, their syntheses, and their functions.

Regulation of cellular metabolism occurs at two levels: the control of enzyme synthesis and the variation of enzyme activity. Control at the level of enzymes synthesis determines many pathways of metabolism. Production of several enzymes belonging to the same metabolic sequence is generally under common regulation. This concerns the rate of synthesis of the specific enzymes in relation to the synthesis rate for total proteins. The rate of synthesis is governed by the transcription frequency of structural genes.

Many enzymes are constantly produced and always present, irrespective of environmental conditions. They are **constitutive** components of the cell and are called constitutive enzymes; the terms **constitutive** genes and **constitutive enzyme** synthesis refer to these.

The synthesis of many catabolic enzymes is regulated by **enzyme induction**. It is economically advantageous for cellular metabolism, that enzymes required for the utilisation of a nutrient and for the entry of its catabolic products into intermediary metabolism, are produced only when the nutrient is present in the medium. In other words, catabolic enzymes that the cell is potentially able to produce are not synthesised when they are not required.

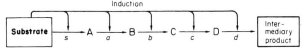

The synthesis of many anabolic enzymes is regulated by **enzyme repression**. Again, metabolic economy is promoted if the enzymes of a biosynthetic pathway are not produced when the respective end product is present in the nutrient medium; the presence or accumulation of an end product thus leads to repression, i.e. decrease in the synthesis rate of all enzymes that are specific components of the biosynthetic chain.

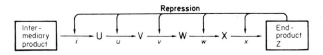

Normally, the enzymes for synthesis of building blocks are constantly produced. Their formation is inhibited (repressed) when the end product is present in excess. This is called **end-product repression**.

Regulation at the level of enzyme activity usually concerns key enzymes in cellular metabolism. The catalytic activity of a particular enzyme in a specific metabolic pathway can undergo variations: it can be increased (by a positive effector) or decreased (by a negative effector). In **end-product inhibition** (feedback inhibition), the end product is inhibitory for the first enzyme in the sequence.

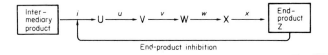

Both types of regulation, induction and repression, on the one hand, and alteration of enzyme activity, on the other hand, have similar effects. They change the material flux through a metabolic pathway. The effects of induction and repression on metabolism are rather slow and they are regarded as 'coarse tuning'. The change in activity of a key enzyme is immediately effective and is regarded as 'fine tuning'.

16.1   Regulation of enzyme synthesis

Many bacteria can grow on a large variety of nutrients. This requires the capacity to produce the necessary enzymes for utilisation of the nutrients, and therefore the possession of the appropriate structural genes. The terms enzyme induction, inducible enzyme, and inducing substrate apply to the situation where a catabolic enzyme (or enzymes) is formed only in response to the presence of its substrate in the nutrient medium and the absence of other (competing) substances. The synthesis of most catabolic enzymes is subject to induction.

On the other hand, synthesis of enzymes involved in synthetic metabolism, for example those for pyrimidine, purine and amino acid synthesis, are regulated by repression. In most cases the signal for repression is the end product of the biosynthetic pathway (hence called end-product repression).

When two catabolic substrates are simultaneously present in the nutrient medium, one is used preferentially in most cases, namely that which supports the fastest growth rate. The formation of catabolic enzymes for the other substrate is repressed, and this is referred to as catabolite repression.

16.1.1   Induction

Induction of β-galactosidase.   The most extensively studied example of enzyme induction is the utilisation of lactose by *Escherichia coli* (Fig. 16.1). Lactose is a disaccharide that must be hydrolysed before it can enter the catabolic pathway for hexoses:

$$\text{lactose} + H_2O \xrightarrow{\ \beta\text{-galactosidase}\ } D\text{-glucose} + D\text{-galactose}$$

Wild-type cells growing on glucose have barely demonstrable β-galactosidase activity. When they are grown on lactose or another galactoside, however, their β-galactosidase level is about 1000-fold higher; almost 3% of the total cellular protein can be present as β-galactosidase. Normally, the enzyme is produced only in the presence of its inducing substrate, lactose. However, analysis of the regulation mechanism was facilitated by use of the substrate analogue, 2-propyl-β-thiogalactoside, which functions as a non-utilisable inducer. The addition of the

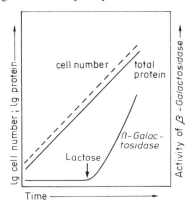

Fig. 16.1. *Induction of β-galactosidase formation.*

Synthesis of β-galactosidase starts after addition of lactose to the nutrient medium.

thiogalactoside results in 'gratuitous induction', i.e. the enzyme is produced but cannot hydrolyse the inducer or make it metabolically useful.

Coordinated and sequential induction.   When the catabolism of a substrate is carried out via a number of intermediates, A, B, C, etc. by enzymes a, b, c, etc.,

$$A \xrightarrow{a} B \xrightarrow{b} C \xrightarrow{c} D \xrightarrow{d} E \xrightarrow{e} I$$

induction of the enzymes can occur according to several theoretical possibilities (Fig. 16.2). (1) Enzyme synthesis can occur sequentially or in steps; each succeeding enzyme is induced by the product of the preceding reaction. (2) All the participating enzymes are coordinately induced, i.e. the substrate A induces all the enzymes a to e, etc. (3) Individual enzymes of sequential reactions (a, b, c) are coordinately induced, whilst the later products (C or D) induce the synthesis of the enzymes in the following sequence (d, e).

Coordinate synthesis of all enzymes involved in the catabolism of a substrate is advantageous for the cell because it enables it to react rapidly in the presence of the substrate. Sequential induction has the effect that conversion of the substrate and hence the growth rate of the cells increases only slowly: the product of the first reaction must reach a threshold concentration in the cell before it can induce the next enzyme. In the regulation of enzymes involved in converging pathways, subdivision into coordinately regulated groups of enzymes that are induced by the product of the preceding group seems appropriate.

$$
\begin{array}{c}
L \longrightarrow M \longrightarrow N \longrightarrow O \\
\\
A \longrightarrow B \longrightarrow C \longrightarrow D \longrightarrow E \longrightarrow F \longrightarrow G \longrightarrow H \longrightarrow I \\
\\
P \longrightarrow Q \longrightarrow R
\end{array}
$$

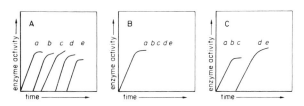

Fig. 16.2. *The time course of the appearance of inducible enzymes.*

(A) Strictly sequential; (B) strictly co-ordinate; (C) sequential induction of co-ordinately regulated enzyme groups. Cultures grown under non-inducing conditions had the inducing substrate added at zero time.

The regulatory patterns of converging metabolic pathways have been extensively investigated in the case of mandelate, 4-hydroxybenzoate and tryptophan catabolism by *Pseudomonas putida*, *Acinetobacter calcoaceticus* and *Alcaligenes eutrophus*; the patterns differ in different species.

Product induction.   Some catabolic enzymes are induced by the product of the first or subsequent reactions in the pathway. A case in point is the breakdown of tryptophan. The pathway goes from tryptophan via formylkynurenine, kynurenine and anthranilate to catechol and is induced by kynurenine. This kind of enzyme induction requires that the basal level of the enzymes converting tryptophan to kynurenine is sufficiently high to yield at least traces of kynurenine in the presence of tryptophan.

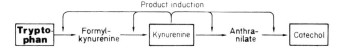

The product induction of tryptophan catabolism can be regarded as a protective mechanism to prevent the induction of catabolic enzymes by endogenously produced tryptophan, which is required for protein synthesis. Tryptophan is catabolised only when it is added to the nutrient medium and present in high concentrations in the cell.

16.1.2   Repression

End-product repression.   The biosynthesis of arginine can be used to show how the repression by an end product of biosynthesis affects the concentration of the biosynthetic enzymes. Arginine synthesis starts from glutamate (Fig. 7.17) and leads via ornithine, citrulline and argininosuccinate to arginine.

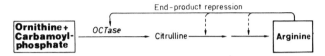

If *E. coli* is grown in minimal medium and the enzyme ornithine carbamoyl transferase (OCTase) is monitored as a representative enzyme of the arginine synthetic pathway, it is found in 'normal' concentrations. Addition of arginine (20 μg/ml) to the minimal medium produced immediate cessation (repression) of OCTase synthesis. During growth of the culture in the presence of arginine, the enzyme was 'diluted out'; that is, its specific activity (activity per unit mass of protein) declined to a very low value. When the repressed cells were freed of arginine, by washing and resuspending in an arginine-free minimal medium, synthesis of the enzyme was immediately derepressed, and the enzyme concentration rapidly increased to many times the value initially present (Figs 16.3, 16.4). Eventually, after the functioning of the biosynthetic enzymes so produced had led to the formation and accumulation of arginine, the specific activity of OCTase gradually declined to the 'normal' level (Fig. 16.3).

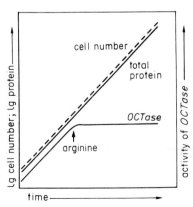

Fig. 16.3. *Repression of ornithine carbamoyl transferase (OCTase).*

Formation of the enzymes for the biosynthetic pathway of arginine is almost instantaneously repressed by the addition of arginine to the nutrient medium.

544   Regulation of metabolism

Fig. 16.4. *Accelerated formation of ornithine carbamoyl transferase (OCTase) by de-repression of the arginine operon.*

A wild-type culture of *Escherichia coli* was grown in a minimal medium that contained excess of arginine. The cells were washed and divided into two parallel cultures which were further incubated with and without arginine. At various time intervals samples were removed and their cell concentration and ornithine carbamoyl transferase activity (as a representative enzyme of the arginine synthesis pathway) were determined. It can be seen that in the culture without arginine the enzyme activity increased rapidly to a level above normal and then gradually declined to the normal level because of dilution by growth. In the presence of arginine in the nutrient medium, no enzyme was produced. (From Gorini, L. & Maas, W. K. (1957). *Biochim. Biophys. Acta*, **25**, 208.)

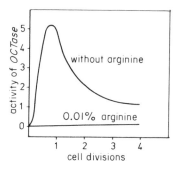

In a chemostat experiment it could be shown, by using mutants with a defect in one of the enzymes of the arginine biosynthetic pathway, that the de-repressed condition could be maintained. When the growth of the mutant was limited by arginine, the specific activity of OCTase remained at 25 times the value of the 'normal' level (Fig. 16.4).

Pattern of regulation in branched biosynthetic pathways.   The formation of enzymes involved in branched biosynthetic pathways is regulated in a complicated manner. Examples are furnished by the aromatic amino acid family, the aspartate family and the pyruvate family (Fig. 7.17). Each end product apparently represses only the formation of enzymes in its specific synthetic pathway. The synthetic enzymes functioning before the branch point are subject to repression by all the end products, i.e. multivalent repression. This means they are repressed only when all the end products are present in the medium; the addition of single end products has no effect.

A very interesting branched pathway is that leading to the synthesis of L-valine, L-isoleucine and L-leucine. Four of the reactions starting from pyruvate and 2-oxobutyrate, respectively, and leading to valine and isoleucine, re-

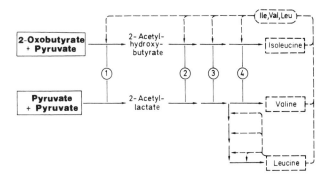

Fig. 16.5. *Regulation by multivalent repression (trivalent) of enzymes in the biosynthesis pathways for* L-*isoleucine,* L-*valine, and* L-*leucine, and* L-*leucine.*

The enzymes acetohydroxic acid synthase (1), acetohydroxyic acid isomeroreductase (2), dihydroxy acid dehydratase (3), and transaminase (4) function in both the isoleucine and valine pathways.

spectively, are catalysed by the same enzymes. Furthermore, 2-oxoisovalerate (2-oxo-3-methylbutyrate) is the precursor of valine and the initial substrate (i.e. the branchpoint) for the synthesis of leucine (Fig. 16.5).

Catabolite repression. Whereas end-product repression applies to the enzymes of biosynthetic pathways, catabolite repression concerns catabolic pathways. It is the cause of the well-known phenomenon of diauxie (Fig. 6.10). The pairs of substrates, glucose and sorbitol, glucose and lactose, or glucose and acetate, are not utilised simultaneously by *E. coli*, but sequentially. Glucose is utilised first and represses the formation of the enzymes for the catabolism of the other substrate (Fig. 16.6).

The situation is more complex when an amino acid serves at the same time as energy and carbon source, and as the nitrogen source. Histidine utilisation by *Enterobacter aerogenes* furnishes a good example of the influence of glucose on the synthesis of the enzymes needed for utilisation of an amino acid. Histidase serves as a representative catabolic enzyme whose concentration in the cell can be monitored (Table 16.1). When glucose and an ammonium salt are present in the nutrient medium, no histidase is formed, even when histidine is also present.

Glucose plus ammonium ions almost completely repress synthesis of histidase. When no ammonium-nitrogen is present, so that the cells are dependent on histidine as their nitrogen source, the repressing effect of glucose on histidase formation is much less severe. This example indicates

Table 16.1. *Histidase content of* Enterobacter aerogenes *cells after growth in different nutrient media*

Addition to basal medium			Histidase per 10 mg cells
Glucose	L-histidine	$(NH_4)_2SO_4$	
+	−	+	< 5
+	+	+	< 5
−	+	−	182
−	+	+	170
+	+	−	70

From Neidhardt, F. C. & Magasanik, B. (1957). *J. Bacteriol.* **73**, 253.

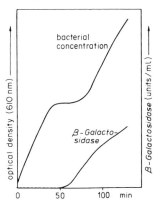

Fig. 16.6.*'Glucose effect' or catabolite repression.*

Delayed formation of β-galactosidase in *Escherichia coli.* The nutrient solution contained 0.4 mg/ml glucose and 0.2 mg/ml lactose. As long as glucose is present, formation of β-galactosidase is repressed. (From Epstein, W., Naono, S. & Gros, F. (1966). *Biochem. Biophys. Res. Commun.* **24**, 588.)

that lack of nitrogen can partially counteract the catabolite repression exerted by glucose. Thus the formation of a catabolic enzyme depends not only on the presence of an inducer and supply of an energy source, but is also determined by the availability of nitrogen in the medium.

Regulation of enzyme concentrations in the central metabolic pathways. The enzymes of amphibolic pathways may also be subject to genetic regulation. In aerobically growing *E. coli*, the enzymes of the tricarboxylic acid cycle are present at high concentrations, whereas in anaerobically growing cells their specific activities are only one tenth or one twentieth of these levels, and the 2-oxoglutarate dehydrogenase is completely repressed. Some of the anaplerotic enzymes, such as malate synthase, isocitrate lyase and glyoxylate carboligase, are found only in cells that require them for the metabolism of their substrates.

16.1.3   Mechanisms of regulation

In theory, enzyme synthesis could be regulated at the level of translation as well as at the level of transcription. It has been discovered, however, that in prokaryotes gene expression is mostly regulated at the transcriptional level. For the majority of genes coding for the structure of polypeptide chains, transcription is subject to regulation. Environmental conditions and the metabolic state of the cell determine whether and at what frequency a structural gene is to be transcribed. This kind of regulation requires that certain signals are transmitted from the metabolic sphere to the DNA. The signal substances, or **effector molecules**, are low molecular weight compounds, such as sugars and their derivatives, amino acids or nucleotides. Since these effectors cannot interact directly with DNA, they each interact with a specific **regulatory protein**. At high intracellular concentrations, an effector binds specifically to its regulatory protein, causing an alteration in conformation, and hence an alteration in the proteins' ability to bind a specific sequence of DNA. A regulatory protein that binds to DNA in the absence of the effector (**inducer**) is called a **repressor**. A regulatory protein that binds to DNA only in the presence of the effector (**co-repressor**) is called an **apo-repressor.**

The regions at which the regulatory proteins bind to DNA are not the structural genes themselves, but neighbouring sequences, known as **promoters** and **operators**. Promoter, operator, and structural gene(s) constitute an **operon**. The promoter is a base sequence that is recognised by the DNA-dependent RNA polymerase. It is the binding site for RNA polymerase and the initiation point of transcription for a given gene or operon. Even genes whose expression is not subject to regulation have promoters. The promoters of genes that are subject to regulation are different in that their initiation properties are modified by binding of regulatory proteins. The **operator** is a base sequence situated between the promoter and the structural genes and it also reacts with a regulatory protein, namely the repressor. The latter determines whether transcription can take place. The term **operon** is used to designate a group of functionally related genes. The proteins determined by the genes of one operon are usually enzymes that catalyse several steps in a metabolic pathway. The transcription of one operon results in the synthesis of one (**polycistronic**) mRNA molecule.

Synthesis of the regulatory proteins is determined by regulatory genes, which are constitutive. They can, but do not need, to be situated in the neighbourhood of the operon that they control. The complete RNA polymerase holoenzyme is necessary for the proper combination with the promoter. RNA polymerase consists of subunits α, β, β', σ and ω. In the absence of the **sigma (σ) factor**, which is easily dissociated, the enzyme has its full catalytic activity but lacks the ability to bind to the promoter. The sigma factor apparently has an important function in the binding of the polymerase to DNA.

The termination of mRNA synthesis at the end of an operon is apparently also determined by a specific DNA sequence, the terminator. The role of the **termination factor** rho (ρ), a tetrameric protein, in the detachment of RNA polymerase from the DNA is still unclear.

In contrast to tRNA and rRNA, most mRNA is labile and short-lived; many kinds of mRNA have a half-life of only 0.5–10 minutes. In this way the concentration of a given mRNA in the cell is governed by the frequency of its transcription. The concentration of mRNA, in its turn, determines the concentration of the protein that it codes.

Operons are also classified as those that are **inducible** and **repressible**. The operons for the breakdown of lactose, galactose and arabinose are inducible; that is, the maximum frequency of their transcription is achieved only when the external effectors (inducers) are present in the medium. The process of induction initiates the synthesis of the (inducible) enzymes coded by inducible operons. On the other hand, operons such as those coding for arginine, histidine or trytophan are called repressible; that is the maximal frequency of their transcription is achieved only when the respective effectors are absent from the medium, or present below a critical threshold concentration. As already mentioned, these effectors are called co-repressors, and the regulatory proteins on which they act are called apo-repressors. The synthesis of enzymes coded by repressible operons is initiated by derepression.

Induction of the lactose operon (negative control).   The lactose (*lac*) operon of *E. coli* comprises the *lac* promoter, the *lac* operator and the structural genes for the three enzymes β-galactosidase, permease and transacetylase (Fig. 16.7). This operon has been investigated in great detail. The DNA has been isolated and the base sequence of the promoter-operator region has been determined. The *lac* repressor (regulatory protein) has also been isolated and analysed.

The operon is subject to **negative control**; this means that the regulatory protein (*lac* repressor) remains attached to the operator and inhibits transcription as long as no inducer is present. Lactose (α-D-galactosyl-β-1,4-D-glucose) functions as the external inducer. It is transported into the cell by the permease and converted to allolactose (α-D-galactosyl-β-1,6-D-glucose), which functions as the internal inducer. The conversion to allolactose is catalysed by β-galactosidase. The two enzymes permease and β-glactosidase are present in non-induced cells, though only at less than one thousandth of the concentrations achieved in fully induced cells. The binding of allolactose to the *lac* repressor causes a

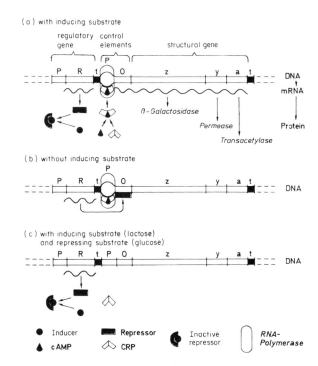

Fig. 16.7. *Model for the regulation of the lactose operon, including induction by substrate and catabolite repression.*

Binding of the cAMP receptor protein (CRP) to the promoter is required for the transcription of the operon. The CRP binds only in the presence of cAMP. Glucose inhibits the formation of cAMP, and hence the transcription of the *lac* operon.

conformational change that lowers the affinity of the repressor for the operator DNA sequence. The inducer-charged *lac* repressor thus frees the operon for transcription.

The *lac* operon is subject to a second, **positive control**. This means that transcription takes place only when a second regulatory protein (called CRP or CAP) is actually bound to the promoter. (The abbreviations CRP, cyclic AMP receptor protein, and CAP, catabolite activator protein, are synonymous). The binding of CRP to the promoter is essential for the attachment of RNA polymerase to the DNA. The affinity of CRP for the promoter is increased by interaction with cyclic AMP (cAMP), and is sufficient for binding only when cAMP is present in high concentration inside the cell.

Catabolite repression of the lactose operon.   As already mentioned, when lactose and glucose are present together in the nutrient medium of *E. coli*, synthesis of the enzymes of the *lac* operon is repressed (Figs 16.6, 16.7). This glucose effect (giving rise to diauxic growth) is due to the low concentration of intracellular cAMP in the presence of glucose. Catabolite repression by glucose (also by fructose and glucose-6-phosphate) is also exerted on other inducible catabolic pathways (namely those for arabinose, galactose, sorbose, glycerol, etc.). The decrease in cAMP concentration by glucose is probably due to the localisation of the cAMP-forming enzyme adenylate cyclase, which converts ATP intracellularly to cAMP.

$$ATP \xrightarrow{\text{adenylate cyclase}} cAMP + pp_i$$

This enzyme is membrane-bound. Its activity is high when the HPr system for sugar transport into the cell is present in the phosphorylated form. The enzyme activity decreases during the phosphorylating transport of sugars, when the HPr system (see Ch. 7.7) consumes a lot of energy, i.e. ATP (via phosphoenolpyruvate).

Induction of the arabinose operon (positive control).   The arabinose (*ara*) operon of *E. coli* (as well as the rhamnose and maltose operons) is subject to positive control. The *ara* operon comprises the structural genes *ara* A, *ara* B and *ara* D for the enzymes converting L-arabinose to D-xylulose-5-phosphate. The expression of the operon is induced by arabinose. As in many other catabolic systems, the operon is subject to regulation at the promoter which binds the cAMP-activated CRP. The operon also has two further control regions: the operator and an initiator. A regulatory protein that is coded by the *ara* C gene binds to the operator. This protein acts as a repressor and its binding to the operator inhibits transcription. However, in the presence of arabinose, this protein is converted to an activator which binds to the promoter and initiates transcription. This operon, therefore, is subject to negative control and also to positive control by a specific regulatory protein (in addition to the CRP–cAMP system).

End-product repression of the tryptophan operon.   The tryptophan operon of *E. coli* comprises the structural genes for the five enzymes involved in the conversion of chorismate to tryptophan, as well as for an operator segment and promoter at the start of the operon. A second, less effective promoter situated within the sequence of structural genes can be ignored here. The detailed investigations on the functioning of this operon have

(a) In absence of end-product

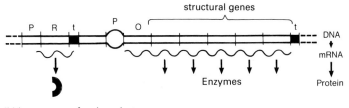

(b) In presence of end-product

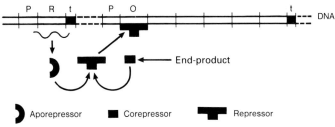

■ Aporepressor   ■ Corepressor   ▬ Repressor

Fig. 16.8. *Model for the regulation of the formation of biosynthetic enzymes by end-product repression.*

Enzyme formation occurs only in the absence of the end product. Formation of the active repressor, which closes the operator, occurs only by binding of the end product i.e. the co-repressor, to the aporepressor.

yielded a picture that corresponds closely to the model formulated by Jacob and Monod in 1961 for the functioning of a repressible operon (Fig. 16.8). The regulatory gene *trp* R, which is situated well away from the operator, codes for an effector protein, the apo-repressor. In the presence of tryptophan, which functions as co-repressor and has a high affinity for the apo-repressor protein, the (holo)repressor prevents transcription. Lowering of the tryptophan concentration leads to dissociation of the repressor and liberation of the operator and hence synthesis of mRNA.

Autogenous regulation. This term characterises regulatory systems in which the product of a gene located within the operon carries out the function of a regulatory protein. The principle of autogenous regulation lies in the possession of a regulatory protein that controls expression of the operon and thereby regulates its own synthesis, irrespective of whether the operon is under positive or negative control. The best understood system regulated in this way is that of histidine utilisation in *Salmonella*. The catabolism of histidine to glutamate and ammonium is catalysed by four enzymes whose structural genes (*(hut* genes) are close together on the chromosome. Their expression is subject to control by a repressor protein. The gene coding for this repressor protein is situated between the structural genes and is thus a part of the operon. The *hut* operon is induced by the first product of the catabolic pathway, urocanate (product induction). Induction of the operon, therefore, leads not only to the formation of the histidine catabolising system but also to accumulation of the repressor protein. This then causes a decrease in transcription of the operon, including the regulatory gene, etc. This autogenous regulation leads to a very smooth control of enzyme formation. Such self-regulating systems are widely distributed in bacteria, eukaryotes and bacteriophages.

Regulation of tRNA and rRNA synthesis.   Whereas the synthesis of mRNA is controlled by induction, repression and catabolite repression, the synthesis of stable RNA is regulated in a completely different manner. As has been known for a long time, wild-type strains of *E. coli*, *Salmonella typhimurium* and *Bacillus subtilis* respond very abruptly to the lack or exhaustion of a required amino acid. The cells immediately cease to synthesise not only proteins but also RNA. This strict (stringent) dependence on the presence of amino acids (i.e protein building blocks) shows that the synthesis of stable RNA is not solely dependent on the presence of its own building blocks (the nucleotides). The isolation of one-step mutants that were not stringent but relaxed in their regulation and could synthesise RNA even in the absence of a required amino acid showed that at least one gene (*rel* A) must be concerned in this regulation. Lack of an amino acid in the wild-type cells leads to the accumulation of unusual nucleotides (ppGpp and pppGpp), but this is not the case in the mutants. It is assumed that the above nucleotides are signals for the cessation of tRNA and rRNA synthesis.

16.2   Enzyme regulation by alteration of catalytic activity

In the preceding sections we have discussed the possibilities the cell has at its disposal for adjusting the intracellular concentrations of enzymes to the demands of metabolism. However, *de novo* synthesis or diluting out of enzymes during growth affords only a gradual adaptation to changes in environmental conditions. A much more rapid adaptation to abrupt changes in metabolic conditions can be brought about by alterations in the catalytic activities of enzymes.

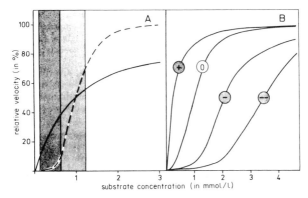

Fig. 16.9. *Substrate saturation curves for 'hyperbolic' and 'sigmoidal' enzymes.*

(A) Substrate saturation of a 'hyperbolic' enzyme (solid line) and a 'sigmoidal' enzyme (broken line). (B) Effectors can alter the course of the substrate saturation curve: positive effectors (+) increase the affinity and negative effectors (−) decrease the affinity of the enzyme for its substrate. The shaded areas indicate the regions of highest sensitivity.

16.2.1   Mechanisms of regulation

The rate of an enzyme-catalysed reaction, usually expressed as amount of substrate converted per unit time (μmol substrate/min) depends on the affinity of the enzymes for the substrate (K_m) and on the maximal velocity (V_{max}), as well as on the concentrations of enzyme (E) and substrate (S) or product (P). The K_m, the so-called Michaelis–Menten constant, defines the substrate concentration at which the enzyme activity exhibits half the maximal velocity ($V_{max}/2$). The maximum velocity of an enzyme is achieved when substrate is present in excess so that the enzyme is 'saturated' with its substrate. K_m and V_{max} are kinetic parameters of an enzyme.

Simple enzymes.   Most enzymes are characterised by a hyperbolic substrate saturation curve; the reaction velocity depends only on the concentrations of substrate and product and increases hyperbolically with increasing substrate concentration: the enzyme obeys the Michaelis–Menten relation. Such enzymes are termed 'hyperbolic' or simple enzymes (Fig. 16.9, solid curve).

It is plausible that an enzyme increases its velocity of substrate conversion with increasing substrate concentration. The sensitivity of an enzyme to alterations in substrate concentration is given by the substrate saturation curve. The steeper the curve, the more pronounced is the change in reaction velocity with only a slight change in substrate concentration. As can be seen in Fig. 16.9, the slope is steepest at low substrate concentrations. These considerations indicate that the velocity of metabolic flux in the cell depends on the concentrations of metabolites. As a rule, enzyme substrates, i.e. metabolites, are present in the cell at concentrations below their K_m values.

Regulatory enzymes. The regulatory enzymes have much more complex properties than the simple enzymes. Most of them are characterised by substrate saturation curves whose course deviates from the hyperbolic and is often sigmoid (Fig. 16.9A, B). Sigmoid substrate saturation curves have a region where the slope is considerably steeper than that of simple enzymes. In this region, between approximately $\frac{1}{2}$ and $1\frac{1}{4}$ of the K_m value, the enzymes are extremely sensitive; very small alterations in substrate concentration are sufficient to produce large changes in reaction velocity.

The sigmoid nature of the curve indicates that the enzyme is composed of subunits that exhibit cooperative interactions. The binding of the substrate to the catalytic centre of one subunit apparently increases the affinities of the other substrate binding sites on the same enzyme molecule. In fact, regulatory enzymes have been found to consist of two or more, most commonly four, subunits.

The regulatory enzymes also possess, besides their catalytic centre(s) which recognise and bind the substrate, other stereospecific sites called allosteric centres. These are the binding sites for the effectors which alter the substrate affinity of the enzymes. There are specific binding sites for positive effectors (activators) and for negative effectors (inhibitors). The effectors alter the sigmoidicity of the enzyme activity curve (Fig. 16.9B). The terms allosteric enzymes, allosteric inhibition, and allosteric effectors are used as well as allosteric centres, and the expressions allosteric enzymes, regulatory enzymes, and sigmoidal enzymes are often used synonymously.

> The degree of cooperativity is expressed by the Hill coefficient or cooperativity coefficient n. This gives the number of mutually dependent binding sites, or rather, the number of cooperatively interacting subunits. When there is no cooperativity $n = 1$. For an allosteric enzyme consisting of four subunits, the value for n lies between > 1 and < 4, according to the degree of positive cooperativity. In negative cooperativity $n < 1$. There are also more complex systems which cannot be dealt with here.

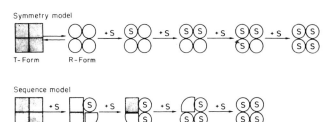

Fig. 16.10. *Symmetry model and sequence model of allosteric enzymes.*
The models are for an enzyme
consisting of four identical subunits.

Models of cooperativity. The cooperativity between enzyme subunits is
recognised by their sigmoid substrate saturation curve and has elicited
two explanatory hypotheses: the symmetry model of Monod, Wyman
and Changeux and the sequence model of Koshland. Both these models
are shown schematically in Fig. 16.10.

Both models are based on the concept that the enzymes can assume
different states or conformations: an active form (with high substrate
affinity) and an inactive form (with low substrate affinity). The precise
relationship between the different forms of the subunits at any time is
dependent on the presence and concentration of the ligands (substrate,
activator and inhibitor molecules). The models differ in their ideas as to
how the conformational changes are brought about.

According to the symmetry model the enzyme has only two alternative conformational states, which are in dynamic equilibrium with each
other. All the subunits of an enzyme molecule are assumed to have the
same conformational state; no mixed states are possible, only symmetrical oligomers (Fig. 16.11). The equilibrium is characterised by the allosteric
constant L. In the absence of ligands, the inactive ground state (T state
for 'tense') predominates over the active R state (R for 'relaxed'). When
ligands are added they react with those enzyme molecules that are in the
appropriate conformational state: inhibitors with molecules in the T
state and substrates and activators with molecules in the R state. Binding of the substrate molecules fixes, or stabilises, the enzyme in the R
state. More enzyme molecules are then converted from the T state to the
R state to maintain the equilibrium between the two conformational
states. This then promotes further binding of the substrate molecules. It
is thought that the binding of substrate to the several binding sites on
each enzyme molecule (i.e. the different subunits) will promote the conversion of an equivalent number of further enzymes molecules to the R

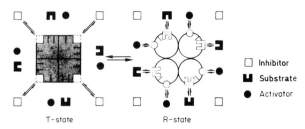

T-state   R-state

☐ Inhibitor
⬛ Substrate
● Activator

Fig. 16.11. *Representation of the equilibrium between a state of low activity and a state of high activity in an allosteric enzyme consisting of four subunits, according to the symmetry model.*

(After Kirschner, K. (1968). *Ergebn. Mikrobiol.* **44**, 123.)

state, where they can react with further substrate molecules. In other words, the binding of only a few substrate molecules facilitates the binding of a larger number of further substrate molecules, thus constituting the cooperative effect and resulting in the sigmoidal dependence of reaction velocity on substrate concentration. A negative effector is assumed to have the same effect in the opposite direction.

According the the **sequence model**, the enzyme will assume the catalytically active conformation only by virtue of its interaction with the substrate (Fig. 16.10). In an enzyme consisting of several subunits, the conformational change of one subunit, induced by interaction with a ligand, is transmitted sequentially to the other subunits so that the binding of further substrate molecules by the subunits is progressively facilitated. This model can accommodate unsymmetrical oligomers (tetramers in Fig. 16.10) with subunits in different conformational states. The presence (binding) of activators facilitates transition to the active form, whilst the presence of inhibitors makes it more difficult.

Allosteric enzymes and effectors. As a rule, regulatory enzymes occur in all biosynthetic pathways and also in some catabolic sequences. In most cases, the allosteric regulatory enzymes are those at the beginning of a specific pathway or in a key position. The allosteric effectors, usually low molecular weight compounds, are either the end products of biosynthetic pathways or substances whose concentrations reflect the metabolic state of the cell; some examples are ATP, ADP, AMP, acetyl-CoA, phosphoenolpyruvate, $NADH_2$, etc.

Alteration of enzyme activity by covalent modification. Another kind of regulatory mechanism has been demonstrated in some enzymes; they can

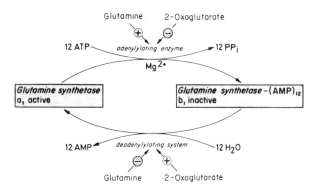

Fig. 16.12. *Regulation of glutamine synthetase in* Escherichia coli *by enzyme-catalysed modification.*

(+), Positive effector (stimulation);   (From Holzer, H. & Duntze, W.
(−), negative effector (inhibition).   (1971). *Ann. Rev. Biochem.* **40**, 345.)

be modified enzymatically. Such changes can result in decrease or increase of enzymatic activities. The modifications (so far discovered) can be adenylylation, phosphorylation and acetylation of the enzyme protein. These modifications exert their effects rapidly. In the mammalian system the glycogen-degrading phosphorylase and the glycogen synthetase are enzymically activated and de-activated. In *E. coli* the formation of glutamine synthetase is repressible, but the activity of the enzyme can also be decreased by 80–90% in a few minutes on addition of NH_4^+ to the medium. This decrease is due to an enzyme-catalysed chemical modification of the active form of the enzyme glutamine synthetase a to the inactive form glutamine synthetase b by adenylylation (Fig. 16.12). The presence of glutamine in the cell stimulates the adenylylating enzyme whilst free 2-oxoglutarate inhibits it. After removal of the NH_4 ions from the medium, glutamine becomes limiting, the adenylylating enzyme loses activity, and glutamine synthetase is reactivated by a de-adenylylating system that removes the adenylic group (AMP).

16.2.2   Specific examples of regulatory patterns

Biosynthetic pathways.   The first enzyme in a biosynthetic pathway is usually a regulatory enzyme. It is inhibited by the end product (end-product or feedback inhibition). On accumulation or overpopulation of an end product in the cell, inhibition of the first enzyme in the biosynthetic

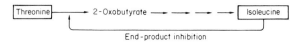

End-product inhibition

pathway leads to an immediate decline in the flow of metabolites through the pathway. An example is threonine deaminase in the biosynthetic pathway from threonine to isoleucine.

Controlled and uncontrolled isofunctional enzymes.   It must be pointed out that not every threonine deaminase is inhibited by isoleucine, even in the same organism. When *E. coli* is grown aerobically on glucose and ammonium salts, only one threonine deaminase is produced. The demonstration that it is subject to allosteric inhibition by isoleucine serves to identify its anabolic function. When the organism is grown anaerobically, however, on a mixture of amino acids (casamino acids, peptone), the anabolic threonine deaminase is repressed, but an isoenzyme with catabolic function is produced; this isoenzyme is only subject to allosteric regulation by AMP and ADP. Another example is the formation of 2-acetyllactate by *Enterobacter aerogenes*. The reaction catalysed by acetylhydroxyacid synthase plays a role in the anaerobic fermentation of glucose to acetoin (catabolism) and it also initiates the synthesis of valine (anabolism). Thus, 2-acetyllactate is the common intermediary product of a branched metabolic pathway.

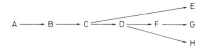

The organism is able to produce two isofunctional enzymes. One of these is formed only when the pH has declined during fermentation and acetoin is being produced as a neutral fermentation product. The other enzyme is also produced at neutral and at slightly alkaline pH; it has a high pH optimum and is allosterically inhibited by valine. These examples show how mutual interference of two metabolic pathways can be avoided by the formation of isofunctional enzymes, one of which is usually strictly regulated and the other regulated in a different manner, or not at all.

Branched biosynthetic pathways.   Special problems arise when the first step(s) in a biosynthetic pathway is common to two or more end products. In a hypothetical reaction sequence converting A to E, G, and H, the first reaction A → B would be inhibited by feedback inhibition when only one of the end products (e.g. H) was accumulated. This would, however, also decrease the synthesis of E and G.

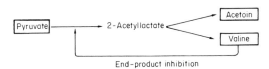

End-product inhibition

These complications resulting from branched biosynthetic pathways have been overcome by different organisms in different ways. Up to now, several strategies have been found for the regulation of enzyme function in divergent or parallel pathways.

(1) The first step is catalysed by a number of isoenzymes each of which is regulated by one of the different end products.

(2) The first step is catalysed by a single enzyme, but (a) this is only inhibited when all the end products are present in excess (concerted inhibition), or (b) each end product participates equally in the inhibition (cumulative inhibition), although the total inhibition can exceed the sum of the inhibitions produced by the individual end products (cooperative inhibition).

The synthesis of the amino acids methionine, lysine, threonine and isoleucine (the aspartate family) is initiated by **isofunctional** enzymes (Fig. 16.13). *E. coli* has three parallel aspartokinases to accomplish the reaction:

$$\text{aspartate} + \text{ATP} \rightarrow \text{aspartate-4-phosphate} + \text{ADP}$$

Their activities are regulated by different end products. Aspartokinase I and homoserine dehydrogenase I are inhibited by threonine. Aspartokinase III is regulated by lysine, whilst aspartokinase II is not subject to allosteric control. The regulation of the aspartokinases is supplemented by a secondary mechanism in which each of the first enzymes specific for a branch of the pathway is subject to end-product inhibition (fig. 16.13).

A regulatory pattern similar to the above is seen in the synthesis of the aromatic amino acid family (Fig. 7.18). The synthesis of the amino acids phenylalinine, tyrosine, tryptophan and 4-aminobenzoate is initiated by the conversion of erthyrose-4-phosphate and phosphoenolpyruvate to 3-deoxy-D-arabineheptulose-7-phosphate (DHAP). *E. coli* has three DHAP synthases. One of these is inhibited by tyrosine, the second is inhibited by phenylalanine, and the third enzyme, which has only low activity, is not subject to end-product inhibition. Further feedback loops then provide for secondary controls.

Phosphofructokinase and the Pasteur effect.   The Pasteur effect, that is, the inhibition of glycolysis by respiration, was convincingly explained by the assumption that the respiratory chain and substrate level phosphory-

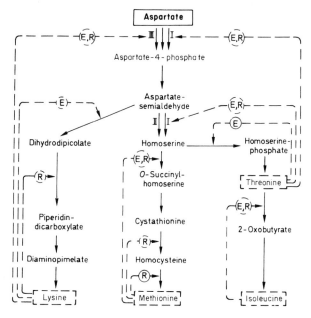

Fig. 16.13. *Regulation of the biosynthesis of amino acids belonging to the 'aspartate family' in* Escherichia coli.

The broken lines indicate enzyme reactions that are subject to end-product inhibition (E). For some enzymes end-product repression (R) has also been demonstrated.

lation compete for ADP and phosphate (Ch. 8.1). According to more recent research, control of hexose catabolism via the fructose-bisphosphate pathway is exerted primarily by the allosteric regulation of phosphofructokinase (Fig. 16.14).

Phosphofructokinase from baker's yeast is subject to allosteric inhibition by ATP. ATP increases the sigmoidicity of the substrate saturation curve. It is striking and significant that the 5'-phosphates of inosine, guanosine and cytidine can serve as phosphate donors in place of ATP, but they cannot function as inhibitors or regulators of the enzyme. This must mean that the allosteric centre is highly specific for ATP and that the signal is clear and singular. By comparison, the specificity of the catalytic centre is low. AMP can act as a positive effector and counteracts the inhibition by ATP. The effects of other mono- and diphosphates are only very slight or zero. In *E. coli*, ADP functions as the positive effector

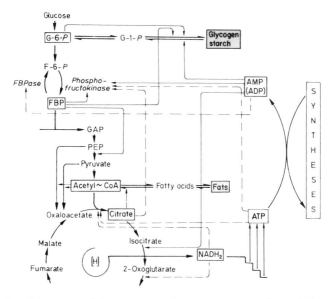

Fig. 16.14. *Some of the interactions between enzymes and metabolites involved in the regulation of hexose catabolism and synthesis of storage materials.*

In this scheme, data obtained from experiments with yeast, animal tissues, and bacteria have been combined. Metabolites with important effector functions have been boxed. The thin black lines with arrows originating from these indicate positive effector function, and the broken lines with arrows indicate negative effector functions.

in place of AMP. Phosphofructokinase is also inhibited by citrate, and this inhibition is enhanced by ATP but decreased by fructose-6-phosphate.

Knowledge of the allosteric properties of phosphofructokinase leads to the following model. When aerobically cultured yeast or tissue cells are deprived of oxygen, and electron-transport phosphorylation is thereby blocked, the cellular concentration of ATP, relative to AMP, declines. This leads to an increase in enzyme (phosphofructokinase) activity and hence a faster flow of metabolites through the fructose-bisphosphate pathway. Determinations of the intracellular concentrations of glucose, glucose-6-phosphate, fructose-6-phosphate, fructose 1,6-bisphosphate, and triose phosphates, before and after transition from anaerobic to aerobic conditions, have confirmed that this pattern of regulation actually occurs in the living cell. The concentrations of glucose-6-phosphate and fructose-6-phosphate increase immediately upon aeration of the cells, whilst the concentrations of fructose-1,6-bisphosphate and triose phosphates are drastically diminished. Phosphofructokinase appears to act like a valve controlled by adenylates and other metabolites; when closed, metabolites situated above (upstream from) the valve accumulate, whereas those lying downstream are further metabolised and, hence, diminish. The decline in the rate of glucose conversion on transition to aerobic conditions (inhibition of glycolysis) can be seen to follow from this model.

Gluconeogenesis. The adenylates ATP, ADP, AMP and acyl-CoA derivatives are involved in the regulation of several reactions of hexose catabolism, intermediary metabolism, and the synthesis of storage products. The regulation of phosphofructokinase apparently represents the main control point that directs substrate flow through the fructose-bisphosphate pathway. In a number of bacteria, the corresponding enzyme that controls catabolism via the 2-keto-3-deoxy-6-phosphogluconate pathway is glucose-6-phosphate dehydrogenase. This is also strongly inhibited by ATP and by $NADH_2$.

The synthesis of glucose from pyruvate or lactate (gluconeogenesis) is important when these serve as carbon source and no carbohydrates are present. The synthesis proceeds via the reactions of the fructose-bisphosphate pathway in reverse, with the exception of three steps which are irreversible (Fig. 16.14). These reactions are catalysed by regulatory enzymes. In animal tissues the production of phosphenolpyruvate from pyruvate is via oxaloacetate. The first step is catalysed by pyruvate carboxylase and is dependent on the presence of acetyl-CoA. It seems that acetyl-CoA here serves as a signal for the saturation of all acetyl-CoA-consuming metabolic routes, especially terminal oxidation via the tricarboxylic acid cycle (TCA). This control mechanism allows glucose synthesis to proceed only when acetyl-CoA is in excess, and it ensures that metabolism is directed to necessary energy gain. Furthermore, the dependence of oxaloacetate formation (from pyruvate) on acetyl-CoA may also be of importance for the delivery of oxaloacetate to the TCA cycle. The second irreversible reaction of glucose catabolism is bypassed in gluconeogenesis by the action of fructose-1,6-bisphosphatase.

fructose-1,6-bisphosphate + $H_2 \rightarrow$ fructose-6-phosphate + P_i

This enzyme is inhibited by AMP, which thus serves as an indicator of the extent to which the cell's requirements for energy-rich compounds can be satisfied; excess of AMP signifies that insufficient ATP is available to satisfy the requirements of the energy-consuming reactions. It seems logical that under these conditions gluconeogenesis should be curbed in favour of glucose catabolism to yield utilisable energy.

The tricarboxylic acid cycle.   In yeast, ATP greatly diminishes the affinity of citrate synthase for acetyl-CoA. In E. *coli* and other bacteria high concentrations of $NADH_2$ are the signal for saturation of the respiratory chain, demanding a decline in the flow through the TCA cycle. 2-Oxoglutarate dehydrogenase, citrate synthase, and pyruvate dehydrogenase are subject to inhibition by $NADH_2$ (Fig. 16.14).

Synthesis of storage lipids.   Reserve materials are usually accumulated when carbon and energy sources are present in excess, whilst lack of nitrogen or sulphur prevents or limits growth. The signal for the formation of fats (fatty acids) and polysaccharides originates predominantly from intermediary metabolites. In yeast, the rate-limiting reaction of fatty acid synthesis is the carboxylation of acetyl-CoA by acetyl-CoA carboxylase:

$$\text{acetyl-CoA} + CO_2 \xrightarrow[\text{biotin enzyme}]{\text{ATP}} \text{malonyl-CoA}$$

This enzyme is the first in the biosynthesis of long-chain fatty acids. Other syntheses starting from acetyl-CoA (carotenoid, steroid, malate and citrate synthesis, etc.) do not require activation by the formation of malonyl-CoA. Acetyl-CoA carboxylase is activated by citrate. An elevated citrate level in the cell, therefore, leads via malonyl-CoA synthesis to the production of long-chain fatty acids and fats (triglycerides). The CoA derivatives of palmitic and other fatty acids function in the opposite direction, as negative effectors. Accumulation of these CoA derivatives thus results in end-product inhibition.

Synthesis of storage polysaccharides.   The synthesis of glycogen and starch begins with glucose-1-phosphate. This is activated by nucleoside triphosphate (NuTP) and transferred to a polyglucose chain.

$$\text{glucose-1-phosphate} + \text{NuTP} \xrightarrow{\text{pyrophosphorylase}} \text{NuDP-glucose} + PP_i$$

$$n \text{ NuDP-glucose} \xrightarrow{\text{glycogen synthetase}} (\text{glucose})_n + \text{NuDP}$$

Whereas **glycogen synthesis** in liver utilises UDP-glucose, starch synthesis in green plants and glycogen synthesis in several bacteria use ADP-glucose. The glycogen synthetase of liver is activated by glucose-6-phosphate. The regulatory systems in bacteria and plants, however, differ profoundly from that of liver cells. They have pyrophosphorylase as the regulatory enzyme. In E. *coli*, *Arthrobacter*, *Rhodospirillum rubrum*, and in spinach leaves, AMP and ADP inhibit, and the precursor (glucose-1-phosphate) stimulates the enzyme. The pyrophosphorylase of E. *coli* is activated by fructose-bisphosphate, glyceraldehyde phosphate, and phosphoenopyruvate. The enzyme of R. *rubrum* has pyruvate as activator, and that of spinach leaves has 3-phosphoglycerate, phosphoenolpyruvate and fructose-bisphosphate as activators. The synthesis of polysaccharides furnishes a good example of different regulatory systems achieving the same effect.

Autotrophic carbon dioxide fixation.   Carbon dioxide fixation via the ribulose-1,5-bisphosphate cycle is one of the most energy-demanding processes in cellular metabolism. It seems logical, therefore, that control mechanisms exist to ensure that the cycle functions at its maximum rate only when the energy supply for the maintenance of the cell (synthesis of monomers and polymers, renewal of enzymes, etc.) is assured. Phosphoribulokinase is subject to an appropriate control. The enzyme is inhibited by AMP (and sometimes by ADP) and its activity is increased by $NADH_2$.

The energy charge of the cell.   The examples cited above confirm the assumption that adenylates have important control functions in the cell. They seem to furnish signals that are common to catabolic and anabolic processes and serve to adjust the rates of energy gain and biosyntheses to each other. The cellular content of ATP, AMP and ADP or, more specifically, the relationship between the adenylates determines the rates of individual reactions and thereby the overall rates of catabolic and anabolic pathways.

> A quantitative expression for the energy charge (E.C.) of the cell has been formulated as follows:
>
> $$E.C. = \tfrac{1}{2} \cdot \frac{2 \ ATP + ADP}{ATP + ADP + AMP} = \frac{ATP + 0.5 \ ADP}{ATP + ADP + AMP}$$
>
> The factor 0.5 is arbitrary and can be conveniently varied between 0 and 1. The energy charge thus states how many energy-rich bonds are present in relation to the total number of adenosine units. The value is 1 when all adenylate is present as ATP and 0 when only AMP is present. In exponentially growing cells, the energy charge is usually about 0.8.

Existing experimental evidence is in agreement with the idea that allosteric enzymes are inhibited or activated by one or other of the adenylates in such a way that the overall metabolism of the cell is kept 'in harmony' (attuned). Thus, if the energy charge of the cell increases, the activities of catabolic enzymes decline and those of synthetic enzymes increase. A decline in the energy charge elicits the opposite enzymic responses.

16.3   Mutants with defective regulation

Elucidation of the regulatory mechanisms for enzyme synthesis and activity is largely due to the isolation of mutants with defects in regulation. Mutants have been and are still being isolated that, for example (1) do not make a functional repressor protein, or that contain it at many times the normal concentration; (2) are operator constitutive because their operator does not bind the repressor protein; (3) lack allosteric sensitivity, i.e. their allosteric enzymes cannot recognise allosteric effectors. Some basic procedures for the isolation of such mutants are described below.

Mutants with constitutive catabolic enzymes.   Mutants that make catabolic enzymes constitutively can be enriched by frequently alternating substrate changes. If cells can produce the enzymes for utilisation of substrate A constitutively, transfer from substrate B to A will allow them to grow immediately at maximum rate, whereas the inducible wild-type cells still must synthesise the enzymes for A and thus undergo a lag phase. After several generations, the culture is again transferred to substrate B and allowed to grow until the enzymes for A have been 'diluted out' in the inducible cells. After a number of repeated transfers of this kind, the mutants that make the enzymes for substrate A constitutively should have outgrown the wild-type inducible cells. *E. coli* mutants that are constitutive for the lactose operon have been isolated in this way. Other selection methods utilise the inhibitory effects of substrate analogues on induction. An example of this is thiomethyl galactoside which inhibits the induction of the *gal* operon by galactose in *E. coli*.

Mutants with constitutive biosynthetic enzymes.   Mutants that form biosynthetic enzymes constitutively or that lack the fine control of biosynthesis (feedback inhibition) can be obtained by the **antimetabolite** method. Many structural analogues or antimetabolites (Ch. 6.6) of normal biosynthetic end products (amino acids, purines, pyrimidines, etc.) have bacteriostatic effects. On the one hand, they mimic the end product and inhibit the synthesis of the normal metabolite and, on the other hand, they can be incorporated into proteins or nucleic acids but render these non-functional. Growth ceases because of the pseudo-end product inhibition (of a necessary biosynthetic pathway) in the absence of the normal end product. Thus if a wild-type population of 10^8–10^{10} cells is streaked out on antimetabolite-containing agar medium, only a few resistant mutants can form colonies.

This resistance to antimetabolites can result from a number of different mutational changes in the physiological properties of the cell. (1) Mutation to loss of allosteric sensitivity. This results in the allosteric

Fig. 16.15. *Mutants resistant to an antimetabolite.*

View of a petri dish with nutrient agar containing an antimetabolite; this has been inoculated with about 108 bacteria. Only colonies of resistant mutants grow at first. The zones of the large colonies (of resistant mutants) indicate that these excrete a metabolite.

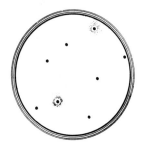

(first) enzyme not being influenced by either the normal metabolite or the antimetabolite so that the production of the end product of the biosynthetic pathway is uncontrolled. (2) Mutation to constitutive derepression. This mutation results in the uncontrolled production of the biosynthetic enzymes for the particular end product. (3) Mutations at the catalytic centers of the metabolite-activating and -converting enzymes; by increasing the specificity of the enzyme, it can lose the ability to bind the antimetabolite, though it is still able to deal normally with the metabolite, so that the antimetabolite loses its bacteriostatic effect. (4) Mutation to a defect in transport mechanisms can result in loss of transport capacity for the antimetabolite into the cell and, hence, its loss of antimetabolite effect. (5) Mutation to a constitutive catabolism of the antimetabolite, by which the antimetabolite is again rendered ineffective.

Only the first two types of mutants are of interest for the selection of cells with defects in regulation. The derepressed synthesis of biosynthetic enzymes as well as the loss of allosteric inhibition often results in over-production and excretion of the biosynthetic end product. This overproduction of the metabolite by a mutant cell leads to the displacement of the antimetabolite from the reaction sites in the cell and, hence, to growth and colony formation. Since the overproduced metabolite is also excreted and diffuses into the agar, it can also counteract the effect of the antimetabolite on wild-type cells in the diffusion zone. These can therefore grow and form small satellite colonies. Thus a ring of secondary or satellite colonies identifies the central colony as a mutant that excretes the metabolite (Fig. 16.15) and, therefore, indicates a defect in regulation. The actual kind of defect that causes accumulation and excretion of a metabolite will require further analysis. A considerable number of mutants with regulatory defects have been isolated by the antimetabolite method. Comparisons between different regulation-defective mutants have shown that the loss of repression has a smaller effect on the rate of end-product synthesis than changes in sensitivity to allosteric inhibition. A mutant that has lost the sensitivity to inhibition of a biosynthetic pathway accumulates the end product inside the cell and often excretes it, even when repression is quite normal. In contrast, mutants with considerable derepression (constitutivity) show only moderate accumulation and excretion of the metabolite, as long as the sensitivity to allosteric inhibition is retained. It would seem that repression is primarily of importance for the economy of mRNA and protein synthesis, whereas the actual synthesis of the metabolite is regulated mainly by end-product inhibition.

Mutants with altered sensitivity to allosteric effectors.   Mutants with altered sensitivity of an allosteric enzyme to its effectors have also been isolated according to another principle; namely, as revertants of auxotrophs (auxotroph method). The procedure is illustrated in the following recipe. First, mutants are isolated that are auxotrophic for the metabolite that is desired as the excreted product. Among these auxotrophic mutants, those whose inability to synthesise the metabolite is due to a defect in an allosteric enzyme of the synthetic pathway are selected. Prototrophic revertants are isolated from these auxotrophic defective mutants. The revertants are no longer dependent on the supply of the end product, i.e. they can synthesis it. From these revertants, mutants that excrete the end-product are selected. These can be recognised by satellite growth or by the method of bioautography described in Ch. 10.2.2

These mutants obtained by two-fold selection can be assumed to have lost the functional capacity at the catalytic centre of an allosteric enzyme in the first mutation. The second, different mutational step would probably concern the structure, i.e. conformation of the whole protein molecule; it would therefore restore its catalytic activity but abolish its allosteric sensitivity.

The employment of several mutation and selection steps, as in this case, may also be necessary for the isolation of a number of other, particular mutants.

Theoretical and applied aspects.   The strategy of mutant selection is of great importance for further elucidation of cell metabolism and identification of regulatory mechanisms. It also has applied aspects, as it points the way to deliberate selection of high performance mutants for the production of any substances that can be achieved by microbiological processes.

17   Microorganisms and the environment

In the preceding chapters, the microorganisms were discussed according to their biochemical and physiological properties, and in many cases their habitats were also mentioned. With the knowledge so obtained, it is now possible and fruitful to consider the relationships of microorganisms to their environments. In what follows, the terminology and basic ideas of ecology will be introduced first. Ecology deals with the behaviour of organisms in their natural habitats and with the relations between different organisms, i.e. with the relationship of organisms and the environment.

The earliest evidence of life on earth goes back some 3×10^9 years and, until about 0.5×10^9 years ago, microorganisms dominated the biosphere of this planet. The prokaryotes, besides having come into being close to the origins of life and being the source for the development of the multiplicity of eukaryotic organisms, have also been present throughout. This means that the higher organisms were never on their own in the course of evolution; they were always supported by, or competed with, unicellular organisms. The higher organisms that achieved dominance must be those that not only competed successfully with their peers but were also able to hold their own against opportunistic microorganisms. In many cases, amiable partnerships, mutual symbioses, developed in the course of evolution. The second part of this chapter will deal with such partnerships between microorganisms, animals, and plants.

Microorganisms were already in existence at the times when the surface of the earth assumed its present form. They were present when the continents migrated, when a number of sediments, 1000 m thick, were formed, when the earth's crust sank and became folded, and when deposits of ores, carbon, petroleum and natural gas were laid down. Microorganisms were even active participants in many of these processes. The third section of this chapter will discuss some geomicrobiological topics.

The earth was inhabited solely by microorganisms for up to 80% of the time that is ascribed to organic evolution. Comparative physiological and biochemical considerations offer sufficient basis for a classification of prokaryotes by their type of metabolism, although only few microfossils have been found. Even so, in the section on the evolution of microorganisms, a number of gaps and speculations will need to be tolerated.

17.1   Ecology of microorganisms

17.1.1   Introduction

Much effort has been expended in the isolation and description of individual microorganisms. Investigations on pure cultures are important to judge the potential abilities and functions of individual species in nature. However, the detailed taxonomic, biochemical, physiological, and genetic investigations have made many microbiologists lose sight of the original aim of their scientific work: namely, to study the behaviour of microorganisms in their natural environment.

Ecology deals with interactions between organisms and relations between organisms and environments. Microbial ecology deals only with a segment of the total ecological system. Ecology is a very complex science and is studied from several aspects by the representatives of the various biological subdisciplines. The use of basic terms and concepts, therefore, is often not uniform. For this reason the following sections will try to define the meanings of common terms used in microbial ecology.

The ecosystem.   The basic unit in ecology is the ecosystem, comprising abiotic as well as biotic components. The biotic element is the community of living organisms, or biocenosis. This usually deals with populations of microorganisms; a population consisting of clones of one or of several species. The abiotic component of the ecosystem comprises the chemical and physical conditions in which the organisms live. The dimensions of microbial ecosystems show enormous variations. An ecosystem could be a pond, a lake, or the root system of a plant. Ecosystems can also be small, such as the oral cavity of man, the rumen of a cow or sheep, or a segment of intestine. On the other hand, the total domain of living organisms on our planet, the biosphere, can also be regarded as a giant ecosystem. The term **environment** is often used in connection with **ecosystems** and, in this sense, concerns an ecosystem's biotic and abiotic components that constitute the immediate surroundings of a given organism.

Habitat.   Within an ecosystem each kind of organism can be ascribed a habitat. The ecological habitat is the place or locality that a given organism (individual or population) normally inhabits. Thus each organism can be assigned at least one habitat where it can normally be found, where it can grow and flourish, and from which it can be isolated. Habitats can be sediments in lakes, fertile humus-rich soils, the nasal cavity, or the intestinal tract of humans, to give some examples. Most microorganisms have just one habitat within a given ecosystem, though some microorganisms can have several different habitats, each in a different ecosystem. Rhizobia, for instance, grow in soil and in the root hairs of leguminous plants; a methanogenic bacterium can have its habitat in the sediment of a lake, the rumen of an animal, or in the sludge tanks of sewage plants. One might say that the habitat defines the street and house number where an organism lives; some organisms may have several addresses.

The ecological niche. In contrast to the habitat, the ecological niche does not refer to the actual location of an organism, but relates to the functioning of a species or population within the community. The ecological niche can be said to characterise the profession or trade of a species or population. Each can be assumed to fulfil certain functions, determined by its nutritional demands, kinetic properties, biochemical abilities, structural features, and by its tolerance towards environmental conditions. The total of these parameters determines its function in a given ecosystem. It is commonly found that the distribution of a species or population is less widespread than could be assumed from its known properties. In other words, the actual ecological niches of an organism are more limited in reality than its potential niches. Quite often, secondary factors determine whether a species can really fulfil a function for which it has the potential capacity.

> This can be illustrated by the following example. Only those cellulolytic bacteria that can degrade cellulose anaerobically and gain their energy by fermentation can maintain themselves and flourish in the rumen. Furthermore, they must be able to tolerate the temperature of the rumen and the presence of fatty acids, enzymes, ammonia, gases, and other products. Finally, the continuous removal of certain fermentation products, for example, hydrogen, must be assured. Thus, an abundance of capacities and tolerances may be required to fulfil certain functions in a given ecosystem.

The inhabitants of an ecosystem. According to a concept first proposed by Winogradsky in 1925, the microorganisms found in an ecosystem can be classified into two categories, **autochthonous** and **allochthonous**. Autochthonous microorganisms are those that are indigenous and always present in a given ecosystem (soil, intestine, etc.). **Autochthonous** organisms of soils are always present, irrespective of any additions of particular nutrients. Their presence is based on the more or less constant supply of nutrients that are typical for the ecosystem. **Allochthonous** (or **zymogenous**) microorganisms are those that are dependent on an occasional increase in concentration of certain nutrients or on the presence of specific nutrients. They are basically strangers to the ecosystem, appearing only occasionally, or persisting in a resting state.

The autochthonous flora of an ecosystem often comprises highly specialised organisms, such as nitrifying types or inhabitants of hot springs and other extreme environments. Many of the ubiquitous soil and aquatic bacteria, on the other hand, belong to the allochthonous flora.

Number and diversity of microorganisms in an ecosystem.   Under normal conditions the flora of soils and waters contains large numbers of species. 'Normal' here means about neutral pH, high nutrient concentrations and water content. As the conditions depart from this 'normality', i.e. as the chemical and physical conditions of an ecosystem become more 'extreme', their species diversity diminishes, but the actual number of individual organisms increases. This kind of relationship between numbers of individuals and species diversity with the 'extremity' of the environment has been observed in many ecosystems: in hot springs, salt lakes, acidic mining effluents, dry soils, and in intestines. In such ecosystems, those organisms that are most completely adapted to their habitat and usually cannot grow under less extreme conditions come to predominate. These highly specialised and adapted organisms are described as 'extreme thermophiles', 'extreme' psychrophiles, 'extreme' halophiles, acidophiles, etc.

Nutrient limitation is the normal state in the natural ecosystem.   In nature, microorganisms living in soil and water are usually faced with extreme nutrient limitation. In aquatic ecosystems concentrations of nutrients often are below 10 μg/l. For most microorganisms, therefore, 'hunger and poverty' are the normal life situation. Very slow growth, or alternating phases of fast growth and no growth are thus normal lifestyles in nature. In many places, generation times can be as long as 100–200 days. Even *E. coli* in the human colon has to put up with a doubling time of 20 hours. Microbial growth studies generally omit to consider that the potential capacities of an organism are being investigated only in the direction of their optimal growth environment and growth rates. The reaction patterns of organisms under conditions of severe nutrient deficiencies is as yet largely unexplored.

Extreme substrate limitations are included in the kind of conditions that are encompassed in the fashionable term 'stress'. 'Heat stress' or 'heat shock' are seen as the cell's reactions to a rise in temperature; in the case of *E. coli*, for instance, from 30 to 42 °C. This leads to the transient synthesis, or increased synthesis, of a number of new proteins, to a partial degradation of RNA and to many other reactions. Similar reactions are induced by substrate deficiency stress. Apparently new catabolic enzymes are produced which have higher substrate affinities than the enzymes produced in nutrient-rich media. The ecologically most important response to substrate deficiency is the development of a **more resistant state** of the cell. Cells that have been exposed to substrate limitations have increased resistance to heat shock, osmotic stress or disinfecting agents.

17.1.2   Aquatic ecosystems

The biosphere of our planet contains a large number of ecosystems in which microorganisms play an important part; some ecosystems are solely inhabited by microorganisms. Since it is clearly impossible to mention all the different ecosystems, the scope of this presentation must be restricted. Soil as an example of terrestrial ecosystems and lakes and oceans as examples of aquatic ecosystems are obvious candidates for selection. Investigations of fertile agricultural soils are very interesting, but, because of the manifold heterogeneities within minimal areas, the ecosystems of soils are exceedingly complex. The following presentation therefore concentrates on aquatic systems, especially as a large part of microbial conversions (in nature) occur in water. Oceans, lakes, ponds, pools and running waters are typical aquatic ecosystems.

Oceans.   Marine microbiology is a part of marine biology and is a very young discipline. The primary producers in the sea are unicellular algae, the phytoplankton. The food chain comprises bacteria, protozoa, arthropods and fish. Although the oceans constitute the largest recipient and reservoir of solar energy, their contribution to food production is small; only 5–10% of the total protein produced on this planet comes from the sea. In addition, the productivity is very unevenly distributed. This heterogeneity in primary and secondary production can be illustrated by data on fish production. The open seas, with 90% of the surface area of the world's oceans, produce 0.7% of its fish; the coastal zones with 9.9% of the ocean surface area produce 54% of the fish, and the upwelling regions with only 0.1% of the ocean surface area contribute 44% of the fish. Fish yields are obviously correlated with total biomass production. Their distribution gives clear indication of the limitations on primary production by availability of nutrients, mainly nitrate and phosphate. Discharge of nutrient-rich effluents into the world's oceans therefore does not cause pollution; rather, it is the precondition for biomass production in the sea. Without constant addition of nutrients, no harvest can be reaped from the oceans.

Interesting bacteriological conversions occur at the edges of the sea, in estuaries, marshlands, salt marshes and zones of brackish water. The universal presence of sulphates in seawater causes the production of hydrogen sulphide by sulphate-reducing bacteria in anaerobic areas, with consequential effects on the rest of the bacterial flora.

Investigations on the halophilic bacteria of coastal areas have so far been less extensive than the subject merits. It would seem advisable for research to take marine bacteria into greater consideration, not only to increase our general knowledge, but also for the solution of practice-orientated problems. At present, considerable microbiological research is concentrated on effluent flora and the degradation of very resistant impurities in effluents and drainage systems. However, effluents are not only contaminated with organic impurities but also contain considerable salt loads, including sulphates. They therefore offer conditions that resemble those of marine ecosystems. Studies on biology of effluents, therefore, emphasise the necessity to give increasing attention to the microbial conversions in marine ecosystems.

Primary production of biomass in deep waters.   The life of practically all heterotrophic organisms is based on the **biomass** produced by photosynthetic plants. Compared to this, the biomass produced by **chemolithoautotrophic** bacteria is quantitatively negligible. An exception is the primary production of biomass in the lightless depths of the ocean. In the shelf areas, where the continents diverged, the resulting fissures are penetrated by magma from below and seawater from above. The water then issuing from the sea bed contains gases (NH_3, H_2S, H_2, CO_2, CH_4) and minerals (Ca^{2+}, Fe^{2+}, Mn^{2+}, Cu^{2+}) (Fig. 17.1). On contact with the oxygen- and sulphate-containing deep waters, these ions form precipitates which cover the emerging water jet with a kind of pall. The description '**black smokers**' refers to the 'smoke trail' that appears when the water jet emerging at 350 °C mixes with the deep-sea water. In the neighbourhood of these 'hot springs' warm water ('warm springs'), also enriched with dissolved gases, emerges from the fissured basalt rock. These regions are noted for their abundance of mussels, crabs and worms which **feed on bacteria**, growing in suspension and on surfaces. Among them H_2S-oxidising organisms predominate; (endosymbiosis between sulphur-oxidising bacteria and worms has already been noted in Ch. 11.2). Thus, in the areas of the lightless depths there exist hot springs and ecosystems whose primary biomass is produced by **chemolithoautotrophy** rather than by photosynthesis (Fig. 17.1).

Lakes.   The science of limnology (study of lakes and ponds) has laid the foundations for our understanding of the various cycles and their integration. Lakes, ponds and pools represent well-defined aquatic systems and can be easily described. They always contain aerobic and anaerobic zones. Such regions are also found in soils, but their very

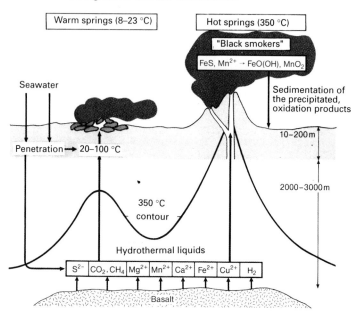

Fig. 17.1. *Hydrothermal vents at the bottom of the ocean.*

Inside the tectonic zones between the continents, geochemical changes cause erosion of the rigid magma (basalt) by seawater. The hot, hydrothermal waters carry dissolved gases and minerals to the deep ocean floor. Chemolithotrophic bacteria, which can utilise H_2S, Fe^{2+} and H_2, provide for primary production and supply the biomass for a species-poor, highly specialised ecosystem.

coexistence in close spatial proximity makes their investigation difficult. In lakes these regions occupy large areas and are much more amenable to analysis. It seems likely, though, that the results of limnological research can be applied in principle to soils and their microheterogeneities.

Biological processes in lakes and ponds are strongly influenced by the physical state of the water. Water has its maximum density at 4 °C. Water temperatures change with increasing depth, and a more or less stable seasonal **stratification** can occur (Fig. 17.2). Stratification is found in two types of lakes. One of these is represented by the freshwater lakes of the temperate zones. In the spring the cold water of the lake is warmed by the sun. The surface layer warms up most and decreases in density. This is called the **epilimnion**, which floats on the colder water layer, the **hypolimnion**. A transition zone, the **thermocline** or **metalimnion**, sepa-

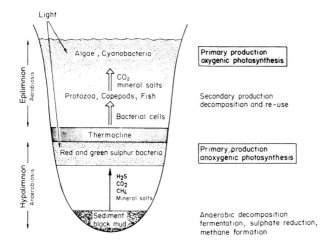

Fig. 17.2. *A vertical section through a eutrophic lake, as an example of an aquatic ecosystem.*

The thermocline (or chemocline) separates the aerobic from the anaerobic body of water. Photosynthetic primary production occurs in both. Anaerobiosis starts with anaerobic degradative processes in the sediment.

rates the layers. The boundaries between the zones can be very abrupt. In deep lakes, these layers may persist throughout the summer. Oxygen-consuming catabolic processes from the sediment render the hypolimnion anaerobic. The epilimnion is in contact with atmospheric oxygen and is stirred and mixed by wind; it therefore remains aerobic as a rule. In this way, the stratification also leads to a gradient of redox relations and chemical parameters. For this reason the thermocline is also called the **chemocline** or **redox discontinuity layer**. In the autumn the epilimnion becomes cooler. A fall of the epilimnion temperature to below that of the hypolimnion leads to mixing of the layers, which is also promoted by autumn gales. This autumnal mixing terminates the stratification. Thus the annual cycle has the effect of bringing the deep water layers to the surface, where they can be enriched with oxygen. In addition, the more nutrient-rich deeper waters become more evenly distributed. Lakes with such a complete circulation cycle are called **holomictic**. During the winter an inverse stratification can develop. The deeper water has a temperature of 4 °C and may be covered by a layer of colder water (which has a lower density) and possibly by ice. When the temperature of the surface water rises to above 4 °C in the spring, this stratification is abolished.

When nutrient-rich deep waters are brought to the surface, they cause a prolific multiplication of cyanobacteria and green algae, the so-called algal bloom. The extent of metabolism and biomass production depends on the 'trophy' (nutrient concentration) of the water. Eutrophic waters undergo pronounced changes of the kind described above, whereas in oligotrophic waters these changes are barely perceptible.

The holomictic lakes are distinguished from **meromictic** and **amictic** waters. In these, mixing of the water layers is incomplete or absent, so that a stable anaerobic hypolimnion (monimolimnion) becomes established and persists independent of seasons. Such permanent stratifications are found mostly in tropical lakes, whose surface waters rarely cool to temperatures below those of the deeper layers. Some meromictic lakes are also found in temperate zones. The stability of stratification in these is mostly due to high salt concentrations (fjords and inlets) or to geographical conditions.

Holomictic lakes can be used as an example for the biological processes that cause the seasonal stratification lasting for several months during the summer. In the epilimnion, which is penetrated by light, the phytoplankton (diatoms, flagellates, green algae and cyanobacteria) produce biomass. As a rule, further organic material also enters the lake from the environment. Some of these organic substances, especially those containing cellulose, tend to sink to the bottom, where they are decomposed. During the initial aerobic stages of degradation, oxygen is consumed and the sediment becomes anaerobic. The further anaerobic catabolism then results in the formation of anaerobic fermentation products and the liberation of H_2, H_2S, CH_4 and CO_2. Since there is no convection, these products enter the body of water rather slowly; only methane, the main product of the anaerobic food chain in the sediment, escapes in the form of gas bubbles. During its rise to the surface, some of the methane is dissolved in the water and it can then be oxidised by methane-utilising aerobic bacteria. The rapid distribution of methane through the water and the growth of methane-oxidising aerobic bacteria lead to rapid consumption of the oxygen present in the hypolimnion, which eventually becomes completely anaerobic. Once the hypolimnion has been rendered anaerobic, anaerobic microbial processes take over. The primary fermentation products are used for the reduction of nitrate and sulphate. By far the largest portion of the hydrogen sulphide (of the lake) is produced by reduction of sulphate in the body of the water (Fig. 17.3). The hypolimnion and the chemocline are the El Dorado of the anaerobic bacteria. When hydrogen sulphide is present and the illumination is suitable, appropriate purple and green sulphur bacteria grow

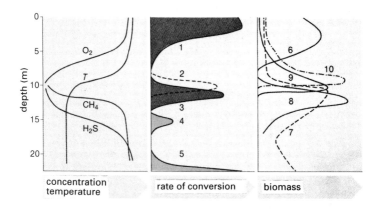

Fig. 17.3. *Idealised vertical profile of a freshwater lake in the temperate zones, showing concentrations, rates of conversion, and biomass.*

(Based on data of Y. I. Sorokin (1970), V. M. Gorlenko, G. A. Dubinina, and S. I. Kuznezow (1977) and of J. Overbeck (1972).) *T*, temperature in °C; O_2, H_2SO and CH_4 in mg/l. Conversion rates in $\mu g/$ (l·d): (1) CO_2 fixation in the light (oxygenic photosynthesis); (2) CO_2 fixation in the dark; (3) CO_2 fixation in the light (anoxygenic photosynthesis); (4) and (5) sulphate reduction; (6) to (10) biomass in mg/ml; (6) algae and cyanobacteria; (7) total bacterial mass; (8) phototrophic bacteria; (9) protozoa; (10) cladocera and copepods.

beneath the chemocline and form a layer of primary biomass production. Genera containing gas cacuoles (*Lamprocystis*, *Amoebobacter*, *Thiodictyon*, *Thiopedia*, *Pelodictyon*, *Ancalochloris*) as well as those propelled by flagella (*Chromatium*, *Thiospirillum*) are found in this zone. The biomass production due to anoxygenic photosynthesis is considerable; this can be seen in the number of ciliates, copepods and cladocera that live immediately above the chemocline and feed on the phototrophic bacteria. The sulphate produced by the purple sulphur bacteria is quickly reduced back to hydrogen sulphide by sulphate-reducing bacteria that can probably utilise excreted products of the phototrophic organisms as hydrogen donors.

The metalimnion is also characterised by vigorous biological activity. Some cyanobacteria that can tolerate hydrogen sulphide and anaerobic conditions flourish in this region; one of these is *Oscillatoria limnetica*. The idealised profile (Fig. 17.3) and the schematic diagram (Fig. 17.2) illustrate the situations described above. They emphasise the remarkable fact that a stratified lake can have two bodies of water in which photosynthetic primary production can occur: namely, oxygenic photosynthesis in the strata near the surface of the epilimnion and anoxygenic photosynthesis in the upper stratum of the hypolimnion.

Running waters (streams, brooks, rivers).   In natural, unpolluted streams the number of unicellular organisms is often so low that the water appears crystal clear. It is to be remembered, though, that a suspension of 10^6 bacteria/ml does not appear turbid to the human eye. As long as pollution remains low, the course of a brook or river several kilometres long is sufficient to mineralise the easily degradable organic materials introduced from neighbouring settlements. The composition of the microflora and fauna of a stream is a good indicator for the extent of pollution. As long as water fleas can be found, the water can be considered clean. The presence of *Sphaerotilus natans* indicates considerable organic pollution, and the smell of hydrogen sulphide is evidence of anaerobic sulphate reduction and should serve as an alerting signal.

Sewage and waste water treatment.   In principle, waste water installations consist of flowing watercourses whose organic load is decomposed aerobically and anaerobically by fungi and bacteria. The pollution of waste waters can be of different kinds according to whether only domestic waste and excrement are collected, or whether abbatoir wastes, liquid manures and industrial wastes are also dealt with. In many cases, heavy metals and persistant organic chemicals may also be found in waste waters. The purification of sewage water has the aim of removing solid and liquid mineral and organic contaminants before draining it into streams and rivers. Special procedures are required for the microbial decomposition of organic contaminants.

> The content of microbially degradable organic material can be estimated as the biological oxygen demand (BOD). That is, the amount of oxygen required for the aerobic oxidation of the organic material. Thus a BOD 5 value indicates the amount of oxygen (in mg) that the microflora consumes during 5 days, for the aerobic oxidation of the organic substances present. The chemical oxygen demand (COD) is the amount of oxygen consumed in the complete chemical oxidation of the organic material to CO_2 and H_2O.

A number of technical processes have been introduced in the purification of waste water. The various operations are based on common principles and they include: (1) removal of easily and moderately sedimentable solids in a grit chamber and sedimentation tank; (2) microbial oxidation of the dissolved organic materials by activated sludge or in a trickling

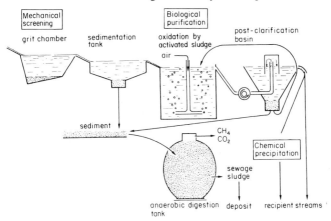

Fig. 17.4. *A sewage plant involving chemical and biological purification.*

filter; (3) anaerobic incubation of the sewage sludge obtained from the pre- and post-clarification basins in an anaerobic digestion tank, which produces methane and a sludge that is easily sedimented. This can be composted after removal of water and used as fertiliser, or it can be burned (Fig. 17.4). The purified clear water can then be drained directly or via screening devices into streams and rivers. It still contains the mineralised products nitrate, phosphate, ammonium and other ions. This can cause such enrichment of the water with nutrients as to increase primary production. To avoid such eutrophication, the water can be conducted through a sewage farm, used for fertilisation of forests, or subjected to an additional procedure to remove at least the nitrogen by denitrification. In addition, a further chemical purification procedure of precipitating the phosphate with iron salts can be applied.

17.2   Microorganisms as symbiotic partners

Interactions of many kinds exist between different microorganisms. In the course of evolution, some mutual or one-sided dependencies have developed which by far exceed the interactions in a food chain. When the prokaryotes and many eukaryotic microorganisms reached the present state of development, and higher forms began to emerge, these also became available as potential habitats. Animals and plants developed in an environment in which practically all prokaryotic types of metabolism were already present. It is therefore readily intelligible that numerous partnership relations developed between microorganisms and animals or plants. Such associations between different kinds of organisms are called **symbiosis**.

Several categories can be distinguished according to the advantages that the partners obtain from the association. If the association is advantageous to both partners it is termed **mutual symbiosis** (or mutualism). When one of the partners is damaged, the association is called **parasitism**. **Commensalism** is an association where one partner gains an advantage but the other is not damaged. In many cases the partners can coexist without any considerable influence on each other; this is called neutralism.

The associations can also differ in their spatial relations. If one of the partners exists outside the cells of the other, the relation is called **ectosymbiosis**; if one partner lives inside the cells of the other, it is called **endosymbiosis**. The larger of the two partners is usually referred to as the host.

The kind of advantage that one or both partners can derive from the association can also serve different functions. The association can have nutritional advantages, for example, fixation of nitrogen, decomposition of cellulose, or supply of basic nutrients or accessory factors. It can also serve recognition functions, as in the symbiosis of fish and luminescent bacteria. In many cases it can simply serve for protection, usually conferred by the host to the ecto- or endosymbiont, though in some cases the host may also derive protection against other parasitic or pathogenic microorganisms (e.g. in the intestinal tract or skin).

17.2.1   Mutualistic symbiosis

Between microorganisms.   There are numerous examples of mutual nutrition or syntrophy between microorganisms. The association between *Desulfuromonas acetoxidans* and *Chlorobium* is a syntrophic one, as is that between *Desulfovibrio* and *Chromatium*. In both these cases the first-named organism supplies hydrogen donors to the second, and the second supplies the first with hydrogen acceptors (Ch. 9.3). Syntrophy can also exist in the supply of vitamins or certain precursors. Both the fungus *Mucor ramannianus* and the yeast *Rhodotorula* depend on the presence of vitamin B_1 (thiamine) in the nutrient medium. The first organism can synthesise the pyrimidine component but not the thiazole; the yeast synthesises the thiazole but not the pyrimidine. During cultivation of the two organisms together, the fungus excretes pyrimidine and the yeast excretes thiazole into the medium, and the vitamin requirements of both are thereby satisfied.

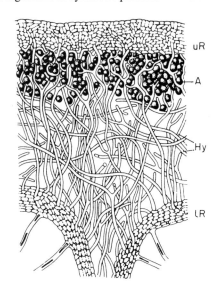

Fig. 17.5. *Section through a lichen thallus.*

A, alga (phycobiont); Hy, fungal hyphae (mycobiont); uR and lR, upper and lower cortical layer.

The **lichens** are examples of highly developed ectosymbiosis between microorganisms. In a lichen a fungus and an alga are so closely associated that they make up a unitary vegetative body (Fig. 17.5). Both partners gain advantage from this association. As a rule, the fungal component of the association, the **mycobiont**, determines the shape. The fungus obtains its organic nutrients from the alga, namely its CO_2 fixation products; in turn it supplies the alga with minerals and protects it from unfavourable conditions, especially from dehydration. The **phycobionts** of lichens can be green algae or cyanobacteria. It is possible to separate the two partners and culture them in isolation, and also to construct artificial (i.e. new) lichens. Lichens colonise extreme ecosystems in which neither of the partners would be able to exist on its own.

Commensalism.   In the production of cheeses from naturally curdled milk (by lactic acid fermentation), a fungus and a bacterium are involved. This association is advantageous only to the bacterium; the fungus oxidises the acid present in the curd and thereby renders it habitable for the bacterium. Another example is the association between aerobes and anaerobes, where the aerobes, by rapidly consuming oxygen, renders the habitat anaerobic and hence suitable for the growth of anaerobes.

Other examples concern microorganisms excreting depolymerases by which polysaccharides, proteins and nucleic acids can be hydrolysed and made accessible, not only for their own nutrition, but also for that of other microorganisms.

Microorganisms and plants.   Very frequently more bacteria are found in the soil surrounding plant roots, the **rhizosphere**, than in soil free of roots. Evidently, growth of bacteria is promoted by organic nutrients excreted by the plant roots. The advantage that such relatively loose associations might offer the plant is not easily recognised. However since many soil bacteria carry out processes that are useful to plants, such as nitrogen fixation and decomposition of almost insoluble salts, mutualistic associations are clearly possible. In recent years several bacteria that are commonly found associated with certain grasses have been recognised as nitrogen-fixing organisms: for example, *Azotobacter paspali* in the rhizosphere of *Paspalum notatum*; *Azospirillum lipoferum* in the root region of *Digitaria* and maize.

The roots of many plants are closely associated with fungi in what are called mycorrhizae. A large number of fungi, including mushrooms, can penetrate plant roots, stimulate their growth by auxin production, and penetrate into the cells. Fungal experts know that many edible mushrooms are found in the vicinity of certain trees (pine, larch, oak, spruce, etc.) that are the host plants of the **mycorrhiza**. The fungi, upon penetrating into the cortical cells, form vesicular and arbuscular mycorrhizae (in the form of vesicles and branched structures, respectively). The advantages to the partners lie in the easy access to assimilation products of the plant for the fungus, and in the highly effective absorption of mineral salts (phosphate, fixed nitrogen) from the soil for the plant.

The association of plants with nitrogen fixing ecto- or endosymbiotic bacteria has already been discussed in Ch. 13.1. The association of *Rhizobium* species in the **root nodules** of leguminous plants belong to the most highly differentiated symbiotic interactions. This root nodule symbiosis is a very good example of the establishment of an endosymbiotic system and furnishes some of the basic assumptions for the endosymbiotic hypothesis relating to the development of eukaryotic cells discussed in Ch. 2.1.

Microorganisms and animals.   The number of symbiotic associations between animals and microorganisms is immense. The rumen symbiosis in ruminants represents one of the few cases where the advantages to both partners are fairly obvious (Ch. 14.1). Research on symbiotic systems, especially those involving lower animals and protozoa, poses many problems, often of methodological difficulties. One of the main questions is whether the microbial flora or fauna that inhabits the intestinal tract provides some protection against pathogenic microorganisms, or whether it performs specific digestive functions. Only a few of the numerous examples will be dealt with here. The symbiosis between giant tube worms (**Pogonophores**) and bacteria has already been dealt with (Ch. 11.2). In the trophosomes of *Riftia pachyptila*, H_2S-oxidising bacteria grow as endosymbionts. They are supplied with oxygen and H_2S by the blood of the host and serve as the sole food for the worm. Recently, small pogonophores were discovered which contain methane-oxidising bacteria as endosymbionts.

Protozoa, both free-living and those ciliates, flagellates, and amoebae that inhabit the intestinal tracts of ruminants, termites and cockroaches, very often are themselves colonised by bacterial ecto- and endo-symbionts.

One of the phenomena that became widely known in the early years of microbial genetics is the 'killer gene' of *Paramecium aurelia*. At first Sonneborn showed that two groups could be distinguished among the strains of this ciliate; the strains of one group liberate a toxin to which they themselves are resistant. The other group is sensitive and the organisms are killed by the toxin. The ability to produce the toxic substance and to kill other cells was found to be cytoplasmic and not determined by nuclear genes. It is thought that the 'killer' ability can be transmitted by conjugation, the sensitive recipient thereby acquiring the killer character. It was found that the killer property was associated with particles that were called 'kappa' (kappa factor); eventually, these were recognised as endosymbiotic bacteria. The killer strains could be cured of the kappa particles by treatment with antibiotics. The kappa particles are easily recognised under the microscope because of the presence of a highly refractive inclusion body, called the R body. The R body apparently consists of a rolled-up protein chain and it is thought that the toxic killer substance may be associated with it. Discovery of phage heads inside the kappa cells has made the system even more complicated; the kappa cells apparently harbour temperate phages. Unfortunately, outside the host, no pure cultures of the undoubtedly endosymbiotic bacteria have so far been obtained. Research on the kappa system has been reactivated by the discovery of R bodies in recently isolated soil bacteria.

Many protozoa are hosts to **methanogenic** bacteria, cyanobacteria and unicellular algae. Among the anaerobic ciliates and amoebae found in sea- and freshwater sediments (and in the rumen), some contain methanogenic bacteria as endosymbionts. These symbionts can be easily demonstrated by fluorescence microscopy because of the fluorescence of their coenzymes (F_{420} and methylpterin). The symbiosis rests on the ability of some protozoa to evolve molecular hydrogen which can be converted to methane by the methanogenic bacteria. (The rumen protozoa include *Endiplodinium*. The sapropelic protozoa include the giant amoeba *Pelomyxa palustris* and several small amoebae, as well as ciliates like *Metopus contortus*. Sapropelic protozoa which contain phototrophic organisms are easily recognised by their pigments.) The green algae are called **zoochlorellae** and the yellow and brown algae **zooxanthellae**. The flagellate *Cyanophora* harbours symbiotic cyanobacteria, known as **cyanellae**.

Many **insects** harbour ciliates, yeasts and bacteria as symbionts, either in the intestinal tract or in special intestinal appendices. The microorganisms are present as ectosymbionts or in the cells of specific tissues as endosymbionts. The function of these microorganisms can be easily surmised in the case of those insects, such as wood-eating termites, that feed on poorly degradable materials (wood cellulose), or in the case of many aphids and heteroptera that have an unbalanced diet (plant juices). The symbionts either carry out digestive functions or supply required accessory nutrients (steroids, vitamins, amino acids, etc.). Morphological-anatomical investigations on insect symbiosis are well advanced, especially by the work of P. Buchner's group. Physiological-biochemical investigations, however, have been frustrated mostly by the inability to culture the symbiotic microorganisms outside the host.

In many insects the organs that harbour the endosymbionts (mycetomes) are derived from continuations or appendices of the hind gut. In contrast, the rumen in ruminants is an organ of the foregut. Hind-gut appendices are also found in mammals. In many herbivorous mammals the digestive action supported by microorganisms takes place in hind-gut appendages. Since the host cannot reap sufficient advantage from this location of the symbiosis, it becomes understandable that some animals eat their own excreta (coprophagy) in order to benefit from the basic and accessory nutrients provided by the microbes.

The composition of the human **intestinal flora** has been discussed already in Ch. 8.4 (see also the accompanying Box). The mutualistic character of the association between humans and their intestinal flora becomes obvious when the relationship is disturbed and the bacterial population is eliminated by antibiotic treatment or chemotherapeutic measures. The function of the intestinal flora is especially clearly recognisable in animals reared under sterile conditions. Although the animals can develop normally provided that they are fed an appropriate diet, their sensitivity to infections is drastically enhanced. It seems that a normal bacterial flora also has an important protective function against pathogenic and opportunistic microorganisms.

Similar relations exist between humans and the **skin flora**. Human skin has a characteristic bacterial flora, consisting primarily of mycobacteria, streptococci, staphylococci, and the propionibacteria, deriving their nutrients from perspiration. The normal skin flora does not have any adverse consequences for man, except for the production (under some circumstances) of odorous substances. The useful functions of

The human gastro-intestinal tract consists of the oesophagus, the stomach, the duodenum, the jejunum and ileum (which constitute the small intestine), the colon and the rectum. The upper part contains only a few bacteria, allochthonous and mouth bacteria, which reach the stomach with the chymus. Most bacteria, including pathogens, do not survive passage through the stomach because of its very low pH (0.5–2.0). There are rarely more than 10 organisms/ml beyond the pylorus,

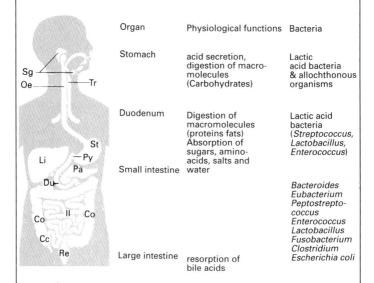

	Organ	Physiological functions	Bacteria
	Stomach	acid secretion, digestion of macro-molecules (Carbohydrates)	Lactic acid bacteria & allochthonous organisms
	Duodenum	Digestion of macromolecules (proteins fats) Absorption of sugars, amino-acids, salts and water	Lactic acid bacteria (*Streptococcus, Lactobacillus, Enterococcus*)
	Small intestine		
	Large intestine	resorption of bile acids	*Bacteroides Eubacterium Peptostrepto-coccus Enterococcus Lactobacillus Fusobacterium Clostridium Escherichia coli*

The human gastrointestinal tract and its bacterial flora. Cc, Caecum (with appendix); Co, colon; Du, duodenum; Il, ileum; Li, liver; Oe, oesophagus; Pa, pancreas; Py, pylorus; Re, rectum; Sg, salivary gland; St, stomach; Tr, trachea.

provided that the food has not been extensively diluted with liquid. Lactic acid bacteria are found in the duodenum. The pH begins to rise in the upper small intestine (jejunum), the food bolus becomes alkaline and the flora changes. Facultative anaerobes (coliforms) provide for the consumption of any oxygen, and strict anaerobes, such as *Bacteroides*, *Eubacterium*, *Peptostreptococcus* and *Bifidobacterium* gain predominance. 10^5 to 10^7 bacteria/ml are found in the food bolus at this stage.

The wall of the small intestine – which, with a length of about 3 m, has an internal surface of 100 m² – is covered with a bacterial lawn. In the large intestine the bacterial density becomes extraordinary, with 10^{11} cells/g, so that they may represent 20–30% (by weight) of the composition of faeces. *Bacteroides*, *Eubacterium* and *Bifidobacterium* are again predominant, though the colon usually also contains coliforms, lactobacteria, clostridia and yeasts. *Escherichia coli*, however, usually represents no more than 1% of the total bacterial mass.

The composition of the food, and resorption by the epithelia of the different intestinal regions, have a decisive influence on the **microbial activity of the intestinal tract**. Water and salts including Na^+, K^+, SO_4^{2-} and NO_3^- are reabsorbed in the upper small intestine. Only 200–300 ml of water per day reach the large intestine. Di- and monosaccharides are also reabsorbed in the upper small intestine, but **alpha-galactosides** are not reabsorbed: humans do not have the appropriate alpha-galactosidases. When excess sugar or alpha-galactosides in the food reach the lower small intestine or the large intestine, they are metabolised by fermentative bacteria with the production of gases (H_2, CO_2 and sometimes CH_4). It is likely that the flatulence that often accompanies the consumption of beans and other pulses is due to their content of alpha-galactosides, such as raffinose, stachyose and verbacose which altogether can account for 5–10% of the weight. The fact that some people produce larger amounts of gas, even without consumption of alpha-galactosides, is probably due to their lower ability to digest some polysaccharides and to absorb sugars. A genetically determined reduced ability to absorb **lactose** is fairly widely distributed among members of non-white races. In these people the lactose reaches the last part of the intestine and leads to microbial gas formation. Only about a third of these people who have been tested produce methane. In the normal human intestine, although many non-reabsorbed metabolites are broken down, little toxic material is produced. Even **nitrate** does not represent a definite danger, because it is largely absorbed in the stomach and upper small intestine and eliminated by the kidneys, before it can be microbially reduced in the lower small intestine or the colon to nitrite and lead to the formation of nitrosamine, which are both known to be carcinogenic.

Research into the reabsorption of food components in the different regions of the intestinal tract is still in its infancy. The best-researched digestive systems are those of ruminants and termites. Because of the very important role of invertebrates in the decomposition of organic substances in soil, elucidation of microbial metabolism in their digestive tracts merits greater attention.

the skin flora, again, are recognised when topical application or excessive internal medication with antibiotics have a growth-inhibitory effect on the skin bacteria. Often, the result is proliferation of pathogenic yeasts (*Candida albicans*) and other pathogenic fungi.

Many marine fish have **organs of luminescence**. These are usually highly differentiated morphologically and are colonised by luminescent bacteria (*Vibrio fischeri*: see Ch. 8.4).

17.2.2   Antagonistic symbiosis

In some symbiotic associations between different microorganisms and between microorganisms and plants or animals, the host suffers more or less pronounced damage. Several kinds of parasitism have already been described, for example, that of the bacterial parasite *Bdellovibrio bacteriovorus* (Ch. 3.14), the obligatory cell parasites rickettsiae and chlamydiae (Ch. 3.18), the causative organisms of plant diseases (*Erwinia, Corynebacterium, Pseudomonas, Uredo, Ustilago, Puccinia, Claviceps*), and those of animal diseases. The disciplines of veterinary and human microbiology and plant pathology deal with the theoretical aspects of parasitism and with the intervention in the equilibria between parasitic microorganisms and their hosts.

Pathogenic bacteria.   Although this textbook does not deal with medical and veterinary aspects of microbiology, nor with immunology, the most important human pathogens – most of which have been mentioned in the text – are collected in Table 17.1.

17.3   Microorganisms and the evolution of the earth

Microorganisms have played an important role in the formation of the earth's crust. The mixtures of elements and compounds that made up the primeaval rocks became partially separated due to the activities of microorganisms.

The deposition of a number of raw materials that are mined and extracted today are solely or partially the result of microbial action.

Deposition of iron.   The largest iron ore deposits are the 'banded iron formations', referred to in short as BIF. The deposition of these iron oxides occurred in the main during the period from $2.8–1.6 \times 10^9$ years ago. Until then the iron solubilised from the magnetic rocks of the ocean floor as Fe^{2+} ions had accumulated in large amounts, together with other

Table 17.1. *Causative organisms of bacterial infections and toxin production*

Organism	Disease	Toxin, target tissue
Bordetella pertusis	Whooping cough	Bronchial epithelium
Bordetella burgdorferi	Borrelliosis	Tissue
Chlamydia trachomatis	Trachoma, eye and venereal disease	
Chlamydia psittaci	Parrot disease	
Clostridium botulinum	Botulism	Neurotoxin
Clostridium histolyticum	Gas gangrene	Proteinases, tissues
Clostridium perfringens	Gas gangrene, food poisoning	Alpha-toxin, connective tissues
Clostridium tetani	Tetanus	Neurotoxin
Corynebacterium diphtheriae	Diphtheria	Diphtheria toxin
Escherichia coli	Gastroenteritis	Enterotoxin
Helicobacter pylori	Gastroenteritis, stomach inflammation	Acid production
Legionella pneumophila	Legionnaire's disease, pneumonia	
Listeria monocytogenes	Listeriosis, general infection	Toxins, macrophages
Mycobacterium leprae	Leprosy	Skin and other tissues
Mycobacterium tuberculosis	Tuberculosis	Lung and other tissues
Neisseria gonorrhoeae	Gonorrhoea	Urethral epithelium
Neisseria meningitidis	Meningitis	Central nervous system
Pseudomonas aeruginosa	Skin and lung infections	Necrotic toxin, exotoxin A
Ricketisia prowazekii	Typhus	Capillaries
Salmonella enteritidis	Gastroenteritis	LPS
Salmonella paratyphi	Paratyphoid	LPS
Salmonella typhi	Typhoid	LPS
Salmonella typhimurium	Gastroenteritis	Endotoxin
Shigella dysenteriae	Dysentery, diarrhoea	Neurotoxin
Staphylococcus aureus	Pus-forming, food poisoning	Alpha-toxin (enterotoxin)

Table 17.1. *contd.*

Streptococcus pneumoniae	Pneumonia	Haemolysin
Streptococcus pyogenes	Scarlet fever	Streptolysins
Treponema pallidum	Syphilis	Tissues
Vibrio cholerae	Cholera	Enterotoxin
Yersinia pestis	Bubonic plague, pneumonic plague	Plague toxin

ions (S^{2-}, Mn^{2+}) in the sea. With the start of oxygenic photosynthesis by cyanobacteria, S^{2-} was oxidised to SO_4^{2+} and Fe^{2+} to Fe^{3+} ions. Precipitation of iron oxide over wide areas occurred when the iron-containing deep waters made contact with oxygen-containing surface waters. In the BIFs, iron oxide layers alternate with flint (0.2–2.0 mm). This layering is interpreted as a result of seasonal rhythms of photosynthesis in the sedimentation basin. Oxygen could accumulate in the atmosphere only when the sulphur and iron oxidation in the oceans was completed, about 1.6×10^9 years ago.

Microorganisms also participated in the mobilisation of the iron contained in granite and its reprecipitation. When the sulphur components of pyrites and mercasite are oxidised to sulphuric acid by *Thiobacillus thiooxidans* and *T. ferrooxidans*, the iron is solubilised as ferrous salt and is then oxidised by *T. ferrooxidans* to Fe^{3+} salts (Ch. 11.4, leaching of ores). On neutralisation of the water, the Fe^{3+} is precipitated as $Fe(OH)_3$. Many deposits of very pure iron ore are probably due to a microbial leaching process occurring over millions of years. In other places the solubilisation of iron may be promoted by organic acids (humic acid). The final oxidation of Fe^{2+} to Fe^{3+} can also be carried out biologically, i.e. by *Gallionella* or *Siderocapsa* (at neutral pH). The results of these conversions are bog iron ore and marsh or swamp ore.

Deposition of calcium carbonate. In many waters calcium is present as $Ca(HCO_3)_2$ or $CaSO_4$. As a result of pH changes and the withdrawal of CO_2 by photosynthesis, bicarbonate is converted to the insoluble calcium carbonate and precipitated. Under anaerobic conditions the reduction of sulphate to hydrogen sulphide by sulphate-reducing bacteria also leads to the precipitation of the original calcium sulphate as calcium carbonate:

$$CaSO_4 + 8[H] + CO_2 \rightarrow CaCO_3 + 3H_2O + H_2S$$

A large part of limestone may have arisen by calcium bicarbonate being transported in tropical waters and being precipitated as $CaCO_3$ when an increase in temperature led to liberation of CO_2.

$$Ca(HCO_3)_2 \rightleftharpoons CaCO_3 + H_2O + CO_2$$

Deposition of sulphur. The deposition of extractable sulphur is due to bacterial sulphate reduction. When organic compounds are decomposed anaerobically in the presence of sulphates, these sulphates are the preferred hydrogen acceptors. The resulting hydrogen sulphide inhibits all other potentially possible anaerobic respiratory processes. Isotope studies have confirmed that sulphur deposits in Texas and Louisiana are of biogenic origin. Sulphur occurs in seawater predominantly as two stable isotopes: 95% as ^{32}S and 4% as ^{34}S. In bacterial sulphate reduction (limited in the main by the supply of hydrogen donors), the light isotope-containing $^{32}SO_4^{2-}$ has a greater chance of being taken up by the cells than the heavier $^{34}SO_4^{2-}$. The resulting H_2S therefore has a lower ^{34}S content than the seawater sulphate. Oxidation of the 'light' H_2S (whether biological or abiotic) produces 'light' sulphur. Thus, the isotope content in the above deposits identified them as biogenic. The isotope content of biogenic sulphur is quite different from that determined for volcanic sulphur.

Discussion of biogeochemical conversions could be continued with respect to the deposition of coal, petroleum, natural gas, bauxite and silica. Microorganisms took part in these processes by their metabolic activities: oxidations, fermentations, acid production, reductions, carbon dioxide assimilation, and the formation of transient products. These reactions have resulted in mineralisation, solubilisations, mobilisation, and immobilisations. The problems associated with the role of microorganisms in the formation, change and disintegration of rocks are dealt with by the discipline of geomicrobiology.

17.4   The evolution of microorganisms

Basic **Molecular** structures and biochemical **reactions** are the same in all living organisms. This conclusion is constantly being confirmed and extended. It was first formulated as the '**unity of biochemistry**' (Ch. 7.1). Compared to this **basic** uniformity, differences and variations in detail appear of minor significance. It can be assumed that all living organisms extant today have gone through a common evolutionary pathway for a considerable portion of their history. Life forms of increasing complexity and specialisation must have arisen from simple forms which did not survive. Their ecological niches were often colonised later by organisms derived from more highly developed forms which had regressed to quasi-primitive properties. The evolution of organisms is one of the central problems in biology; in the words of Dobzhansky, 'Nothing in Biology makes sense except in the light of evolution'.

The primitive atmosphere of the earth.   It is thought that the earth originated in a collision of interstellar material, and the consequent heating and melting of the earth's core then pressed water and gases to the surface. Experts assume that the original atmosphere of the earth had a composition similar to the present gaseous atmosphere of the planets Mars or Venus: namely, about 3% N_2, 96% CO_2, 0.1% H_2O, and less than 1% oxygen. Photolysis of the water vapour present in the earth's atmosphere might have produced oxygen, but this would be quickly reduced by ferrous iron and hydrogen sulphide. The oxygen-free atmosphere provided favourable conditions for chemical evolution.

Chemical evolution.   The hypothesis that life might have arrived on this planet from other sources is hardly under serious discussion at the present time. Self-reproducing biological units must have arisen on Earth. According to the model proposed by Haldane and Oparin, large amounts of organic materials must have accumulated in the earliest period. At that time there were no organisms that could utilise the organic compounds and mineralise them. Since the experimental demonstration – originally by Miller and by many others since – that simple organic molecules can be synthesised from inorganic substances (H_2, CO_2, CH_4, NH_3, H_2O, etc.) under appropriate conditions, there is no longer any doubt about the occurrence of chemical evolution on Earth. It is assumed that in a reduced, oxygen-free atmosphere, organic compounds were formed under the influence of chemically effective radiations by the sun and electrical discharges; that these then became adsorbed on clay-like minerals (montmorillonite) and pyrites and accumulated in water. Such minerals with extended surface areas may have played an important role in the structuring and polymerisation of building blocks. A most interesting hypothesis is based on the discovery that iron (II) sulphide can react with H_2S under strictly anaerobic conditions to form pyrite and hydrogen.

$$FeS + H_2S \rightarrow FeS_2 + H_2; \Delta G = -38.4 \text{ kJ/mol}$$

This reaction is exergonic and yields energy as well as a structured and positively charged surface. It therefore fulfils the prerequisite for the orderly polymerisation of organic building blocks. It can be assumed that large quantities of organic compounds plus structured cationic and anionic surfaces supplied the external conditions under which chemical evolution could advance to the emergence of the first self-reproducing life forms.

Biological evolution.   The transition from non-living organic material to a living cell must have occurred in a relatively short period. There is consensus that the Earth originated $4.5–4.6 \times 10^9$ years ago; stromatolites have been found in the oldest (about 3.5×10^9 years old) sedimentary rocks so far discovered. Sedimentary rocks in which organic carbon (C_{org}) could be demonstrated are of a similar age. Stromatolites and C_{org} are universally accepted as the first life clues and as a sign that autotrophy must have predominated among the earliest living forms.

> The arguments supporting this assumption are as follows. (1) The **archaic stromatolites** present extensive similarities to more recent forms. Stromatolites are by definition organo-sedimentary structures (biogenic) which are formed by the binding and precipitation of sediment-forming minerals in the course of the growth and metabolism of microorganisms. At the present time stromatolites are formed by filamentous cyanobacteria. Their autotrophic CO_2 fixation produces an alkaline environment which precipitates calcium carbonate. This results in a chalky matrix with manifold tubules. The organisms involved in formation of (the older) stromatolites must (have) be(en) filamentous, autotrophic gliding bacteria. Since cyanobacteria fulfil all these conditions, it has to be assumed that the archaic stromatolites bear witness to oxygenic photosynthesis carried out by cyanobacteria as long as 3.5×10^9 years ago. The participation of autotrophic bacteria remains undisputed. Carbon dioxide-fixing autotrophic bacteria occur among anoxygenic phototrophs as well as among anaerobically respiring (methanogenic and H_2S-forming) chemolithautotrophs. Filamentous forms also occur among these.
>
> (2) The second argument in favour of the assumption that the organic carbon found in archaic sediments is derived from autotrophic bacteria is based on **isotope** data. The organic carbon (C_{org}) isolated from sediments is in the form of an acid-insoluble, highly polymerised end product of the conversion of organic material into sediment, the so-called 'kerogen'. Carbon, like many other bioelements, occurs as a mixture of the two isotopes, ^{12}C and ^{13}C. All known pathways of autotrophic CO_2 fixation lead to enrichment of the synthesised cellular substance with the lighter isotope, ^{12}C. This has been found in numerous measurements of current CO_2-fixing bacteria. Since the archaic 'kerogen' is found to have almost the same isotopic composition as the mass of recent autotrophic bacteria, it seems logical that the formation of the archaic 'kerogen' must be due to autotrophic bacteria.

The evolution of prokaryotes.   On the basis of established facts and some controversial assumptions, a highly speculative model can be proposed for the sequence in which different metabolic types developed

(Fig. 1.3). The question whether the first bacteria carried out autotrophic or heterotrophic metabolism was the subject of extensive arguments for a long time. However, there are no reasons to exclude the possibility that **heterotrophic fermentors** and **autotrophic, anaerobically respiring** bacteria developed **simultaneously**; especially in view of the easy exchange of genetic material at the early stages of evolution. The abundantly present organic compounds may have allowed the early development of metabolic processes which are now found in contemporary fermenting organisms and play a predominant role in central metabolic pathways.

The availability of CO_2, sulphur, sulphite, ferric iron and molecular hydrogen (the latter provided by de-gassing of magma and basalt as well as the formation of pyrites and the photolysis of water) would have allowed the development of the metabolic processes that we know in anaerobic respiration (Ch. 9.2, 9.3, 9.4). Thus, an efficient electron transport system with the production of a proton potential, which could drive ATP regeneration, could have evolved. At this stage the iron- and nickel-containing porphyrins and carbon autotrophy may have developed. The **reductive acetyl-CoA pathway** is undoubtedly the first pathway of autotrophic carbon dioxide fixation. Present-day representatives of this type are the methanogenic and acetogenic bacteria, and the sulphidogenic, sulphur and sulphite-respiring organisms. The now well-known 'horizontal transfer' of hereditary information by bacteriophages, plasmids or free DNA make it likely that similar mechanisms allowed information exchange in archaic times, and provided the possibility of rapid evolution.

Following the invention of electron-transport phosphorylation, development of photosystem I made it possible to utilise **light as an energy source**. Magnesium porphyrins (**chlorophyll**) served as reaction centres. The first phototrophic organisms probably assimilated organic substances in the light, as do the Rhodospirillaceae. Acquisition of the ability to fix carbon dioxide via the ribulose-bisphosphate cycle, and to utilise inorganic hydrogen donors (H_2, H_2S, S) resulted in the type of metabolism found in the purple sulphur bacteria (Chromatiaceae). The development of the second photosystem made the organisms even less dependent on exogenous electron donors such as H_2 and H_2S, or organic compounds. Photosystem II allows an open-chain electron transport with water as the electron donor. This process is obligatorily linked to the liberation of oxygen. Oxygenic photosynthesis initiated the development of an aerobic atmosphere on earth. These first oxygen-producing photosynthetic organisms were the cyanobacteria.

Autotrophy.   Three pathways of **autotrophic carbon dioxide fixation** are now known: the ribulose-bisphosphate cycle, the reductive tricarboxylic acid cycle and the reductive acetyl-CoA pathway. The fixation of CO_2

and its conversion to metabolites is a reductive process. In the absence of oxygen, where re-oxidation of metabolites can be excluded, a sequential arrangement of completely reversible enzyme reactions would be sufficient – under such anoxic conditions – to produce reduced carbon compounds with a minimal expenditure of energy. These arguments give a plausible explanation for the widespread occurrence of the reductive acetyl-CoA pathway among strictly anaerobic bacteria. When oxygen is present, however, the reduction of CO_2 needs a sequence of enzyme reactions containing irreversible steps. Such a sequence is the **Calvin cycle**. This is expensive in energy and probably evolved from central sugar metabolism. Only the oxygenic and anoxygenic photosynthetic organisms and some chemolithoautotrophs derived from the purple bacteria possess this pathway. It has not been found in any of the Archaebacteria. This supports the assumption that the development of the Calvin cycle occurred after the division into Archaebacteria and Eubacteria. On the other hand, the acetyl-CoA pathway seems to be most widely distributed among the Archaebacteria, and is found in Eubacteria only among desulphurisers, acetogenic clostridia and in *Acetobacterium*.

The **transition from the original reduced atmosphere to the oxygen-containing atmosphere** was undoubtedly the greatest upheaval in the evolution of living organisms and of minerals. The development of cytochrome into terminal oxidases and the utilisation of oxygen as electron acceptor led to the type of metabolism of the aerobic respiring bacteria. It is thought that all phototrophic and aerobically respiring prokaryotes that are known today were already present 2.1×10^9 years ago. According to geological evidence, a small amount of oxygen was present already 2.7×10^9 years ago, and since about 1.2×10^9 years ago, the whole of life on earth has been based on biological photosynthesis and the oxygen-producing plants.

The aerobic oxidation of metals and minerals has meant that the evolution of living organisms also played a part in the evolution and development of today's rock structures.

Until about 0.6×10^9 years ago, the oxygen content of the atmosphere probably reached only about 2%. Colonisation of the land masses by green plants led to dense plant coverage and brought a rapid increase in the oxygen concentration of the atmosphere, to reach the present value of 21%. This production of oxygen was accompanied by deposition of carbon in the form of coal, gas and petroleum, as well as carbon-rich sedimentary rocks.

Fossil evidence from the early Precambrian is very sparse. Because of their small size and lack of hard components, fossils of primitive living forms could survive only under very special conditions. Structures about

2.7×10^9 years old, seen in some sediments from Minnesota, have been interpreted as bacteria and cyanobacteria. South African sediments that also appear to contain some bacteria-like structures are even older: about 3.1×10^9 years. These are the oldest known traces of living matter.

Bacteria can be regarded as the surviving living witnesses to the early evolution of organisms. Many bacteria and cyanobacteria types that were successful and widely distributed in earlier times lead a modest and spartan existence nowadays; anaerobic bacteria, for example, have survived only in ecosystems that offer them the appropriate conditions.

The evolution of eukaryotes.   Eukaryotes seem to have evolved only from the time sufficient oxygen for aerobic life became available. Practically all eukaryotes, with very few exceptions, are aerobes. The prokaryotes had already occupied many ecological niches. Their development of metabolic–physiological diversity was probably due to their simple cell structure, high growth rate, well-developed regulatory systems, and their multiple mechanisms for gene transfer. Further evolutionary development, however, was probably limited by such factors as their small genome size, small cell size, and the predominantly haploid state of the genome. The new environment, namely aerobic conditions, allowed higher energy yields. Exploitation of these energy yields, however, needed larger-sized cells with potential for greater structural differentiation and, hence, a genome several times larger to store more information. A genome size of 5×10^9 seems to be the upper limit for one double-stranded bacterial chromosome. Further development required a new model.

The differences between a prokaryotic and a eukaryotic cell are enormous. The most important features specific to eukaryotic cells can be summarised again. (1) Separation of the DNA-information store from the metabolic space by a nuclear membrane. (2) The consequent uncoupling of transcription (in the nuclear space) from translation (in the cytoplasm). (3) Division of the genome into a number of portions, i.e. several linear chromosomes in place of one circular one. (4) DNA replication limited to the interphase; each chromosome has several replicons and the daughter chromosomes are separated by mitosis. (5) Intracellular mechanisms of motility by means of actin microfilaments and tubulin microtubules (to enable chromosomes to move during mitosis, meiosis, nuclear pairing) and the development of vesicles (lysosomes, peroxisomes and other microbodies). (6) Split genes in DNA and gene splicing in RNA. (7) Nucleosome structure, i.e. association of DNA on bead-like arrangements of histone complexes. (8) Meiosis, that is, pairing of chromosomes and reduction of the diploid to the haploid number; this made possible the development of sexual combination with new combinations of genes and alternation between haplophase and diplophase during vegetative growth. (9) Exocytosis: exoenzymes need not be made at or in the cytoplasmic membrane and simultaneously exported, but can be synthesised on intracellular membranes (the ER), transported into cisternae, and emptied to the outside. (10) Endocytosis as phagocytosis and pinocytosis, as well as the ability to maintain endosymbionts. (11) Mitochondria and chloroplasts for energy (ATP) regeneration. (12) 9 + 2 cilial structure.

Thus the eucyte differs from the protocyte by a multiplicity of structures and functions. Although a few eukaryotes are known that lack one or the other of these features, there are no primitive forms that could indicate the sequence in which these new characters developed. It seems probable that individual steps (in the changes leading to a novel feature) conferred only slight selective advantage, especially when compared to the next, better-endowed organism. The 'missing links' have not survived and were probably so unstable that even intermediate forms with analysable functional differences were not preserved in the fossil record. Very few recent organisms could be regarded as forms derived from 'missing links'. Any possibility of constructing a sequence for the appearance of the features listed above seems remote. It can be assumed, however, that during the early stages of eukaryotic evolution, several models of cellular organisation had arisen before the multicellular organisms appeared.

Surviving monopolies of eukaryotes.   It is noteworthy that the eukaryotes specialised in photosynthesis and aerobic life and left many essential ecological functions to the prokaryotes. Some of these functions are nitrogen fixation, nitrification, denitrification, sulphate respiration, sulphur and metal oxidations, and methane formation and utilisation. The nitrogen and sulphur cycles in nature are either entirely or predominantly the domains of prokaryotes. Thus the prokaryotes collectively, and without participation of the eukaryotes, can accomplish the elementary cycles of our planet and maintain the biosphere, but the eukaryotes are unable to do this on their own.

Whereas the prokaryotes developed on their own for thousands of millions of years, eukaryotes were never the only organisms on earth. They always had to deal with prokaryotes. They afforded new ecological niches and protection to the prokaryotes and also served as prey. The highly developed defence, protection and survival mechanisms of multicellular organisms might, in part, have arisen in response to aggressive properties of prokaryotes. On the other hand, the eukaryotes also learned to draw benefits from their association with prokaryotes and 'took them into service' as it were, as ectosymbionts (in the intestinal tract and rumen and on the skin) and as endosymbionts (for nitrogen fixation, biomass production via photosynthesis, or utilisation of H_2S and removal of H_2). The evolution of organisms presents fascinating problems. Their elucidation has only just commenced.

Reading list

It has become impossible, due to space limitations, to continue citation of the epoch-making original papers. The following list gives an overview of the literature, citing textbooks, monographs, review articles, and reference works. Recent reports on specific problems or groups of organisms are found in the periodicals and review journals (i.e. Advances ..., Annual Reviews, Symposia, Progress in ..., etc.) listed at the end. Some references are given in the legends to figures and tables and have not been included here. To keep a breast of current developments in research, it is necessary to resort to frequent and regular consultation of the journals listed at the end (and many others).

I General textbooks of microbiology

Atlas, R. M. (1984). *Microbiology, Fundamentals and Applications.* New York: Macmillan.

Brock, T. D. & Madigan, M. T. (1991). *Biology of Microorganisms*, 6th edn. Englewood Cliffs, NJ: Prentice-Hall.

Davis, B. D., Dulbecco, R., Eisen, H. N. & Ginsberg, H. S. (1990). *Microbiology*, 4th edn. New York: Harper & Row.

Jawetz, E., Melnick, J. L. & Adelberg, E. A. (1991). *Review of Medical Microbiology*, 19th edn. Los Altos, CA: Lange.

Pelczar, M. J., Jr., Reid, R. D. & Chan, E. C. S. (1986)). *Microbiology*, 5th edn. New York: McGraw-Hill.

Stanier, R. Y., Adelberg, E. A. & Ingraham, J. L. (1986). *General Microbiology*, 5th edn. London: Macmillan.

II The cell and its structure

Alberts, B., Bray, D., Lewis, J., Raff, M., Roberts, K. & Watson, J. D. (1990). *Molecular Biology of the Cell.* New York: Garland Publishing.

Carlile, M. J. (1980). From prokaryote to eukaryote: gains and losses. *Symp. Soc. Gen. Microbiol.* **30**, 1.

Cavalier-Smith, T. (1981). The origin and early evolution of the eukaryotic cell. *Symp. Soc. Gen. Microbiol.* **32**, 33.

Gunsalus, I. C. *et al.* (1960–86). *The Bacteria*, Vols I–X. New York: Academic Press

Kandler, O. (1982). Cell wall structures and their phylogenetic implications. *Zentbl. Bakt. Parasitkde.*, Abt. 1, Orig. C, **3**, 149.

Kelly, D. P. & Carr, N. G (ed.) (1984). The Microbe. *Symp. Soc. Gen. Microbiol.* **36**, II.

Lodish, H., Darnell, J. & Baltimore, D. (1986). *Molecular Cell Biology.* New York: Sci. Am. Books Inc.

Mayer, F. (1988). *Methods in Microbiology*, Vol. 20. London: Academic Press.

Neidhardt, F. C., Ingraham, J. L. & Schaechter, M. (1990). *Physiology of the Bacterial Cell: A Molecular Approach.* Sunderland, MA: Sinauer Associates.

III The grouping system of prokaryotes

Krieg, N. R. & Holt, J. G. (1984–9). *Bergey's Manual of Systematic Bacteriology*, Vols 1–4. Baltimore: Williams & Wilkins.

Lapage, S. P., Sneath, P. A. M., Lessel, E. F., Jr, Skerman, V. B. D., Seeliger, H. P. R. & Clark, W. A (1975). *International Code of Nomenclature of Bacteria.* Washington, DC: American Society for Microbiology.

Rippka, R., Dernelles, J., Waterbury, J. B., Herdman, M. & Stanier, R. Y. (1979). Generic assignments, strain histories and properties of pure cultures of Cyanobacteria. *J. gen. Microbiol.* **111**, 1.

Schleifer, K. H. & Stackebrandt, E. (1983). Molecular systematics of prokaryotes. *Ann. Rev. Microbiol.* **37**, 143.

Sneath, P. H. A. & Sokal, R. R. (1973). *Numerical Taxonomy: The Principles and Practice of Numerical Classification.* San Francisco: W. H. Freeman.

Starr, M. P., Stolp, H., Trüper, H. G., Balows, A. & Schlegel, H. G. (ed.). (1981). *The Prokaryotes: A Handbook on Habitats, Isolation and Identification of Bacteria*, Vols I & II. Heidelberg: Springer.

Woese, C. R. (1987). Bacterial Evolution. *Microbiol. Rev.* **51**, 221–72.

IV The viruses: distribution and structure

Davis, B. D., Dulbecco, R., Eisen, H. N. & Ginsberg, H. S. (1990). *Microbiology*, 4th edn. New York: Harper & Row.

Fraenkel-Conrat, H., Kimball, P. C. & Levy, J. A. (1988). *Virology*, 2nd edn. Engelwood Cliffs, NJ: Prentice-Hall.

Glass, R. E. (1982). *Gene Function:* E. coli *and its heritable elements.* London: Croom Helm.

Luria, S. E., Darnell, J. E., Jr, Baltimore, D. & Campbell, A. (1978). *General Virology*, 3rd edn. New York: Wiley.

Martin, S. J. (1978). *The Biochemistry of Viruses.* Cambridge University Press.

Watson, J. D., Hopkins, N. H., Roberts, J. W., Steitz, J. A. & Weiner, A. M. (1987). *Molecular Biology of the Gene*, 4th edn Menlo Park, CA: The Benjamin/Cummings Publ. Corp, Inc.

V The fungi: mycota

Esser, K. (1982). *Cryptograms: Cyanobacteria, Algae, Fungi, Lichens.* London: Cambridge University Press.

Smith, J. E. & Berry, D. R. (1975). *The Filamentous Fungi*, Vol. I, *Industrial Mycology*. London: E. Arnold.

Smith, J. E. & Berry, D. R. (1976). *The Filamentous Fungi*, Vol. II, *Biosynthesis and Metabolism*. London: E. Arnold.

Smith, J. E. & Berry, D. R. (1978). *The Filamentous Fungi*, Vol. III, *Developmental Mycology*. London: E. Arnold.

Webster, J. (1980). *Introduction to Fungi*, 2nd edn. London: Cambridge University Press.

IV Growth of microorganisms

Ingraham, J. L., Maaloe, O. & Neidhardt, F. C. (1983). *Growth of the Bacterial Cell.* Sunderland, MA: Sinauer Associates.

Mandelstam, J., McQuillen, K. & Dawes, J. (ed.) (1982). *Biochemistry of Bacterial Growth*, 3rd edn. Oxford: Blackwell.

Nierlich, D. P. (1978). Regulation of bacterial growth, RNA and protein synthesis. *Ann. Rev. Microbiol.* **32**, 393–432.

Starr, M. P., Stolp, H., Trüper, H. G., Balows, A. & Schlegel, H. G. (ed.) (1981). *The Prokaryotes: A Handbook on Habitats, Isolation and Identification of Bacteria.* Heidelberg: Springer.

Stouthamer, A. M. (1977). Energetic aspects on the growth of microorganisms. In *Microbial Energetics*, ed. B. A. Haddock & W. A. Hamilton. London: Cambridge University press.

Veldkamp, H. (1976). *Continuous Culture in Microbial Physiology and Ecology.* Durham: Meadowfield Press.

VII Basic mechanisms of metabolism and energy conversion

Crosa, J. H. (1989). Genetics and molecular biology of siderophore-mediated iron transport in bacteria. *Microbiol. Rev.* **53**, 517-30.

Gottschalk, G. (1981). The anaerobic way of life of prokaryotes. In *The Prokaryotes*, ed. M. P. Starr *et al.* Heidelberg: Springer.

Gottschalk, G. (1986). *Bacterial Metabolism*, 2nd edn. Heidelberg: Springer.

Harold, F. M. (1986). *The Vital Force: A study of Bioenergetics.* New York: W. H. Freeman.

Harwood, J. L. & Russell, N. J. (1984). *Lipids in Plants and Microbes.* London: George Allen & Unwin.

Ingledew, W. J. & Poole, R. K. (1984). The respiratory chains of *Escherichia coli. Microbiol. Rev.* **48**, 222.

Jones, C. W. (1984). *Bacterial Respiration and Photosynthesis.* Walton-on-Thames: Nelson.

Lehninger, A. L. (1988). *Principles of Biochemistry*, 6th edn. New York: Worth.

Stryer, L. (1990). *Biochemistry*, 4th edn. San Francisco: Freeman.

VII Special fermentations

Brown, C. M. & Campbell, I. (1985). *Introduction to Biotechnology.* Oxford: Blackwell.

Gunsalus, I. C. *et al.* (ed.) (1986). *The Bacteria,* Vol. II. New York: Academic Press.

Reed, G. (ed.) (1982). *Prescott & Dunn's Industrial Microbiology.* Westpoint: The AVI Publishing Company, Inc.

Rehm, H. J. (1980). *Industrielle Mikrobiologie.* Berlin: Springer.

Thauer, R. K. L. & Morris, J. G. (1984). Metabolism of chemotrophic anaerobes: old views and new aspects. *Symp. Soc. Gen. Microbiol.* **36** (II), 123.

Zehnder, A. J. B. (ed.) (1988). *Biology of Anaerobic Microorganisms.* New York: Wiley.

Ziegler, M. M. & Baldwin, T. O. (1981). Biochemistry of bacterial bioluminescence. *Curr. Top. Bionerg.* **12**, 65.

IX Electron transport under anaerobic conditions

Blaut, M. & Gottschalk, G. (1984). Coupling of ATP synthesis and methane formation from methanol and molecular hydrogen in *Methanosarcina barkeri. Eur. J. Biochem.* **141**, 217.

Crawford, R. L. & Hanson, R. S. (ed.) (1984). *Microbial Growth on C_1 compounds.* Washington, DC: American Society for Microbiology

Large, P. J. (1983). *Methylotrophy and Methanogenesis.* Wokingham: Van Nostrand Reinhold (UK).

Lundgren, D. G. & Wilver, M. (1980). Ore leaching by bacteria. *Ann. Rev. Microbiol.* **34**, 263–83.

Postgate, J. R. (1984). *The Sulphate-reducing Bacteria,* 2nd edn. London: Cambridge University Press.

Thauer, R. K. & Morris, J. G. (1984). Metabolism of chemotrophic anaerobes: old views and new aspects. *Symp. Soc. Gen. Microbiol.* **36** (II), 123.

Zehnder, A. J. B. (ed.) (1988). *Biology of Anaerobic Microorganisms.* New York: Wiley.

X Incomplete oxidations and microbial biotechnology

Demain, A. L. & Solomon, N. A. (ed.) (1986). *Manual of Industrial Microbiology and Biotechnology.* Washington, DC: American Society for Microbiology.

Kieslich, K. (1976). *Microbial Transformations.* Stuttgart: Thieme.

Mann, J. (1978). *Secondary Metabolism.* Oxford: Clarendon Press.

Moo-Young, M. (1984). *Comprehensive Biotechnology,* Vols I–IV. Oxford: Pergamon Press.

Peppler, H. J. & Perlman, D. (1979). *Microbial Technology,* vols. I & II. New York: Academic Press.

Präve, P., Faust, U., Sittig, W. & Sukatsch, D. A. (1982). *Handbuch der Biotechnologie.* Wiesbaden: Akad. Verlagsges (being translated into English).

Rose, A. H. (1979). *Secondary Products of Metabolism.* London: Academic Press.

Sutherland, I. W. (1982). Biosynthesis of microbial exopolysaccharides. *Adv. Microb. Physiol.* **23**, 79.

XI Chemo- and phototrophic bacteria

Clayton, R. K. & Sistrom, W. R. (ed.) (1978).*The Photosynthetic Bacteria.* New York: Plenum Press.

Collins, V. G. (1978). Isolation, cultivation and maintenance of autotrophs. In *Methods in Microbiology*, Vol. 3B, ed. J. R. Norris & D. W. Ribbons. London: Academic Press.

Jones, C. W. (1982). *Bacterial Respiration and Photosynthesis.* Walton-on-Thames: Nelson.

Jones, O. T. G. (1977). Electron transport and ATP synthesis in the photosynthetic bacteria. In *Microbial Energetics*, ed. B. A. Haddock & W. A. Hamilton. Cambridge: Cambridge University Press.

Matin, A. (1978). Organic nutrition of chemolithotrophic bacteria. *Ann. Rev. Microbiol.* **32**, 433.

Schlegel, H. G. & Bowien, B. (ed.) (1989). *Autotrophic Bacteria.* Madison & Heidelberg: Science Techn/Springer-Verlag.

Shively, J. M. & Barton, L. L. (1991). *Variations in Autrotrophic Life.* London: Academic Press.

XII Nitrogen fixation

Bothe, H., De Bruijn, F. J. & Newton, W. E. (ed.) (1988). *Nitrogen Fixation: A Hundred Years After.* New York: Gustav Fischer Verlag.

Fenchl, T. & Blackburn, J. H. (1979). *Bacteria and Mineral Cycling* London: Academic Press.

Hardy, R. W. F., Bottomley, F. & Burns, R. C. (ed.) (1979). *A Treatise on Dinitrogen Fixation.* New York: Wiley.

Postgate, J. R. (1982). *The Fundamentals of Nitrogen Fixation.* London: Cambridge University Press.

Sprent, J. I. (1979). *The Biology of Nitrogen-fixing Organisms.* London: McGraw-Hill.

XIII Degradation of naturally occurring materials

Alexander, M. (1977). *Introduction to Soil Microbiology.* New York: John Wiley & Sons.

Campbell, R. (1983). *Microbial Ecology*, 2nd edn. Oxford: Blackwell.

Gibson, D. T. (ed.) (1984). *Microbial Degradation of Organic Compounds.* New York: Marcel Decker Inc.

Gray, T. R. G. & Parkinson, D. (ed.) (1967). *The Ecology of Soil Bacteria.* Liverpool: Liverpool University Press.

Hungate, R. E. (1966). *The Rumen and its Microbes.* London: Academic Press.

Watkinson, R. J. (ed.) (1978). *Developments in Biodegradation of Hydrocarbons*. London: Applied Science Publishers, Ltd.

White, R. E. (1979). *Introduction to the Principles and Practice of Soil Science*. Oxford: Blackwell.

XIV Constancy, change and transfer of genetic characters

Bachmann, B. J. (1990). Linkage map of *Escherichia coli* K12. *Microbiol. Rev.* **54**, 130–97.

Bainbridge, B. W. (1980). *Genetics of Microbes*. Glasgow: Blackie & Sons.

Birge, E. A. (1981). *Bacterial and Bacteriophage Genetics: An Introduction*. Heidelberg: Springer.

Broda, P. (1979). *Plasmids*. Bristol: Freeman.

Freifelder, D. (1987). *Microbial Genetics*. Boston: Jones & Bartlett Publ.

Glass, R. E. (1982). *Gene Function: E. coli and its heritable elements*. London: Croom Helm.

Lewin, B. (1984). *Genes*. London: Wiley.

Lewin, B. (1974, 1977 & 1990). *Gene Expression*, Vols I–IV. New York: Wiley and London: Oxford University Press.

Maniatis, T., Fritsch, E. F. & Sambrook, J. (1989). *Molecular Cloning: A Laboratory Manual*. Cold Spring Harbour, NY: Cold Spring Harbor Laboratory.

Old, R. W. & Primrose, S. B. (1985). *Principles of Gene Manipulation.*3rd edn. Oxford: Blackwell.

Smith, H. O., Danner, D. B. & Deich, R. A. (1981). Genetic transformation. *Ann. Rev. Biochem.* **50**, 41.

Stent, G. S. & Calendar, R. (1978). *Molecular Genetics: An Introductory Narrative.*San Francisco: Freeman.

Winnaker, E. L. (1987). *From Genes to Clones: Introduction to Gene Technology*. Weinheim: VCH Verlagsgesellschaft.

XV Regulation of metabolism

Axel, R., Maniatis, T. & Fox, C. F. (1979). *Eukaryotic Gene Regulation.* New York: Academic Press.

Miller, J. H. & Reznikoff, W. S. (Ed.) (1978). *The Operon*. Cold Spring Harbor, NY: Cold Spring Harbor Laboratory.

Neihardt, F. C. (ed.) (1987). Escherichia coli *and* Salmonella typhimurium*: Cellular and Molecular Biology*. Washington, DC: American Society of Microbiology.

Ullman, A. & Danchin, A. (1980). Role of cyclic AMP in regulatory mechanisms of bacteria. *Trends in Biochem. Sci.* **5**, 95–6.

Umbarger, H. E. (1978). Amino acid biosynthesis and its regulation. *Ann. Rev. Biochem.* **47**, 533.

XVI Microorganisms and the environment

Alexander, M. (1977). *Introduction to Soil Microbiology*. New York: Wiley.

Atlas, R. M & Bartha, R. (1987). *Microbial Ecology: Fundamentals and Applications*, 2nd edn. Reading, MA: Addison-Wesley Publishing Company.

Brock, T. D. (1978). *Thermophilic Microorganisms and Life at High Temperatures*. New York: Springer.

Broda, E. (1975). *The Evolution of the Bioenergetic Processes*. Oxford: Pergamon.

Campbell, R. (1983). *Microbial Ecology*. Oxford: Blackwell.

Ehrlich, H. L. (1980). *Geomicrobiology*. New York: Marcel Dekker.

Fletcher, M. & Gray, T. R. G. (ed.) (1987). *Ecology of Microbial Communities*. Symp. Soc. Gen. Microbiol. 41.

Holland, H. D. & Schidlowski, M. (ed.) (1982). *Mineral Deposits and the Evolution of the Biosphere*. Report of Dahlem Workshop on Biospheric Evolution and Precambrian Metallogeny, Berlin 1980. Heidelberg: Springer.

Kushner, D. J. (ed.) (1978). *Microbial Life in Extreme Environments*. New York: Academic Press.

Rheinheimer, G. (1980). *Aquatic Microbiology* 2nd edn. London: Wiley.

Riley, M. & Anilionis, A. (1978). Evolution of the bacterial genome. *Ann. Rev. Microbiol.* **32**, 519.

Savage, D. C. (1977). Microbial ecology of the gastrointestinal tract. *Ann. Rev. Microbiol.* **31**, 107.

Schlegel, H. G. & Jannasch, H. W. (1981). Prokaryotes and their habitats. In *Prokaryotes: A Handbook on Habitats, Isolation and Identification of Bacteria*, ed. M. P. Starr *et al.* New York: Springer.

Schleifer, K. H. & Stackebrandt, E. (ed.) (1985). *Earth's Earliest Biosphere: Its Origin and Evolution*. Princeton, NJ: Princeton University Press.

Schopf, J. W. (ed.) (1983). *Earth's Earliest Biosphere, its Origin and Evolution.* Princeton, NJ: Princeton University Press.

Shilo, M. (ed.) (1979). *Strategies of Life in Extreme Environments*: Dahlem Konferenzen, Berlin. Weinheim: Verlag Chemie.

Skinner, F. A. & Carr, J. G. (ed.) (1978). *The Normal Microbial Flora of Man.* Symposia of Society of Applied Bacteriology. London: Academic Press.

Woese, C. R. (1987). Bacterial evolution. *Microbiol. Rev.* **51**, 221.

Useful reference works and handbooks

Bergmeyer, H. U. (ed.) (1974–84). *Methods of Enzymatic Analysis,* 3rd edn. Vols I–VI. Weinheim: Verlag Chemie.

Gerhardt, P. (ed.) (1981). *Manual of Methods for General Microbiology*. Washington, DC: American Society for Microbiology.

Gunsalus, I. C. *et al.* (ed.) (1960–86). *The Bacteria*, Vols I–X. New York: Academic Press.

Krieg, N. R. & Holt, J. G. (1984–9). *Bergey' s Manual of Systematic Bacteriology*, Vols 1–4. Baltimore: Williams & Wilkins.

Maniatis, T., Fritsch, E. F. & Sambrook, J. (1989). *Molecular Cloning: A Laboratory Manual.* Cold Spring Harbor, NY: Cold Spring Laboratory.

Meynell, G. G. & Meynell, E. (1970). *Theory and Practice in Experimental Bacteriology.* London: Cambridge University Press.

Norris, J. R. & Ribbons, D. W. (ed.) (1970–) *Methods in Microbiology.* New York: Academic Press.

Starr, M. P., Stolp, H., Trüper, H. G., Balows, A. & Schlegel, H. G. (ed.) (1981). *The Prokaryotes: A Handbook on Habitats, Isolation and Identification of Bacteria,* Vols I & II. Heidelberg: Springer.

Historical

De Kruif, P. (1954). *The Microbe Hunters.* New York: Harcourt Brace.

Dobell, C. (1958). *Antonie van Leeuwenhoek and His Little Animals.* New York: Russel & Russel.

Lechevalier, H. A. & Solotarovsky, M. (1974). *Three Centuries of Microbiology.* New York: Dover Publishers.

Nicolle, J. (1961). *Louis Pasteur, the Story of His Major Discoveries.* New York: Basic Books.

Watson, J. D. (1976). *Molecular Biology of the Gene*, 3rd edn. New York: Benjamin.

Periodicals

Advances in Applied Microbiology
Advances in Microbial Physiology
Annual Review of Biochemistry
Annual Review of Genetics
Annual Review of Microbiology
Critical Reviews in Biochemistry
Critical Reviews in Microbiology
Current Topics in Cellular Regulation
Developments in Industrial Microbiology
Ergebnisse der Biologie
Symposia of the Society for General Microbiology

Journals

Antonie van Leeuwenhoek, Journal of Microbiology and Serology
Applied Microbiology
Archives of Microbiology
Biotechnology and Bioengineering
Canadian Journal of Microbiology

Current Microbiology
European Journal of Applied Microbiology
FEMS Microbiology Ecology
FEMS Microbiology Letters
FEMS Microbiology Reviews
International Journal of Systematic Bacteriology
Journal of Applied Bacteriology
Journal of Bacteriology
Journal of General and Applied Microbiology
Journal of General Microbiology
Journal of General Virology
Journal of Molecular Biology
Journal of Virology
Microbiological Reviews
Microbiological Sciences
Molecular and General Genetics
Mycologia
Process Biochemistry
Trends in Biochemical Sciences
Trends in Microbiological Sciences (TIMS)
Virology
Zentralblatt für Bakteriologie und Parasitenkunde, I, II, and III

Vocabulary

F = French; G = Greek; L = Latin.

A

aboriri (abortus) L – perish (premature birth)

abortivus L – aborted development

accipio L – accept

acetum L – vinegar

acidus L – sour (acid)

aer, aeros G – air

aerugo L – verdigris

aes aeris L – ore

aggregare L – increase, accumulate

agilis L – mobile, quick

aktis, aktinos G – ray

allos G – different

ambo L – both

amphi G – surrounding

ampulla L – small flask

amylon G – starch

anabaino G – climb up

anapleroo G – replenish

angeion G – vessel

annulo, annulare L – cancel (annul)

anthos G – flower

anthrax G – coal

apex, apicis L – point (of a cone)

aphanizo G – make invisible

applanatus L – flattened

arthron G – limb

aqua L – water

archaios G – originally

armilla L – bracelet

askos G – tube

aspergillum L – fan for spraying

aspergo L – spraying

aster G – star

attenuare L – to weaken

attrahere L – attract

aureus L – golden

autos G – self

auxano, auxanein G – multiply

axon G – axis

B

bacillum L – small rod

baeo G – dwarf

backterion G, – small rod

ballo, ballein G – throw

bdallo, bdallein G – to milk, suck

bdella G – leech

bifidus L – divided in two

bini L – each two

bioo, bioun G – live

bios g – life

bis L – twice

blepharon G – eyelid, lash

bolos G – throw

bos, bovis L – cattle

botulus L – sausage, intestine

bradys G – slow

brevis L – short

C

caedo, caedere L – cut down, kill

cancer L – crab

capsa L – box, capsule

carbo L – coal

caseus L – cheese

caulis L – stem, twig

cereus L – smear, waxen

cerevisia L – beer, yeast

chaite G – hair, bristle

cheo G – pour

chimaera G – dragon, monster

chimaira G – goat

chiton G – robe

chlamys G – cloak, dress

chloros G – light green, bleached
choane G – funnel
chondros G – lump, gristle
chroma G – colour
chronos G – time
chryos G – gold
chthon, onos G – soil, earth
chytra G – pot
cilium L – eyelid, lash
cinereus L – ash grey
cinnabaris L – red colour
circino, circinare L – to make circular
circulo, circulare G – to circle
cisterna L – cistern
clatratus L – barred, wired in, enclosed
clavis L – key
coccum L – berry, kernel
coelum L – sky, weather
colo, colere L – inhabit
columella L – small culumn
complere L – to fill up
confluere G – flow together
coniungere L – connect
cornutus L – horned
corrodere L – gnaw, eat away
cortex L – skin, envelope
crassus L – thick, dense
cremor L – slime
cribrum L – sieve
crista L – comb, ridge

D

daktylos G – finger
deiknymi G – to show
delere L – destroy
deletio L – destruction
dendron G – tree
derma G – skin
deuteros G – second
dexter L – right, right hand
dicha G – divided in two
diktyon G – net
diplous G – double
dis G – twice
diskos G – plate
dispergere L – scatter, distribute
divaricare L – to spread

duro, durare L – hardening, enduring

E

edaphos G – soil
eikosi G – twenty
ekleipo G – release
ektos G – outside
endon G – inside
enteron G – entrails, intestines
epi G – on
eremos G – empty, naked
ergon G – work, deed
erythros G – red
eu G – good
excidere G – to cut out
extra L – outside, in addition to

F

facio, facere L – to make, do
facultas L – possibility
faex, faecis L – sediment, yeast
fasciare L – to wind round
fermentum L – yeast, sourdough
ferrugineus L – rust coloured
ferrum L – iron
fervere L – to cook, boil
fervidus L – boiling, fiery
figere l – tighten
filum L – thread, tissue
fimbria L – thread, fringe
fimum L – dung
flectere L – to bend
flos, floris L – flower
fluor L – river, stream
fuligo L – soot, blacking
fulvus L – yellow-red
fusus L – thread, spindle

G

galla L – gall
gamos G – wedding, marriage
ganos G – gloss, radiance
gaster G – stomach
gigno, gignere L – produce, originate
gignomai, gignesthai, gegona G – to become
genesis G – originate, arise from
globare L – to round up

globus ʟ – lump, round mass
gloios ɢ – sticky mass
glykys ɢ – sweet
gonos ɢ – sprout, offspring
gossypium ʟ – cotton
grandis ʟ – large
grapho ɢ – write
gratis ʟ – free, without payment
griseus ʟ – grey
gyne, gynaikos ɢ – woman
gyros ɢ – ring, circle

H

haima ɢ – blood
helix ɢ – spiral, turning
helveticus ʟ – swiss
helvus ʟ – honey coloured
hepta ɢ – seven
herpeton ɢ – crawling animal
heteros ɢ – the other (of two)
heurisko ɢ – to find
hexadeka ɢ – sixteen
hirsutus ʟ – thorny, spinous, bristly
holos ɢ – entire
homoioa ɢ – similar
hormao, horman ɢ – start moving
hyalos ɢ – glass
hydor ɢ – water
hymen ɢ – thin skin
hyper ɢ – excessive
hyphos ɢ – tissue
hypo ɢ – less, lower (as prefix)

I

ictus ʟ – push
immunis ʟ – undamaged
inducere ʟ – lead, to cause
infestare ʟ – endanger
inficere ʟ – to colour, to poison
integratio ʟ – restoration
intra ʟ – inside
isos ɢ – same

K

karpos ɢ – fruit
karyon ɢ – nut, kernel
kata ɢ – lower, downwards
kephale ɢ – head

kineo ɢ – move
klados ɢ – branch, twig
kleio ɢ – shut
klino ɢ – lean, bow, incline
koinos ɢ – together
koleon ɢ – limit, sheath
kollybos ɢ – small coin
konis ɢ – dust
kopros ɢ – dung
kormos ɢ – tree trunk
koryne ɢ – club, stick
krypto ɢ – hide
kyanos ɢ – blue colour
kybos ɢ – dice
kyklos ɢ – circle
kyon ɢ – dog
kystis ɢ – blister, bladder
kytos ɢ – cell, cave

L

labor, labi ʟ – glide, fall
laevus ʟ – left, left side
lampros ɢ – light, clear
latere ʟ – to be hidden
latus, lateris ʟ – side
latus ʟ – wide
legnon ɢ – border, edge
leichen ɢ – moss, lichen
leptos ɢ – fine, thin
letalis ʟ – mortal, lethal
leukos ɢ – white
lignum ʟ – wood
limicola ʟ – inhabitant of sediment
limus ʟ – mud, sediment
linere ʟ – to cover, smear
lipos ɢ – fat, tallow
lithos ɢ – stone
lobos ɢ – rag, lobe
logos ɢ – work, precept
lophos ɢ – hill, mound
lux ʟ – light
luna ʟ – light
lyo, lyein ɢ – loosening, dissolve

M

macerare ʟ – to soften
marcescere ʟ – to rot
megas ɢ – great, large

meion G – less
mel, mellis L – honey
melas G – black
meninx G – membrane, film
mensa L – table
merismos G – division
meros G – part
mesos G – the middle one
meta G – changed (prefix)
mikros G – small
mitos G – thread
mixis G – mixture
monile L – collar
monos G – single, singular
morphe G – shape, figure
mucor G – mould, mildew
murus L – wall
mutare L – to change, alter
mutatic L – change, alteration
mutuus L – reciprocal, mutual
mykes G – fungus
myon G – muscle
myxa G – slime

N

nanus L – dwarf
natare L – to swim
necare L – to kill
nectere L – to knot
nema G – thread
neura G – sinew, chord
nidulans L – making a small nest
nidus L – nest
niger L – black
nomos G – law
notare L – to mark
novellus L – new
novus L – new
nucleus L – kernel, core

O

ochros G – pale, yellow
oculus L – eye
oikos G – house, household
okto G – eight
oligos G – little

oma G – swelling
omnis L – all, every
onkos G – swelling
oon G – egg
operor L – to work, do something
opsis G – sight, seeing
organon G – tool
oryza L – rice
oscillum L – the swing
osmos G – push, impetus
ouron G – urine

P

pagus L – place, region
pallidus L – pale
palluster L – swampy
panus L – swelling
par L – same, similar
parare L – to prepare
partiri L – divide
patior, pati L – tolerate
pecten L – comb
pelos G – mud
pente G – five
perficere L – to finish, complete
peri G – around
permeare L – to go through, penetrate
perone G – needle
petra G, L – rock
phagein G – eat
phaino G – to show
phaios G – grey, slightly brown
phero G – carry
philos G – friend
phleos G – reed
phoebeo G – frighten, be fearful
phormos G – basket
photos G – light
phthora G – destruction
phykos G – seaweed
phyllon G – leaf
physis G – nature, growth
phyton G – plant
pikros G – sharp, bitter
pilum G – spear
pilus L – hair

pix, picis L – pitch, tar
planes L – wander
planus L – flat
plaque F – plate, shield
plasma G – formation, product
platto G – to form, produce
pleko G – plait, braid
plico, plicare L – to pleat
pneuma G – breath, exhalation
poieo G – to make, produce
polos G – pivot
polys G – much, many
pous, podos G – foot
prodigiosus L – unnatural, miraculous
promovere L – to advance, increase
pros G – in addition to (prefix)
prostheka G – appendage
proteus G – greek god
protos G – the first
pseudo G – false, deceiving
psittakos G – parrot
psychros G – cold, cool
purpureus L – purple-coloured
putidus L – rotting, decomposing
pyon G – pus
pyr, pyros G – fire
pyren G – kernel

Q

quintus L – the fifth

R

racemus L – berry, grape
radius L – ray, rod
radix L – root
ramiger L – carrying branches
ramus L – branch, twig
repellere L – to push back
repreimere L – to restrain, stop
restringere L – to limit, restrain
reticulum L – small network
revertere L – to return
rhage G – tear, rupture
rhiza G – root
rhodon G – rose
rivus L – brook, small stream

ruber, rubrum L – red
rufus L – red
rugosis L – pleated, folded
ruminare L – chew the cud

S

sacculus L – little sack
saeptum L – enclosure, enclosed place
sal L – salt
salivarius L – slimy
sapros G – rotted
sarcina L – package, bundle
sarcos G – meat, flesh
schizo G – split
secale L – a type of cereal
selene G – moon
semi L – half
sentire L – to feel, to take notice
sepo G – to leave to rot
sideros G – iron
skleros G – hard, rough
skopeo G – to regard, view
skotos G – darkness
socius L – companion
soma G – body
sordes L – dirt
soros G – vessel, heap
speira G – convolution, turn
spheira G – sphere
staphyle G – grape, bunch of grapes
spira L – turn winding
sporos G – sowing, seed
stear G – tallow
sterigma G – support
stele G – column
stereos G – fast, firm
sto, stare L – to stand
stolo L – root tip
stratum L – layer
strepho G – to turn
stringere L – draw together
stroma G – base, support
stylos G – column, support
styptikos G – closing, stoppering
substerno, (substratus) L – being the
    base

subtilis L – fine, thin
sucus L – juice
supplere L – to fill up
supprimere L – to hold back, depress
symbiosis G – live together
syn G – together with
synecho G – keep together, keep
  closed

T

tachys G – fast
taxis G – order, arrangement
teichos G – wall
telos G – end
tenax L – obstinate, standfast
tenuis L – delicate
tettares G – four
thallos G – green twig
theion G – sulphur
theke G – box
therion G – animal
thermos G – warm
thrix, thrichos G – hair
thylakos G – sack
tithemi G – sit, stand, lie
tolype G – skein, coil
tomaculum L – sausage
tome G – cut
tonos G – tension
toxikon G – poison
treis, tria G – three
tremere L – tremble
trepo G – turn away
trope G – alteration, change
trophe G – food
tropos G – direction, diversion
tuber L – swelling, bump
tubulus L – small tube
tumor L – swelling
turbare L – entangle
typhos G – fever

U

ubique L – everywhere
ultra L – beyond
undula L – small wave
uredo L – mildew, blight
uro, usus L – burnt
utilis L – useful
uva L – grape

V

valere L – to value, be valued
variare L – to change, alter
varius L – different, mixed
ventriculus L – small stomach
venus L – beauty, attraction
versi-colour L – many-coloured
versus L – altered
vertere L – turn, turning
vesicula L – small bubble, vesicle
vinosus L – vinous
viridescere L – to become green
viridis L – green
virulentus L – poisonous
virus L – poison, juice
viscidus L – tough, sticky
vitis L – vine
vitreus L – glassy
vitrum L – glass
vivus L – alive, lively
voluto, volutare L – to roll, rotate
voro, vorare L – to devour

X

xylon G – wood

Z

zoon G – living organism
zyme G – yeast, sourdough
zygos G – yoke, pair

Index